I0056592

Principles and Practice of Intensive Care

Principles and Practice of Intensive Care

Edited by Rafael Nash

hayle
medical

New York

Hayle Medical,
750 Third Avenue, 9th Floor,
New York, NY 10017, USA

Visit us on the World Wide Web at:
www.haylemedical.com

© Hayle Medical, 2019

This book contains information obtained from authentic and highly regarded sources. Copyright for all individual chapters remain with the respective authors as indicated. All chapters are published with permission under the Creative Commons Attribution License or equivalent. A wide variety of references are listed. Permission and sources are indicated; for detailed attributions, please refer to the permissions page and list of contributors. Reasonable efforts have been made to publish reliable data and information, but the authors, editors and publisher cannot assume any responsibility for the validity of all materials or the consequences of their use.

ISBN: 978-1-63241-594-3

Trademark Notice: Registered trademark of products or corporate names are used only for explanation and identification without intent to infringe.

Cataloging-in-Publication Data

Principles and practice of intensive care / edited by Rafael Nash.
p. cm.
Includes bibliographical references and index.
ISBN 978-1-63241-594-3
1. Critical care medicine. 2. Emergency medicine. 3. Intensive care units.
I. Nash, Rafael.
RC86.7 .P75 2019
616.025--dc23

Table of Contents

Preface

The main aim of this book is to educate learners and enhance their research focus by presenting diverse topics covering this vast field. This is an advanced book which compiles significant studies by distinguished experts in the area of analysis. This book addresses successive solutions to the challenges arising in the area of application, along with it; the book provides scope for future developments.

Patients who require dedicated care and monitoring along with life-saving support are treated within the domain of intensive care medicine. It is a technologically advanced, expensive and resource-intensive area of medical care. A daily plan comprising of observation, intervention and impression with respect to the vital systems of a patient is implemented in an intensive care strategy. Such care is provided in critical care units. Some of the equipment used in such units are hemodynamic and cardiac monitoring systems, ventricular assist devices, intra-aortic balloon pumps, extracorporeal membrane oxygenation circuits, continuous renal replacement equipment, etc. Such equipment facilitate mechanical ventilation, hemofiltration, drug infusion and total parenteral nutrition, among others. Nutrition in the intensive care unit is another significant aspect of such care. This book is a compilation of chapters that discuss the most vital principles and practices of intensive care. From theories to research to practical applications, case studies related to all contemporary topics of relevance to this field have been included in this book. It includes contributions of experts and scientists, which will provide innovative insights into this field.

It was a great honour to edit this book, though there were challenges, as it involved a lot of communication and networking between me and the editorial team. However, the end result was this all-inclusive book covering diverse themes in the field.

Finally, it is important to acknowledge the efforts of the contributors for their excellent chapters, through which a wide variety of issues have been addressed. I would also like to thank my colleagues for their valuable feedback during the making of this book.

Editor

Derivation and validation of a prognostic model for postoperative risk stratification of critically ill patients with faecal peritonitis

Ascanio Tridente[1]*[iD], Julian Bion[2], Gary H. Mills[3], Anthony C. Gordon[4], Geraldine. M. Clarke[5], Andrew Walden[6], Paula Hutton[7], Paul A. H. Holloway[4], Jean-Daniel Chiche[8], Frank Stuber[9], Christopher Garrard[7], Charles Hinds[10] and On behalf of the GenOSept and GAinS Investigators

Abstract

Background: Prognostic scores and models of illness severity are useful both clinically and for research. The aim of this study was to develop two prognostic models for the prediction of long-term (6 months) and 28-day mortality of postoperative critically ill patients with faecal peritonitis (FP).

Methods: Patients admitted to intensive care units with faecal peritonitis and recruited to the European GenOSept study were divided into a derivation and a geographical validation subset; patients subsequently recruited to the UK GAinS study were used for temporal validation. Using all 50 clinical and laboratory variables available on day 1 of critical care admission, Cox proportional hazards regression was fitted to select variables for inclusion in two prognostic models, using stepwise selection and nonparametric bootstrapping sampling techniques. Using Area under the receiver operating characteristic curve (AuROC) analysis, the performance of the models was compared to SOFA and APACHE II.

Results: Five variables (age, SOFA score, lowest temperature, highest heart rate, haematocrit) were entered into the prognostic models. The discriminatory performance of the 6-month prognostic model yielded an AuROC 0.81 (95% CI 0.76–0.86), 0.73 (95% CI 0.69–0.78) and 0.76 (95% CI 0.69–0.83) for the derivation, geographic and temporal external validation cohorts, respectively. The 28-day prognostic tool yielded an AuROC 0.82 (95% CI 0.77–0.88), 0.75 (95% CI 0.69–0.80) and 0.79 (95% CI 0.71–0.87) for the same cohorts. These AuROCs appeared consistently superior to those obtained with the SOFA and APACHE II scores alone.

Conclusions: The two prognostic models developed for 6-month and 28-day mortality prediction in critically ill septic patients with FP, in the postoperative phase, enhanced the day one SOFA score's predictive utility by adding a few key variables: age, lowest recorded temperature, highest recorded heart rate and haematocrit. External validation of their predictive capability in larger cohorts is needed, before introduction of the proposed scores into clinical practice to inform decision making and the design of clinical trials.

Keywords: Faecal peritonitis, Outcome, Prognostication, GenOSept, GAinS, Sepsis

Background

Prognostic scores and models of illness severity are useful both clinically and for research. They support critical care physicians in decision making through more accurate prognostication; they describe and summarise case mix, and inform health economic evaluations of cost-effectiveness. Many types of models exist, and their roles are not mutually exclusive, as their combined use may afford better prognostic reliability [1]. These tools are usually insufficiently accurate to be useful for predicting individual survival and are generally reserved for benchmarking

*Correspondence: ascanio.tridente@doctors.org.uk
[1] Whiston Hospital Prescot, Merseyside and Department of Infection, Immunity and Cardiovascular Disease, The Medical School, University of Sheffield, Sheffield, UK
Full list of author information is available at the end of the article

quality of care and for research studies [2–4], for example when examining heterogeneity of treatment effect in clinical trials [5].

When considering prognostication in the context of the wide ranging spectrum of intra-abdominal infections, complexity is increased by the heterogeneity of aetiology, clinical manifestations and pathophysiological mechanisms. The International Sepsis Forum Consensus Conference on Definitions of Infection in the Intensive Care Unit describes intra-abdominal infections as a "very heterogeneous group of infectious processes that share an anatomical site between the diaphragm and the pelvis" [6]. The anatomical, clinical and pathophysiological heterogeneity of these infections, together with their varied aetiology and prognosis, have given rise to a range of prognostic instruments tailored to specific populations.

Generic "peritonitis" prognostic tools (aimed at peritonitis of any origin), such as the Mannheim Peritonitis Index (MPI) or the Peritonitis Index of Altona II (PIA II), rely on factors such as age, degree of organ failure, origin of sepsis and intra-operative findings to risk-stratify different types of peritonitis, but, given the considerable heterogeneity of intra-abdominal infections, these scoring systems may not be sufficiently specific in terms of aetiology [7, 8]. Other scoring systems have been devised to explicitly address the issue of prognostication in selected forms of peritonitis, such as the left colonic Peritonitis Severity Score (PSS), developed for patients with distal large bowel peritonitis of various origins [9]. The physiological and operative severity score for the enumeration of mortality and morbidity (POSSUM) is another risk adjustment model, developed in 1991 for use in surgical patients [10]. A modification of this prognostic model, obtained by excluding some of the physiological factors of the original POSSUM, was developed for use specifically in patients undergoing surgery for colorectal cancer (CR-POSSUM) [11]. Importantly, all of these scores incorporate intra-operative findings and are either designed to cater for, and include, the whole heterogeneous spectrum of peritoneal infections (such as the MPI and PIA II), or to focus on a very narrow subset of peritonitis, identified by location (left colonic, in the case of PSS) or aetiology (colorectal malignancy, as in CR-POSSUM).

To date no prognostic score has been developed for the critically ill patient with faecal peritonitis (FP) in the postoperative phase. We therefore aimed to specifically study critically ill patients suffering from FP, in the postoperative phase, and quantify their mortality risk at 28 days and 6 months. International multicentre prospectively collected patient datasets, such as The GenOSept and GAinS cohorts, provided an opportunity to develop and evaluate such prognostic systems.

Methods

Aim, design and setting

The Genetics of Sepsis and Septic Shock in Europe (GenOSept) and Genomic Advances in Sepsis (GAinS) are prospectively gathered cohorts of critically ill septic patients with FP recruited from multiple centres in Europe. They include data from patients with various degrees of illness severity, including potential risk modifiers and confounding factors (such as comorbidities, indices of acute physiological derangement, organ support, radiological and laboratory findings, origin of FP) [12, 13]. These diagnostically homogeneous cohorts of FP patients, gathered primarily for the purposes of studying genetic epidemiology in sepsis, also provide high-quality data well suited to the development and testing of a prognostic model specific to this postoperative patient population.

The primary aim of this study was to develop and validate a prognostic modelling tool able to stratify postsurgical critically ill patients with FP, by quantifying their mortality risk in the short- (28 day) and long-term (6 month), independently from intra-operative surgical findings, using prospectively collected data from the GenOSept and GAinS cohorts.

Recruitment criteria

The same inclusion and exclusion criteria were used for both cohorts. Inclusion criteria: adult patients (>18 years) admitted to a High Dependency Unit (HDU) or Intensive Care Unit (ICU) with FP, defined as visible inflammation of the serosal membrane that lines the abdominal cavity, secondary to contamination by faeces, as diagnosed by the operating surgeon at laparotomy. All critically ill patients in this cohort, therefore, were recruited after the diagnosis was established during surgical source control. Exclusion criteria: peritonitis due to gastric or upper GI-tract perforation (e.g. gastric or duodenal ulcer perforation, small bowel perforation), patient or legal representative unwilling or unable to give consent; patient pregnant; advanced directive to withhold or withdraw life-sustaining treatment or admitted for palliative care only; patient already enrolled in an interventional research study of a novel/ unlicensed therapy (patients enrolled in interventional studies examining the clinical application or therapeutic effects of widely accepted, "standard" treatments, were not excluded); patient immunocompromised (known regular systemic corticosteroid therapy, exceeding 7 mg/ kg/day of hydrocortisone or equivalent, within 3 months of admission and prior to acute episode; known regular therapy with other immunosuppressive agents, e.g. azathioprine; known to be HIV positive or have acquired immunodeficiency syndrome as defined by the Centre for Disease Control; neutrophil count less than 1000 mm^{-3}

due to any cause, including metastatic disease and haematological malignancies or chemotherapy, but excluding severe sepsis; organ or bone marrow transplant receiving immunosuppressive therapy).

The definition of sepsis was based on the International Consensus Criteria: "the clinical syndrome defined by the presence of both infection and a systemic inflammatory response" [14]. Patients were followed for up to 6 months from enrolment or until death.

Database and quality assurance

The case report form (CRF) was developed and tested by CH, CG, AG, JDC and Dr J. Millo, together with other members of the GenOSept Consortium. Variables recorded included demographic, clinical and outcome data. A specific electronic case report form (eCRF) was developed by Lincoln, Paris, France, using software developed in collaboration with JDC. The database was password-protected, allowing investigators to enter data into the eCRF online, and included audit trail capability for data entry and subsequent modifications. To minimise errors, logical range checks were in place so that the investigators would be alerted if an attempt was made to enter data values outside the expected ranges.

Quality assurance (QA) was performed by P.H., C.G., A.W., A.G. and C.H, who systematically reviewed all data. Data queries (DQs) were generated within the eCRF for missing or erroneous data and sent electronically to the relevant investigators for action, where necessary. Up to the end of January 2011, an estimated 3986 valid DQs had been generated, with a response rate by the investigators of approximately 92%. Common reasons for DQs were missing information, particularly the Charlson Index, antimicrobial use, estimated day of onset of FP before ICU admission, information about circumstances of GCS assessment and outcome data.

All patients' eCRFs were reviewed by experienced critical care physicians. Where the patient's eligibility for inclusion in the relevant cohort was unclear, clarification was sought from the investigators. Regular QA reports were provided to the relevant Management Committee for review; the National Investigators were contacted regarding quality issues if necessary.

Statistical analyses
Prognostic model
In order to build the prognostic model, patients recruited up to January 2011 (included in the GenOSept cohort) were divided into two subsets of patients: one for derivation and the other for external geographic validation. To limit the effect of potentially unmeasured and unaccounted confounding factors, related to possible differences in national systems of healthcare provision among participating countries across Europe, these patients were divided into UK (derivation) and non-UK (geographic validation) sub-cohorts, with the aim of optimising homogeneity in the datasets and decreasing potential background noise. Subsequent patients recruited in the UK between January 2011 and March 2015 (included in the GAinS cohort) were included in the temporal validation cohort.

We evaluated all 50 clinical and laboratory variables available on admission to critical care (day 1) (for a full list, see Additional file 1). The primary outcome was 6-month mortality risk with the secondary outcome being 28-day mortality risk. To select the variables to include in the model, Cox proportional hazards regression analysis for 6-month mortality was fitted, using stepwise backwards selection, to determine the predictors to be included in the models from 50 bootstrapped samples derived from the derivation subset (nonparametric bootstrap procedure). Increasing the number of bootstrap replications did not alter the model significantly. The p value cut-off used was 0.05. The same predictor variables were employed to construct a prognostic tool for the secondary outcome, 28-day mortality.

The procedure of bootstrapping is a re-sampling method which relies on random sampling with replacement of the available observations. This procedure allows evaluation of the characteristics of an estimator (such as its variance) by measuring those properties when obtaining multiple samples from the original dataset (and of size equal to the observed dataset) [15, 16].

A final Cox proportional hazards regression analysis for both 6-month and 28-day mortalities was fitted using the set of variables found to be significant in the majority of bootstrap replications.

We confirmed that the proportional hazards assumption was met by drawing Kaplan–Meier Curves and Nelson Aalen plots for the covariates after categorisation. Predictors which satisfy the proportional hazard assumption show very similar curves, with the separation between them remaining proportional across analysis time [17]. We also tested the correctness of this assumption testing on the basis of Schoenfeld residuals [18].

In order to assess for the presence of collinearity (which happens when two variables are almost perfect linear combinations of one another), we calculated the variance inflation factors (VIFs). It is generally accepted that variables with VIFs greater than 10 merit further investigation [19].

The two models obtained were evaluated using area under the receiver operating characteristic curve (AuROC) analysis, which plots sensitivity against 1-specificity to describe the accuracy of a diagnostic test [20, 21] and to compare the performance of different tests [22].

Nonparametric bootstrapping and prognostic model derivation for 6-month mortality

The bootstrapping procedure was performed using 50 repetitions based on the UK derivation cohort. A final Cox proportional hazards regression analysis for 6-month mortality was fitted using the set of variables found to be significant in the majority of bootstrap replications. Saturation was reached after 50 bootstrap replications, with additional replications not yielding significantly different results.

A set of 5 variables assessed on day 1 met this criterion (age, SOFA score, lowest temperature, highest heart rate, haematocrit). The Cox proportional hazards model estimates for those risk variables are presented in Table 1.

The same five variables were employed to formulate the 6-month mortality prognostic tool by entering the estimates obtained from the Cox proportional hazards model in the following equation:

$$\text{FP score (6 month)} = \left(10^3\right) * \exp\left((0.0447387 * A\right)$$
$$+ (0.1812872 * S) + (-0.2767377 * T)$$
$$+ (0.0114629 * HR) + (-0.0313029 * H))$$

where A = age at admission to critical care, S = SOFA score day 1, T = lowest recorded temperature (as °C) on day 1, HR = highest recorded heart rate on day 1, H = haematocrit (as percentage points) on day 1.

The model coefficients used for prediction of 6-month mortality were adjusted for the 28-day mortality outcome. To achieve this, a separate Cox proportional

Table 1 Variables found to be significant in the majority of bootstrap replications run on the UK derivation cohort for the two outcomes

Variable	HR	HR 95% CI	coeff	coeff 95% CI	p
6 month mortality					
Age	1.05	1.03–1.07	0.045	0.02–0.06	<0.001
SOFA score	1.20	1.12–1.28	0.18	0.11–0.25	<0.001
Low temperature	0.76	0.63–0.91	[−0.28]	[−0.46]-[−0.09]	0.004
High heart rate	1.01	1.01–1.02	0.01	0.01–0.02	0.007
Haematocrit	0.97	0.94–0.99	[−0.031]	[−0.059]-[−0.003]	0.028
28-day mortality					
Age	1.05	1.03–1.08	0.049	0.03–0.07	<0.001
SOFA score	1.22	1.12–1.33	0.2	0.11–0.29	<0.001
Low temperature	0.70	0.55–0.88	[−0.36]	[−0.59]-[−0.13]	0.002
High heart rate	1.01	1–1.02	0.01	[−0.001]-0.2	0.07
Haematocrit	0.99	0.95–1.02	[−0.013]	[−0.047]-0.022	0.47

HR hazard ratio; *95% CI* 95% confidence interval, *coeff* coefficient, *SOFA* Sequential Organ Failure Assessment; the use of the square brackets [] indicates negative values

hazards regression analysis was fitted for 28-day mortality, utilising the same set of five variables. The resulting model estimates are presented in Table 1. The estimates were utilised to construct the 28-day mortality prognostic tool as described in the following equation:

$$\text{FP score (28 day)} = \left(10^4\right) * \exp\left((0.048728 * A\right)$$
$$+ (0.2005776 * S) + (-0.3591817 * T)$$
$$+ (0.0098462 * HR) + (-0.0125259 * H))$$

While haematocrit and high heart rate did not offer independent predictive power in the 28-day mortality model, they were useful in explaining variability when retained in the model.

Comparison of the prognostic models with preexisting scores

Comparison of the prognostic models with SOFA and APACHE II was performed graphically by drawing the superimposed ROC curves and testing the underlying AuROC obtained, taking into account that the data are correlated, using a nonparametric approach as suggested by DeLong et al. [23].

For all statistical analyses, Stata version 10.0 was used (StataCorp, Texas, USA; http://www.stata.com).

Results

Baseline and outcome data

The derivation cohort included 462 patients with FP recruited in the UK. Their median (inter-quartile range, IQR) age was 69.4 (58.6–77.2) years. The geographic validation (non-UK) cohort included 515 FP patients recruited to the GenOSept study from the other European countries. Their median (IQR) age was 69.1 (58–77) years. The temporal validation cohort included 323 FP patients recruited in the UK between January 2011 and March 2015. Their median (IQR) age was 68.3 (57.6–77.2) years. For details of the recruiting centres, please see Additional file 1.

The baseline characteristics and the outcomes of the three cohorts are presented in Tables 2 and 3, respectively.

The age distribution was not significantly different across the cohorts, although the derivation cohort had a higher proportion of patients aged over 75. Males predominated in all cohorts. The racial distribution was more heterogeneous in the geographic validation cohort, while the derivation and the temporal validation cohorts were almost entirely Caucasian. Among the comorbidities diabetes, previous serious infections and other illnesses were more prevalent in the geographic validation cohort, compared to the other cohorts. The underlying causes for FP varied across cohorts, with anastomotic breakdown being particularly common in the geographic

Table 2 Patients' baseline characteristics for the derivation, geographic and temporal external validation sub-cohorts

Cohort	Derivation (UK until Jan 2011)		Geographic validation (non-UK)		Temporal validation (UK post-Jan 2011)	
Total number of patients	462		515		323	
Characteristics	Median or n	IQR or %	Median or n	IQR or %	Median or n	IQR or %
Age						
Available data	462	100%	515	100%	323	100%
18–34	11	2.4%	25	4.9%	11	3.4%
35–44	15	3.3%	18	3.5%	16	5%
45–54	54	11.7%	52	10.1%	38	11.8%
55–64	93	20.1%	98	19%	73	22.6%
65–74	113	24.5%	151	29.3%	88	27.2%
75–84	149	32.3%	149	28.9%	75	23.2%
85–95	27	5.8%	22	4.3%	22	6.8%
Gender						
Available data	462	100%	515	100%	323	100%
Male	236	51.1%	304	59%	171	52.9%
Female	226	48.9%	211	41%	152	47.1%
Race						
Available data	460	99.6%	510	99%	323	100%
Caucasian	454	98.7%	502	98.4%	315	97.5%
Asian	4	0.9%	7	1.4%	3	0.9%
African	1	0.2%	1	0.2%	3	0.9%
Mixed	1	0.2%	0	0%	2	0.6%
Medical comorbidities						
Available data	462	100%	515	100%	323	100%
Heart and vascular disease	187	40.6%	202	39.2%	117	36.2%
Respiratory disease	111	24.1%	133	25.8%	97	30%
Neurological disease	48	10.4%	57	11.1%	24	7.4%
Severe renal disease	39	8.6%	21	4.3%	16	5%
Gastrointestinal disease	98	21.3%	132	25.7%	76	23.5%
Malignancy	135	29.3%	160	31.1%	84	26%
Diabetes	61	13.2%	102	19.8%	44	13.6%
Previous serious infection[a]	8	1.7%	25	4.9%	5	1.6%
Other illness	130	28.2%	210	40.8%	83	25.7%
Severe exercise restriction	3	0.7%	6	1.2%	1	0.3%
Chronic dialysis	5	1.1%	8	1.6%	5	1.6%
Chronic steroids use[b]	2	0.4%	9	1.8%	5	1.6%
Cause of FP						
Available data	461	99.8%	511	99.2%	323	100%
Perforated diverticulum	137	29.7%	175	34.3%	89	27.6%
Anastomotic breakdown	115	25%	187	36.6%	61	18.9%
Malignancy	65	14.1%	64	12.5%	35	10.8%
Trauma	22	4.8%	45	8.8%	16	5%
Other	122	26.5%	40	7.8%	124	38.4%
Time to surgery (days)	1	1–3	1	1–3	1	1–3

Table 2 continued

Characteristics	Median or n	IQR or %	Median or n	IQR or %	Median or n	IQR or %
Acute physiology						
Available data	461	99.8%	513	99.6%	321	99.4%
APACHE II score	15	12–20	17	13–22	16	12–21
SOFA score	7	5–9	7	5–11	6	5–8
Acute renal failure	129	32.7%	214	42.8%	70	21.8%
Renal replacement therapy	81	21%	105	21.3%	26	8.1%
Mechanical ventilation	346	75.1%	397	77.4%	228	71%

APACHE Acute Physiology and Chronic Health Evaluation, *SOFA* Sequential Organ Failure Assessment

[a] Serious infection was defined as a serious, prolonged or recurrent infection

[b] Chronic steroid use was defined as taking corticosteroids below the immunosuppression dose (>7 mg/kg/days hydrocortisone), which would exclude patient from inclusion in the study

Table 3 Outcomes for the derivation, geographic and temporal external sub-cohorts

Cohort	Derivation (UK until Jan 2011)		Geographic validation (non-UK)		Temporal validation (UK post-Jan 2011)	
Total number of patients	462		515		323	
Characteristics						
Length of stay (days)	Median	IQR	Median	IQR	Median	IQR
Available data	462	100%	515	100%	322	99.7%
ICU	7	4–14	14	7–29	6	3–11
Hospital	26	14–47	30	17–54	29	18–47
Mortality	*n*	%	*n*	%	*n*	%
Available data	462	100	515	100	321	99.4
6 month	124	26.8	185	35.9	64	19.9
ICU	73	15.8	131	25.4	24	7.5
Hospital	109	23.6	171	33.2	29	9.8
28 day	79	17.1	171	33.2	40	12.4

validation cohort. Baseline Sequential Organ Failure Assessment (SOFA) and Acute Physiology and Chronic Health Evaluation II (APACHE II) scores and prevalence of mechanical ventilation on day one were comparable across the cohorts. The occurrence of acute renal failure on day one was more frequent in the geographic validation cohort, with differences with the other cohorts (32.7, 42.8 and 23.3% for the derivation, geographic and temporal validation cohorts, respectively), accompanied by a difference in the utilisation of renal replacement therapy (21, 21.3 and 7.5% for the derivation, geographic and temporal validation cohorts, respectively) on day one. The geographic validation cohort was characterised by higher mortality rates (at all time points) and longer ICU stay, compared to the other two cohorts; this latter feature was also reflected, although to a lesser extent, in the length of hospital stay.

Performance of the prognostic tools

When evaluated using a receiver operating characteristics (ROC) curve, the discriminatory performance of the 6-month prognostic model in the UK derivation sub-cohort yielded an AuROC of 0.81 (95% CI 0.76–0.86) as indicated in Fig. 1a. At geographic validation in the non-UK sub-cohort, the 6-month prognostic model produced an AuROC of 0.73 (95% CI 0.69–0.78; Fig. 1b). At temporal validation, the 6-month model yielded an AuROC of 0.76 (95% CI 0.69–0.83; Fig. 1c).

The 28-day prognostic tool also performed similarly, yielding an AuROC 0.82 (95% CI 0.77–0.88; Fig. 2a) for the derivation UK sub-cohort. At geographic validation in the non-UK sub-cohort, the 28-day prognostic model produced an AuROC of 0.75 (95% CI 0.69–0.80; Fig. 2b). In the temporal validation cohort, the 28-day model yielded an AuROC of 0.79 (95% CI 0.71–0.87; Fig. 2c).

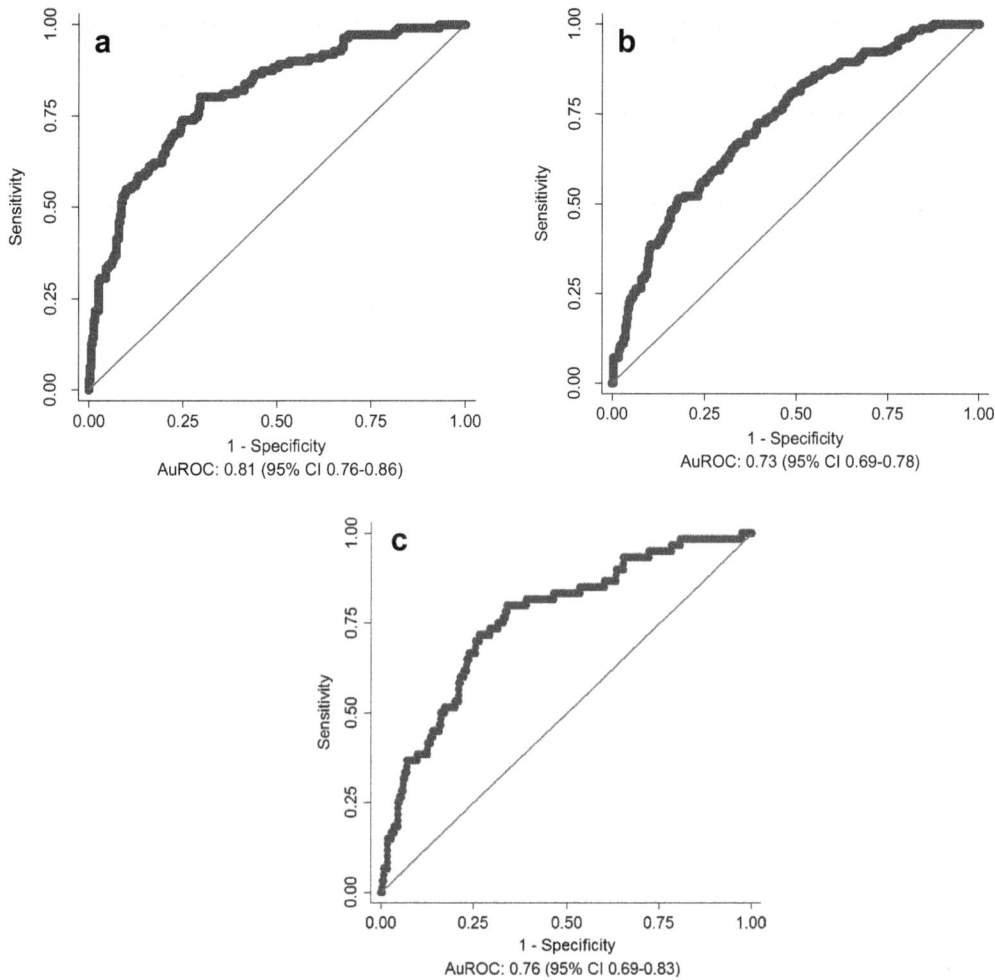

Fig. 1 Receiver operating characteristics (ROC) curve obtained when applying the 6-month prognostic model to the derivation (**a**), geographic validation (**b**) and temporal validation sub-cohorts (**c**) respectively; *AuROC* area under the receiver operating characteristic curve, *CI* confidence interval

The 6-month FP prognostic score produced numerical values which can be stratified within 5 intervals (0–2; above 2–4; above 4–6; above 6–12; above 12) corresponding to five levels of 6-month mortality risk. The 28-day mortality FP score produces values classified within 5 intervals, corresponding to different risk categories for the outcome (0–2; above 2–4; above 4–8; above 8–16; above 16). The observed mortality rates corresponding to each class of risk for the two scoring systems are presented in Table 4 for all three cohorts (Additional file 1: Figs. S1 and S2 display the corresponding histograms of mortality). A 6-month FP score above 12 is consistently associated with a greater than 50% mortality risk at 6 months across all cohorts. A 28-day FP score above 16 is associated with a greater than 40% mortality risk for the 28-day outcome for the derivation and geographic

validation cohorts, but not for the temporal validation cohort, in which the highest observed mortality risk was around 22%.

The discriminatory capabilities of the FP prognostic tools versus the SOFA and APACHE II scores in the FP cohorts

To assess how the FP models compare, as prognostic tools, to the routinely used SOFA and APACHE II scores, we calculated AuROCs for these scoring systems, to predict 6-month and 28-day mortality, in order to compare each tool across all cohorts and for both outcomes. For 6-month mortality, the SOFA score produced AuROCs of 0.73 (95% CI 0.68–0.78), 0.68 (95% CI 0.63–0.72) and 0.62 (95% CI 0.54–0.7) in the derivation, geographic and temporal external validation cohorts, respectively, while the APACHE II score yielded AuROCs of 0.74 (95% CI

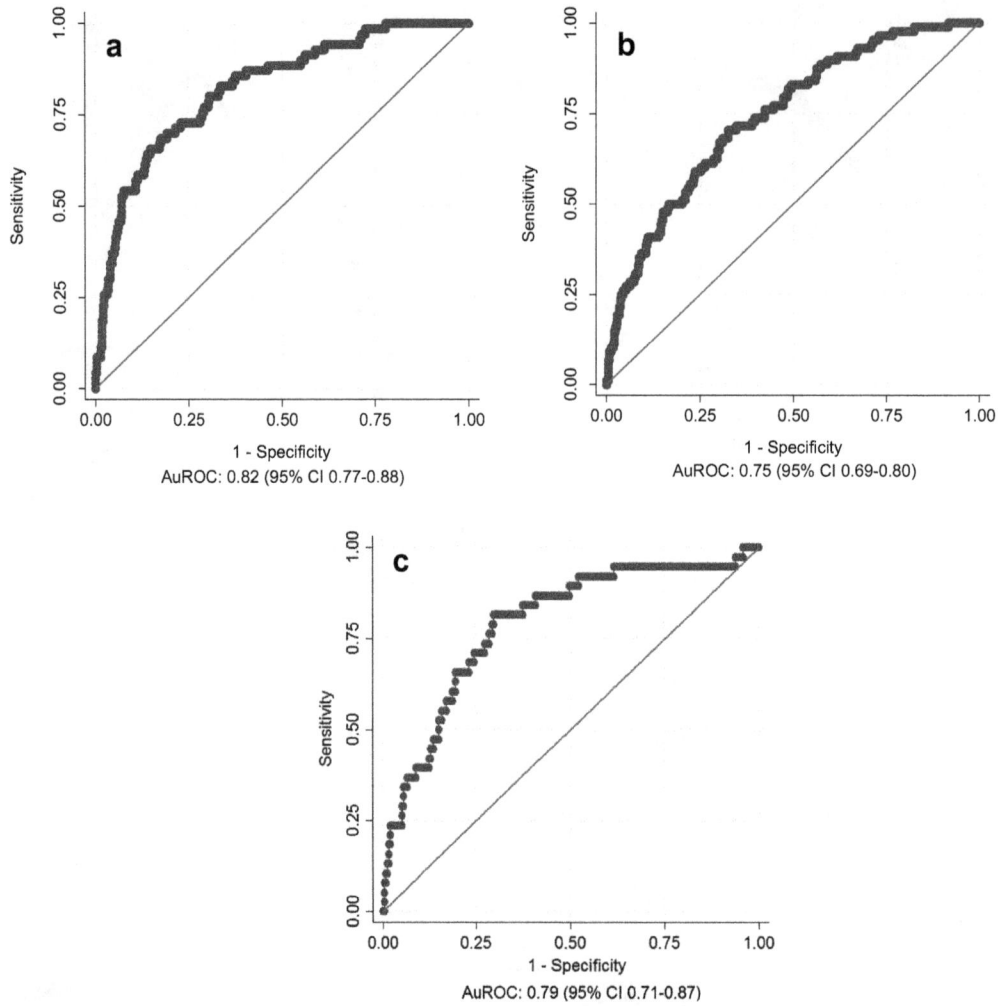

Fig. 2 Receiver operating characteristics (ROC) curve obtained when applying the 28 day prognostic model to the derivation (**a**), geographic validation (**b**) and temporal validation sub-cohorts (**c**) respectively; *AuROC* area under the receiver operating characteristic curve, *CI* confidence interval

Table 4 Observed 6-month and 28-day mortality rates for the derivation, geographic and temporal external validation sub-cohorts, stratified by FP score interval

Cohort	Derivation (UK until Jan 2011)	Geographic validation (non-UK)	Temporal validation (UK post-Jan 2011)
FP score	Deceased	Deceased	Deceased
6-month mortality			
0–2	3 (3.7%)	14 (13.7%)	5 (6.3%)
>2–4	11 (10.8%)	25 (22.5%)	7 (10.5%)
>4–6	14 (20%)	29 (36.3%)	12 (26.1%)
>6–12	29 (31.9%)	44 (40.7%)	15 (28.9%)
>12	67 (57.3%)	73 (64%)	22 (59.5%)
28-day mortality			
0–2	0 (0%)	10 (9.9%)	2 (2.7%)
>2–4	8 (8.3%)	12 (12%)	3 (5.4%)
>4–8	10 (9.5%)	17 (15.3%)	8 (11.1%)
>8–16	14 (16.5%)	27 (26.2%)	12 (22.2%)
>16	47 (45.6%)	42 (42%)	15 (22.4%)

0.7–0.79), 0.71 (95% CI 0.66–0.75) and 0.69 (95% CI 0.62–0.77) for those cohorts, respectively. For the 28-day mortality outcome, the SOFA score produced AuROCs of 0.76 (95% CI 0.7–0.82), 0.66 (95% CI 0.6–0.73) and 0.67 (95% CI 0.58–0.77) in the derivation, geographic and temporal external validation cohorts, respectively, while the same AuROCs for the APACHE II score were 0.71 (95% CI 0.64–0.77), 0.69 (95% CI 0.63–0.75) and 0.75 (95% CI 0.67–0.83), respectively.

The AuROCs obtained using the FP scores were consistently superior to those obtained with the SOFA score, with statistical significance across all cohorts (derivation, geographic and temporal external validation) and for both 6-month and 28-day mortality outcomes (Additional file 1: Figs. S3 and S4, respectively).

The AuROCs obtained using the FP scores were also superior to those derived using the APACHE II score for both outcomes, although statistical significance was not consistently achieved across all cohorts (Additional file 1: Figs. S5 and S6, for 6-month and 28-day mortality, respectively).

Discussion

Faecal peritonitis continues to be associated with a high mortality. Approximately one out of five critically unwell patients with FP in Europe will die in the intensive care unit; this mortality rate increases to over 30% at 6 months.

As we previously reported, and perhaps unexpectedly, the presence of co-morbidities, the time from presumed onset of symptoms to surgery, the underlying cause of FP and the degree of organ support needed in critical care did not appear to influence survival significantly in these postoperative critically ill patients [24, 25]. We are not aware of any prognostic tool designed to assess the risk of long-term mortality specifically in the critically ill postsurgical FP patient. The risk prediction models described in our study aim to improve the SOFA score's predictive power for mortality at 6 months and 28 days, by adding just a few key variables: age, lowest recorded temperature, highest recorded heart rate and haematocrit on admission to intensive care.

The 6-month mortality model demonstrates AuROCs of 0.81 (0.76–0.86), 0.73 (0.69–0.78) in the derivation and geographic validation cohorts, respectively, while the 28-day prognostic tool yielded AuROCs of 0.82 (0.77–0.88) and 0.75 (0.69–0.80) for the same cohorts. An area under the ROC curve over 0.8 is generally regarded as indicating a good discriminatory capacity [26]. In the temporal validation cohort, the 6-month and 28-day mortality models yielded AuROC of 0.76 (95% CI 0.69–0.83) and 0.79 (0.71–0.87), respectively. The models, therefore, retained reasonable discriminatory capability,

and systematically outperformed the other scoring systems tested (SOFA and APACHE II), in these cohorts.

This FP prognostic tool may, therefore, be useful to complement the currently used risk scores and bedside clinical assessment, enhancing the critical care clinician's capacity to predict long-term outcome, thereby supporting the clinical decision making process in the postoperative phase.

The prognostic models presented here have some strengths, particularly as they have been derived and internally validated using large, homogeneous and recently gathered cohorts of FP patients (hence reflecting current practices and therapies).

Biondo and colleagues have recently evaluated the performance of the MPI as a predictor of immediate postoperative mortality, demonstrating an AuROC of 0.72 (95% CI 0.65–0.79), while, for the more specific left colonic Peritonitis Severity Score (PSS), the AuROC was 0.79 (95% CI 0.72–0.85) for this outcome [27].

We have previously reported that factors such as age, acute renal dysfunction, hypothermia, lower haematocrit and thrombocytopaenia are associated with an increased risk of death from FP [24, 25], and a number of other studies have evaluated the prognostic relevance of the individual components of our proposed prognostic models.

SOFA

The SOFA score was developed in a mixed (medical and surgical) ICU population [28] and has been subsequently externally validated in various populations [1], such as cardiac surgical patients [29] and critically ill burn patients [30].

While the SOFA score was originally developed for the purpose of describing the evolution of organ dysfunction, rather than for prognostic purposes, we previously found that both admission SOFA and trends in the global SOFA scores were closely associated with mortality [25]. Many studies have reported the use of the SOFA score both in isolation [31–35] and in combination with other variables [36, 37], for the purpose of outcome prediction. In our study, neither the SOFA nor the APACHE II scores, when used in isolation, performed as well as the tools developed here. Furthermore, day one SOFA performed particularly poorly in the temporal validation group, while the APACHE II risk model (which was developed for the purpose of outcome prediction) performed more consistently across the three cohorts, both for the 6-month and the 28-day outcome. This finding suggests that the value of SOFA lies primarily in describing temporal changes in organ function. Nevertheless, a single SOFA score can be successfully integrated with other parameters, to provide a prognostic tool with improved accuracy [36, 37], as we have done for day one SOFA in these analyses. While the confidence intervals for the AuROCs were relatively wide, when the FP models were compared to SOFA, statistically significant differences were found across all cohorts. This was not always the case for comparisons with APACHE II, further highlighting the superior prognostic accuracy of this severity score compared to an isolated, day one SOFA score.

Hypothermia

The adverse effect of hypothermia on the outcome of critically ill patients has been described by other authors, although data on the relevance of hypothermia to outcomes remain conflicting [38, 39]. Laupland and co-authors studied 10,962 medical, non-scheduled and scheduled surgical patients admitted to critical care with varying degrees of hypothermia and fever. Hypothermia was, after controlling for confounding factors, significantly and independently associated with mortality in medical patients [38]. Tiruvoipati et al. reported data from 175 elderly ICU patients, identifying lower temperatures and the Simplified Acute Physiology Score II (SAPS II) during the first day of ICU admission as being independently associated with higher hospital mortality [39, 40]. An association between severe hypothermia and the risk of ICU acquired infections has also been reported among medical patients [41].

Highest recorded heart rate

An increased heart rate is a physiological response to infection and sepsis, and part of the systemic inflammatory response syndrome (SIRS). Sprung and colleagues found that the presence of SIRS predicts infection, severity of illness, organ failure and outcome, with the two most common SIRS criteria met during ICU stay being respiratory rate (82%) and heart rate (80%) [42]. Morelli and co-workers randomised a total of 154 septic shock patients to receive a continuous infusion of esmolol (targeting a heart rate of 80–94 bpm) or standard treatment in an open label trial. The patients in the esmolol arm achieved lower heart rates, without an increase of adverse events. Interestingly, an improvement in survival and other secondary outcomes was also reported [43]. Others have found that a high daily mean heart rate was a significant predictor of ICU mortality [44].

Haematocrit

Anaemia in surgical patients undergoing both cardiac and non-cardiac procedures has previously been reported to be associated with worse outcomes [45–49]. Beattie and co-workers performed a retrospective observational study of 7759 non-cardiac surgical patients to establish the relationship between preoperative anaemia

and postoperative mortality and found that preoperative anaemia was common and strongly linked with postoperative mortality, even after adjustment for major confounders [49].

All of the patients with FP included in the analyses reported here underwent laparotomy (the diagnosis of FP was based on the intra-operative finding of faecal soiling of the peritoneal cavity). In addition, a significant proportion of patients (40%) were documented to have cardiovascular co-morbidity, a group in which anaemia has been shown to be associated with worse survival and major adverse cardiovascular events. Although anaemia may be associated with a poor outcome, data on the effects of blood transfusion are conflicting, with most reports not demonstrating benefit from transfusion aimed at achieving a higher haemoglobin threshold [50, 51].

Limitations

One limitation of the current study is that we were unable to test the performance of other scoring systems such as the colorectal POSSUM, the MPI, PIA II or the PSS in our dataset, as these systems all require some intra-operative or preoperative findings, which were not available to us. On the other hand, the fact that our scores do not require any intra-operative findings could be viewed as an advantage.

A further limitation is the lack of comparison with alternative and more recent versions of severity scores, such as the Simplified Acute Physiology Score (SAPS) 3, the APACHE III or IV or the Mortality Prediction Model (MPM) III. We consider this unlikely to have a significant impact on the validity of our results, as multiple studies have shown that the performance of such tools, even in their more recent versions, is not significantly improved [52]. A pragmatic decision was made to rely on the APACHE II (rather than more recent versions of APACHE) in view of its practicality, the fact that it is the only available non-proprietary version in widespread clinical use [1, 2, 4] and the comparator of choice in multiple other recently published studies [53, 54].

The SOFA score may be a less than ideal comparator, as the SOFA was not originally developed for prognostication. Multiple previous studies have, however, reported using the SOFA score, both in isolation [31–35] and in combination with other parameters [36, 37], for outcome prediction.

Another limitation is that our study was not designed to evaluate the influence on outcome of the timing and adequacy of source control or antibiotic treatment. All patients included in the study reported here received source control via surgical laparotomy prior to recruitment and the overwhelming majority of the patients

(91.8%) received antimicrobial therapy deemed to be adequate [24].

Although the homogeneity of the patient population within our cohorts represents a methodological strength of the study, it may also be considered a potential weakness, as some *real-world* critically ill patients with FP would have not been included in our analyses.

Mortality differed markedly between the cohorts, even though they were recruited using the same inclusion and exclusion criteria. Whilst it is impossible to identify with certainty which factors explain these differences, multiple potential reasons can be postulated. Firstly, the variation in mortality rates strongly correlates with the occurrence of acute renal failure on day one. Acute renal dysfunction and deteriorating renal function have both been consistently associated with poor outcome in this specific subset of patients [24, 25]. The effects of random variability and the fact that in the UK the centres recruiting to GenOSept and those recruiting to GAinS were not always the same may have also contributed. Finally, improvements in the management of sepsis over the years may have influenced the incidence of renal failure and outcomes.

Conclusions

The present study describes the development of two prognostic models for the risk of 6-month and 28-day mortality in critically ill septic patients with FP, following laparotomy for source control. The tools incorporate five of the major independent risk factors identified in previous studies (SOFA score, age, heart rate, temperature and haematocrit) and combine them to produce a numerical value associated with mortality risk over 6 months or 28 days. Although, in the setting of postoperative FP patients admitted to critical care, the tools appeared to be superior to other existing scoring systems, such as SOFA and APACHE II, these findings should not be considered definitive. External validation in larger cohorts, such as the NELA (National Emergency Laparotomy Audit) or other databases [55], of their predictive capability is needed before introduction of the scores into clinical practice to inform decision making and the design of clinical trials.

Abbreviations
APACHE: Acute Physiology and Chronic Health Evaluation; ARF: acute renal failure; bpm: beats per minute; CI: confidence interval; CPAP: continuous positive airways pressure; CVS: cardiovascular; CXR: chest radiography; eCRF: electronic case report form; FP: faecal peritonitis; GCS: Glasgow Coma Scale; HR: hazard ratio; ICU: Intensive Care Unit; IQR: interquartile range; MAP: mean arterial pressure; MOSF: multiple organ system failure; N: number of non-missing observations; paO2: arterial partial pressure of oxygen; paCO2: arterial partial pressure of carbon dioxide; P:F: ratio of partial pressure arterial oxygen and fraction of inspired oxygen; RRT: renal replacement therapy; SBP: systolic blood pressure; SOFA: Sequential Organ Failure Assessment; WCC: white cell count.

Authors' contributions
AT conducted statistical analyses on the database, appraised the background literature, prepared the first draft of the manuscript and coordinated subsequent revisions; GMC prepared and quality-assured the database for analysis and contributed to revise the manuscript; AW contributed to drafting and reviewing the manuscript; ACG contributed to reviewing the manuscript; PH prepared and quality-assured the database for analysis and contributed to revise the manuscript; J-DC contributed to revise the manuscript; PAHH contributed to revise the manuscript; GHM contributed to revise the manuscript; JB conceived the study, contributed to drafting and reviewing the manuscript; FS conceived the study, contributed to reviewing the manuscript; CG conceived the study, contributed to quality assurance of the database, contributed to drafting and reviewing the manuscript; CH conceived the study, contributed to drafting and reviewing the manuscript; all authors read and approved the final manuscript.

Author details
[1] Whiston Hospital Prescot, Merseyside and Department of Infection, Immunity and Cardiovascular Disease, The Medical School, University of Sheffield, Sheffield, UK. [2] School of Clinical and Experimental Medicine, University of Birmingham, Birmingham, UK. [3] University of Sheffield, Sheffield, UK. [4] Imperial College, London, UK. [5] The Wellcome Trust Centre for Human Genetics, University of Oxford, Oxford, UK. [6] Intensive Care Unit, Royal Berkshire Hospital, Reading, UK. [7] Intensive Care Unit, John Radcliffe Hospital, Oxford, UK. [8] Hospital Cochin, Paris, France. [9] Department of Anaesthesiology and Pain Medicine, Bern University Hospital and University of Bern, Bern, Switzerland. [10] Barts and the London Queen Mary School of Medicine, London, UK.

Acknowledgements
Mr. Graham Paul Copeland, of the Department of Surgery, Warrington Hospital, Warrington, UK, provided us with very valuable insights into the development and evaluation of a scoring system.

The authors of this manuscript wish to thank all GenOSept and GAinS Investigators, as listed in Additional file 1.

Competing interests
The authors declare that they have no competing interest.

Funding
GenOSept (Genetics Of Sepsis and Septic Shock in Europe) is a pan-European part-FP6-funded study conceived by the European Critical Care Research Network of the European Society for Intensive Care Medicine to investigate the potential impact of genetic variation on the host response and outcomes in sepsis (https://www.genosept.eu/).

CIBERES is a Spanish research network which was used to identify investigators and contributed to funding through supporting logistics. A grant in partial support of FP6 projects was provided by the Spanish minister of Health.

References
1. Vincent J-L, Moreno R. Clinical review: scoring systems in the critically ill. Crit Care [Internet]. 2010 [cited 2015 Mar 16];14:207. Available from: http://www.pubmedcentral.nih.gov/articlerender.fcgi?artid=2887099&tool=pmcentrez&rendertype=abstract.
2. Eachempati SR. Critical care scoring systems [Internet]. Merck Man. 2014 [cited 2016 Aug 1]. Available from: http://www.merckmanuals.com/professional/critical-care-medicine/approach-to-the-critically-ill-patient/critical-care-scoring-systems#.
3. Breslow MJ, Badawi O. Severity scoring in the critically ill: Part 1—interpretation and accuracy of outcome prediction scoring systems. Chest. 2012;141:245–52.
4. Bouch DC, Thompson JP. Severity scoring systems in the critically ill. Contin Educ Anaesth Crit Care Pain [Internet]. Oxford University Press; 2008 [cited 2016 Aug 1];8:181–5. Available from: http://bjarev.oxfordjournals.org/lookup/doi/10.1093/bjaceaccp/mkn033.
5. Iwashyna TJ, Burke JF, Sussman JB, Prescott HC, Hayward RA, Angus DC. Implications of heterogeneity of treatment effect for reporting and

analysis of randomized trials in critical care. Am J Respir Crit Care Med [Internet]. 2015 [cited 2016 Sep 12];192:1045–51. Available from: http://www.ncbi.nlm.nih.gov/pubmed/26177009.

6. Calandra T, Cohen J. The international sepsis forum consensus conference on definitions of infection in the intensive care unit. Crit Care Med. [Internet]. 2005 [cited 2014 Apr 28];33:1538–48. Available from: http://www.ncbi.nlm.nih.gov/pubmed/16003060.

7. Wacha H, Linder M, Feldman U, Wesch G, Gundlach E, Steifensand R. Mannheim peritonitis index—prediction of risk of death from peritonitis: construction of a statistical and validation of an empirically based index. Theor Surg. 1987;1:169–77.

8. Wittmann DH, Teichmann W, Muller M. 176. Entwicklung und Validierung des Peritonitis-Index-Altona (PIA II). Langenbecks Arch Chir Chir [Internet]. 1987 [cited 2015 May 26];372:834–5. Available from: http://link.springer.com/10.1007/BF01297960.

9. Biondo S, Ramos E, Deiros M, Ragué JM, De Oca J, Moreno P, et al. Prognostic factors for mortality in left colonic peritonitis: a new scoring system. J Am Coll Surg [Internet]. 2000 [cited 2015 Dec 13];191:635–42. Available from: http://www.ncbi.nlm.nih.gov/pubmed/11129812.

10. Copeland GP, Jones D, Walters M. POSSUM: a scoring system for surgical audit. Br J Surg [Internet]. 1991 [cited 2015 Dec 23];78:355–60. Available from: http://www.ncbi.nlm.nih.gov/pubmed/2021856.

11. Tekkis PP, Prytherch DR, Kocher HM, Senapati A, Poloniecki JD, Stamatakis JD, et al. Development of a dedicated risk-adjustment scoring system for colorectal surgery (colorectal POSSUM). Br J Surg [Internet]. 2004 [cited 2015 Dec 23];91:1174–82. Available from: http://www.ncbi.nlm.nih.gov/pubmed/15449270.

12. European Society of Intensive Care Medicine—GenOSept study [Internet]. Available from: http://www.esicm.org/research/other-studies/genosept.

13. UK Critical Care Genomics group—GAinS study [Internet]. Available from: http://www.ukccg-gains.org/index.htm.

14. Bone RC, Balk RA, Cerra FB, Dellinger RP, Fein AM, Knaus WA, et al. Definitions for sepsis and organ failure and guidelines for the use of innovative therapies in sepsis. The ACCP/SCCM Consensus Conference Committee. American College of Chest Physicians/Society of Critical Care Medicine. Chest [Internet]. 1992 [cited 2014 Apr 28];101:1644–55. Available from: http://www.ncbi.nlm.nih.gov/pubmed/1303622.

15. Chen CH, George SL. The bootstrap and identification of prognostic factors via Cox's proportional hazards regression model. Stat Med [Internet]. 1985 [cited 2015 May 2];4:39–46. Available from: http://www.ncbi.nlm.nih.gov/pubmed/3857702.

16. Harrell FE, Lee KL, Mark DB. Multivariable prognostic models: issues in developing models, evaluating assumptions and adequacy, and measuring and reducing errors. Stat Med [Internet]. 1996 [cited 2015 Jul 26];15:361–87. Available from: http://www.ncbi.nlm.nih.gov/pubmed/8668867.

17. Hess KR. Graphical methods for assessing violations of the proportional hazards assumption in Cox regression. Stat Med [Internet]. 1995 [cited 2016 Aug 5];14:1707–23. Available from: http://www.ncbi.nlm.nih.gov/pubmed/7481205.

18. Therneau TM, Grambsch PM. Modeling survival data: extending the cox model [Internet]. Berlin: Springer; 2000 [cited 2015 May 26]. Available from: https://books.google.com.my/books/about/Modeling_Survival_Data_Extending_the_Cox.html?id=9kY4XRuUMUsC&pgis=1.

19. Slinker BK, Glantz SA. Multiple regression for physiological data analysis: the problem of multicollinearity. Am J Physiol [Internet]. 1985 [cited 2016 Aug 5];249:R1–12. Available from: http://www.ncbi.nlm.nih.gov/pubmed/4014489.

20. Metz CE. Basic principles of ROC analysis. Semin Nucl Med [Internet]. 1978 [cited 2014 Apr 28];8:283–98. Available from: http://www.ncbi.nlm.nih.gov/pubmed/112681.

21. Hanley JA, McNeil BJ. The meaning and use of the area under a receiver operating characteristic (ROC) curve. Radiology [Internet]. 1982 [cited 2014 Dec 5];143:29–36. Available from: http://www.ncbi.nlm.nih.gov/pubmed/7063747.

22. Zweig MH, Campbell G. Receiver-operating characteristic (ROC) plots: a fundamental evaluation tool in clinical medicine. Clin Chem [Internet]. 1993 [cited 2014 Apr 28];39:561–77. Available from: http://www.ncbi.nlm.nih.gov/pubmed/8472349.

23. DeLong ER, DeLong DM, Clarke-Pearson DL. Comparing the areas under two or more correlated receiver operating characteristic curves: a nonparametric approach. Biometrics [Internet]. 1988 [cited 2016 Jul 18];44:837–45. Available from: http://www.ncbi.nlm.nih.gov/pubmed/3203132.

24. Tridente A, Clarke GM, Walden A, McKechnie S, Hutton P, Mills GH, et al. Patients with faecal peritonitis admitted to European intensive care units: an epidemiological survey of the GenOSept cohort. Intensive Care Med. 2014;40:202–10.

25. Tridente A, Clarke GM, Walden A, Gordon AC, Hutton P, Chiche J-D, et al. Association between trends in clinical variables and outcome in intensive care patients with faecal peritonitis: analysis of the GenOSept cohort. Crit Care [Internet]. 2015 [cited 2015 Nov 2];19:210. Available from: http://www.pubmedcentral.nih.gov/articlerender.fcgi?artid=4432819&tool=pmcentrez&rendertype=abstract.

26. Tape TG. University of Nebraska Medical Center: interpreting diagnostic tests—the area under an ROC curve [Internet]. Univ. Nebraska Med. Cent. webpage. 2016. Available from: http://gim.unmc.edu/dxtests/roc3.htm.

27. Biondo S, Ramos E, Fraccalvieri D, Kreisler E, Ragué JM, Jaurrieta E. Comparative study of left colonic Peritonitis Severity Score and Mannheim Peritonitis Index. Br J Surg [Internet]. 2006 [cited 2015 Dec 13];93:616–22. Available from: http://www.ncbi.nlm.nih.gov/pubmed/16607684.

28. Vincent JL, Moreno R, Takala J, Willatts S, De Mendonça A, Bruining H, et al. The SOFA (Sepsis-related Organ Failure Assessment) score to describe organ dysfunction/failure. On behalf of the Working Group on Sepsis-Related Problems of the European Society of Intensive Care Medicine. Intensive Care Med [Internet]. 1996 [cited 2014 Apr 28];22:707–10. Available from: http://www.ncbi.nlm.nih.gov/pubmed/8844239.

29. Ceriani R, Mazzoni M, Bortone F, Gandini S, Solinas C, Susini G, et al. Application of the sequential organ failure assessment score to cardiac surgical patients. Chest [Internet]. 2003 [cited 2015 May 18];123:1229–39. Available from: http://www.ncbi.nlm.nih.gov/pubmed/12684316.

30. Lorente JA, Vallejo A, Galeiras R, Tómicic V, Zamora J, Cerdá E, et al. Organ dysfunction as estimated by the sequential organ failure assessment score is related to outcome in critically ill burn patients. Shock [Internet]. 2009 [cited 2015 Apr 4];31:125–31. Available from: http://www.ncbi.nlm.nih.gov/pubmed/18650779.

31. Hynninen M, Wennervirta J, Leppäniemi A, Pettilä V. Organ dysfunction and long term outcome in secondary peritonitis. Langenbecks Arch Surg [Internet]. 2008 [cited 2014 Jun 11];393:81–6. Available from: http://www.ncbi.nlm.nih.gov/pubmed/17372753.

32. van Ruler O, Kiewiet JJS, Boer KR, Lamme B, Gouma DJ, Boermeester MA, et al. Failure of available scoring systems to predict ongoing infection in patients with abdominal sepsis after their initial emergency laparotomy. BMC Surg [Internet]. 2011 [cited 2014 Apr 28];11:38. Available from: http://www.pubmedcentral.nih.gov/articlerender.fcgi?artid=3268736&tool=pmcentrez&rendertype=abstract.

33. van Ruler O, Lamme B, Gouma DJ, Reitsma JB, Boermeester MA. Variables associated with positive findings at relaparotomy in patients with secondary peritonitis. Crit Care Med [Internet]. 2007 [cited 2014 Apr 28];35:468–76. Available from: http://www.ncbi.nlm.nih.gov/pubmed/17205025.

34. Sumi T, Katsumata K, Katayanagi S, Nakamura Y, Nomura T, Takano K, et al. Examination of prognostic factors in patients undergoing surgery for colorectal perforation: a case controlled study. Int J Surg [Internet]. 2014 [cited 2014 Jun 11];12:566–71. Available from: http://www.ncbi.nlm.nih.gov/pubmed/24709571.

35. Jones AE, Trzeciak S, Kline JA. The Sequential Organ Failure Assessment score for predicting outcome in patients with severe sepsis and evidence of hypoperfusion at the time of emergency department presentation. Crit Care Med [Internet]. 2009 [cited 2015 Mar 2];37:1649–54. Available from: http://www.pubmedcentral.nih.gov/articlerender.fcgi?artid=2703722&tool=pmcentrez&rendertype=abstract.

36. Zügel NP, Kox M, Lichtwark-Aschoff M, Gippner-Steppert C, Jochum M. Predictive relevance of clinical scores and inflammatory parameters in secondary peritonitis. Bull Soc Sci Med Grand Duche Luxemb [Internet]. 2011 [cited 2014 Jun 11];41–71. Available from: http://www.ncbi.nlm.nih.gov/pubmed/21634221.

37. Matsumura Y, Nakada T, Abe R, Oshima T, Oda S. Serum procalcitonin level and SOFA score at discharge from the intensive care unit predict post-intensive care unit mortality: a prospective study. PLoS One [Internet]. 2014 [cited 2015 Mar 2];9:e114007. Available from: http://www.pubmed-central.nih.gov/articlerender.fcgi?artid=4252062&tool=pmcentrez&rendertype=abstract.

38. Laupland KB, Zahar J-R, Adrie C, Minet C, Vésin A, Goldgran-Toledano D, et al. Severe hypothermia increases the risk for intensive care unit-acquired infection. Clin Infect Dis [Internet]. 2012 [cited 2014 Apr 28];54:1064–70. Available from: http://www.ncbi.nlm.nih.gov/pubmed/22291110.

39. Tiruvoipati R, Ong K, Gangopadhyay H, Arora S, Carney I, Botha J. Hypothermia predicts mortality in critically ill elderly patients with sepsis. BMC Geriatr [Internet]. 2010 [cited 2014 Apr 28];10:70. Available from: http://www.pubmedcentral.nih.gov/articlerender.fcgi?artid=2955035&tool=pmcentrez&rendertype=abstract.

40. Le Gall JR, Lemeshow S, Saulnier F. A new Simplified Acute Physiology Score (SAPS II) based on a European/North American multicenter study. JAMA [Internet]. 1994 [cited 2015 May 24];270:2957–63. Available from: http://www.ncbi.nlm.nih.gov/pubmed/8254858.

41. Laupland KB, Zahar J-R, Adrie C, Schwebel C, Goldgran-Toledano D, Azoulay E, et al. Determinants of temperature abnormalities and influence on outcome of critical illness. Crit Care Med [Internet]. 2012 [cited 2014 Apr 28];40:145–51. Available from: http://www.ncbi.nlm.nih.gov/pubmed/21926588.

42. Sprung CL, Sakr Y, Vincent J-L, Le Gall J-R, Reinhart K, Ranieri VM, et al. An evaluation of systemic inflammatory response syndrome signs in the Sepsis Occurrence in Acutely Ill Patients (SOAP) study. Intensive Care Med [Internet]. 2006 [cited 2016 Jan 24];32:421–7. Available from: http://www.ncbi.nlm.nih.gov/pubmed/16479382.

43. Morelli A, Ertmer C, Westphal M, Rehberg S, Kampmeier T, Ligges S, et al. Effect of heart rate control with esmolol on hemodynamic and clinical outcomes in patients with septic shock: a randomized clinical trial. JAMA [Internet]. 2013 [cited 2016 Sep 11];310:1683–91. Available from: http://www.ncbi.nlm.nih.gov/pubmed/24108526.

44. Park S, Kim D-G, Suh GY, Park WJ, Jang SH, Hwang Y Il, et al. Significance of new-onset prolonged sinus tachycardia in a medical intensive care unit: a prospective observational study. J Crit Care [Internet]. 2011 [cited 2016 Jan 24];26:534.e1–8. Available from: http://www.ncbi.nlm.nih.gov/pubmed/21376521.

45. Shander A, Knight K, Thurer R, Adamson J, Spence R. Prevalence and outcomes of anemia in surgery: a systematic review of the literature. Am J Med [Internet]. 2004 [cited 2014 Apr 28];116 Suppl:58S–69S. Available from: http://www.ncbi.nlm.nih.gov/pubmed/15050887.

46. Qiu M, Yuan Z, Luo H, Ruan D, Wang Z, Wang F, et al. Impact of pretreatment hematologic profile on survival of colorectal cancer patients. Tumour Biol [Internet]. 2010 [cited 2014 Apr 28];31:255–60. Available from: http://www.ncbi.nlm.nih.gov/pubmed/20336401.

47. Vignot S, Spano J-P. [Anemia and colorectal cancer]. Bull Cancer [Internet]. 2005 [cited 2014 Apr 28];92:432–8. Available from: http://www.ncbi.nlm.nih.gov/pubmed/15932806.

48. Halm EA, Wang JJ, Boockvar K, Penrod J, Silberzweig SB, Magaziner J, et al. The effect of perioperative anemia on clinical and functional outcomes in patients with hip fracture. J Orthop Trauma [Internet]. 2004 [cited 2014 Apr 28];18:369–74. Available from: http://www.pubmedcentral.nih.gov/articlerender.fcgi?artid=1454739&tool=pmcentrez&rendertype=abstract.

49. Beattie WS, Karkouti K, Wijeysundera DN, Tait G. Risk associated with preoperative anemia in noncardiac surgery: a single-center cohort study. Anesthesiology [Internet]. 2009 [cited 2014 Apr 28];110:574–81. Available from: http://www.ncbi.nlm.nih.gov/pubmed/19212255.

50. Hébert PC, Wells G, Blajchman MA, Marshall J, Martin C, Pagliarello G, et al. A multicenter, randomized, controlled clinical trial of transfusion requirements in critical care. N Engl J Med [Internet]. 1999 [cited 2016 Sep 11];340:409–17. Available from: http://www.nejm.org/doi/abs/10.1056/NEJM199902113400601.

51. Holst LB, Petersen MW, Haase N, Perner A, Wetterslev J. Restrictive versus liberal transfusion strategy for red blood cell transfusion: systematic review of randomised trials with meta-analysis and trial sequential analysis. BMJ [Internet]. Br Med J Publ Group; 2015 [cited 2016 Sep 11];350:h1354. Available from: http://www.ncbi.nlm.nih.gov/pubmed/25805204.

52. Lee H, Shon Y-J, Kim H, Paik H, Park H-P. Validation of the APACHE IV model and its comparison with the APACHE II, SAPS 3, and Korean SAPS 3 models for the prediction of hospital mortality in a Korean surgical intensive care unit. Korean J Anesthesiol [Internet]. 2014 [cited 2016 Jul 18];67:115–22. Available from: http://www.ncbi.nlm.nih.gov/pubmed/25237448.

53. Donnino MW, Salciccioli JD, Dejam A, Giberson T, Giberson B, Cristia C, et al. APACHE II scoring to predict outcome in post-cardiac arrest. Resuscitation [Internet]. 2013 [cited 2016 Aug 1];84:651–6. Available from: http://www.ncbi.nlm.nih.gov/pubmed/23178739.

54. Naeini AE, Abbasi S, Haghighipour S, Shirani K. Comparing the APACHE II score and IBM-10 score for predicting mortality in patients with ventilator-associated pneumonia. Adv Biomed Res [Internet]. Medknow Publications; 2015 [cited 2016 Aug 1];4:47. Available from: http://www.ncbi.nlm.nih.gov/pubmed/25789273.

55. Odor PM, Grocott MPW. From NELA to EPOCH and beyond: enhancing the evidence base for emergency laparotomy. Perioper. Med. (London, England) [Internet]. BioMed Central; 2016 [cited 2016 Nov 27];5:23. Available from: http://www.ncbi.nlm.nih.gov/pubmed/27594991.

2

Occurrence of marked sepsis-induced immunosuppression in pediatric septic shock: a pilot study

Solenn Remy[1] [ID], Karine Kolev-Descamps[1], Morgane Gossez[2], Fabienne Venet[2,3], Julie Demaret[2], Etienne Javouhey[1] and Guillaume Monneret[2,3*]

Abstract

Background: While the process of sepsis-induced immunosuppression is now well described in adults, very little information is available on immune functions in pediatric sepsis. The current study investigated this in children with septic shock by performing immunomonitoring, including both innate (monocyte human leukocyte antigen-DR, mHLA-DR, expression) and adaptive immunity (lymphocyte subsets count), as well as cytokine concentrations (IL-6, IL-8, IL-10, IL-1Ra, TNF-α, IFN-γ). Subsequent objectives were to assess the associations between inflammatory response, potential immunosuppression and secondary acquired infection occurrence.

Methods: Single-center prospective observational study, including children aged between 1 month and 18 years admitted to pediatric intensive care unit (PICU) for septic shock. Age-matched controls were children hospitalized for elective surgery without any infectious criteria. Blood was sampled at day 1–2, 3–5, and 7–9 after sepsis onset. mHLA-DR and lymphocyte subsets count were measured by flow cytometry and cytokine concentrations by Luminex technology.

Results: A total of 26 children and 30 controls were included. Patients had lymphopenia, and mHLA-DR levels were significantly lower than controls at each time point ($p < 0.0001$). All cytokines peaked at day 1–2. Children with secondary acquired infection had lower day 3–5 mHLA-DR and higher pro-inflammatory cytokine concentrations (IL-6, IL-8 and TNF-α) at day 1–2 compared to children without secondary acquired infection.

Conclusions: The higher initial inflammatory cytokine production was, the more innate immunity was altered, while evaluated by low mHLA-DR expression. Children with decreased mHLA-DR expression developed more secondary acquired infections. Upon confirmation in multicenter cohorts, these results pave the way for immunostimulation for the most immunosuppressed children in order to prevent nosocomial infections in PICU.

Keywords: Septic shock, Immunosuppression induced, Children

Background

Despite advances in critical care management, septic shock remains one of the most important causes of mortality and morbidity in children worldwide [1]. As for adults, the inability of adjunctive therapies to mitigate the deleterious effects of this condition indicates that it is likely that initial hypotheses for sepsis pathophysiology have been inadequately addressed [2]. In adults, it is now agreed that sepsis deeply perturbs immune balance by inducing a strong systemic inflammatory response and a concomitant anti-inflammatory process, acting as a negative feedback. This compensatory response may secondarily become harmful as most immune functions are compromised, and thus sepsis-induced immune alterations may play a major role in the decreased resistance

*Correspondence: guillaume.monneret@chu-lyon.fr
[2] Hospices Civils de Lyon, Immunology Laboratory, E. Herriot Hospital, 69003 Lyon, France
Full list of author information is available at the end of the article

to secondary acquired infections in patients who initially survive [3]. This immunosuppressive state is characterized by both abnormal innate and adaptive immune responses. In particular, patients mostly present with marked lymphopenia and decreased expression in monocyte human leukocyte antigen-DR (mHLA-DR). The latter remains, to date, the key parameter of patient monitoring and its diminished expression has been reported to be associated with increased mortality and nosocomial infection rate in adults [4–6]. In this context, and as it is already the case for cancer immunotherapy, targeted treatments aimed at rejuvenating immune responses in adult septic patients (e.g., GM-CSF, Interleukin-7, anti-PD-1/-L1) are now envisaged [7–10]. In comparison with adults, data are very scarce in children with septic shock. The impact of this altered immune response on secondary infections is poorly reported in children affected by septic shock. In order to envisage therapeutic interventions to restore immune function in children, a reliable biomarker is required to identify children at highest risk of secondary acquired infection or mortality. Such a marker is currently lacking in children. Most pediatric results are rarely specific of septic shock. They refer, as a whole, to various pediatric intensive care unit (PICU) admission causes (surgery, organ dysfunctions) [11–14], or are limited to particular cases of preterm neonates [15, 16]. Thus, the objective of the present prospective observational study was to investigate whether pediatric septic shock patients present immune alterations similar to those seen in adults. For this, immunomonitoring was performed during the first week after sepsis onset. This monitoring included mHLA-DR, lymphocyte subsets count, and phenotyping as well as measurement of plasma cytokine concentrations: interleukin-6 (IL-6), interleukin-8 (IL-8), interleukin-10 (IL-10), tumor necrosis factor-α (TNF-α), interferon-γ (IFN-γ), and interleukin-1 receptor antagonist (IL-1Ra). As control values may depend on age, and in the absence of mHLA-DR reference range in pediatrics, healthy children were also investigated to explore mHLA-DR expression during the first years of life.

Methods

Study population

This single-center, prospective study was held in PICU from a tertiary academic hospital (23 beds mixed medical-surgical unit, > 1100 admissions/year). Children, aged from 1 month to 18 years, were included prospectively during 24 h of PICU admission, if they presented septic shock, defined by "Surviving Sepsis Campaign" and Goldstein's criteria [17, 18]. Exclusion criteria were: non-septic shock, chronic inflammatory disease, long-term corticosteroid treatment, transplantation and/or immunosuppressive therapy, immunodeficiency syndrome, malignant tumors. Opposition from the child and/or parent/holder of parental authority also constituted exclusion criteria. Controls were age-matched to the case group and identified among outpatients admitted for a scheduled surgery, without any criteria of infection. Exclusion criteria were the same as the case group. Three age subgroups were defined: 1 month to 2, 2–8, and > 8 years, according to the physiological age-based development of immunity in children [19].

Clinical data and definitions

Clinical data were collected prospectively and obtained from the electronic medical record. At admission (day 1), severity of illness was evaluated using the pediatric index of mortality 2 (PIM2) [20]. Organ failure was assessed by the measurement of PEdiatric Logistic Organ Dysfunction Score, version 2 (PELOD-2) at day 1, 3, and 7 [21]. Vasoactive treatments during hospitalization in PICU were determined by the cumulative vasopressor index (CVI) [22]. We also collected incidence of secondary acquired infection, mortality (death occurring within 28 days after the onset of shock), number of mechanical ventilation-free days, and number of PICU-free days in the first 30 days. Secondary acquired infection was defined by Center for Disease Control criteria, included any new bacterial or fungal infection, distinct from initial infection, occurring more than 48 h after sepsis onset, during the first 30 days after sepsis onset [23]. Determination of secondary acquired infection was performed prospectively by one physician (SR), blinded to immunological data.

Blood sampling for immunomonitoring

Blood samples were collected within the first 48 h after the onset of infection, again between day 3–5, and day 7–9. Samples were not available if patients were no longer in PICU. Blood was collected in EDTA tubes, transported rapidly at 4 °C to the Cellular Immunology Laboratory, and analyzed within less than 4 h. The amount of blood sample did not exceed 2.4 ml/kg, in accordance with European recommendations. At each time point, the following parameters were determined by flow cytometry: mHLA-DR, total lymphocytes and lymphocytes subpopulations (CD4$^+$ and CD8$^+$ T cells, natural killer [NK] cells, regulatory T cells [Treg], and B cells). In addition, after completion of cellular analysis, plasma was obtained after centrifugation and stored at − 80 °C for subsequent quantification of following circulating cytokines: IL-6, IL-8, IL-10, IL-1RA, TNF-α, and IFN-γ. For the control group, blood was sampled in the operating room immediately after induction of general anesthesia with sevoflurane, before start of surgery.

Flow cytometry

Quantification of mHLA-DR on circulating monocytes was performed using a standardized flow cytometric assay as previously described [24.] The median fluorescence intensity of the entire monocyte population was then transformed to number of antibodies bound per cell (ABC) using calibrated PE beads (BD QuantiBRITE™ PE Beads, Becton–Dickinson San Jose, CA, USA). The following lymphocyte subsets were analyzed by flow cytometry as previously described [25, 26]: total T lymphocytes ($CD45^+$ $CD3^+$), $CD4^+$ T lymphocytes ($CD45^+$ $CD4^+$ $CD3^+$), $CD8^+$ T lymphocytes ($CD45^+$ $CD8^+$ $CD3^+$), total B cells ($CD45^+$ $CD19^+$), NK cells ($CD45^+$ $CD3^-$ $CD56^+$), and Treg ($CD4^+$ $CD25^+$ $CD127^-$). Results were expressed as numbers of cells per microliter of blood for lymphocyte subsets and as percentage of positive cells among total $CD4^+$ lymphocyte population for Treg.

Cytokine measurement

IL-6, IL-8, IL-10, IL-1RA, TNF-α, and IFN-γ were quantified with a single panel (Milliplex® MAP Human Cytokine/Chemokine Magnetic Bead Panel, Merck Millipore) using the fluorescent bead-based multiplexed Luminex xMAP technology [27]. Analyses were performed on Bio-Plex 200 Luminex instrument using Bio-Plex software (Bio-Rad, Hercules, CA, USA).

Statistical analysis

Results are expressed as median and interquartile range [IQR]. Comparisons between groups were analyzed using the Man–Whitney U test for continuous nonparametric variables; the independent paired t test for continuous parametric variables and the Chi-square test for categorical data. Correlation analyses were performed using the Pearson test for variables following a normal distribution, and Spearman for nonparametric variables. Kaplan–Meier analyses were performed using Youden's index to stratify groups of patients. A p value < 0.05 was considered to represent significant statistical difference. Data were analyzed by using Prism6 software (GraphPad Inc., La Jolla, CA, USA).

Results

Subjects

Between September 2014 and July 2016, 73 children were screened for septic shock. Among these, 47 were excluded (toxic shock syndrome, non-infectious shock, known immunosuppression, or chronic inflammatory disease). A total of 26 children were included and analyzed (Fig. 1). Demographic data are presented in Table 1. Nine children (35%) presented a complex chronic condition. The most frequent was prematurity ($n=4$), but all children presented a corrected age greater than 1 month.

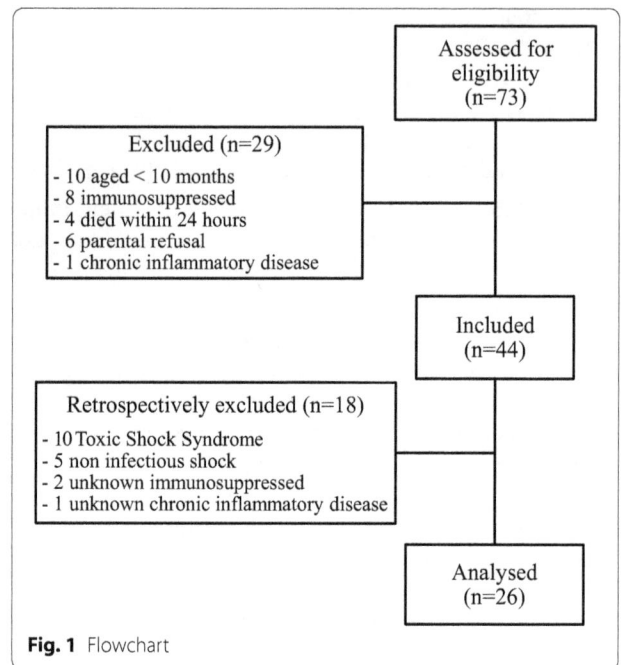

Fig. 1 Flowchart

Others presented psychomotor delay ($n=2$), polymalformative disease ($n=2$), and sickle cell disease ($n=1$). Two children died: one precociously at day 2, due to refractory shock with multi-organ failure; and the second one at day 32, with withdrawal treatment for major brain damage after meningitis. A total of 30 healthy children were included as controls. They were age-matched with children in septic shock ($p=0.3$, Mann–Whitney): 11 were aged between 1 month and 2 years, 14 between 2 and 8 years, and 5 > 8 years.

mHLA-DR expression

In healthy control children, mHLA-DR was > 25,000 ABC; among those aged between 1 month to 2 years it was (median [IQR]) 25,477 ABC [20,478–39,143], among those aged 2–8 years it was 34,295 ABC [25,763–43,368], and among those older than 8 years it was 29,597 ABC [26,636–41,939]; there was no significant difference between age subgroups ($p=0.35$; ANOVA, Fig. 2a). There was also no correlation between age and mHLA-DR ($r=0.018$).

In children with septic shock, mHLA-DR was 6066 ABC [3737–16,310] at day 1–2, 6308 ABC [3185–8965] at day 3–5, and 9323 ABC [6384–12,738] at 7–9; at each time point values were significantly different to that found in healthy control children ($p<0.0001$; Fig. 2b). There was no correlation between mHLA-DR and PIM2 or PELOD-2 scores, at any time point, while a significant correlation was found between day 3–5 mHLA-DR and CVI ($r=-0.50$; $p=0.031$; Fig. 2c).

Table 1 Characteristics of the 26 children with septic shock included in the study

	Septic shock (n = 26)
Age (years)	2.12 [0.47–4.60]
Male gender [n (%)]	11 (42)
Complex chronic conditions [n (%)]	9 (35)
Primary nosocomial infection	1 (3.9)
Site of initial infection [n (%)]	
Blood	3 (11.5)
Lung	4 (15.4)
Abdomen	8 (30.8)
Multi-site	9 (34.6)
Others	1 (3.9)
No documentation	1 (3.9)
Microbiology	
Gram-negative bacteria	
Neisseria meningitidis	8 (30.8)
Escherichia coli	3 (11.5)
Klebsiella species	2 (7.7)
Enterobacter species	2 (7.7)
Campylobacter jejuni	1 (3.8)
Haemophilus influenzae	1 (3.8)
Gram-positive bacteria	
Streptococcus pneumoniae	3 (11.5)
Streptococcus pyogenes	2 (7.7)
Staphylococcus aureus	1 (3.8)
Viruses	
Parainfluenzae virus	1 (3.8)
PIM2 admission (%)	8.1 [3.2–17.4]
PELOD-2	
Day 1	9.5 [2.75–12.0]
Day 3	4.0 [0.0–10.0]
Day 7	0.0 [0.0–5.0]
CVI	4.0 [0.0–7.0]
ICU-free days in 30 days	23.0 [19.0–26.0]
Secondary acquired infections [n (%)]	8 (30)
Mortality [n (%)]	2 (7)

Values are expressed as median [interquartile range], or a number (percentage)

PIM2 pediatric index of mortality 2, PELOD-2 PEdiatric Logistic Organ Dysfunction score, version 2, CVI cumulative vasopressor index

Cytokines

For all cytokines, maximal elevated values were measured on early time point. Then, they presented a gradual decrease on following days but remained significantly elevated in comparison with normal values (Table 2). At day 1–2, IL-6 and IL-8 levels were significantly correlated with PELOD-2 ($r = 0.52$, $p = 0.012$ and $r = 0.43$, $p = 0.048$, respectively) and with CVI ($r = 0.65$, $p = 0.001$ and $r = 0.51$, $p = 0.015$, respectively). No correlation between initial cytokines concentrations and PIM2 score was found. Also, there was no correlation between initial cytokines levels and mHLA-DR at day 1–2. However, IL-8, IL-10, IL-1ra and TNF-α levels at day 1–2 were significantly negatively correlated with mHLA-DR at day 3–5 ($r = -0.84$, $p < 0.0001$; $r = -0.59$, $p = 0.0198$; $r = -0.58$, $p = 0.023$; $r = -0.69$, $p = 0.0042$, respectively).

Lymphocyte subsets

Lymphocyte subsets from healthy control children are presented in Table 3. Among septic patients the total lymphocyte count was significantly lower than in healthy control children at day 1–2 and day 3–5; there was no significant difference at day 7–9 (Fig. 3a). Similar results were observed for CD4$^+$ (Fig. 3b) and CD8$^+$ T cell (Fig. 3c) subsets. The median total NK cell count was significantly lower as compared to healthy control children over the whole monitoring period (Fig. 3d). In contrast and, although diminished, B cells were modestly affected (Fig. 3e). The median proportion of Treg was initially similar to that found in healthy control children; this increased at day 3–5, and became significantly greater at day 7–9 (Fig. 3f). Of note, we did not find any correlation between lymphocytes subsets and CVI (data not shown).

Secondary acquired infections

A secondary acquired infection was diagnosed in eight children (Additional file 1: Tables S1 and S2). The median time to onset of these infections was 13.5 days (range: [9–25]). Compared to children who did not developed secondary acquired infection, the sole difference was a longer length of hospital stay for children who presented secondary acquired infection ($p = 0.009$; Additional file 1: Table S1). Between these two groups, no difference was observed concerning duration of invasive equipment, PICU staying, complex chronic condition and severity scores. No significant difference in lymphocyte subset was observed between children with or without secondary acquired infections. No association was found between persistent lymphopenia (defined as an absolute lymphocyte count of < 1000 cells/μl for 3 days) and development of secondary acquired infection. At day 1–2, there was no significant difference in mHLA-DR values; at day 3–5 those with secondary acquired infection had a significantly lower level of mHLA-DR (4398 ABC [2437–6212]) than those without (8474 ABC [5904–10,844], $p = 0.022$; Fig. 2d). At day 1–2, children with secondary acquired infection had higher concentrations of IL-6, IL-8, and TNF-α than those without (Additional file 1: Table S1). There was no significant difference in cytokine concentrations at other time points. The area under the curve from receiver operating curve (ROC) analysis for the risk to develop a secondary acquired infection were all significantly > 0.8 for these four significant parameters

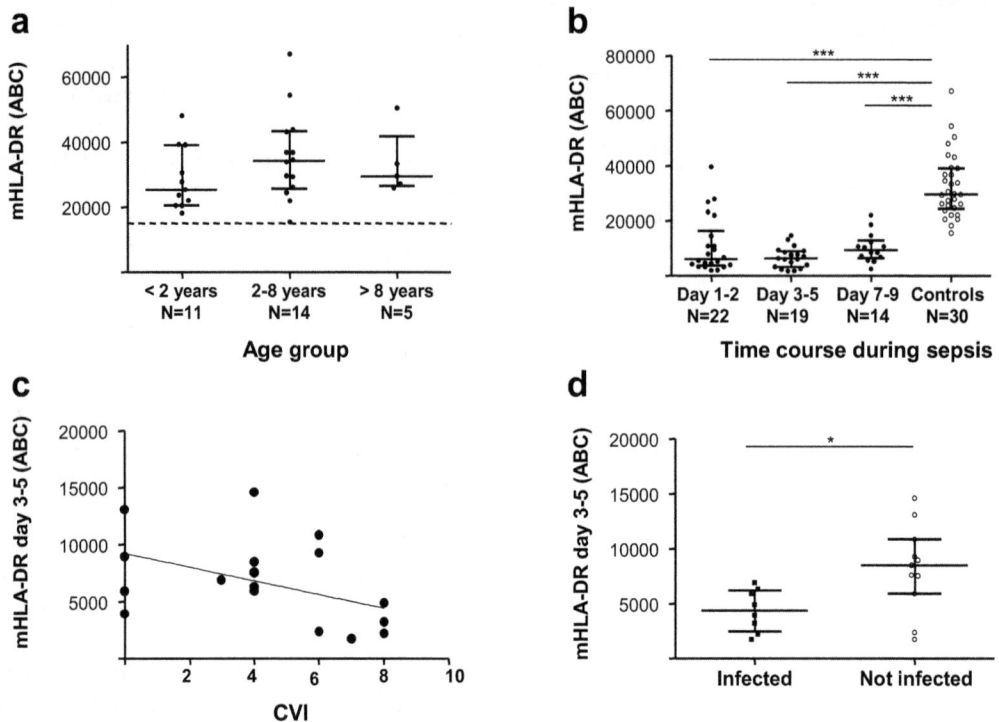

Fig. 2 mHLA-DR measurements in pediatric septic shock. **a** mHLA-DR expression in healthy children: no difference according to age groups ($p = 0.35$; ANOVA). Dashed line depicts usual threshold to define normal values in adults. **b** mHLA-DR was significantly decreased at each time point during septic shock, than controls ($p < 0.001$; Mann–Whitney). **c** mHLA-DR at day 3–5 was significantly negatively correlated with cumulative vasopressor index, CVI ($r = -0.50$; $p = 0.031$; Spearman). **d** mHLA-DR was significantly lower in children with secondary acquired infection than those without ($p = 0.022$; Student t test)

Table 2 Plasma cytokines levels from healthy children and children with septic shock

	Healthy controls	Children with septic shock		
		Day 1–2	Day 3–5	Day 7–9
IL-6	0.0 [0.0–0.36]	178.5 [25.77–3311]	18.13 [12.92–172.5]	17.97 [3.30–33.08]
IL-8	2.05 [0.43–5.06]	51.72 [19.07–145.7]	21.45 [11.42–56.36]	15.00 [7.98–37.98]
IL-10	0.36 [0.0–4.44]	43.37 [17.11–331.6]	8.26 [3.44–21.66]	11.83 [1.70–23.73]
IL1-RA	0.0 [0.0–17.16]	136.9 [23.72–647.8]	48.02 [0.0–153.2]	56.54 [0.0–121.3]
TNF-α	4.91 [3.35–7.11]	25.13 [14.52–40.47]	8.37 [5.34–14.62]	10.15 [4.10–15.43]
INF-γ	4.98 [1.82–6.45]	15.81 [6.55–24.22]	8.07 [2.78–11.45]	10.92 [4.65–23.70]

Values (pg/ml) are expressed as median [IQR]. All cytokine values in children with septic shock at all-time points were different from those of healthy controls

(mHLA-DR at day 3–5, and IL-6, IL-8 and TNF-α at day 1–2, Additional file 1: Table S3). In line with this, mHLA-DR at day 3–5 was negatively correlated with cytokines (except IFN-γ). Owing to the sample size, no multivariate regression could be performed to test independence between mHLA-DR and cytokines for the prediction of risk of secondary acquired infection occurrence.

We next performed Kaplan–Meier analyses associating mHLA-DR values and each cytokine level separately, which found that children with lowest values of mHLA-DR and highest cytokine levels were significantly more likely to be infected. Those with mHLA-DR above the threshold remained uninfected, independently of cytokine level (Additional file 1: Fig. S1).

Table 3 mHLA-DR and lymphocytes subsets depending on age in healthy and septic children

	0–2 years		2–8 years		>8 years	
	Healthy (n = 11)	Septic (n = 11)	Healthy (n = 14)	Septic (n = 6)	Healthy (n = 5)	Septic (n = 2)
mHLA-DR (ABC)	25,477 [20,478–39,143]	6302 [2187–9278]	34,295 [25,763–43,368]	5913 [2977–8911]	29,597 [26,636–41,939]	7927 [6888–8965]
Total lymphocytes (absolute count; cells/µl)	5934 [4148–8572]	2736 [1962–3550]	3623 [2940–4358]	1680 [897–2453]	2374 [1831–3298]	1047 [403–1691]
CD4+ T cells (absolute count; cells/µl)	2187 [1566–2738]	1186 [939–1640]	1184 [968–1583]	574 [236–478]	895 [682–1100]	332 [187–478]
CD8+ T cells (absolute count; cells/µl)	1033 [910–1380]	487 [311–591]	758 [631–1264]	365 [155–608]	689 [467–924]	161 [51–270]
NK cells (absolute count; cells/µl)	645 [392–753]	58 [25–124]	424 [295–576]	96 [35–156]	315 [191–645]	60 [4–117]
B cells (absolute count; cells/µl)	1811 [1326–2750]	901 [648–1397]	729 [563–988]	622 [288–791]	352 [273–508]	422 [150–693]
Regulatory T cells (% among CD4+)	7.67 [5.39–8.24]	7.72 [5.1–9.0]	6.29 [5.29–8.31]	8.83 [7.1–10.3]	6.80 [6.10–8.48]	7.9 [5.8–10.1]

Values are expressed as median [IQR] according to age group. Septic children values were obtained at day 3

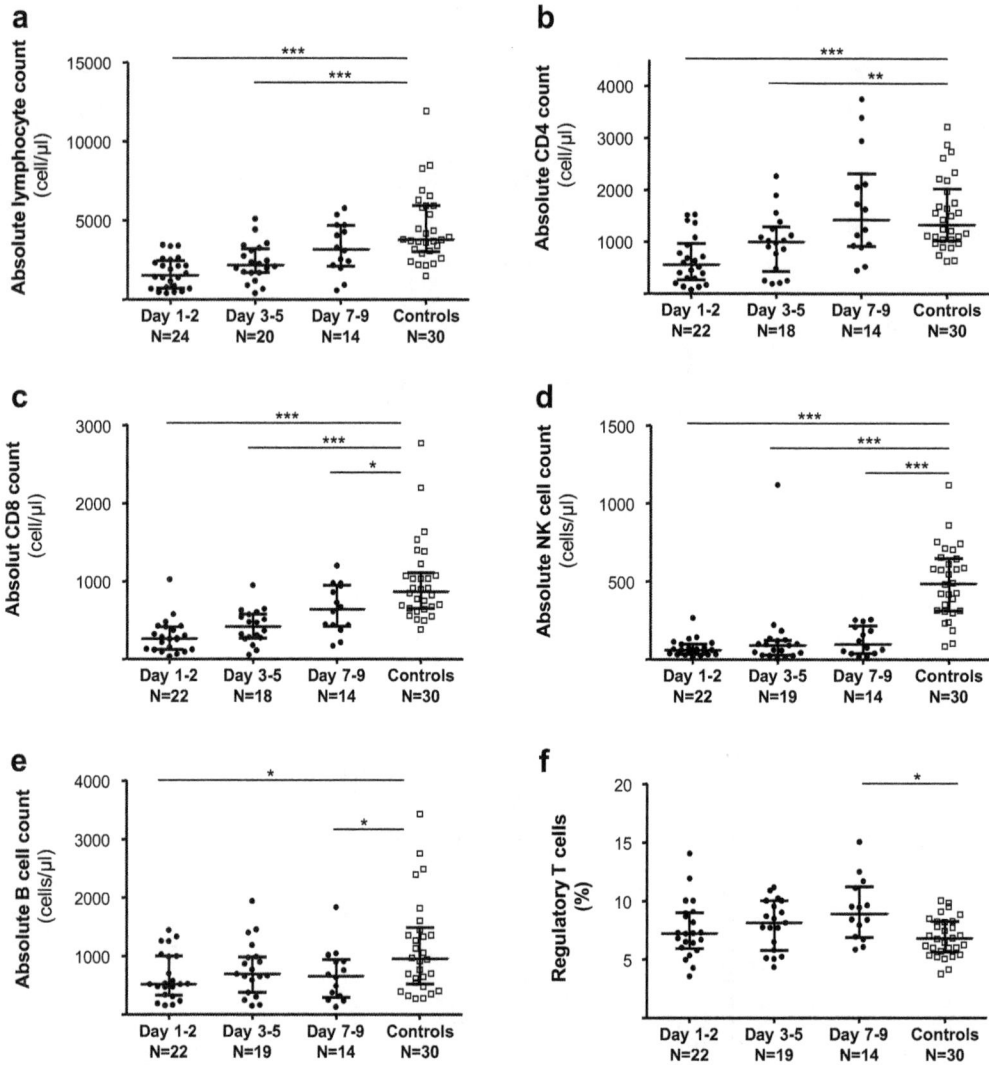

Fig. 3 Time course of lymphocytes' subsets during septic shock. **a** Total lymphocytes, **b** CD4+ T cells, **c** CD8+ T cells, **d** NK cells, **e** B cells (from **a** to **e**, results as cell number/µl), **f** proportion of regulatory T cells (among CD4 + lymphocytes). *$p < 0.05$; **$p < 0.01$; ***$p < 0.0001$

Discussion

The present investigation is, to the best of our knowledge, the first prospective pediatric study reporting a wide immune monitoring, specifically in septic shock. However, the first important result of this study is the values of mHLA-DR expression in healthy children. There was no variation according to age (between 6 months and 17 years) and, furthermore, the values are not different to those reported in adults [28]. These results strongly suggest that there is no difference between healthy adults and children in terms of mHLA-DR expression. Important fall in mHLA-DR during pediatric septic shock seems to be similar to those observed during adult septic shock.

The cytokine storm reported herein, involving both pro and anti-inflammatory cytokines, was found in the initial period after shock (day 1–2). At the same time, children who later developed a secondary acquired infection had higher plasma cytokine concentrations (i.e., IL-6, IL-8, and TNF-α). This is in agreement with observations from genomic studies that have found that early mRNA expression modulations of cytokines and apoptotic genes were associated with deleterious outcomes (mortality, secondary infections) [29, 30]. Moreover, to the best of our knowledge, this is the first pediatric study which reported correlation between initial cytokine storm and alteration of innate immunity, represented by loss of mHLA-DR.

Concerning adaptive immunity, B and T lymphocytes were diminished initially, but less impacted and corrected faster than mHLA-DR alteration. The modest diminution of B cells constitutes a difference with that found in adults, for instance Monserrat et al. [31] described severe abnormality of circulating B lymphocytes associated with mortality. Concerning NK cells, Halstead et al. [32] observed a decrease at the beginning of sepsis in children. The present study provides supplementary data since a deep and prolonged alteration of circulating NK cells was found. Although we did not explore this side, NK cell alterations could promote infections by opportunistic viral pathogens [33]. In contrast with the study reported by Muszynski et al. [14], an increase in Treg proportion during the first week was observed herein. This kinetic seems similar to that described in adult septic shock, where an increased proportion of Treg was associated with poor outcome [34]. Here, as for other lymphocyte parameters, no association with nosocomial infections was found. Additional functional testing (proliferation, intracellular cytokine production) would be likely informative and deserves to be further investigated. At this stage, the present lymphocyte data seem to indicate that altered lymphocyte count rapidly self-resolves, in contrast with observations made in adults.

With regards to innate immunity, loss of mHLA-DR has emerged as a gold standard biomarker owing to its association with altered monocyte functionality, increased mortality, and nosocomial infection rate after adult septic shock [6, 35]. In accordance, we report here a significant fall in mHLA-DR in children. Importantly, the lowest values at day 3–5 were found in patients who developed secondary acquired infections. At this time point, all patients with forthcoming infections presented mHLA-DR below 8000 ABC (i.e., the usual threshold for defining the most severely immunosuppressed adult patients [36]). Most pediatric studies have used ex vivo LPS-induced TNF-α production by monocytes to assess innate immunity function. However, Drewry et al. [35] presented recently mHLA-DR as a better predictor of deleterious outcomes than LPS-stimulated TNF-α production. Add to our results, these data reinforced the idea to use mHLA-DR as biomarker of altered innate immunity in pediatric studies. Due to low number of deaths in the present cohort, we did not investigate the potential association with mortality. Although not all obtained using a standardized measurement protocol, the pediatric mHLA-DR data available in the literature are in agreement with that reported herein. For example, Manzoli et al. [13] found the extent of mHLA-DR level reduction during the first week after sepsis onset to be associated with mortality (23% mortality), and Genel et al. [16] also reported lower levels of mHLA-DR among infected neonates who did not survive compared to those who did (20% mortality). Decreased mHLA-DR has also been described in pediatric surgery and was associated with later sepsis and pneumonia [37, 38]. In addition, Hall et al. [11] reported that, in children with multiple organ dysfunction syndrome, persistent decreased TNF-α release (that reflects monocyte functionality) over 5 days was associated with development of secondary infection. In addition, some in vitro and animal studies suggest potential role of norepinephrine in the development of sepsis-induced immunosuppression [39]. These data reinforced our significant correlation between day 3-5 mHLA-DR and CVI.

Collectively, this indicates that, as in adults, mHLA-DR presents potential for the identification of the most severe immunosuppressed children. The next step would, of course, be to perform multivariate analysis in a larger patient sample to explore the independence of each parameter in predicting deleterious outcomes. That given, Kaplan–Meier analyses found that although different markers (i.e., day 3–5 mHLA-DR and early elevated cytokines) were associated with secondary acquired infections, the weight of mHLA-DR was more important. Interestingly, as observed in adult trauma patients, association between early cytokines production and low day 3–5 mHLA-DR appeared as the poorest scenario in pediatric septic shock [40].

Furthermore, secondary acquired infections represent a major economic burden by significantly extending length of hospital stay [41, 42], and concordantly herein the length of hospitalization in those with secondary infection doubled (and this difference was significant). Taken together, these data reinforce the idea that most immunosuppressed septic children might benefit from immunostimulation as an adjunctive therapy [43]. Clinical trials are in progress with GM-CSF (NCT02361528) or IL-7 (NCT02640807/NCT02797431) in adults, and standardized tools are currently used to stratify patients in those trials. This progressively paves the way for this kind of approach in pediatrics, especially for innate immunity that seems to be more affected.

The study does, however, have some limitations. First, the relatively small number of included children precluded multivariate analyses to be performed. Second, some children were discharged from PICU before all samples were obtained, and therefore the time course of different immune parameters in less severe children was not determined. Due to the relatively short follow-up period, we cannot conclude on the long-term outcome of these children treated for septic shock. In addition, functional testing should be performed in next studies. Theses aspects need to be further explored, and ideally in a multicenter study.

Conclusion

As in adults, septic shock in pediatric patients induced marked alterations in immune parameters in accordance with the occurrence of a state of immunosuppression. The present results, in particular the association between low mHLA-DR expression and deleterious outcomes, deserves to be assessed and confirmed in multicenter studies.

Abbreviations

ABC: antibodies bound per cell; CVI: cumulative vasopressor index; IFN-γ: interferon-γ; IL-1Ra: interleukine-1 receptor antagonist; IL-6: interleukine-6; IL-8: interleukine-8; IL-10: interleukine-10; mHLA-DR: monocyte human leukocyte antigen-DR; NK cells: natural killer cells; PELOD-2: PEdiatric Logistic Organ Dysfunction Score, version 2; PICU: pediatric intensive care unit; PIM2: pediatric index of mortality 2; TNF-α: tumor necrosis factor-α; Treg: regulatory T cells.

Authors' contribution

EJ and GM conceptualized and designed the study, and reviewed and revised each draft of the manuscript. SR collected clinical data, performed biological analysis, designed and conducted the statistical analysis, drafted the initial manuscript and reviewed and revised the manuscript. KK-D collected clinical data, reviewed and revised the manuscript. JD, MG and FV performed biological analysis, participated in statistical analysis, and reviewed and revised the manuscript. All authors read and approved the final manuscript.

Author details

[1] Hospices Civils de Lyon, Paediatric Intensive Care Unit, Mother and Children University Hospital, 59 Boulevard Pinel, 69500 Bron, France. [2] Hospices Civils de Lyon, Immunology Laboratory, E. Herriot Hospital, 69003 Lyon, France. [3] EA 7426, Pathophysiology of Injury-Induced Immunosuppression, University Claude Bernard Lyon 1, BioMérieux Hospices Civils de Lyon, E. Herriot Hospital, 69003 Lyon, France.

Acknowledgements

The authors acknowledge technical staff from Cellular Immunology Laboratory for realization of biological analysis. The authors also thank the Clinical Investigation Center, EPICIME – Lyon, for help in study's organization.

Competing interests

The authors declare that they have no competing interests.

Funding

This study was supported by Hospices Civils de Lyon and University of Lyon. In addition, it was also funded by a research grant from the French Intensive Care Society (Société de Réanimation de Langue Française, SRLF) awarded to KKD. The sponsors of the study had no role in study design, data collection, analysis and interpretation, or writing of the report.

References

1. Schlapbach LJ, Straney L, Alexander J, MacLaren G, Festa M, Schibler A, et al. Mortality related to invasive infections, sepsis, and septic shock in critically ill children in Australia and New Zealand, 2002–13: a multicentre retrospective cohort study. Lancet Infect Dis. 2015;15(1):46–54.
2. Bilgin K, Yaramiş A, Haspolat K, Taş MA, Günbey S, Derman O. A randomized trial of granulocyte-macrophage colony-stimulating factor in neonates with sepsis and neutropenia. Pediatrics. 2001;107(1):36–41.
3. Hotchkiss RS, Monneret G, Payen D. Immunosuppression in sepsis: a novel understanding of the disorder and a new therapeutic approach. Lancet Infect Dis. 2013;13(3):260–8.
4. Venet F, Lukaszewicz A-C, Payen D, Hotchkiss R, Monneret G. Monitoring the immune response in sepsis: a rational approach to administration of immunoadjuvant therapies. Curr Opin Immunol. 2013;25(4):477–83.
5. Landelle C, Lepape A, Voirin N, Tognet E, Venet F, Bohé J, et al. Low monocyte human leukocyte antigen-DR is independently associated with nosocomial infections after septic shock. Intensive Care Med. 2010;36(11):1859–66.
6. Monneret G, Lepape A, Voirin N, Bohé J, Venet F, Debard A-L, et al. Persisting low monocyte human leukocyte antigen-DR expression predicts mortality in septic shock. Intensive Care Med. 2006;32(8):1175–83.
7. Hotchkiss RS, Monneret G, Payen D. Sepsis-induced immunosuppression: from cellular dysfunctions to immunotherapy. Nat Rev Immunol. 2013;13(12):862–74.
8. Hotchkiss RS, Moldawer LL. Parallels between cancer and infectious disease. N Engl J Med. 2014;371(4):380–3.
9. Delano MJ, Ward PA. The immune system's role in sepsis progression, resolution, and long-term outcome. Immunol Rev. 2016;274(1):330–53.
10. Meisel C, Schefold JC, Pschowski R, Baumann T, Hetzger K, Gregor J, et al. Granulocyte-macrophage colony-stimulating factor to reverse sepsis-associated immunosuppression: a double-blind, randomized, placebo-controlled multicenter trial. Am J Respir Crit Care Med. 2009;180(7):640–8.
11. Hall MW, Knatz NL, Vetterly C, Tomarello S, Wewers MD, Volk HD, et al. Immunoparalysis and nosocomial infection in children with multiple organ dysfunction syndrome. Intensive Care Med. 2011;37(3):525–32.
12. Muszynski JA, Nofziger R, Greathouse K, Nateri J, Hanson-Huber L, Steele L, et al. Innate immune function predicts the development of nosocomial infection in critically injured children. Shock (Augusta Ga.). 2014;42(4):313–21.
13. Manzoli TF, Troster EJ, Ferranti JF, Sales MM. Prolonged suppression of monocytic human leukocyte antigen-DR expression correlates with mortality in pediatric septic patients in a pediatric tertiary Intensive Care Unit. J Crit Care. 2016;33:84–9.
14. Muszynski JA, Nofziger R, Greathouse K, Steele L, Hanson-Huber L, Nateri J, et al. Early adaptive immune suppression in children with septic shock: a prospective observational study. Crit Care Lond Engl. 2014;18(4):R145.
15. Wisgrill L, Groschopf A, Herndl E, Sadeghi K, Spittler A, Berger A, et al. Reduced TNF-α response in preterm neonates is associated with impaired nonclassic monocyte function. J Leukoc Biol. 2016;100(3):607–12.
16. Genel F, Atlihan F, Ozsu E, Ozbek E. Monocyte HLA-DR expression as predictor of poor outcome in neonates with late onset neonatal sepsis. J Infect. 2010;60(3):224–8.
17. Dellinger RP, Levy MM, Rhodes A, Annane D, Gerlach H, Opal SM, et al. Surviving Sepsis Campaign: international guidelines for management of severe sepsis and septic shock, 2012. Intensive Care Med. 2013;39(2):165–228.
18. Goldstein B, Giroir B, Randolph A, International Consensus Conference on Pediatric Sepsis. International pediatric sepsis consensus conference: definitions for sepsis and organ dysfunction in pediatrics. Pediatr Crit Care Med J Soc Crit Care Med World Fed Pediatr Intensive Crit Care Soc. 2005;6(1):2–8.
19. Shearer WT, Rosenblatt HM, Gelman RS, Oyomopito R, Plaeger S, Stiehm ER, et al. Lymphocyte subsets in healthy children from birth through 18 years of age: the pediatric AIDS clinical trials group P1009 study. J Allergy Clin Immunol. 2003;112(5):973–80.
20. Slater A, Shann F, Pearson G, Paediatric Index of Mortality (PIM) Study Group. PIM2: a revised version of the Paediatric Index of Mortality. Intensive Care Med. 2003;29(2):278–85.

21. Leteurtre S, Duhamel A, Deken V, Lacroix J, Leclerc F, Groupe Franco-phone de Réanimation et Urgences Pédiatriques. Daily estimation of the severity of organ dysfunctions in critically ill children by using the PELOD-2 score. Crit Care Lond Engl. 2015;19:324.

22. Trzeciak S, McCoy JV, Phillip Dellinger R, Arnold RC, Rizzuto M, Abate NL, et al. Early increases in microcirculatory perfusion during protocol-directed resuscitation are associated with reduced multi-organ failure at 24 h in patients with sepsis. Intensive Care Med. 2008;34(12):2210–7.

23. Horan TC, Andrus M, Dudeck MA. CDC/NHSN surveillance definition of health care-associated infection and criteria for specific types of infections in the acute care setting. Am J Infect Control. 2008;36(5):309–32.

24. Demaret J, Walencik A, Jacob M-C, Timsit J-F, Venet F, Lepape A, et al. Inter-laboratory assessment of flow cytometric monocyte HLA-DR expression in clinical samples. Cytometry B Clin Cytom. 2013;84(1):59–62.

25. Venet F, Davin F, Guignant C, Larue A, Cazalis M-A, Darbon R, et al. Early assessment of leukocyte alterations at diagnosis of septic shock. Shock (Augusta Ga.). 2010;34(4):358–63.

26. Saison J, Maucort-Boulch D, Chidiac C, Demaret J, Malcus C, Cotte L, et al. Increased regulatory T-cell percentage contributes to poor CD4(+) lymphocytes recovery: a 2-year prospective study after introduction of antiretroviral therapy. Open Forum Infect Dis. 2015;2(2):ofv063.

27. de Jager W, te Velthuis H, Prakken BJ, Kuis W, Rijkers GT. Simultaneous detection of 15 human cytokines in a single sample of stimulated peripheral blood mononuclear cells. Clin Diagn Lab Immunol. 2003;10(1):133–9.

28. Döcke W-D, Höflich C, Davis KA, Röttgers K, Meisel C, Kiefer P, et al. Monitoring temporary immunodepression by flow cytometric measurement of monocytic HLA-DR expression: a multicenter standardized study. Clin Chem. 2005;51(12):2341–7.

29. Wong HR, Cvijanovich N, Wheeler DS, Bigham MT, Monaco M, Odoms K, et al. Interleukin-8 as a stratification tool for interventional trials involving pediatric septic shock. Am J Respir Crit Care Med. 2008;178(3):276–82.

30. Peronnet E, Nguyen K, Cerrato E, Guhadasan R, Venet F, Textoris J, et al. Evaluation of mRNA biomarkers to identify risk of hospital acquired infections in children admitted to paediatric intensive care unit. PLoS ONE. 2016;11(3):e0152388.

31. Monserrat J, de Pablo R, Diaz-Martín D, Rodríguez-Zapata M, de la Hera A, Prieto A, et al. Early alterations of B cells in patients with septic shock. Crit Care Lond Engl. 2013;17(3):R105.

32. Halstead ES, Carcillo JA, Schilling B, Greiner RJ, Whiteside TL. Reduced frequency of CD56 dim CD16 pos natural killer cells in pediatric systemic inflammatory response syndrome/sepsis patients. Pediatr Res. 2013;74(4):427–32.

33. von Muller L, Klemm A, Durmus N, Weiss M, Suger-Wiedeck H, Schneider M, et al. Cellular immunity and active human cytomegalovirus infection in patients with septic shock. J Infect Dis. 2007;196(9):1288–95.

34. Monneret G, Debard A-L, Venet F, Bohe J, Hequet O, Bienvenu J, et al. Marked elevation of human circulating CD4 + CD25 + regulatory T cells in sepsis-induced immunoparalysis. Crit Care Med. 2003;31(7):2068–71.

35. Drewry AM, Ablordeppey EA, Murray ET, Beiter ER, Walton AH, Hall MW, et al. Comparison of monocyte human leukocyte antigen-DR expression and stimulated tumor necrosis factor alpha production as outcome predictors in severe sepsis: a prospective observational study. Crit Care Lond Engl. 2016;20(1):334.

36. Bo L, Wang F, Zhu J, Li J, Deng X. Granulocyte-colony stimulating factor (G-CSF) and granulocyte-macrophage colony stimulating factor (GM-CSF) for sepsis: a meta-analysis. Crit Care Lond Engl. 2011;15(1):R58.

37. Gessler P, Pretre R, Bürki C, Rousson V, Frey B, Nadal D. Monocyte function-associated antigen expression during and after pediatric cardiac surgery. J Thorac Cardiovasc Surg. 2005;130(1):54–60.

38. Hoffman JA, Weinberg KI, Azen CG, Horn MV, Dukes L, Starnes VA, et al. Human leukocyte antigen-DR expression on peripheral blood monocytes and the risk of pneumonia in pediatric lung transplant recipients. Transpl Infect Dis. 2004;6(4):147–55.

39. Stolk RF, van der Poll T, Angus DC, van der Hoeven JG, Pickkers P, Kox M. Potentially inadvertent immunomodulation: norepinephrine use in sepsis. Am J Respir Crit Care Med. 2016;194(5):550–8.

40. Gouel-Chéron A, Allaouchiche B, Guignant C, Davin F, Floccard B, Monneret G, et al. Early interleukin-6 and slope of monocyte human leukocyte antigen-DR: a powerful association to predict the development of sepsis after major trauma. PLoS ONE. 2012;7(3):e33095.

41. Field-Ridley A, Dharmar M, Steinhorn D, McDonald C, Marcin JP. ICU-acquired weakness is associated with differences in clinical outcomes in critically ill children. Pediatr Crit Care Med J Soc Crit Care Med World Fed Pediatr Intensive Crit Care Soc. 2016;17(1):53–7.

42. Carcillo JA, Dean JM, Holubkov R, Berger J, Meert KL, Anand KJS, et al. Inherent risk factors for nosocomial infection in the long stay critically ill child without known baseline immunocompromise: a post hoc analysis of the crisis trial. Pediatr Infect Dis J. 2016;35(11):1182–6.

43. Pfortmueller CA, Meisel C, Fux M, Schefold JC. Assessment of immune organ dysfunction in critical illness: utility of innate immune response markers. Intensive Care Med Exp. 2017;5(1):49.

3

Patient–ventilator asynchrony during conventional mechanical ventilation in children

Guillaume Mortamet[1,2,3], Alexandrine Larouche[1,3], Laurence Ducharme-Crevier[1,3], Olivier Fléchelles[4], Gabrielle Constantin[1,3], Sandrine Essouri[3,5], Amélie-Ann Pellerin-Leblanc[6], Jennifer Beck[7,8,9], Christer Sinderby[7,9,10], Philippe Jouvet[1,3] and Guillaume Emeriaud[1,3]* ⓘ

Abstract

Background: We aimed (1) to describe the characteristics of patient–ventilator asynchrony in a population of criti-cally ill children, (2) to describe the risk factors associated with patient–ventilator asynchrony, and (3) to evaluate the association between patient–ventilator asynchrony and ventilator-free days at day 28.

Methods: In this single-center prospective study, consecutive children admitted to the PICU and mechanically venti-lated for at least 24 h were included. Patient–ventilator asynchrony was analyzed by comparing the ventilator pressure curve and the electrical activity of the diaphragm (Edi) signal with (1) a manual analysis and (2) using a standardized fully automated method.

Results: Fifty-two patients (median age 6 months) were included in the analysis. Eighteen patients had a very low ventilatory drive (i.e., peak Edi < 2 μV on average), which prevented the calculation of patient–ventilator asynchrony. Children spent 27% (interquartile 22–39%) of the time in conflict with the ventilator. Cycling-off errors and trigger delays contributed to most of this asynchronous time. The automatic algorithm provided a NeuroSync index of 45%, confirming the high prevalence of asynchrony. No association between the severity of asynchrony and ventilator-free days at day 28 or any other clinical secondary outcomes was observed, but the proportion of children with good synchrony was very low.

Conclusion: Patient–ventilator interaction is poor in children supported by conventional ventilation, with a high frequency of depressed ventilatory drive and a large proportion of time spent in asynchrony. The clinical benefit of strategies to improve patient–ventilator interactions should be evaluated in pediatric critical care.

Keywords: Diaphragm function, Mechanical ventilation, Patient–ventilator asynchrony, Patient–ventilator interaction, Pediatric intensive care unit, Pediatrics

Background

Mechanical ventilation is commonly used in pediatric intensive care units (PICUs) [1]. Maintaining the patient's own spontaneous breathing effort during ventilation is key. Assisted (or patient-triggered) ventilation may improve ventilation perfusion matching and forestall the

development of ventilator-induced diaphragmatic dys-function [2]. As the patient contributes in the ventilation, good interaction between the patient and the ventilator is essential.

Children have higher respiratory rates, smaller tidal volumes, and weaker inspiratory efforts when compared with adults, and patient–ventilator synchrony is diffi-cult to achieve in pediatric patients [3]. These can lead to a mismatch between the patient and the ventilator, defined as a patient–ventilator asynchrony (PVA). PVA

*Correspondence: guillaume.emeriaud@umontreal.ca
[1] Pediatric Intensive Care Unit, CHU Sainte-Justine, 3175 Côte Sainte-Catherine, Montreal, QC, Canada
Full list of author information is available at the end of the article

includes the inspiratory and expiratory timing errors (delays between patient demand and ventilator response), efforts undetected by the ventilator, assist delivered in the absence of patient demand, and double triggering (two rapidly successive assists following a single effort).

In critically ill adults, asynchronies occur frequently and are associated with prolonged ventilator support, sleep disorders, poor lung aeration, longer stay in the intensive care unit and mortality [4–9]. Pediatric data in this field are lacking. PVA seems frequent in PICU [10–13], but little is known about the risk factors of PVA and the association with patient outcome.

In the present study, we aimed to describe the characteristics of PVA in critically ill children, to identify risk factors associated with PVA, and to evaluate the association between PVA and patient outcome.

Methods

This prospective observational study was conducted in the PICU of CHU Sainte-Justine, a university-affiliated pediatric hospital, from August 2010 to October 2012. The study protocol was approved by the ethics committee of CHU Sainte-Justine. Written informed consent was obtained from the parents or legal tutor.

Patients

Consecutive children aged between 7 days and 18 years admitted to the PICU and mechanically ventilated for at least 24 h were eligible. The screening was performed daily by a research assistant. Eligible patients reached inclusion criteria when the presence of spontaneous breathing was evidenced by clinical respiratory efforts or by a respiratory rate sustainably higher than the set ventilator rate. Patients were excluded if they had one of the following criteria: chronic respiratory insufficiency with prior ventilatory support longer than 1 month, tracheostomy, neuromuscular disease, contraindications to nasogastric tube exchange (i.e., local trauma, recent local surgery, or severe coagulation disorder), suspected bilateral diaphragm paralysis, immediate postcardiac surgery period, expected death in the next 24 h, or a limitation of life support treatment.

No modification of the ventilator settings was done for the study. The attending physicians set the ventilator mode and settings according to the local practices. Patients were ventilated with the Evita XL (Dräger, Lubeck, Germany) or the Servo-I ventilator (Maquet, Solna, Sweden). Sedation and analgesia were decided by the treating team and usually involved a combination of benzodiazepines and opioids. There was no local written protocol regarding the ventilator management or the sedation during the study. The ventilation support

was reassessed every 1 or 2 h by respiratory therapists according to local practice. At the time of the study, neurally adjusted ventilatory assist (NAVA) was not routinely used in clinical practice in our unit.

Protocol

PVA was recorded at two different times during the PICU stay. We obtained a first 30-min recording in acute phase, i.e., as soon as possible after inclusion in the study, and an esophageal catheter was installed to record the electrical activity of diaphragm (Edi). The second (pre-extubation) recording was performed during 15 min in the 4 h preceding extubation, if the Edi catheter was still in place.

Data recording

PVA was analyzed by comparing the ventilator pressure curve and the Edi signal. Edi was recorded using a specific nasogastric catheter (Edi catheter, Maquet, Solna, Sweden) connected to a dedicated Servo-I ventilator (Maquet, Solna, Sweden). This ventilator was used only to continuously process and record the Edi signal, the patient being ventilated with his own ventilator as before the study. The catheter was positioned according to the recommendations of the manufacturer as previously described [12, 14].

Demographic data and patient's characteristics, including age, gender, weight, time of measurements, admission diagnostic and comorbidities, Pediatric Index of Mortality (PIM) II and Pediatric Logistic Organ Dysfunction (PELOD) scores, were collected. The sedation score was calculated for the 4-h period preceding the first recording, as suggested by Randolph et al. [15], using a score for which one point was given for the amount of each drug that would be equivalent to 1 h of sedation in a nontolerant subject. The Comfort B scale was used to determine the level of comfort (comfort is better when score is lower).

Clinical outcomes

The primary outcome was the number of ventilator-free days at day 28 (since intubation). Patients who died were considered having zero ventilation-free day. The secondary clinical outcomes were first extubation success (no need for invasive ventilation support within 48 h of extubation), duration of mechanical ventilation, and length of PICU stay.

PVA manual analysis

As previously described [12, 16, 17], for each recording, Edi and ventilator pressure curves were analyzed in a breath-by-breath manner over a continuous 5-min period exempt of artifacts linked to agitation or patient care. Timings of the beginning and the end of inspiration and expiration phases on the Edi and the ventilatory pressure signals were semiautomatically identified: Main timings were automatically identified, and a visual inspection was performed breath by breath, permitting to validate and/or adjust the timing cursors if necessary. All analyses were performed by two independent investigators. By comparing the ventilator and Edi timings, PVA was identified, including wasted efforts (clear effort observed on Edi with no ventilator assist), auto-triggered breath (ventilator assist delivered in the absence of Edi increase), double triggering (two rapidly successive assists following a single effort), and inspiratory trigger and cycling-off errors. As the response of the ventilator for triggering or cycling off could be frequently either retarded or premature [12], we reported both types of asynchrony.

The main PVA variable of interest was the percentage of time spent in asynchrony, calculated from the total duration spent in each type of PVA (wasted efforts, auto-triggering, double triggering, trigger and cycling off errors) divided by the duration of the recording. A priori, we defined severe PVA when the percentage of time spent in asynchrony was superior to the 75th percentile of the entire cohort, i.e., the quarter of patients with the worst synchrony.

In order to facilitate the comparison with other studies [18], we also calculated the asynchrony index (AI), defined as the number of asynchronous events (i.e., the sum of wasted efforts, ineffective triggering, double triggering, and cycles with important trigger and cycling-off errors) divided by the total respiratory rate (i.e., the sum of ventilator cycles and wasted efforts), and expressed as a percentage. Important trigger and cycling-off errors were considered when the error (i.e., premature or delayed response) exceeded 33% of inspiratory and expiratory times, respectively. An AI > 10% was considered as a high incidence of asynchrony [5, 18].

PVA automatic analysis

Asynchrony was also analyzed using a standardized automated method over the same period, to prevent interobserver variability and to avoid observer subjectivity [19]. Inspiratory and expiratory timings were fully automatically detected on ventilator pressure and Edi signals based on predetermined thresholds (0.5 µV for Edi amplitude). Asynchrony was quantified using the NeuroSync index, a global index considering both inspiratory and cycling-off errors. A higher NeuroSync index reflects worse asynchrony, and synchrony can be considered as poor when NeuroSync index exceeds 20% [20, 21].

Sample size calculation

Based on studies conducted in adults, we expected a difference in ventilator-free days of 6 days. With a group distribution of 3/1 and a type-1 error risk of 0.05, the inclusion of 56 patients was necessary to achieve a power of 80%. We planned to enroll a sample of 60 patients to take into account the attrition risk.

Statistical analysis

Data are expressed as median values (with interquartiles, IQR) for continuous variables, and number and/or frequency (%) for categorical data. Differences in categorical variables were tested using Chi-square or Fisher's exact test. Differences in continuous variables were assessed by the nonparametric Mann–Whitney test, the paired t test, or the Wilcoxon test.

Patients with peak inspiratory Edi < 2 µV were a posteriori excluded from PVA analysis (both manual and automated) because the reality of the spontaneous activity in those patients appeared questionable, and the identification of PVA is complex. intraclass correlation coefficient (ICC, two-way random model) was calculated to assess interobserver reproducibility for manual PVA analysis and to compare the results from the manual and the automatic methods. After confirmation of an excellent interobserver agreement (ICC > 0.75), the averages of the two observer's results were calculated and used in further analysis.

The association of potential risk factors with severe PVA was studied by univariate logistic regression analysis. Noncollinear factors associated with a univariate association with p < 0.05 were included in a multivariate logistic regression. The relationship between PVA and clinical outcomes was described using univariate analysis.

All p values are two-tailed and considered significant if p < 0.05. Statistical analyses were performed using SPSS 24.0 (SPSS, Inc, Chicago, IL).

Results

Study population

During the study period, 2090 patients were admitted to the PICU. Among the 406 eligible patients, 60 patients reached inclusion criteria and were enrolled (Fig. 1). Exploitable signals were finally available in 52 patients, who were included in the analysis. Median age of eligible patients who were not included was 8 (1–48) months old, which is similar to analyzed patients (p = 0.96). Twenty-two of these patients also had a second recording in the pre-extubation period. The patient characteristics are presented in Table 1. They were studied 4 (IQR: 1–10) days after PICU admission.

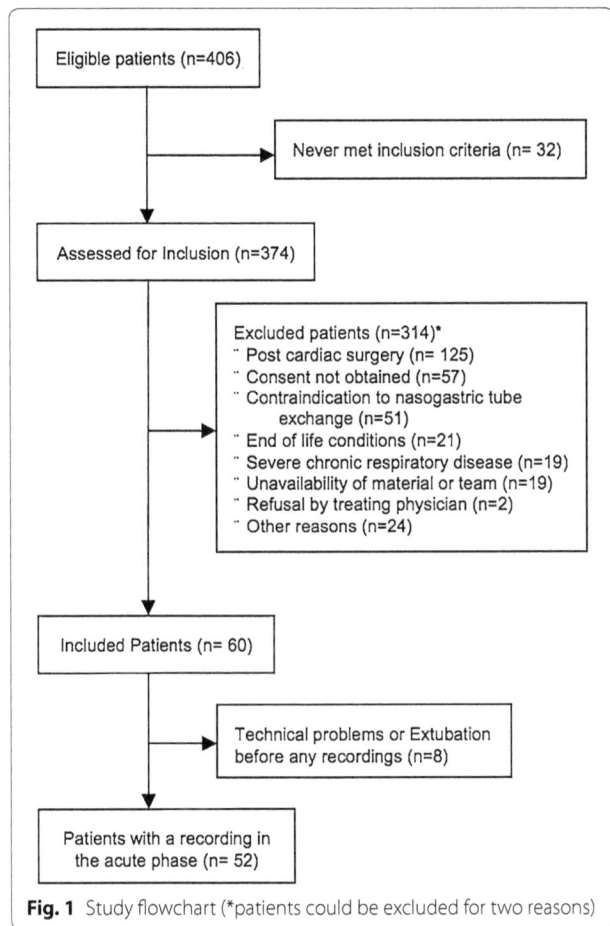

Fig. 1 Study flowchart (*patients could be excluded for two reasons)

Eighteen patients had a very low ventilatory drive (peak Edi < 2 μV on average), which prevented the calculation of PVA. As detailed in Table 1, these patients tended to be older, were affected less frequently by a respiratory disease, and had a lower $PaCO_2$ and a lower comfort score as compared to patients with higher drive.

Magnitude of PVA
A total of 9806 breaths were analyzed with the manual method, with a median of 168 (IQR: 123–258) breaths analyzed per recording. The interrater agreement for PVA manual analysis was excellent, with ICC > 0.85 for all PVA parameters. The total proportion of time spent in PVA was 27% (IQR: 22–39) of the time. As illustrated in Fig. 2, cycling-off errors and trigger delays contributed to most of this asynchronous time 12% (IQR: 8–15) and 11% (IQR: 8–16), respectively. Auto-triggered cycles, wasted efforts, and double triggering were also highly prevalent, with two (IQR: 0–3), two (IQR: 1–10), and one (IQR: 0–5) events per minute, respectively.

The median AI was 25% (IQR: 18–35), and 33 (97%) patients had an AI greater than 10%.

Characteristics of patients with severe asynchrony
Nine patients were considered as severely asynchronous, with a proportion of time spent in asynchrony > 75th percentile, i.e., > 39% of time (Table 2). Patients with severe asynchrony were younger (p = 0.007), had more frequently a narrower and noncuffed ETT (p = 0.001 and p = 0.019, respectively), and were less frequently ventilated in pressure-support ventilation (PSV, p = 0.034). All but one of these patients were admitted for a respiratory failure as a first reason, and five of them had bronchiolitis. In the multivariate logistic regression model in which age, presence of a cuffed ETT, and PSV mode were tested, none of these variables were independently associated with severe PVA (all p > 0.17).

The patients with severe asynchrony were enrolled earlier in the PICU course (2 days (1–5) vs 8 (2–11), p = 0.054), which must be considered while looking at the relationship between PVA and length of stay or ventilation duration.

Evolution of PVA
As illustrated in Fig. 3, when comparing the recordings from acute phase and pre-extubation phase, the level of PVA tended to decrease over time (p = 0.01), and both period data were correlated (R^2 = 0.41). Peak Edi increased between the two phases (p = 0.01).

Automatic analysis of PVA
The automatic algorithm provided a NeuroSync index of 45% (32–70%), confirming the high prevalence of asynchrony. As shown in Fig. 4, a good correlation was observed between NeuroSync index and the percentage of time spent in asynchrony derived from the manual analysis, with an ICC of 0.88.

Outcome
We did not observe any association between the level of asynchrony and neither ventilator-free days at day 28, nor the secondary outcomes (Table 2). This holds true with the manual classification as severe PVA or not (Table 2), as well as with the automated NeuroSync index (correlation with ventilation duration: R^2 = 0.12; p = 0.58). None of the patient characteristics were associated with the duration of mechanical ventilation.

Discussion
The incidence of PVA is very high during pediatric conventional ventilation. As a whole, children spend about one-third of the time in conflict with their ventilator. We described an a priori defined group with severe PVA, but marked PVA was present even in the other children, and the proportion of children which could be considered as "well synchronized" is low. Besides, an unexpected form

Table 1 Characteristics of population (n = 52)

	Total $n = 52$	Peak Edi < 2 μV $n = 18$	Peak Edi > 2 μV $n = 34$
Age (months)	10 (2–42)	21 (1–135)	6 (2–29)
Weight (kg)	6.5 (4.3–17.4)	11 (4.8–38.4)	5.3 (4.0–12.0)
Male, n (%)	31 (60%)	11 (61%)	20 (59%)
Days between admission and inclusion	4 (1–10)	3 (1–7)	4 (1–10)
Days between MV initiation and inclusion	3 (1–7)	2 (1–6)	4 (2–7)
Main reasons for PICU admission, n (%)			
Respiratory failure	31 (60%)	5 (28%)	26 (76%)*
Including bronchiolitis	11 (21%)	1 (6%)	10 (29%)
Hemodynamic failure	3 (6%)	2 (11%)	1 (3%)
Neurologic disorder	9 (17%)	6 (33%)	3 (9%)
Metabolic disorder	2 (4%)	0 (0%)	2 (6%)
Trauma	2 (4%)	2 (11%)	0 (0%)
Postoperative admission	5 (10%)	3 (17%)	2 (6%)
Chronic condition, n (%)			
Respiratory disease	8 (15%)	2 (11%)	6 (18%)
Cardiac disease	9 (17%)	3 (17%)	6 (18%)
Neurological disease	11 (21%)	4 (22%)	7 (21%)
Immuno-oncologic disease	3 (6%)	0 (0%)	3 (9%)
Clinical status			
PIM-2 score	1.7 (0.8–4.3)	2.3 (0.9–4.5)	1.6 (0.8–4.4)
PELOD score	2 (1–1)	1 (1–11)	1 (1–11)
Set respiratory rate, min^{-1}	25 (20–35)	23 (14–38)	31 (25–42)*
Measured respiratory rate, min^{-1}	29 (20–36)	20 (15–29)	34 (28–40)*
pH	7.40 (7.35–7.42)	7.40 (7.36–7.43)	7.39 (7.34–7.43)
$PaCO_2$, mmHg	46 (42–53)	42 (38–47)	48 (45–57)*
HCO_3^-, mmHg	28 (24–32)	27 (23–30)	30 (25–33)
PEEP, cmH_2O	5 (5–6)	5 (5–5)	5 (5–6)
FiO_2	0.35 (0.29–0.41)	0.30 (0.24–0.35)	0.35 (0.30–0.50)
Comfort score	13 (10–15)	11 (8–13)	15 (12–16)*
Score sedation	11 (6–21)	10 (1–14)	15 (6–25)
Edi analysis			
Peak inspiratory Edi, μV	3.6 (1.2–7.6)	1.1 (0.6–1.3)	6.6 (3.8–11.5)
Tonic expiratory Edi, μV	0.7 (0.4–1.9)	0.4 (0.3–0.5)	1.1 (0.7–2.5)

Data are expressed as median (interquartile range) or n (%)

Edi electrical activity of the diaphragm, *MV* mechanical ventilation, *PICU* pediatric intensive care unit, *PEEP* positive end-expiratory pressure

*Significant difference between the two groups (p < 0.05)

of bad interaction was observed, with the high prevalence of low ventilatory drive.

The magnitude of PVA that we observed is in agreement with that previously described [10–12]. In a recent study conducted in a PICU, Blokpoel et al. [10] showed that PVA occurred in 33% of breaths. These authors identified PVA using the analysis of ventilator waveforms, a method which has a low sensitivity [6]. We used the Edi signal which clearly facilitates the detection of PVA, in particular the calculation of timing errors for triggering or cycling off [3, 12, 13, 17, 22, 23]. We were therefore able to show that most of the time spent in asynchrony results from delayed or premature reactions of the ventilator. These timing errors are important, especially when the normal inspiratory time is frequently around 400 ms in this population. We hypothesize that this delay in ventilator response is the consequence of small tidal volumes and short inspiratory and expiratory times in children as compared to adults. Although considered as the classical method [12, 17, 24], the breath-by-breath manual analysis of PVA could be criticized because of its dependency on an investigator, as well as being highly time

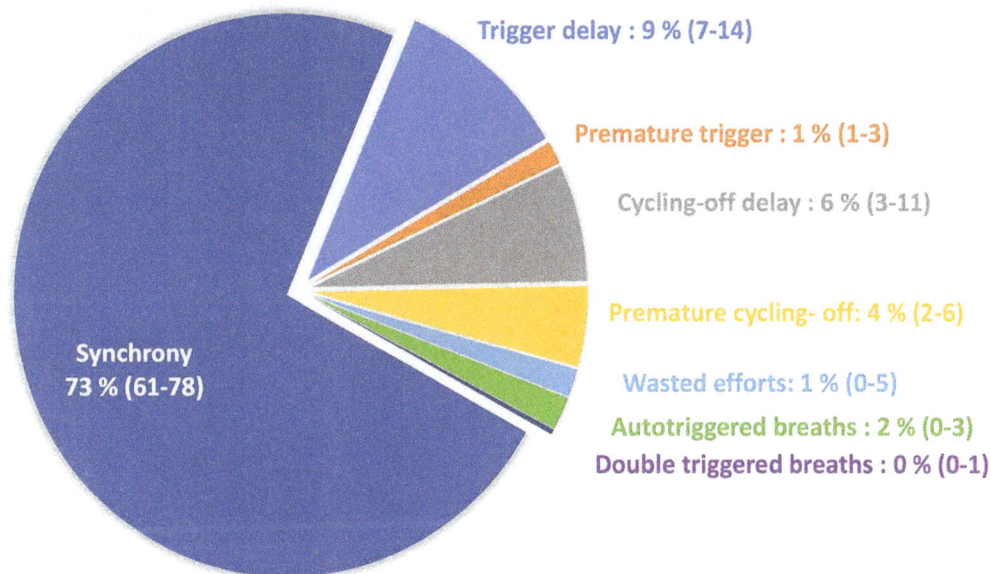

Fig. 2 Contribution of the different types of asynchrony in the total time spent in conflict with the ventilator

consuming. However, our findings were supported by the good agreement between the two independent investigators, and by the concordance also observed between the automatically calculated NeuroSync index and the manually calculated PVA.

To date, no definition of severe PVA in children had been standardized. Some authors use the specific index described in adults by Thille et al. [5, 25] and others the percentage of asynchronous breaths [3, 10, 12]. In the present study, we primarily assessed the magnitude of PVA according to the time spent in asynchrony, because it illustrates well the burden of asynchrony while taking into account different types of patient–ventilator conflict [17]. As expressed using the AI, our results confirm the severity of PVA, a huge proportion of the patients having an AI > 10%. A recent meta-analysis reported that the mean reported AI varied from 13 to 37% in adults, and from 38 to 74% in children during conventional ventilation, while a significant decrease in AI was observed with NAVA [18]. Consistent with the other PVA indices, only two patients in our series had a NeuroSync index < 20%, which corresponds to an adequate synchrony [20, 21]. The nonsevere group can therefore not be assumed as "well synchronized." In agreement with Blokpoel et al. [10], who observed that only 20% children had an acceptable level of PVA, our study highlights that PVA is a major problem in PICU and concerns more than three-quarters of the children, as opposed to one-quarter of adult patients.

Younger age, smaller tracheal tubes, and absence of a cuff on the tracheal tube were associated with severe PVA, and PSV mode was more frequent in patients with less severe PVA. The smaller size and the absence of cuff may suggest that increased leaks could have played a role, as suggested by Blokpoel et al. [10]. The magnitude of the leaks was not different between the two groups, but the precision of this measure is not perfect [26]. None of the patients ventilated in PSV was classified as severe PVA. We may hypothesize that the patients ventilated in PSV have a stronger ventilatory drive, leading to a better detection of the breathing efforts by the ventilator [5]. However, a confounding factor may also explain this association, PSV being mostly used in our unit in older and less sedated patients.

Overall, we did not observe any association between severe asynchrony and adverse outcomes during the PICU course, in contrast to studies in adults [4, 5, 7]. Similarly, Blokpoel et al. did not observe prolonged ventilation in patients with higher levels of asynchrony. While this may be the consequence of the limited power of these two pediatric studies, several explanations could be hypothesized to explain this difference with adult studies. In adults, adverse outcome was observed in severe PVA groups, while the remaining patients were appropriately synchronized [4, 5, 7]. In contrast, the number of children with good patient–ventilator interaction is quite low. In our study, patients with severe PVA frequently had diseases usually associated with good outcome (e.g.,

Table 2 Characteristics of patients depending on the level of asynchrony (in patients with Edi > 2 µV, $n = 34$)

	% time spent in asynchrony < 39% ($n = 25$)	% time spent in asynchrony > 39% ($n = 9$)	p value
Age (m)	14 (2–40)	2 (1–3)	0.007
Weight (kg)	7.0 (4.5–17.3)	4.3 (3.6–5.4)	0.049
Male, n (%)	14 (56%)	6 (67%)	0.70
Days between admission and inclusion	8 (2–11)	2 (1–5)	0.054
Main reasons for PICU admission, n (%)			0.56
Respiratory failure	18 (72%)	8 (89%)	0.40
Including bronchiolitis	5 (20%)	5 (56%)	0.08
Hemodynamic failure	1 (4%)	0 (0%)	1
Neurologic disorder	3 (12%)	0 (0%)	0.55
Metabolic disorder	1 (4%)	1 (11%)	0.46
Trauma	0 (0%)	0 (0%)	1
Post-surgery	2 (8%)	0 (0%)	1
Chronic condition, n (%)			
Respiratory disease	5 (20%)	1 (11%)	1
Cardiac disease	6 (24%)	0 (0%)	0.16
Neurological disease	6 (24%)	1 (11%)	0.64
Immuno-oncologic disease	3 (12%)	0 (0%)	0.55
Clinical status			
PIM-2 score	2.5 (0.9–4.4)	0.9 (0.5–7.0)	0.40
PELOD score	1 (1–11)	11 (1–12)	0.38
pH	7.40 (7.33–7.42)	7.37 (7.33–7.42)	0.63
HCO_3^-, mmHg	30.0 (25.1–32.9)	28.8 (24.9–32.0)	0.84
$PaCO_2$, mmHg	48.0 (44.4–53.4)	48.9 (45.8–57.5)	0.57
Hb, g/dL	10.2 (7.3–10.7)	10.4 (7.9–12.3)	0.33
Lactate, mmol/L	1.5 (0.8–2.1)	1.5 (1.2–1.9)	1
Comfort score	15 (13–16)	15 (11–17)	0.95
Sedation score	11 (6–23)	21 (11–39)	0.15
ETT size	4.0 (3.5–4.5)	3.5 (3.5–3.5)	0.013
Cuffed ETT	17 (68%)	2 (22%)	0.019
Ventilatory settings			
Set RR	25 (20–35)	30 (28–38)	0.13
Measured RR	34 (28–40)	35 (29–40)	0.92
Mode PSV	10 (40%)	0 (0%)	0.034
Mode ACV-P	4 (16%)	3 (33%)	0.35
Mode IACV-P	7 (28%)	3 (33%)	1
Mode ACV-V	0 (0%)	0 (0%)	1
Mode IACV-V	1 (4%)	2 (22%)	0.16
Mode PRVC	3 (12%)	1 (11%)	1
PEEP, cmH_2O	5 (5–5)	6 (5–7)	0.06
FiO_2	0.35 (0.26–0.44)	0.35 (0.30–0.60)	0.45
Leaks (%)	7 (4–15)	2 (0–7)	0.17
Analysis			
Peak inspiratory Edi, µV	7.2 (3.8–15.3)	5.5 (3.4–7.2)	0.20
Tonic expiratory Edi, µV	0.9 (0.6–2.4)	2.0 (1.1–2.9)	0.058
Type of asynchrony			
Wasted Efforts, % of breath analyzed	4.5 (1.6–15.8)	30.6 (18.7–39.8)	0.002
Auto-triggering, % of breath analyzed	6.1 (1.3–9.9)	8.4 (0.9–23.3)	0.36
Double triggering, % of breath analyzed	2.1 (0.0–3.2)	0.0 (0.0–0.8)	0.08
Trigger error, ms	136 (104–176)	284 (190–302)	0.008

Table 2 continued

	% time spent in asynchrony < 39% (n = 25)	% time spent in asynchrony > 39% (n = 9)	p value
Cycling-off error, ms	64 (40–131)	255 (184–297)	0.018
Time spent in asynchrony			
Total time spent in asynchrony, %	24 (17–28)	47 (43–50)	< 0.001
Wasted Effort, %	0.6 (0.2–3.5)	5.3 (2.8–13.6)	0.03
Auto-triggering, %	1.6 (0.3–2.4)	2.3 (0.3–4.7)	0.40
Double triggering, %	0.1 (0.0–0.4)	0.0 (0.0–0.1)	0.053
Trigger error			
Delay, %	7.6 (7.6–11.2)	15.5 (12.2–19.1)	0.001
Premature, %	0.8 (0.5–2.1)	2.3 (1.4–2.9)	0.058
Cycle-off error			
Delay, %	3.8 (1.8–6.3)	15.0 (10.2–17.5)	< 0.001
Premature, %	4.1 (2.2–5.9)	3.2 (2.0–6.7)	0.98
NeuroSync index, %	38 (31–47)	81 (69–83)	< 0.001
Outcome			
Death in PICU	1 (4.0%)	1 (11.1%)	1
Days in PICU	14 (5–22)	7 (4–14)	0.17
Days in PICU after inclusion	6 (4–12.5)	5 (3–6)	0.66
Days on MV	9 (4–15)	4 (3–12)	0.23
Days on MV after inclusion	2.5 (1–6.5)	3 (1–4)	0.9
NIV post extubation	4 (16.0%)	1 (11.1%)	1
Reintubation	5 (20.0%)	1 (11.1%)	1

Edi electrical activity of the diaphragm, *PICU* pediatric intensive care unit, *RR* respiratory rate, *PSV* pressure-support ventilation, *ACV-P* pressure-regulated assist control ventilation, *IACV-P* pressure-regulated intermittent assist control ventilation, *ACV-V* volume-regulated assist control ventilation, *IACV-V* volume-regulated intermittent assist control ventilation, *PRVC* pressure-regulated volume control ventilation, *PEEP* positive end-expiratory pressure, *ETT* endo-tracheal tube, *MV* mechanical ventilation, *NIV* noninvasive ventilation

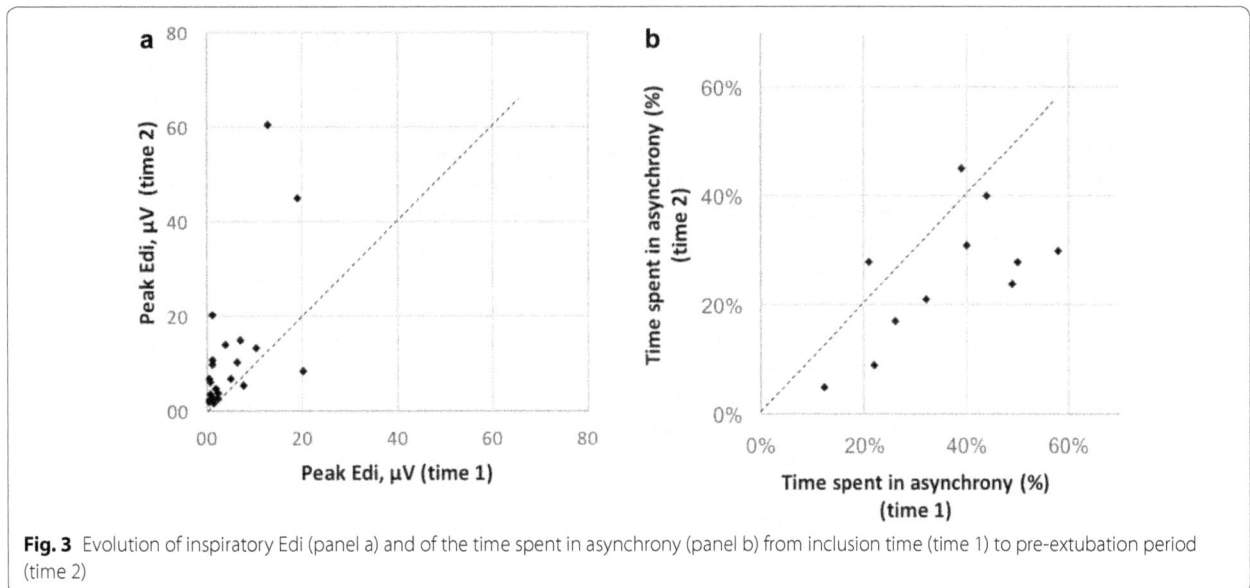

Fig. 3 Evolution of inspiratory Edi (panel a) and of the time spent in asynchrony (panel b) from inclusion time (time 1) to pre-extubation period (time 2)

bronchiolitis). It is also important to note that the patients with more severe PVA were recorded earlier in the PICU course. This baseline discrepancy makes it difficult to assess the relationship between PVA and ventilation duration.

The question remains whether those children would have a better outcome providing the PVA was improved. Only a controlled interventional trial, for example using a specific mode like NAVA, could confirm the independent role of PVA on outcome. Such evidence remains limited

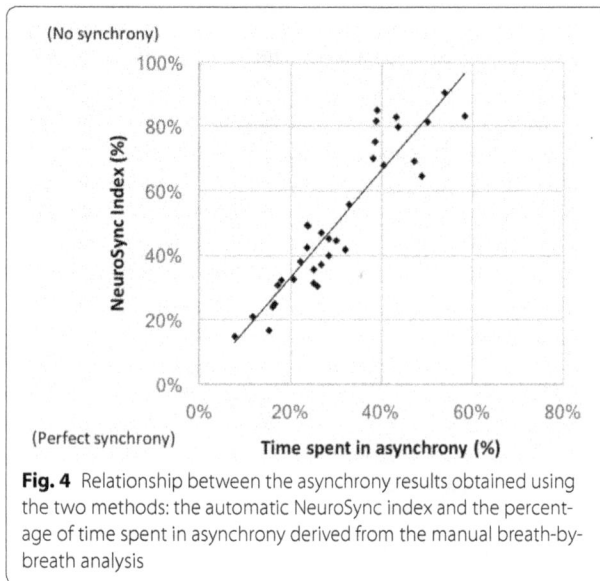

Fig. 4 Relationship between the asynchrony results obtained using the two methods: the automatic NeuroSync index and the percentage of time spent in asynchrony derived from the manual breath-by-breath analysis

in PICU. In a crossover trial conducted in 12 children, De la Oliva et al. [13] observed that the improvement in PVA with NAVA was associated with an improvement in comfort score. This has been supported by another study by Piastra et al. [27]. This finding is interesting when sedation is sometimes needed in cases of severe asynchrony. In the present study, we were not able to confirm that a better synchrony leads to a better comfort for the patient, as similar comfort score was observed in both groups. However, the patient with sever asynchrony tended to require more sedatives, as illustrated by higher sedation score (21 (11–39) vs 11 (6–23), although this difference did not reach significance (p = 0.15). An improved synchrony might have the potential to reduce sedation needs and its associated side effects. In a large randomized controlled trial, Kallio et al. [28] observed an interesting trend for shorter ventilation and ICU length of stay using NAVA (p = 0.03 and p = 0.07, respectively).

Finally, some authors hypothesize that improved PVA could also have deleterious effects that counterbalance the benefits [29]. It is, however, difficult to retain this hypothesis here while very few patients had good synchrony.

Interestingly, the peak Edi in the present study was relatively low (IQR 1.2–7.6) as compared to values observed in extubated children, which usually are between 5 and 30 mcV, depending on the lung condition [30, 31]. Many patients had low respiratory drive after several days of intubation, while they were deemed to be actively breathing. We consider this finding as a new form of poor patient–ventilator interaction, although not an asynchrony. This low respiratory activity has previously been reported [14, 32]. It could be the consequence of overassistance, oversedation, their combination, or more rarely of an abnormal output by the central respiratory center or by bilateral phrenic nerve palsy [33, 34]. In this study group, many patients were admitted for nonrespiratory reasons. Even low level of ventilator support can be sufficient in such conditions to suppress the patient breaths [35]. We previously reported that the ventilatory drive increased in these patients after the extubation, so the central or peripheral neurological explanation seems unlikely [31]. Oversedation may have contributed, as suggested by higher degree of comfort observed in these patients. As described by Vaschetto et al., the combination of overassistance and sedation has a synergistic impact on the drive suppression. More attention should be paid to this frequent complication, especially since such respiratory behavior has clearly been linked to diaphragm dysfunction [30, 36, 37].

Several limitations of our study need to be discussed. We included in the analysis fewer patients than expected. It is possible that our study was underpowered in particular to conduct subgroup analysis or to truly assess the impact on patient outcome. This is a single-center study, and the results may have been influenced by the local practice, especially regarding ventilator settings. NAVA was not used in routine practice during the study period in our PICU. NAVA can improve patient–ventilator interactions [12, 18, 38], and the results of our study would probably be different in population treated with this mode. Many patients were not included, which could limit the external validity of our findings. Certain medical conditions, as chronic respiratory insufficiency with prior ventilatory support, tracheostomy or neuromuscular disease, were a priori excluded, preventing us to generalize our findings to these patients. Two ventilators (Evita XL and Servo-I) were used during the study. Similar studies are necessary to confirm our findings with other ventilators. Due to the study design and the need to observe active breathing for considering patient inclusion, patients were not recorded at the same time after admission. Although the degree of PVA did not seem to change so much over the PICU course, this difference in inclusion timing made it difficult to interpret the relationship between asynchrony and outcome.

Conclusion

Patient–ventilator interaction is poor in critically ill children supported by conventional ventilation. The study did not permit to ascertain if these poor interactions have important clinical consequence. But the magnitude of PVA and the prevalence of low ventilatory drive warrant further studies to assess whether strategies to optimize patient–ventilator interactions can improve the outcome of PICU patients.

Abbreviations
Edi: electrical activity of the diaphragm; ETT: endotracheal tube; NAVA: neurally adjusted ventilatory assist; PICU: pediatric intensive care unit; PSV: pressure support ventilation; PVA: patient–ventilator asynchrony.

Authors' contributions
AL, GE, OF, SE, and PJ designed the study. GM, AL, GC, AAPL, OF, JB, CS, and GE performed the analysis and carried out the chart review and data collection. GM, JB, CS, PJ, and GE wrote the manuscript, which was reviewed, edited, and approved by all authors. As the corresponding author, GE has full access to all the data in the study and has final responsibility for the decision to submit for publication. All authors read and approved the final manuscript.

Author details
[1] Pediatric Intensive Care Unit, CHU Sainte-Justine, 3175 Côte Sainte-Catherine, Montreal, QC, Canada. [2] INSERM U 955, Equipe 13, Créteil, France. [3] CHU Sainte-Justine Research Center, Université de Montréal, Montreal, Canada. [4] Pediatric Intensive Care Unit, CHU Fort-de-France, Fort-de-France, France. [5] Department of Pediatrics, CHU Sainte-Justine, Montreal, QC, Canada. [6] Queen's University, Kingston, Canada. [7] Keenan Research Centre for Biomedical Science, Li Ka Shing Knowledge Institute, St. Michael's Hospital, Toronto, ON, Canada. [8] Department of Pediatrics, University of Toronto, Toronto, Canada. [9] Institute for Biomedical Engineering and Science Technology (iBEST), Ryerson University and St-Michael's Hospital, Toronto, Canada. [10] Department of Medicine, University of Toronto, Toronto, Canada.

Acknowledgements
The authors are indebted to the patients and their families for their willingness to participate in our study. We thank Mariana Dumitrascu, Laurence Bertout, and Noémie Loron for their help in the screening and enrollment process, Lucy Clayton for the study management support, the respiratory therapists for their logistic help, the PICU fellows, attending healthcare providers, and PICU nurses for their collaboration, and Norman Comtois for his invaluable support regarding signal recording and analysis. This work was performed in CHU Sainte-Justine, Pediatric Intensive Care Unit, Montreal, Quebec, Canada.

Competing interests
GM, LDC, OF, GC, SE, and AAPL have no conflict of interest to declare. GE's research program is supported by a scholarship award by the Fonds de Recherche du Québec – Santé. He is currently leading a feasibility study in neonatal ventilation, which is financially supported by Maquet Critical Care. PJ is supported by a scholarship award by the Fonds de Recherche du Québec – Santé, Ministry of Health and Sainte-Justine Hospital. He was a consultant for Sage Therapeutic inc. and was invited to a congress by Medunik Inc and Covidien. JB and CS have made inventions related to neural control of mechanical ventilation that are patented. The patents are assigned to the academic institution(s) where inventions were made. The license for these patents belongs to Maquet Critical Care. Future commercial uses of this technology may provide financial benefit to JB and CS through royalties. JB and CS each own 50% of Neurovent Research Inc (NVR). NVR is a research and development company that builds the equipment and catheters for research studies. NVR has a consulting agreement with Maquet Critical Care. Neurovent research Inc. provided a recording device. Maquet Critical Care provided the ventilator and catheters for the study. This company was not involved in the result analysis and reporting.

Funding
The study was supported by a Young Investigator Award of the Respiratory Health Network of the Fonds de la Recherche du Québec–Santé and by an operating grant for applied clinical research of CHU Sainte-Justine and Sainte-Justine Research Center.

References
1. Payen V, Jouvet P, Lacroix J, Ducruet T, Gauvin F. Risk factors associated with increased length of mechanical ventilation in children. Pediatr Crit Care Med. 2012;13(2):152–7.
2. Petrof BJ, Hussain SN. Ventilator-induced diaphragmatic dysfunction: what have we learned? Curr Opin Crit Care. 2016;22(1):67–72.
3. Beck J, Reilly M, Grasselli G, Mirabella L, Slutsky AS, Dunn MS, et al. Patient–ventilator interaction during neurally adjusted ventilatory assist in low birth weight infants. Pediatr Res. 2009;65(6):663–8.
4. de Wit M, Miller KB, Green DA, Ostman HE, Gennings C, Epstein SK. Ineffective triggering predicts increased duration of mechanical ventilation. Crit Care Med. 2009;37(10):2740–5.
5. Thille AW, Rodriguez P, Cabello B, Lellouche F, Brochard L. Patient–ventilator asynchrony during assisted mechanical ventilation. Intensive Care Med. 2006;32(10):1515–22.
6. Colombo D, Cammarota G, Alemani M, Carenzo L, Barra FL, Vaschetto R, et al. Efficacy of ventilator waveforms observation in detecting patient–ventilator asynchrony. Crit Care Med. 2011;39(11):2452–7.
7. Blanch L, Villagra A, Sales B, Montanya J, Lucangelo U, Lujan M, et al. Asynchronies during mechanical ventilation are associated with mortality. Intensive Care Med. 2015;41(4):633–41.
8. Bosma K, Ferreyra G, Ambrogio C, Pasero D, Mirabella L, Braghiroli A, et al. Patient–ventilator interaction and sleep in mechanically ventilated patients: pressure support versus proportional assist ventilation. Crit Care Med. 2007;35(4):1048–54.
9. Kacmarek RM, Villar J, Blanch L. Cycle asynchrony: always a concern during pressure ventilation! Minerva Anestesiol. 2016;82(7):728–30.
10. Blokpoel RG, Burgerhof JG, Markhorst DG, Kneyber MC. Patient–ventilator asynchrony during assisted ventilation in children. Pediatr Crit Care Med. 2016;17(5):e204–11.
11. Vignaux L, Grazioli S, Piquilloud L, Bochaton N, Karam O, Jaecklin T, et al. Optimizing patient–ventilator synchrony during invasive ventilator assist in children and infants remains a difficult task*. Pediatr Crit Care Med. 2013;14(7):e316–25.
12. Bordessoule A, Emeriaud G, Morneau S, Jouvet P, Beck J. Neurally adjusted ventilatory assist improves patient–ventilator interaction in infants as compared with conventional ventilation. Pediatr Res. 2012;72(2):194–202.
13. de la Oliva P, Schuffelmann C, Gomez-Zamora A, Villar J, Kacmarek RM. Asynchrony, neural drive, ventilatory variability and COMFORT: NAVA versus pressure support in pediatric patients. A non-randomized cross-over trial. Intensive Care Med. 2012;38(5):838–46.
14. Ducharme-Crevier L, Du Pont-Thibodeau G, Emeriaud G. Interest of monitoring diaphragmatic electrical activity in the pediatric intensive care unit. Crit Care Res Pract. 2013;2013:384210.
15. Randolph AG, Wypij D, Venkataraman ST, Hanson JH, Gedeit RG, Meert KL, et al. Effect of mechanical ventilator weaning protocols on respiratory outcomes in infants and children: a randomized controlled trial. JAMA. 2002;288(20):2561–8.
16. Larouche A, Massicotte E, Constantin G, Ducharme-Crevier L, Essouri S, Sinderby C, et al. Tonic diaphragmatic activity in critically ill children with and without ventilatory support. Pediatr Pulmonol. 2015;50:1304–12.
17. Ducharme-Crevier L, Beck J, Essouri S, Jouvet P, Emeriaud G. Neurally adjusted ventilatory assist (NAVA) allows patient–ventilator synchrony during pediatric noninvasive ventilation: a crossover physiological study. Crit Care (London, England). 2015;19:44.
18. Sehgal IS, Dhooria S, Aggarwal AN, Behera D, Agarwal R. Asynchrony index in pressure support ventilation (PSV) versus neurally adjusted ventilator assist (NAVA) during non-invasive ventilation (NIV) for respiratory failure: systematic review and meta-analysis. Intensive Care Med. 2016;42(11):1813–5.
19. Sinderby C, Liu S, Colombo D, Camarotta G, Slutsky AS, Navalesi P, et al. An automated and standardized neural index to quantify patient–ventilator interaction. Crit Care (London, England). 2013;17(5):R239.
20. Doorduin J, Sinderby CA, Beck J, van der Hoeven JG, Heunks LM. Assisted ventilation in patients with acute respiratory distress syndrome: lung-distending pressure and patient–ventilator interaction. Anesthesiology. 2015;123(1):181–90.
21. Doorduin J, Sinderby CA, Beck J, van der Hoeven JG, Heunks LM. Automated patient–ventilator interaction analysis during neurally adjusted non-invasive ventilation and pressure support ventilation in

chronic obstructive pulmonary disease. Crit Care (London, England). 2014;18(5):550.

22. Beck J, Tucci M, Emeriaud G, Lacroix J, Sinderby C. Prolonged neural expiratory time induced by mechanical ventilation in infants. Pediatr Res. 2004;55(5):747–54.

23. Vignaux L, Grazioli S, Piquilloud L, Bochaton N, Karam O, Levy-Jamet Y, et al. Patient–ventilator asynchrony during noninvasive pressure support ventilation and neurally adjusted ventilatory assist in infants and children. Pediatr Crit Care Med. 2013;14(8):e357–64.

24. Piquilloud L, Vignaux L, Bialais E, Roeseler J, Sottiaux T, Laterre PF, et al. Neurally adjusted ventilatory assist improves patient–ventilator interaction. Intensive Care Med. 2011;37(2):263–71.

25. Azoulay E, Kouatchet A, Jaber S, Lambert J, Meziani F, Schmidt M, et al. Noninvasive mechanical ventilation in patients having declined tracheal intubation. Intensive Care Med. 2013;39(2):292–301.

26. Kim P, Salazar A, Ross PA, Newth CJ, Khemani RG. Comparison of tidal volumes at the endotracheal tube and at the ventilator. Pediatr Crit Care Med. 2015;16(9):e324–31.

27. Piastra M, De Luca D, Costa R, Pizza A, De Sanctis R, Marzano L, et al. Neurally adjusted ventilatory assist vs pressure support ventilation in infants recovering from severe acute respiratory distress syndrome: nested study. J Crit Care. 2014;29(2):312e1-5.

28. Kallio M, Peltoniemi O, Anttila E, Pokka T, Kontiokari T. Neurally adjusted ventilatory assist (NAVA) in pediatric intensive care—a randomized controlled trial. Pediatr Pulmonol. 2015;50(1):55–62.

29. Richard JC, Lyazidi A, Akoumianaki E, Mortaza S, Cordioli RL, Lefebvre JC, et al. Potentially harmful effects of inspiratory synchronization during pressure preset ventilation. Intensive Care Med. 2013;39(11):2003–10.

30. Beck J, Emeriaud G, Liu Y, Sinderby C. Neurally adjusted ventilatory assist (NAVA) in children: a systematic review. Minerva Anestesiol. 2016;82:874–83.

31. Emeriaud G, Larouche A, Ducharme-Crevier L, Massicotte E, Flechelles O, Pellerin-Leblanc AA, et al. Evolution of inspiratory diaphragm activity in children over the course of the PICU stay. Intensive Care Med. 2014;40(11):1718–26.

32. Alander M, Peltoniemi O, Pokka T, Kontiokari T. Comparison of pressure-, flow-, and NAVA-triggering in pediatric and neonatal ventilatory care. Pediatr Pulmonol. 2012;47(1):76–83.

33. Szczapa T, Beck J, Migdal M, Gadzinowski J. Monitoring diaphragm electrical activity and the detection of congenital central hypoventilation syndrome in a newborn. J Perinatol. 2013;33(11):905–7.

34. Liet JM, Dejode JM, Joram N, Gaillard Le Roux B, Pereon Y. Bedside diagnosis of bilateral diaphragmatic paralysis. Intensive Care Med. 2013;39(2):335.

35. Khemani RG, Smith LS, Zimmerman JJ, Erickson S. Pediatric acute respiratory distress syndrome: definition, incidence, and epidemiology: proceedings from the Pediatric Acute Lung Injury Consensus Conference. Pediatr Crit Care Med. 2015;16(5 Suppl 1):S23–40.

36. Levine S, Nguyen T, Taylor N, Friscia ME, Budak MT, Rothenberg P, et al. Rapid disuse atrophy of diaphragm fibers in mechanically ventilated humans. N Engl J Med. 2008;358(13):1327–35.

37. Jaber S, Petrof BJ, Jung B, Chanques G, Berthet JP, Rabuel C, et al. Rapidly progressive diaphragmatic weakness and injury during mechanical ventilation in humans. Am J Respir Crit Care Med. 2011;183(3):364–71.

38. Demoule A, Clavel M, Rolland-Debord C, Perbet S, Terzi N, Kouatchet A, et al. Neurally adjusted ventilatory assist as an alternative to pressure support ventilation in adults: a French multicentre randomized trial. Intensive Care Med. 2016;42(11):1723–32.

4

Comparison between a nurse-led weaning protocol and weaning based on physician's clinical judgment in tracheostomized critically ill patients: a pilot randomized controlled clinical trial

Nazzareno Fagoni[1,2†], Simone Piva[1*†], Elena Peli[1], Fabio Turla[1], Elisabetta Pecci[1], Livio Gualdoni[3], Bertilla Fiorese[1], Frank Rasulo[1,3,4‡] and Nicola Latronico[1,3,4‡]

Abstract

Background: Weaning protocols expedite extubation in mechanically ventilated patients, yet the literature investigating the application in tracheostomized patients remains scarce. The primary objective of this parallel randomized controlled pilot trial (RCT) was to assess the feasibility and safety of a nurse-led weaning protocol (protocol) compared to weaning based on physician's clinical judgment (control) in tracheostomized critically ill patients.

Results: We enrolled 65 patients, 27 were in the protocol group and 38 in the control group. Of 27 patients in the protocol group, 1 (3.7%) died in the ICU, 24 (88.9%) were successfully weaned from tracheostomy, and 2 (7.4%) were transferred still on the ventilator. Of 38 patients in the control group, 2 (5.3%) died in the ICU, 22 (57.9%) were successfully weaned from tracheostomy, and 14 were transferred still on the ventilator (36.8%). Risk of being discharged from the ICU on the ventilator was higher in the control group (relative risk: 1.5, IC 95% 1.14–2.01). Concerning safety and feasibility, no patients were excluded after randomization. There was no crossover between the two study arms nor missing data, and no severe adverse event related to the study protocol application was recorded by the staff. Weaning time and rate of successful weaning were not different in the protocol group compared to the control group (long-rank test, $p = 0.31$ for MV duration, $p = 0.45$ for weaning time). Based on our results and assuming a 30% reduction of the weaning time for the protocol group, 280 patients would be needed for a RCT to establish efficacy.

Conclusions: In this pilot RCT we demonstrated that a nurse-led weaning protocol from tracheostomy was feasible and safe. A larger RCT is justified to assess efficacy.

Keywords: Tracheostomy, Weaning, Mechanical ventilation, Nurse-led weaning protocol

Background

Tracheostomy is a common practice in the intensive care unit (ICU), particularly in acutely ill neurological patients and those predicted to have long-term mechanical

*Correspondence: simone.piva@unibs.it
†Nazzareno Fagoni and Simone Piva contributed equally to this paper
‡Frank Rasulo and Nicola Latronico contributed equally to this paper
[1] Department of Anesthesia, Critical Care and Emergency, Spedali Civili University Hospital, Piazzale Ospedali Civili, 1, 23123 Brescia, Italy
Full list of author information is available at the end of the article

ventilation (MV) [1, 2]. Tracheostomy eliminates the risk of extubation failure and re-intubation, but may leave unaffected the process of withdrawing MV. Withdrawing MV can be difficult in these patients because those submitted to tracheostomy often have high-severity disease, complicated clinical course and predicted prolonged MV and ICU stay [1]. Therefore, improving weaning from tracheostomy can be a relevant clinical outcome. Weaning from MV is challenging and represents 40–50% of the duration of MV in patients with tracheal intubation and MV [3–5]. Weaning protocols [4, 6–8], automated systems [9] and daily spontaneous breathing trial (SBT) [10–13] have been proven to significantly reduce the duration of the weaning period and the total number of days on MV [4, 14–18]. However, very few efficacy studies have assessed therapeutic strategies to improve weaning from tracheostomy in the ICU. Vaschetto et al. [19] compared a systematic approach based on daily screening of meaningful physiologic and clinical variables followed by SBT with direct disconnection from the ventilator based on the sole physician's judgment in reducing the rate of reconnection to the ventilator within 48 h; however, the trial was prematurely interrupted due to a high rate of reconnections. Jubran et al. [20] compared pressure support with unassisted breathing through an oxygen-delivery device in tracheostomized patients, but the trial was performed after patient discharge from the ICU to a long-term acute care hospital.

In our center, we strongly support the identification of strategies to improve ICU staff communication and coordination of care delivery as a key translational research priority for critical care [21, 22]. Weaning has been a top research priority in respiratory nursing for many years. Hence, the local weaning working group established that a nurse-led tracheostomy weaning protocol would be a clinically relevant, achievable goal. We therefore conducted the present pilot study to address whether an RCT concerning a nurse-led weaning protocol in tracheostomized patients represents an appropriate trial design, and whether it is feasible to decrease the weaning time and the duration of MV compared to weaning based on the physician's clinical judgment alone. The feasibility objectives were: (1) ability of the ICU team to recruit a sufficient number of patients, (2) the rate of crossover between the two study arms, (3) the ability of the study team to collect data, (4) any severe adverse event during protocol application and (5) providing data to estimate the parameters required to design a definitive RCT. Other clinically relevant secondary outcomes evaluated were: the weaning time, duration of MV, successful weaning rate and the ICU length of stay (ICU-LOS).

Methods
Study design
This single-center parallel randomized controlled clinical pilot trial (ClinicalTrials.gov Identifier: NCT01877850) was conducted from May 2013 to May 2014 at the general and neurological ICU of the Department of Anesthesia, Critical Care and Emergency of the Spedali Civili of Brescia, a large regional university-affiliated hospital. The ICU has 10 beds, 6 general and 4 neurological. The daytime staffing of the unit consists of 1 medical coordinator, 1 attending physician, 2 residents (fourth- and

fifth-year residents of the School of Specialty in Anesthesia and Critical Care Medicine) and 6 critical care nurses. The nightshift team consists of 1 attending physician, 1 resident and 4 nurses. Physical therapists are not dedicated exclusively to the ICU and provide general and respiratory physical therapy for 5 days a week based on a physiatrist-activated written protocol. We do not have respiratory therapists in the ICU.

Patients and those who performed the statistical analyses were blinded to the treatment assignment. The study was conducted in accordance with the Declaration of Helsinki. Ethical approval was obtained from the local ethics committee (registration number 1351/2013). Detailed written information was provided to the patients and family members about the study, and written informed consent to participate in the study was obtained from the patient whenever possible. In case of altered consciousness, the ethics committee waived the requirement for consent; according to Italian laws relatives are not regarded as legal representatives of the patient in the absence of a formal designation [23]. Written informed consent was subsequently requested from all surviving patients as soon as they regained their mental competency. The study conforms to CONSORT extension for pilot studies [24].

Study participants
ICU patients were included if they were ≥ 18 years and had received a tracheostomy during their ICU stay. We excluded patients who were expected to die soon, for whom simple weaning was predicted, those already tracheostomized at ICU admission and those with pre-existing central and peripheral nervous system degenerative diseases with an increased risk of permanent home ventilation.

All patients on MV through an orotracheal tube and the patients in the control group were managed by the attending physician using standard care [25]. In particular (Additional file 1: eFigure 1), after spontaneous awakening trial (SAT), the attending physician performed an SBT screening and started the SBT trial. If SBT trial (using a T-piece) was passed, the patient was extubated; otherwise, the patient was reconnected to the ventilator with the previous setting. When the safety screen (Additional file 1: eFigure 1) was not met, the attending physician attempted to reduce the ventilator settings based on his/her clinical judgment.

Patients predicted to have: (1) prolonged MV (more than 21 days), (2) difficult weaning from the ventilator or (3) prolonged weaning (as defined by the Statement of the Sixth International Consensus Conference on Intensive Care Medicine [26]), received a tracheostomy. The medical ICU staff (medical coordinator and attending physician) was responsible for providing the indication for tracheostomy based on accurate clinical evaluation (admission diagnosis, severity, patients demographic characteristics) and in consideration of the current available literature [27–30].

Study procedures

All tracheostomized patients enrolled into the study were randomly assigned either to the nurse-led weaning group (protocol group) or to the weaning group based on physician's clinical judgment (control group). Randomization sequence was created using Excel 2013 (Microsoft, Redmond, WA, USA) with simple allocation [31] to the two study groups. The allocation sequence was concealed from the researcher enrolling and assessing participants in sequentially numbered, opaque, sealed and stapled envelopes and securely stored.

Interventions

Routine care was no different between the two groups. Nurse training was necessary before starting the clinical trial, consisting of four 2-h meetings with simulated cases

and during routine care; the ICU staff was also provided with written instructions for proper weaning protocol procedure (Fig. 1).

In the protocol group, clinical stability was assessed using a modified version of the Burns Wean Assessment Program score (M-BWAP, see Additional file 1: note and eTable 1) [32, 33] and the respiratory system performance using the Tobin Index (TI, ratio between respiratory rate and tidal volume, in liters) [34]. In the M-BWAP we did not consider the negative inspiratory pressure ≤ 20 cmH$_2$O, the positive expiratory pressure ≥ 30 cmH$_2$O, the vital capacity and the PaCO$_2$ of approximately 40 mmHg with minute ventilation < 10 L/min, which were impractical to measure systematically at bedside in the ICU [35, 36]. Patients randomized to the protocol group began ventilator weaning if a M-BWAP score was > 15, or if the M-BWAP was between 10 and 15 with a concurrently measured TI of < 100. Once the M-BWAP score was judged to be adequate, the nurses took charge of the weaning process as dictated by the protocol (Fig. 1). The protocol consisted of gradually decreasing *pressure support ventilation* (PSV) by

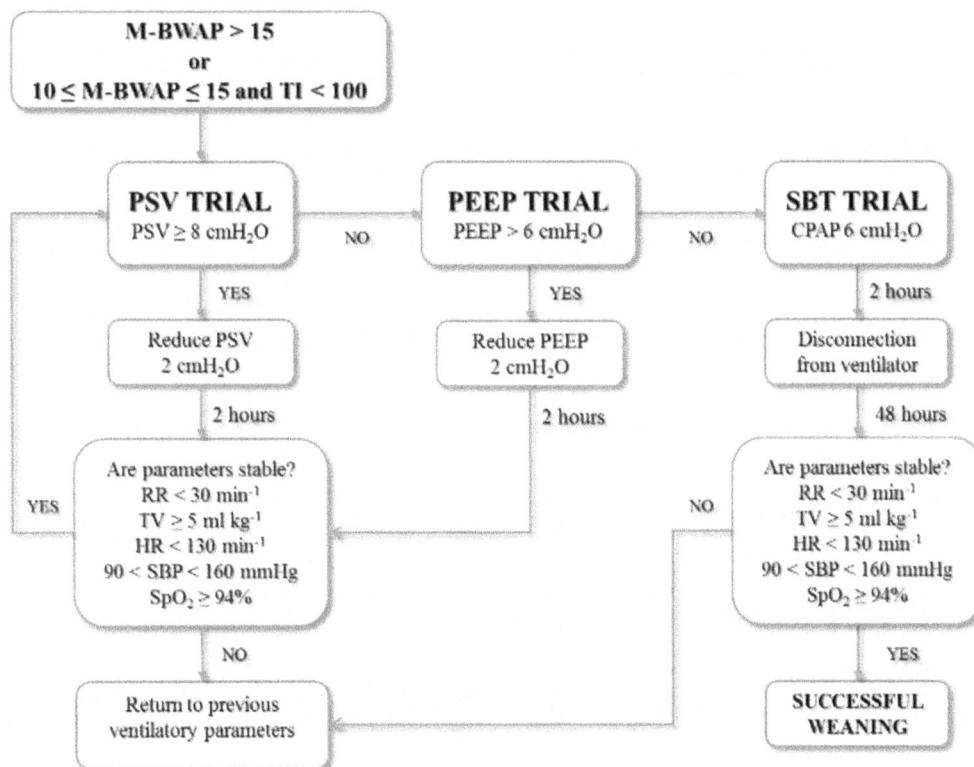

Fig. 1 The nurse-led weaning protocol for tracheostomized critically ill patients. The figure shows the pressure support ventilation (PSV) trial, positive end-expiratory pressure (PEEP) trial and spontaneous breathing trial (SBT). *CPAP* continuous positive airway pressure, *HR* heart rate, *M-BWAP* modified Burns Wean Assessment Program, *SBP* systolic blood pressure, *SpO₂* pulse oximeter oxygen saturation, *TI* Tobin Index (respiratory rate/tidal volume)

2 cmH$_2$O, with a maximum of two steps per day (Fig. 1, PSV trial). When a patient tolerated a PSV < 8 cmH$_2$O for at least 2 h, the nurse reduced the *positive end-expiratory pressure* (PEEP) by 2 cmH$_2$O, with a maximum of two steps per day (Fig. 1, PEEP trial). Once the patient reached PSV < 8 cmH$_2$O and PEEP < 8 cmH$_2$O, the SBT took place, consisting of *continuous positive airways pressure* ventilation with 6 cmH$_2$O for at least 2 h followed by disconnection from ventilator. At the end of the two steps, the respiratory rate, tidal volume, heart rate, blood pressure and peripheral oxygen saturation were monitored, and if one or more of these parameters were impaired, the ventilatory settings previously modified were restored.

Blood gas analysis was performed two times per day in both groups, in the morning, before starting any modifications of the MV, and in the evening.

Feasibility outcome

Concerning the feasibility objectives, the primary outcome of the study, the ability of the ICU team to recruit the patients was evaluated by tracking all patients admitted to the ICU and reporting the number of patients screened by the study team and the percentage of the enrolled patients. Data concerning the rate of crossover between the study arms were also collected. The ability of the study team to collect data was assessed by measuring the missing value of the recorded variables at the end of the study. Any severe adverse event judged as being directly correlated to the protocol application—any major cardiac events (cardiac arrest, hemodynamically significant arrhythmias, acute coronary syndrome), or respiratory event (respiratory arrest)—was eventually recorded.

Secondary outcomes (clinical outcomes)

Secondary clinical outcomes were the weaning time and the total duration of mechanical ventilation. Weaning time was defined as the number of days between the start of the weaning process and patient's disconnection from the ventilator. In the protocol group, the weaning process started when the M-BWAP was > 15 or the M-BWAP was between 10 and 15 with the TI < 100; in the control group, the weaning process started when the on-call physician reduced PSV or PEEP on the ventilator for the first time with a declared intention to start weaning.

Weaning was considered successful when patients could breathe without ventilator assistance for at least 48 h; otherwise, the weaning was considered failed. In this case, the subject remained in the same study arm to which he was initially allocated; as soon as the clinical condition improved, a new weaning process took place.

In case of weaning failure, the weaning time was computed until withdrawing from MV.

Duration of MV was defined as the difference between the beginning and the end of MV. The beginning of MV corresponded to the first day of orotracheal intubation. If a patient died or was discharged while still ventilated, the duration of weaning and that of MV were calculated up to the last day in the ICU.

Statistical analysis

The following variables were recorded in an e-CRF and compared between groups: gender, age, the cause of ICU admission and the Simplified Acute Physiology Score II score at ICU admission; PaO$_2$/FiO$_2$ ratio, PSV value, PEEP value and M-BWAP score at the study enrollment for both groups. In the protocol group, the M-BWAP was calculated for each weaning trial (in case of weaning failure). Data were analyzed using R (version 3.3.3). All data analysis was carried out according to a pre-established intention-to-treat analysis plan. Data are presented as median (interquartile range) for ordinal variables or non-normally distributed continuous variables or as mean (standard deviation) for the normally distributed continuous variables. Normality was assessed by Kolmogorov–Smirnov test. Dichotomous data were compared by two-tailed χ^2 test with the Yates correction or Fisher's exact test when appropriate. Continuous variables were compared using the Mann–Whitney U test or t test as appropriate. A two-sided significance test was set at $p < 0.05$.

As primary analysis, we performed a Kaplan–Meier with log-rank test for weaning time and duration of MV, censoring the patients discharged from the ICU still ventilated or dead in ICU. Since we did not record follow-up data after ICU discharge, and hence we could not define the weaning outcome of those patients discharged while still ventilated, we performed a secondary analysis considering the patients still ventilated at ICU discharge as weaned. Since patients still ventilated when discharged from the ICU were less common among the study group, this categorization favored controls. Therefore, we hypothesized that if a significant reduction in the weaning time could be observed in the study arm, this would not be a chance finding.

Results

Of 655 patients admitted to the ICU, 86 (13.1%) received a percutaneous tracheostomy and were screened for eligibility. Of these, 65 (77%) met the inclusion criteria and were randomized to the protocol group (27) or to the control group (38) (Fig. 2). The baseline characteristics of the studied population are presented in Table 1: no significant differences were found between the two groups.

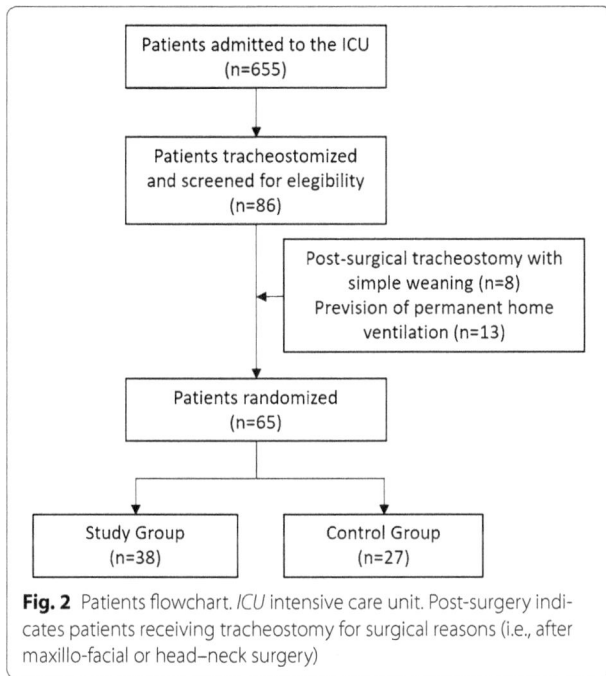

Fig. 2 Patients flowchart. *ICU* intensive care unit. Post-surgery indicates patients receiving tracheostomy for surgical reasons (i.e., after maxillo-facial or head–neck surgery)

Table 1 Characteristics of the study population

	Protocol group	Control group	p value
Number of patients	27	38	
Gender males (%)	22 (81.5%)	25 (65.8%)	0.27
Age	61.3 (13.6)	61.7 (15.2)	0.91
Pathologies at admission			
Neurological (%)	14 (51.9%)	23 (60.5%)	
Cerebral hemorrhage	5	8	0.66
Cardiac arrest	3	5	
Head trauma	3	3	
CNS infections	1	2	
Ischemic stroke	1	2	
Others	1	3	
Non-neurological (%)	13 (48.1%)	15 (39.5%)	
Urgent surgery	6	2	
Respiratory failure	2	6	
Septic shock	2	2	
Polytrauma	1	4	
Others	2	1	
SAPS II, mean (SD)	47.7 (15.3)	49.8 (14.8)	0.66

CNS central nervous system

Of 27 patients in the protocol group, 1 (3.7%) died in the ICU, 24 (88.9%) were successfully weaned from tracheostomy (16 at first attempt) and transferred to the ward, other ICU or rehabilitation, and 2 (7.4%) were transferred still on the ventilator (Table 2). Of 38 patients in the control group, 2 (5.3%) died in the ICU, 22 (58%)

were successfully weaned from tracheostomy (12 at first attempt) and transferred to the ward, other ICU or rehabilitation, and 14 were transferred still on the ventilator (36.8%).

Concerning the feasibility results, no patients were excluded after randomization. There was no crossover between the two study arms. We did not have any missing data, and no severe adverse event related to the study protocol application was recorded by the staff.

Start of weaning timing and M-BWAP scores, TI, PSV, PEEP and PaO_2/FiO_2 at recruitment did not differ between groups. Control group patients had a significantly higher risk of being discharged from the ICU while still mechanically ventilated compared to protocol group (2 of 26 ICU survivors versus 14 of 26; relative risk: 1.5, IC 95% 1.14–2.01). No differences were found concerning the ICU-LOS (Table 3).

The Kaplan–Meier curves censoring patients who died in the ICU or who were discharged still ventilated [16 (42.1%) patients in the control group and 3 (11.1%) patients in the protocol group] showed no difference between the two study groups regarding weaning time ($p = 0.45$) and duration of MV ($p = 0.31$) (Fig. 3). In the secondary analysis, where the patients still ventilated at ICU discharge were considered as weaned, the weaning time and duration of MV were significantly shorter and successful weaning rate was significantly higher in the protocol group compared to the control group (Additional file 1: eTable 2).

Based on our results and assuming a 30% reduction of the weaning time for the protocol group, a study power of 90% and α error of 0.05, 280 patients would be needed for a RCT to establish efficacy.

Discussion

The present pilot RCT demonstrated that a nurse-led weaning protocol compared to weaning based on physician's clinical judgment could reduce the weaning time and the total duration of MV, and increased successful weaning rate in tracheostomized critically ill patients. Moreover, a multicenter RCT would be feasible and would require 280 patients to prove efficacy.

Feasibility was established based on the ability of the ICU team to recruit a sufficient number of patients and collect data, to have a low crossover rate between the two study arms, and good safety of protocol application. We had no crossovers nor any missing data, despite the complexity of the M-BWAP, probably due to the strong motivation of nurses to complete the data collection. There were no severe adverse events indicating that the protocol was safely implemented.

We enrolled 65 patients in 1 year, which is a good result considering the estimated 280 patients needed

Table 2 Outcome of the study population

	Protocol group (*n* = 27)	Control group (*n* = 38)	*p* value
Discharged to the ward (all weaned)	21 (77%)	17(45%)	0.031*
Discharged to other ICU			
Weaned	2 (7%)	2 (5%)	
Not weaned	1 (4%)	0 (0%)	
Discharged to rehabilitation			
Weaned	1 (4%)	3 (8%)	
Not weaned	1 (4%)	14 (37%)	
Patients dead in the ICU	1 (4%)	2 (5%)	
ICU length of stay (days), mean (SD)	19.0 (7.5)	21.1 (9.2)	0.35

ICU intensive care unit

*$p < 0.05$ compared to protocol group

Table 3 Measured parameters of the mechanical ventilation and weaning process

	Protocol group (*n* = 27)	Control group (*n* = 38)	*p* value
Timing of tracheostomy (days after ICU admission), median (IQR)	7 (4–8.5)	5 (4-7)	0.23
Weaning start (days after tracheostomy), mean (SD)	2.4 (2.4)	3.8 (3.5)	0.416
M-BWAP at recruitment, mean (SD)	14.7 (2.0)	14.5 (2.4)	0.71
Tobin Index at recruitment, mean (SD)	53 (26)	67 (38)	0.33
PSV at recruitment (cmH_2O), mean (SD)	10.2 (2.6)	11.2 (2.6)	0.16
PEEP at recruitment (cmH_2O), mean (SD)	9.0 (2.0)	9.3 (2.1)	0.59
PaO_2/FiO_2 at recruitment, mean (SD)	277 (67)	290 (75)	0.46

M-BWAP modified Burns Weaning Assessment Program, *PSV* pressure support ventilation, *PEEP* positive end-expiratory pressure

*$p < 0.05$ compared to protocol group

for a large RCT to definitely prove efficacy. Vaschetto et al. [20] showed similar rate in the only other RCT performed in tracheostomized critically ill patients by enrolling 168 patients in a 3-year period in a single ICU in Italy. An RCT of adequate power could be completed in 18 months with participation of six ICUs with comparable case mix and tracheostomy policy, each enrolling 50 tracheostomized patients per year. These results support the feasibility and acceptability of conducting a larger randomized controlled trial including outcome missing in the present study: the decannulation rate, the ventilator-free days, along with 28- and 90-day mortality of the patient discharged from the ICU. Although no statistical differences were found in the ICU-LOS, 2-day difference is what resulted from the data concerning the weaning period.

Considering the secondary outcome, we could notice a reduced MV duration and weaning time in the protocol group compared to the control group, although non-statistically significant. In fact, our conclusion is based on the Kaplan–Meier with log-rank test, censoring all patients died in ICU or discharged still ventilated from the ICU. This approach leads to a reduced number of patients analyzed, under powering our trial. In

the sensitivity analysis, considering patients discharged still ventilated as weaned, giving a greater advantage to the control group where those patients are more represented (16 patients vs. 2 patients in the protocol group), the differences in MV duration and weaning time became highly significant.

Vaschetto et al. [19] conducted their RCT in a population of critically ill neurological and neurosurgical patients and found no difference in reconnection rate to MV comparing daily screening of readiness for SBT based on physiologic and clinical variables followed by SBT with direct disconnection from the ventilator based on physician's judgment, the same control arm we adopted in our trial. The study was interrupted after inclusion of 168 patients because reconnection rates were much higher than anticipated (29% instead of 16%), and the authors estimated that a further trial should overall enroll 790 patients. This is a substantially higher than our estimation of 280 patients. Sample size calculation is greatly influenced by the predicted effect size of the treatment under study compared to the control treatment on the outcome [37], suggesting that the proposed nurse-led weaning protocol might be superior to daily screening of clinically relevant variables. The M-BWAP

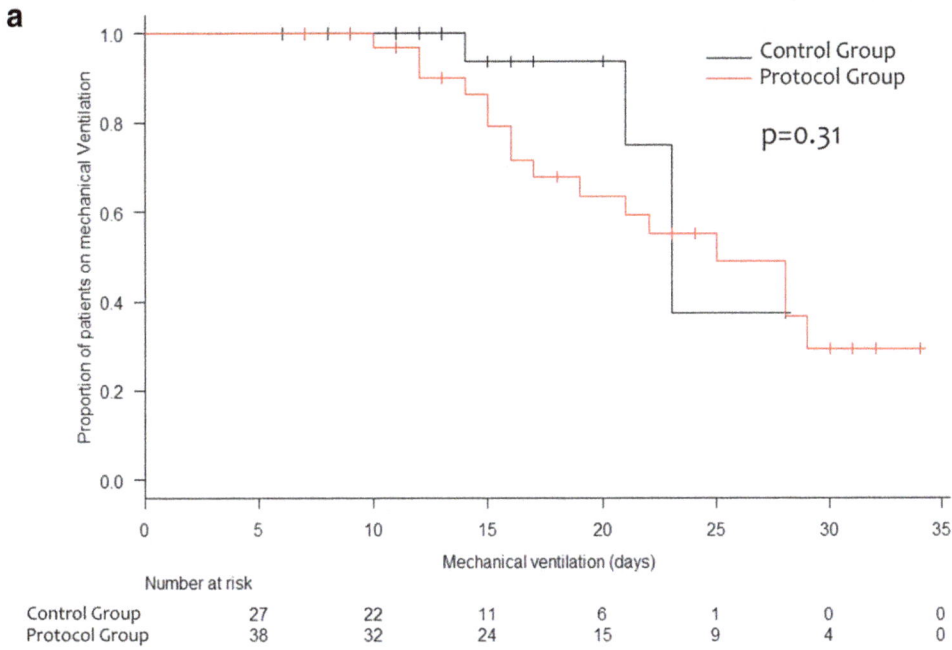

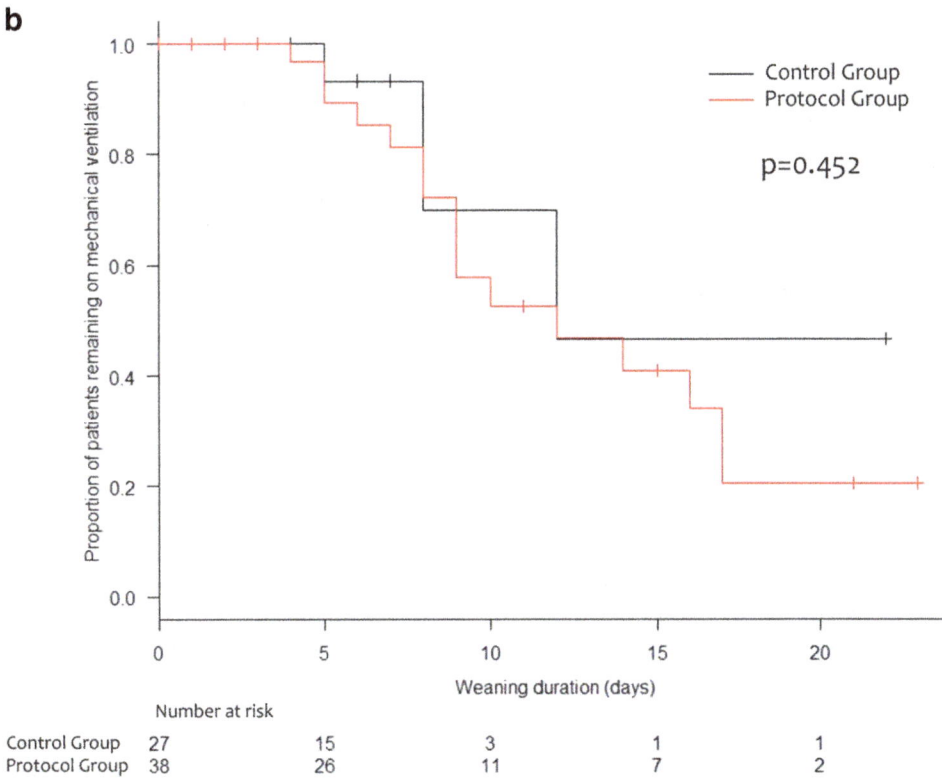

Fig. 3 Kaplan–Meier and log-rank test for MV duration (**a**) and weaning time (**b**) in the two study groups. Patients discharged from the ICU still ventilated or dead were censored

is a comprehensive clinical weaning checklist and scoring instrument; moreover, once the M-BWAP was judged as adequate, the nurse took charge of the entire weaning process with strict patient follow-up at the bedside allowing fine-tuning and timely modification of pressure support ventilation and PEEP in accordance with the protocol steps.

Weaning process was started a mean of 1.6 days earlier in the protocol group than in the control group, although this difference was not statistically significant. We speculated that stricter application of the M-BWAP score in the protocol group may have played a role, because the weaning process started immediately after a predetermined score was reached, whereas in control group physicians started the weaning by clinical judgments whenever it was considered appropriate.

The nurses judged the protocol as being easy to implement. We did not perform a formal survey to explore this aspect, but nurse performance was good as they completely adhered to the protocol without any loss of patient data nor crossover.

A note has to be made regarding the early tracheostomy approach we have adopted in our patients. Although the time to tracheostomy was not an outcome in our study, we should notice the short period between the start of MV and tracheostomy with a median (IQR) of 7 (4–8.5) days in the protocol group and 5 (4–7) days in the control group. Even if the literature is not conclusively in favor to an early approach to the tracheostomy, we have traditionally adopted this approach as standard of care mainly because the unit admits large numbers of neurocritical care patients (up to one-fourth in the control group), in whom incidence of VAP is high [38], and early tracheostomy may provide some benefits [39]. Over the years, this approach has been extended to non-neurological patients since early tracheostomy has been associated with lower incidence of ventilator-associated pneumonia and a significant reduction of MV duration [40]. A recent Cochrane's review with meta-analysis [41] confirmed these results, although not conclusively.

Moreover, we based the clinical decision to perform a tracheostomy on the prevision of prolonged MV or a prevision of difficult and prolonged weaning. Although our decision was not based on a precise protocol, the attitude of the ICU physician coordinator regarding the tracheostomy has been based on the literature. In particular, pneumonia, acute respiratory distress syndrome (ARDS), neuromuscular disease, head trauma and intracerebral hemorrhage patients have a longer mechanical ventilation [42]. Age and obesity are the main demographic characteristics related to prolonged MV, and history of COPD, PaO_2/FiO_2 at intubation, lung injury severity score (LIS) [43] and SOFA [28] at admission, are the main

variables related to prolonged MV. COPD [30, 43], age [30, 43], SOFA at admission, the presence of pneumonia and sepsis, ARDS and high level of PEEP during the first failed SBT [30], are the variables associated with a prolonged and difficult weaning.

Last consideration should be made on the applicability of a weaning protocol by nurses; considered all together, the results of our study demonstrated that a well-designed and shared protocol could be entrust to the nurses, especially in countries where the respiratory therapists are not available.

Limitation of the study

Firstly, the study was not blinded to treatment allocation. Thus, nurses might have been motivated to wean patients assigned to the protocol group; however, this effect might be counterbalanced by similar motivations in physicians for the control group. At the same time, physicians and nurses were aware that they were being observed and might have been more diligent in managing their patients. In fact this 'trial effect' is well described as the phenomenon of improved health outcome in patients treated with standard of care on trial compared to those receiving standard of care outside of a clinical trial setting [38]. A cluster RCT with randomization of participating ICUs to protocol or control would be an option for future RCT, as this would make blinding useless. Moreover, cluster RCTs are suggested to be the best choice whenever the intervention might be a treatment that requires health professionals to change their behavior to impact patient outcomes. However, a cluster RCT would require a larger sample size than that of a non-cluster trial. Hence, researchers should balance the advantage of blinding and homogeneous behavior with the shortcoming of increased resource demand.

Secondly, the patients' observation period did not extend outside the ICU, with 16 patients (2 in the protocol and 14 in the control group) still on the ventilator at the time of ICU discharge. This is *per sé* a proof of efficacy because patients in the protocol group were more frequently weaned than patients in the control group despite comparable weaning start timing and duration of ICU stay. Further, we considered these patients as weaned in the sensitivity analysis, thus favoring the control group.

Future studies should consider extending the observation period until effective withdrawing from MV. Effective patient decannulation and three-month mortality rate would also be worth considering in a future RCT.

Moreover, we enrolled a mixed population of neurological and non-neurological ICU patients. Indication for tracheostomy and causes of failed weaning may differ in these two populations. However, demonstration of protocol efficacy in these diverse populations would strengthen generalizability of results.

A specific protocol to perform early tracheostomy was not adopted, and the decision was based on a consensus between ICU physicians as previously stated, mainly based on clinical prediction of prolonged MV or difficult or prolonged weaning [26], although the actual condition of the patients did not met the criteria (frequently leading to an early tracheostomy). Moreover, the M-BWAP is a non-validated score. The points 20–21–23–25 of the original BWAP were not considered, since these variables required patient's collaboration, which is often lacking in the acute stage of critical illness. The choice of M-BWAP > 15 and BWAP 10–15 with a Tobin Index < 100 was arbitrary and never compared with the performance of the BWAP. We would like to propose a simple tool to be applied by nurses. To be more conservative, before starting the weaning process, we decided that at least 70% of the items should be met before starting the weaning process (M-BWAP > 16).

A note should be made on the sample size calculation for a future RCT, since the number resulted (280 patients) is based on the result of the present pilot study with the above-mentioned limitations, in particular the application of an early tracheostomy and an absence of post-ICU data.

As a last limitation, although a computer-based simple allocation was used, the number of patients per arms resulted unbalanced.

Conclusions

With this pilot study we demonstrated that a protocolled approach to weaning tracheostomized patients could be able to reduce the weaning time and the total duration of MV, and increased successful weaning rate in tracheostomized critically ill patients. Moreover, a larger multicenter RCT comparing a nurse-led weaning protocol with a weaning based on physician's clinical judgment would be feasible and would require 280 patients to definitely prove efficacy.

Abbreviations

BWAP: Burns Wean Assessment Program score; ICU: intensive care unit; ICU-LOS: intensive care unit length of stay; M-BWAP: modified Burns Wean Assessment Program score; MV: mechanical ventilation; PEEP: positive end-expiratory pressure; PSV: pressure support ventilation; RCT: randomized controlled trial; SAT: sedation awakening trial; SBT: spontaneous breathing trial; TI: Tobin Index; TV: tidal volume; VAP: ventilator-associated pneumonia.

Authors' contributions

NF and SP equally contributed to the study. All authors conceived of the study and participated in its design and coordination and helped to draft the manuscript. NF, SP, EPeli, FT, EPecci, LG, BF collected study data. NF, SP and EPeli drafted the manuscript. NF and SP performed statistical analysis. NL and FR participated in study design and coordination and contributed to the final paper draft correction. All authors read and approved the final manuscript.

Author details

[1] Department of Anesthesia, Critical Care and Emergency, Spedali Civili University Hospital, Piazzale Ospedali Civili, 1, 23123 Brescia, Italy. [2] Department of Molecular and Translational Medicine, University of Brescia, Brescia, Italy. [3] School of Specialty in Anesthesia, Intensive Care and Pain Medicine, University of Brescia, Brescia, Italy. [4] Department of Medical and Surgical Specialties, Radiological Sciences and Public Health, University of Brescia, Brescia, Italy.

Competing interests

The authors declare that they have no competing interests.

Funding

The present study was self-founded. The funders had no role in the design and conduct of the study; collection, management, analysis and interpretation of the data; preparation, review or approval of the manuscript; and decision to submit the manuscript for publication.

References

1. Cox CE, Carson SS, Holmes GM, Howard A, Carey TS. Increase in tracheostomy for prolonged mechanical ventilation in North Carolina, 1993–2002. Crit Care Med. 2004;32(11):2219–26.
2. Boles J-M, Bion J, Connors A, Herridge M, Marsh B, Melot C, et al. Weaning from mechanical ventilation. Eur Respir J. 2007;29:1033–56.
3. Esteban A, Anzueto A, Frutos F, Alia I, Brochard L, Stewart TE, et al. Characteristics and outcomes in adult patients receiving mechanical ventilation: a 28-day international study. JAMA. 2002;287(3):345–55.
4. Ely EW, Baker AM, Dunagan DP, Burke HL, Smith AC, Kelly PT, et al. Effect on the duration of mechanical ventilation of identifying patients capable of breathing spontaneously. N Engl J Med. 1996;335(25):1864–9.
5. Esteban A, Ferguson ND, Meade MO, Frutos-Vivar F, Apezteguia C, Brochard L, et al. Evolution of mechanical ventilation in response to clinical research. Am J Respir Crit Care Med. 2008;177(2):170–7.
6. Kollef MH, Shapiro SD, Silver P, St John RE, Prentice D, Sauer S, et al. A randomized, controlled trial of protocol-directed versus physician-directed weaning from mechanical ventilation. Crit Care Med. 1997;25(4):567–74.
7. Vitacca M, Vianello A, Colombo D, Clini E, Porta R, Bianchi L, et al. Comparison of two methods for weaning patients with chronic obstructive pulmonary disease requiring mechanical ventilation for more than 15 days. Am J Respir Crit Care Med. 2001;164(2):225–30.
8. Rose L, Schultz MJ, Cardwell CR, Jouvet P, McAuley DF, Blackwood B. Automated versus non-automated weaning for reducing the duration of mechanical ventilation for critically ill adults and children: a Cochrane systematic review and meta-analysis. Crit Care. 2015;19:48.
9. Burns KE, Lellouche F, Nisenbaum R, Lessard MR, Friedrich JO. Automated weaning and SBT systems versus non-automated weaning strategies for weaning time in invasively ventilated critically ill adults. Cochrane Database Syst Rev. 2014;(9):CD008638.
10. Brochard L, Rauss A, Benito S, Conti G, Mancebo J, Rekik N, et al. Comparison of three methods of gradual withdrawal from ventilatory support during weaning from mechanical ventilation. Am J Respir Crit Care Med. 1994;150(4):896–903.
11. Esteban A, Frutos F, Tobin MJ, Alía I, Solsona JF, Valverdú I, et al. A comparison of four methods of weaning patients from mechanical ventilation. N Engl J Med. 1995;332(6):345–50.
12. Godard S, Herry C, Westergaard P, Scales N, Brown SM, Burns K, et al. Practice variation in spontaneous breathing trial performance and reporting. Can Respir J. 2016;2016:9848942.
13. Wysocki M, Cracco C, Teixeira A, Mercat A, Diehl JL, Lefort Y, et al. Reduced breathing variability as a predictor of unsuccessful patient separation from mechanical ventilation. Crit Care Med. 2006;34(8):2076–83.
14. Blackwood B, Alderdice F, Burns K, Cardwell C, Lavery G, O'Halloran P. Use of weaning protocols for reducing duration of mechanical ventilation in critically ill adult patients: Cochrane systematic review and meta-analysis. BMJ. 2011;342:c7237.
15. Hoffman LA, Miller TH, Zullo TG, Donahoe MP. Comparison of 2 models for managing tracheotomized patients in a subacute medical intensive care unit. Respir Care. 2006;51(11):1230–6.

16. Krishnan JA, Moore D, Robeson C, Rand CS, Fessler HE. A prospective, controlled trial of a protocol-based strategy to discontinue mechanical ventilation. Am J Respir Crit Care Med. 2004;169(6):673–8.

17. Navalesi P, Frigerio P, Moretti MP, Sommariva M, Vesconi S, Baiardi P, et al. Rate of reintubation in mechanically ventilated neurosurgical and neurologic patients: evaluation of a systematic approach to weaning and extubation. Crit Care Med. 2008;36(11):2986–92.

18. Perren A, Domenighetti G, Mauri S, Genini F, Vizzardi N. Protocol-directed weaning from mechanical ventilation: clinical outcome in patients randomized for a 30-min or 120-min trial with pressure support ventilation. Intensive Care Med. 2002;28(8):1058–63.

19. Vaschetto R, Frigerio P, Sommariva M, Boggero A, Rondi V, Grossi F, et al. Evaluation of a systematic approach to weaning of tracheotomized neurological patients: an early interrupted randomized controlled trial. Ann Intensive Care. 2015;5(1):54.

20. Jubran A, Grant BJ, Duffner LA, Collins EG, Lanuza DM, Hoffman LA, et al. Effect of pressure support vs unassisted breathing through a tracheostomy collar on weaning duration in patients requiring prolonged mechanical ventilation: a randomized trial. JAMA. 2013;309(7):671–7.

21. Piva S, Dora G, Minelli C, Michelini M, Turla F, Mazza S, et al. The Surgical Optimal Mobility Score predicts mortality and length of stay in an Italian population of medical, surgical, and neurologic intensive care unit patients. J Crit Care. 2015;30(6):1251–7.

22. Schaller SJ, Anstey M, Blobner M, Edrich T, Grabitz SD, Gradwohl-Matis I, et al. Early, goal-directed mobilisation in the surgical intensive care unit: a randomised controlled trial. Lancet. 2016;388(10052):1377–88.

23. Zamperetti N, Latronico N. Clinical research in critically ill patients: the situation in Italy. Intensive Care Med. 2008;34(7):1330–2.

24. Eldridge SM, Chan CL, Campbell MJ, Bond CM, Hopewell S, Thabane L, et al. CONSORT 2010 statement: extension to randomised pilot and feasibility trials. Pilot Feasibility Stud. 2016;2:64.

25. Barr J, Fraser GL, Puntillo K, Ely EW, Gélinas C, Dasta JF, et al. Clinical practice guidelines for the management of pain, agitation, and delirium in adult patients in the intensive care unit. Crit Care Med. 2013;41(1):263–306.

26. Boles JM, Bion J, Connors A, Herridge M, Marsh B, Melot C, et al. Weaning from mechanical ventilation. Eur Respir J. 2007;29(5):1033–56.

27. Papuzinski C, Durante M, Tobar C, Martinez F, Labarca E. Predicting the need of tracheostomy amongst patients admitted to an intensive care unit: a multivariate model. Am J Otolaryngol. 2013;34(5):517–22.

28. Figueroa-Casas JB, Dwivedi AK, Connery SM, Quansah R, Ellerbrook L, Galvis J. Predictive models of prolonged mechanical ventilation yield moderate accuracy. J Crit Care. 2015;30(3):502–5.

29. Funk GC, Anders S, Breyer MK, Burghuber OC, Edelmann G, Heindl W, et al. Incidence and outcome of weaning from mechanical ventilation according to new categories. Eur Respir J. 2010;35(1):88–94.

30. Peñuelas O, Frutos-Vivar F, Fernández C, Anzueto A, Epstein SK, Apezteguía C, et al. Characteristics and outcomes of ventilated patients according to time to liberation from mechanical ventilation. Am J Respir Crit Care Med. 2011;184(4):430–7.

31. Altman DG, Bland JM. Statistics notes. Treatment allocation in controlled trials: why randomise? BMJ (Clinical Research Ed). 1999;318(7192):1209.

32. Zhu B, Li Z, Jiang L, Du B, Jiang Q, Wang M, et al. Effect of a quality improvement program on weaning from mechanical ventilation: a cluster randomized trial. Intensive Care Med. 2015;41(10):1781–90.

33. Burns SM, Earven S, Fisher C, Lewis R, Merrell P, Schubart JR, et al. Implementation of an institutional program to improve clinical and financial outcomes of mechanically ventilated patients: one-year outcomes and lessons learned. Crit Care Med. 2003;31(12):2752–63.

34. Burns SM, Marshall M, Burns JE, Ryan B, Wilmoth D, Carpenter R, et al. Design, testing, and results of an outcomes-managed approach to patients requiring prolonged mechanical ventilation. Am J Crit Care. 1998;7(1):45–57 **(quiz 8-9)**.

35. Burns SM, Fisher C, Earven Tribble SS, Lewis R, Merrel P, Conaway MR, et al. Multifactor clinical score and outcome of mechanical ventilation weaning trials: Burns Wean Assessment Program. Am J Crit Care. 2010;19:431–9.

36. Burns SM, Fisher C, Tribble SE, Lewis R, Merrel P, Conaway MR, et al. The relationship of 26 clinical factors to weaning outcome. Am J Crit Care. 2012;21(1):52–8 **(quiz 9)**.

37. Latronico N, Metelli M, Turin M, Piva S, Rasulo FA, Minelli C. Quality of reporting of randomized controlled trials published in Intensive Care Medicine from 2001 to 2010. Intensive Care Med. 2013;39(8):1386–95.

38. Acquarolo A, Urli T, Perone G, Giannotti C, Candiani A, Latronico N. Antibiotic prophylaxis of early onset pneumonia in critically ill comatose patients. A randomized study. Intensive Care Med. 2005;31:510–6.

39. Shibahashi K, Sugiyama K, Houda H, Takasu Y, Hamabe Y, Morita A. The effect of tracheostomy performed within 72 h after traumatic brain injury. Br J Neurosurg. 2017;31(5):564–8.

40. Siempos II, Ntaidou TK, Filippidis FT, Choi AMK. Effect of early versus late or no tracheostomy on mortality and pneumonia of critically ill patients receiving mechanical ventilation: a systematic review and meta-analysis. Lancet Respir Med. 2015;3(2):150–8.

41. Andriolo BNG, Andriolo RB, Saconato H, Atallah ÁN, Valente O. Early versus late tracheostomy for critically ill patients. Cochrane Database Syst Rev. 2015;1:CD007271.

42. Seneff MG, Zimmerman JE, Knaus WA, Wagner DP, Draper EA. Predicting the duration of mechanical ventilation. The importance of disease and patient characteristics. Chest. 1996;110(2):469–79.

43. Papuzinski C, Durante M, Tobar C, Martinez F, Labarca E. Predicting the need of tracheostomy amongst patients admitted to an intensive care unit: a multivariate model. Am J Otolaryngol. 2013;34(5):517–22.

5

Delayed cerebral thrombosis complicating pneumococcal meningitis: an autopsy study

Joo-Yeon Engelen-Lee[1], Matthijs C. Brouwer[1]🅾, Eleonora Aronica[2,3] and Diederik van de Beek[1*]

Abstract

Background: Delayed cerebral thrombosis (DCT) is a devastating cerebrovascular complication in patients with excellent initial recovery of pneumococcal meningitis. The aetiology is unknown, but direct bacterial invasion, activation of coagulation or post-infectious immunoglobulin deposition has been suggested.

Methods: We studied histopathology of 4 patients with pneumococcal meningitis complicated by DCT. Results were compared with 8 patients who died of pneumococcal meningitis without DCT and 3 non-meningitis control cases. Furthermore, we evaluated vascular immunoglobulin depositions (IgA, IgG and IgM) and the presence of pneumococcal capsules by immunofluorescence.

Results: Patients who died after pneumococcal meningitis showed inflammation in the meninges and blood vessels with extensive infarction and thrombosis. We did not observe gross differences between DCT and non-DCT patients, except that 2 of 4 DCT patients had a basilar artery aneurysm compared to none of the non-DCT patients. We observed high density of IgM and IgG deposition in meningitis cases as compared to controls, but no difference between DCT and non-DCT patients. Immunofluorescence staining of pneumococci demonstrated the presence of bacterial capsules in the meninges of all meningitis patients, even 35 days after the initiation of antibiotic treatment.

Conclusion: The aetiology of DCT complicating pneumococcal meningitis seems to be of multifactorial aetiology and includes vascular inflammation, thromboembolism of large arteries and infectious intracranial aneurysms. Pneumococcal cell wall components can be observed for weeks after pneumococcal meningitis and may be a source of resurging inflammation after the initial immunosuppression by dexamethasone.

Keywords: Pneumococcal meningitis, Histopathology, Vascular inflammation

Background

Bacterial meningitis is a severe infection of the central nervous system that is most commonly caused by *Streptococcus pneumoniae* (pneumococcus; 70% of cases) [1, 2]. During invasive disease, bacterial nasopharyngeal epithelial adhesion is followed by bloodstream invasion [3]. After crossing the blood–brain barrier (BBB), bacteria multiply freely and trigger activation of immune cells, leading to a massive inflammatory response causing cerebral infarction or seizures and eventually death [4]. In a randomized controlled study, adjunctive anti-inflammatory treatment with dexamethasone was shown to reduce unfavourable outcome with 10% [5, 6]. Implementation of this therapy led to a nationwide decrease in unfavourable outcome of 10% in the Netherlands [7–10]. Nevertheless, case fatality is high (18–25%) and neurological sequelae occur in half of surviving patients [1, 11].

In 2009, we described 6 patients with an excellent initial recovery after pneumococcal meningitis who suddenly deteriorated 7–14 days after admission due to multiple cerebral infarctions [12]. Autopsy in one patient showed an arterial thrombosis in the posterior circulation after which the complication was described as

*Correspondence: d.vandebeek@amc.uva.nl
[1] Department of Neurology, Academic Medical Center, University of Amsterdam, Amsterdam Neuroscience, PO Box 22660, 1100 DD Amsterdam, The Netherlands
Full list of author information is available at the end of the article

"delayed cerebral thrombosis". Further research showed that this delayed cerebral thrombosis (DCT) is a rare but devastating complication of bacterial meningitis occurring in 2–4% of patients with pneumococcal meningitis [12, 13]. DCT has been reported in 19 patients of whom 18 had pneumococcal meningitis and adjunctive dexamethasone therapy seems to be a predisposing condition [12, 14]. The theory was postulated that the immunosuppressive effect by dexamethasone during the first 4 days of meningitis treatment wears off after 7–14 days and bacterial fragments cause a resurgence of the inflammatory response. Besides this theory, other aetiologies have been suggested including direct bacterial invasion, activation of coagulation or a post-infectious immunoglobulin deposition [12, 13, 15–18]. To get more insights in the aetiology of this complication, we performed neuropathological examination of brains of four patients with delayed cerebral thrombosis.

Methods

Patients

Patients with community-acquired pneumococcal meningitis in whom autopsy was performed between 1985 and 2016 were identified from two nationwide prospective cohort studies and in the neuropathology database of the Academic Medical Center, Amsterdam [5]. The pathology specimens and clinical data of these patients have been collected by MeninGene–PATH Biobank following the methods previously described [19]. Clinical information was studied by two neurologists for case selection of DCT (MCB and DvdB). Next, 8 pneumococcal meningitis patients were selected in whom autopsy was performed after at least 7 days of admission without the typical clinical presentation of initial improvement and deterioration thereafter were selected from the previous study (from here on referred to as non-DCT cases) [19]. For controls of the immunoglobulin staining, non-meningitis control cases without neuropathological abnormalities were chosen from the database of the Department of Neuropathology of the Academic Medical Center, Amsterdam. Histology slides, tissue blocks and autopsy reports were obtained. All the brain autopsies were carried out after receiving informed consent and tissue was obtained and used in accordance with the AMC Research Code and the Declaration of Helsinki.

Histopathology

The local pathologists examined the brains macroscopically. All brain slices were examined thoroughly with extra attention to areas with known abnormality from clinical and radiological investigation. Standard brain samples were taken according to the local protocol, and extra samples were taken from clinically relevant areas

and grossly abnormal areas. Brain tissue samples were formalin-fixed and paraffin-embedded, followed by cutting and haematoxylin–eosin (HE) staining at the local institutes. All available slides and paraffin blocks were collected at the AMC. The availability of sampled brain regions (cortex, hippocampus, basal ganglia, brainstem, spinal cord, sagittal venous sinus, large vessels and meninges) for individual cases was documented. The slides were re-evaluated for meningeal and parenchymal infiltration of inflammatory cells, infarction, haemorrhage, abscess, inflammation of medium–large arteries in the meninges, small parenchymal vessels, thrombosis of arterial, venous and small vascular. These evaluations were scored as described in our previous study [19]. The age and extension of infarction and haemorrhage are documented in the brain areas concerned. For the histological evaluation, a Zeiss Axioskop light microscope with 6 object lenses of magnification of 2×, 4×, 10×, 20×, 40× and 100× and LED light source was used.

Immunohistology immunoglobulins

Paraffin blocks were cut in 5 μm thickness and mounted on the slides (StarFrost), followed by deparaffinization and rehydration. Blocking of endogenous peroxidase is performed in 0.3% hydrogen peroxide in methanol for 15 min. After antigen retrieval by boiling in 10 mM sodium citrate pH 6 for 10 min, the slides were incubated with 150 μl primary antibodies (rabbit, DAKO, IgA and IgG 1:32,000, IgM 1:16,000) for 60 min. The slides were then incubated for 30 min at room temperature with the ready-for-use PowerVision peroxidise system (HRP, Immunologic), followed by 10 min incubation with chromogen 3.3′-diaminobenzidine (DAB, Sigma), counterstaining with haematoxylin for 10 min and mounting with the coverslip. The slides were scanned with D. Sight fluo scanner/microscope (A. Menarini, Florence, Italy). The same arteries of consecutive slide sections were chosen to compare the amount of deposition of IgA, IgG and IgM immunoglobulins in the arterial layers of tunica intima, media and adventitia.

Immunofluorescence pneumococcal capsule

Paraffin blocks were cut in 6 μm thickness and mounted on the slides (StarFrost), followed by deparaffinization and rehydration. Blocking of endogenous peroxidase is performed in 0.3% hydrogen peroxide in methanol for 15 min. After antigen retrieval by boiling in 10 mM sodium citrate pH 6 for 10 min, slides were incubated with 150 μl primary antibody (Omni serum, 1:800 diluted, rabbit, Statens Serum Institute, Denmark) for 60 min. The slides were then incubated with 1:400 diluted fluorescent dye (Abcam, anti-rabbit) for 30 min. The slides were washed, air-dried and mounted with the coverslip with a DAPI mounting medium (Vectashield). The slides were visualized with D. Sight fluo scanner/ microscope (A. Menarini, Florence, Italy).

Results

Case descriptions

Patient 1 was a 39-year-old male who presented with fever, headache, aphasia and right-sided hemiparesis in 2003 (Table 1) [13]. He was treated with penicillin and dexamethasone. Cerebrospinal fluid (CSF) examination was consistent with bacterial meningitis, and CSF culture grew pneumococci, susceptible to penicillin. He showed an excellent clinical recovery with a normal neurological examination. However, at day 14 he developed headache and decreased level of consciousness prompting intubation and ICU admission. Cranial MRI showed multiple areas of cerebral infarction, including the thalami, brain stem and the parietal and occipital lobes. MRA of cerebral arteries shows dilatation of the basilar artery. Supportive care was withdrawn at day 32 after initial admission, after which the patient died.

Patient 2 was a 52-year-old male who presented with fever, headache and altered consciousness in 2006. He was treated with amoxicillin and dexamethasone. CSF examination was consistent with bacterial meningitis, and CSF culture grew pneumococci, susceptible to penicillin. The patient gradually improved over 1 week. On day 10 the patient suddenly deteriorated with a decreased level of consciousness prompting intubation and ICU admission. Cranial MRI showed extensive infarction of the brain stem, cerebellum, basal ganglia and temporal lobes with normal flow in the basilar artery. Supportive care was withdrawn at day 12, and the patient died.

Patient 3 was a 73-year-old male who presented with earache, fever and altered consciousness in 2008 [13]. On admission, he had neck stiffness, global aphasia and gaze deviation to the left. He was treated with penicillin and dexamethasone. CSF examination was consistent with bacterial meningitis, and CSF culture grew pneumococci, susceptible to penicillin. Over the next few days, the patient improved. On day 6, he was awake, alert and ambulating. However, on day 7, fever recurred and he developed gait impairment. On day 8, his level of consciousness started to fluctuate, with intermittent dysconjugate eye movements. On day 12, cranial MRI showed multiple areas of cerebral infarction in brainstem and cerebral hemispheres. Supportive care was withdrawn at day 25, and the patient died.

Patient 4 was a 68-year-old female who presented with a shoulder pain, fever and altered consciousness in 2016. She was treated with ceftriaxone, amoxicillin and dexamethasone. CSF examination showed normal leucocyte count, with low glucose and high protein levels.

CSF culture grew pneumococci, susceptible to penicillin. She completely recovered on a week. On day 6, she deteriorated with a decreased level of consciousness. Cranial MRI showed cerebral infarctions in brain stem, thalamus and on several locations in both cerebral hemispheres. MRA taken on the same day demonstrated convolution of basilar artery. Supportive care was withdrawn at day 16, and the patient died.

Histopathology of cases

We had an average number of 16 brain slides per DCT case, range 17–20 slides. In all cases, cortex, basal ganglia (except patient 3), hippocampus, cerebellum, mesencephalon, pons and medulla oblongata were sampled. In two cases, large cerebral arteries including the basilar artery were sampled. The mean age of the non-DCT meningitis patients was 70 years (range 46–88; 4 women) which was comparable with DCT patients (median 54; range 39–73). The cause of death among non-DCT meningitis patients was known in 7 patients and attributed to systemic complications in 6 patients (86%). Three died due to respiratory failure or pneumonia, and myocardial infarction, ruptured aneurysm of the abdominal aorta and septic shock were the cause of death in 1 patient each. Histopathology of brains of these patients has been described previously [19]. We had an average number of 13 slides of these non-DCT meningitis patients (range 11–15). As non-meningitis controls, 3 cases were selected who all died of ischaemic heart disease.

Histopathology in patient 1 showed minor chronic meningeal inflammation with scanty presence of macrophages, old infarctions in temporal/parietal cortex, basal ganglia, thalamus, mesencephalon, pons, medullar oblongata and cerebellum with clearance by macrophages and no active vascular inflammation (Table 2). Thrombosis with organization was seen, but only in small arteries (Fig. 1a). The basilar artery of this patient showed dilatation with irregular thickening of endothelial layer and disruption of elastic layer without inflammation (Fig. 1b). There were small focal haemorrhages.

In patient 2 active inflammation of the meninges was seen with a predominance of neutrophils (Fig. 1c). There were recent infarctions in the basal ganglia (Fig. 1d), brainstem and cerebellum with only focal minor infiltration of neutrophils. The meningeal arteries in the brainstem and cerebellum were severely inflamed with neutrophil infiltration, often with profound vascular destruction (Fig. 1c). Thrombosis in the arteries was observed with vascular inflammation and small focal haemorrhages. A small abscess (diameter 2 mm) in basal ganglia and focal neutrophil infiltration of ventricle were seen.

Table 1 Clinical characteristics of four patients with delayed cerebral thrombosis complicating pneumococcal meningitis

Characteristic	Patient 1	Patient 2	Patient 3	Patient 4
Age (years)	39	52	73	68
Gender	Male	Male	Male	Female
Predisposing conditions				
Otitis or sinusitis	Present	Absent	Present	Absent
Immunocompromised	No	Yes	No	No
Glasgow Coma Scale score	11	11	11	13
Neck stiffness	Yes	Yes	Yes	Yes
CSF leucocyte count (cells/mm^3)	1780	51	17,700	9
Time to secondary deterioration (days)	14	10	7	6
Cranial imaging	MRI: infarction of the thalami, brain stem and cerebral hemispheres MRA: dilatation of the basilar artery	MRI: infarction of the brain stem, cerebellum, basal ganglia and temporal lobes	MRI: infarction in brainstem and cerebral hemispheres	MRI: infarction of the brain stem, thalamus and cerebral hemispheres MRA: convolution of basilar artery
Time to death (days)	32	12	25	16

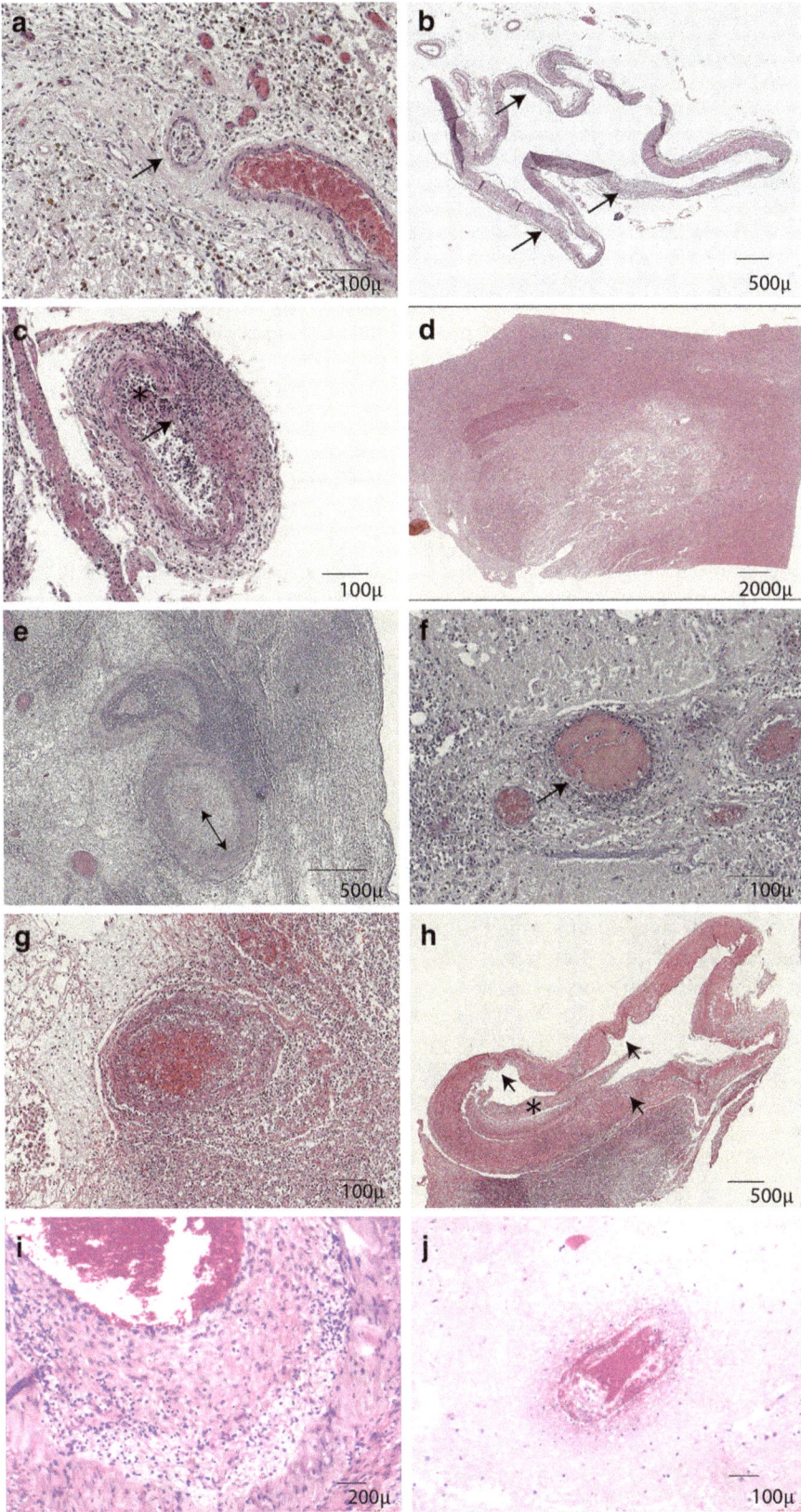

(See figure on previous page.)
Fig. 1 Histology of the four DCT cases. Case 1 (**a** and **b**): **a** small arteries with organized thrombosis are occasionally observed (**a**). **b** The basilar artery showed no active inflammation and was dilated with irregular thickening of endothelial layer (arrow) and disruption of elastic layer. Case 2 (**c** and **d**): **c** the arteries showed still active inflammation with disruption of elastic layer (arrow) and thrombosis (star). **f** Infarction in basal ganglia. Case 3 (**e** and **f**): **e** larger meningeal arteries show often circumferential thickening of intima (arrow) and active inflammation in the media (arrow). **f** Many smaller arteries in the vicinity of the inflamed or destructed arteries show thrombosis with neutrophil infiltrates. Case 4 (**g** and **h**): **g** a severely inflamed artery with vascular destruction and obstruction in the meningeal pus pocket at the frontal lobe showing organization. **h** The basilar artery showed chronic active inflammation and dilatation with disruption of elastic layer (arrows), partially obstructed by thromboembolus (star) with leucocyte clearance. Similarly observed pathologies in non-DCT control meningitis cases (**i** and **j**): **i** active vascular inflammation of a meningeal artery with thickening of intima and inflammation of tunica media. **j** thrombosis of small parenchymal vessel

Patient 3 showed chronic active inflammation in meninges with mixed population of neutrophils and macrophages. There were extensive infarctions in the cortex, basal ganglia, cerebellum, hippocampus and mesencephalon, both recent and of older date. Severe inflammation of larger meningeal arteries with circular thickening of intima (Fig. 1e) was seen with vascular obstruction and destruction and small focal haemorrhages. The smaller arteries showed thrombosis with inflammation (Fig. 1f). Ventricles showed focal infiltration of neutrophils.

Patient 4 showed chronic active inflammation in meninges with the presence of neutrophils mixed with macrophages. There were infarctions present in the frontal lobe, basal ganglia, thalamus, internal capsule, mesencephalon, pons and cerebellum. Meningeal arteries at the sites of meningeal pus pockets in the frontal lobe and cerebellum showed severe inflammation, destruction and obstruction (Fig. 1g). The basilar artery was heavily inflamed with dilatation, irregular thickening of endothelial layer and disruption of elastic layer, infiltrated by neutrophils, macrophages and lymphocytes, and thromboembolism was present with small focal haemorrhages (Fig. 1h). The left medial cerebral artery showed thrombosis and focal mild neutrophil infiltration in intima.

Pathological findings identified in the DCT cases were compared with non-DCT meningitis (Table 2) [12, 13]. All had leucocyte infiltrations, arterial inflammation (except for DCT patient 1), cerebral haemorrhage and infarction. Arterial thrombosis was present in both groups, and extensive infarction in the brainstem, basal ganglia and posterior circulation area were observed in 4 of 4 DCT patients (100%) versus 4 of 8 (50%) of the non-DCT meningitis cases. Two of the 4 DCT patients had basilar artery dilation. None of the non-DCT patients was reported to have basilar artery dilation at original autopsy. Total meningitis pathology scores ranged from 10 to 35 for DCT patients (median, 16) and from 7 to 30 for non-DCT patients (median, 18).

Immunohistology immunoglobulins
To explore whether delayed cerebral thrombosis is mediated by immune complex deposition, we performed an IgG, IgM and IgA staining. The non-meningitis control cases showed variable immune complex deposition with no deposition in the first non-meningitis control (Fig. 2a–c), IgG deposition in tunica intima and adventitia in the arteries in a second non-meningitis control case (Fig. 2d–f) and deposition of IgG in all layers and IgM and IgA in the intima and adventitia in the third non-meningitis control (Fig. 2g–i). There was no difference in immunoglobulin deposition patterns between the non-DCT meningitis and DCT cases. All meningitis cases showed deposition of IgM, IgG and IgA, in the tunica intima and adventitia and occasionally also in the media. The highest density was seen with IgM, whereas IgG density was less and IgA was weak or absent in meningitis cases (Fig. 2j–l). The immunoglobulin deposition was present in the arteries with inflammation, but it was also observed in the arteries without inflammation, occasionally in all three arterial layers (Fig. 2m–o).

Immunofluorescence staining of pneumococcal capsule
The presence of pneumococcal capsule was seen in the meninges of all four DCT cases, represented by circular enhancement in immunofluorescent (IF) staining. In the meninges, one patient (patient 2, Fig. 3a) showed abundance of pneumococcal capsules, two patients moderate amount (patient 3 and 4, Fig. 3b, c) and one case sporadic presence of pneumococcal capsule (case 1, Fig. 3d). The pneumococcal capsules were located either isolated or as groups in the cytoplasm of inflammatory cells or extracellularly. The pneumococcal capsules were identified abundantly in the thromboembolism of basilar artery of case 4 (Fig. 3e). A variable amount of pneumococcal capsules was observed in the non-DCT meningitis cases, ranging from abundant (Fig. 3f) to almost none, with the majority of cases demonstrating a moderate amount.

Discussion
We present four patients with pneumococcal meningitis complicated by DCT. All DCT patients made a good or excellent recovery in the first week of admission and subsequently deteriorated. Histopathology showed arterial inflammation in all patients and multiple cerebral infarcts in cortex, basal ganglia, cerebellum and brain stem.

Table 2 Neuropathological findings of patients with pneumococcal meningitis

Type	Age yrs (M/F)	Days admission-autopsy	DXM	Parenchymal infiltration	Meningeal artery inflammation	Arterial thrombosis	Infarction	Area infarction	Bleeding	Area bleeding	Total pathology score
DCT 1	52, M	10	+	+++	+++	++	+++	Basal ganglia, cerebellum, brainstem	+	Focal minor	19
DCT 2	39, M	35	+	+	++	-	+++	Cortex, basal ganglia, cerebellum, brainstem	+	Focal minor	10
DCT 3	73, M	24	+	+	++	+++	+++	Cortex, cerebellum	+	Focal minor	17
DCT 4	68, F	15	+	+	+++	++	+++	Cortex, basal ganglia, cerebellum, brainstem	+	Focal minor	15
Control	46, M	7	-	++	+++	+++	++	Cortex, basal ganglia, brainstem	+++	Cortex, brainstem, cerebellum	22
Control	78, F	18	+	++	+++	+	+++	Cortex, basal ganglia, cerebellum, brainstem	+++	?	19
Control	73, F	21	+	++	++	++	++	Cortex, basal ganglia, brainstem	+	Brainstem, cerebellum	14
Control	48, F	30	+	++	+++	-	++	Cortex, basal ganglia, cerebellum, brainstem	+++	Basal ganglia	16
Control	88, F	30	?	++	-	++	+	Cortex, cerebellum, brainstem	++	Brainstem, cerebellum	15
Control	75, M	30	?	++	+++	++	+++	Cortex	+	?	19
Control	79, M	12	-	-	+	++	++	Cortex	-	-	14
Control	71, F	15	?	-	+	-	++	Cortex	+	?	6

DCT delayed cerebral thrombosis, *DXM* dexamethasone

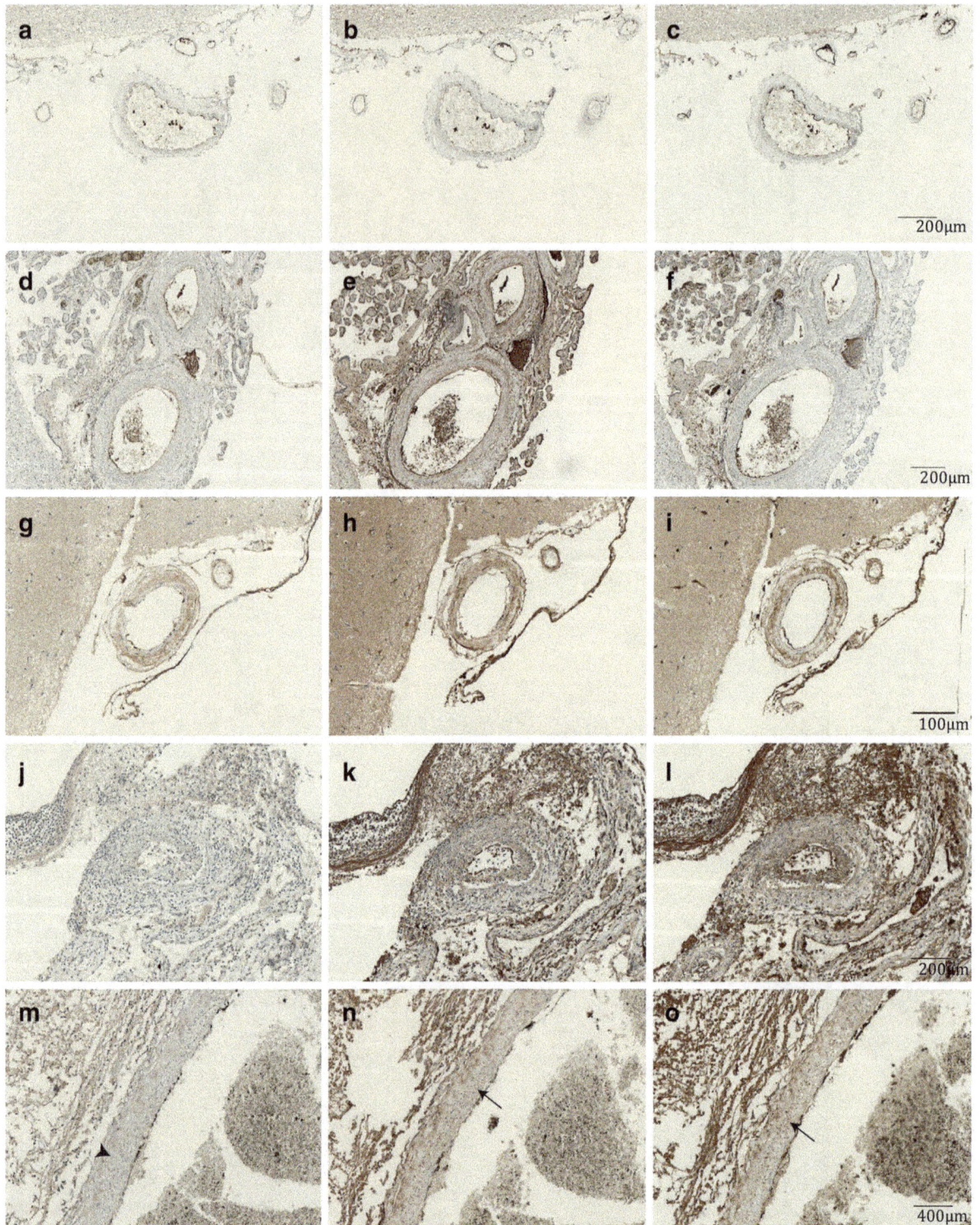

Fig. 2 Immunoglobulin staining of control patients, control meningitis patients and DCT patients. **a–c** A non-meningitis control case without immunoglobulin deposition. IgA (**a**), IgG (**b**) and IgM (**c**). **d–f** A non-meningitis control case with deposition of IgG (**e**). No IgA (**d**) and IgM (**f**) deposition is seen. **g–i** A non-meningitis control case with deposition of IgA (**g**), IgG (**h**) and IgM (**i**). IgG is also deposited in tunica media (arrow). **j–l** Representative image of immune globulin deposition in both DCT and control meningitis cases. IgG (**k**) and IgM (**l**) deposition can be seen in all three arterial layers. There was stronger IgM stain observed than IgG. IgA (**j**) was in most cases absent. **m–o** Immunoglobulin deposition in artery without inflammation. IgG (**n**) and IgM (**o**) were seen in all three arterial layers including media of a non-DCT meningitis case (arrows). Little IgA (**m**) was observed only in tunica adventitia (arrow head)

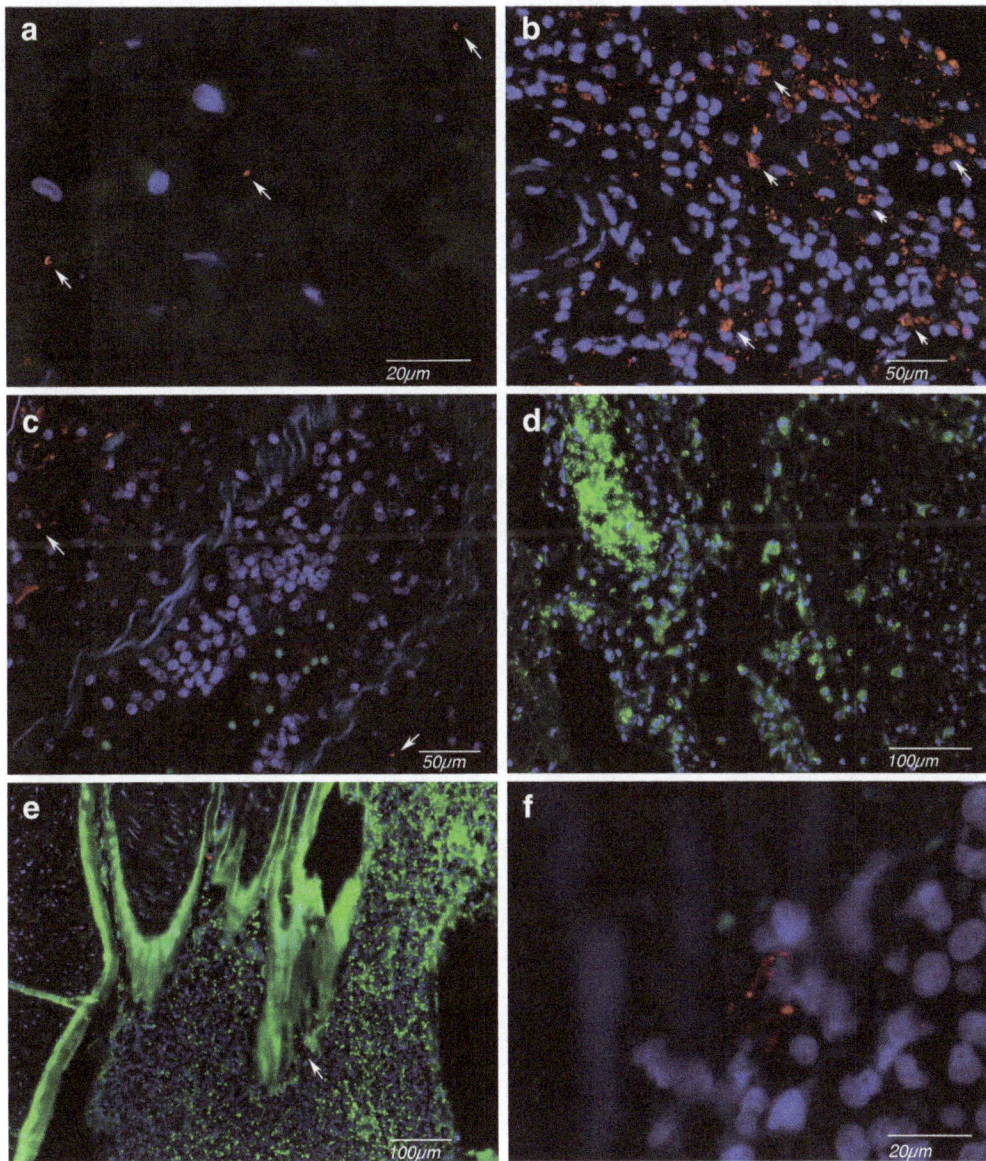

Fig. 3 Immunofluorescent analysis pneumococcal capsules of DCT patients and control meningitis patients. **a–e** DCT cases with the presence of various amount of intact pneumococcal capsules (a arrow). In case 1 (**a**), pneumococcal capsules were present sporadically. In case 2 (**b**), abundant presence of pneumococcal capsules was observed. In case 3 (**c**) and case 4 (**d**), a moderate amount was seen. In the thromboembolus of the basilar artery of the case 4 (**e**), large groups of bacteria were present (arrow) in addition to isolated bacteria (with mix of macrophages and neutrophils). The group of bacteria was enlarged in inlet. **f** Abundant presence of pneumococcal capsules in a control meningitis case

Half of DCT patients had basilar artery dilatation, an unusual finding in bacterial meningitis that was not observed in the non-DCT cases. The fusiform basilar artery dilatation in the course of bacterial meningitis found in two DCT cases is consistent with the diagnosis of infectious intracranial aneurysm, also known as mycotic aneurysm [20]. Infectious intracranial aneurysms are rare, localized, cerebrovascular lesions that make up 0.7–5.4% of all intracranial aneurysms [21]. The

majority of cases (65%) occur in the context of bacterial infectious endocarditis, and meningitis is estimated to be the cause of 5% of infectious intracranial aneurysms [20]. There are few case reports of infectious intracranial aneurysms in pneumococcal meningitis which describe both saccular and fusiform aneurysms [22, 23]. One of our DCT cases showed thrombosis in the basilar aneurysm and its branches which caused the infarction. The origin of the thrombosis cannot be traced, but an embolus or

even spontaneous thrombosis of intracranial aneurysm could be suspected [24], especially in the setting of vascular inflammation [25].

Previously published cases describe bleeding from the aneurysm during the course of bacterial meningitis as cause of secondary deterioration, which was not observed in our DCT cases. Our observation stresses the need of imaging using MR angiography to detect infectious aneurysms or more generalized cerebral vasculopathy in patients with bacterial meningitis and clinical deterioration. Described treatment for DCT so far mostly consisted of high-dose steroids to suppress the supposed resurging inflammatory response [12, 13]. Although platelet aggregation inhibitors could be suggested to reduce the risk of thrombosis in all meningitis patients, it is difficult to test whether this treatment is beneficial in such a rare complication. Anticoagulant treatment has previously been associated with increased risk of cerebral haemorrhage in bacterial meningitis and should be avoided [26].

Histopathological findings of delayed cerebral thrombosis resembled arterial inflammation in acute necrotizing vasculitis with fibrinoid necrosis seen in type III hypersensitivity vasculitis [27]. Type III hypersensitivity occurs when there is accumulation of immune complexes (antigen–antibody complexes) that have not been adequately cleared by innate immune cells, giving rise to an inflammatory response and attraction of leucocytes. Indeed, immunoglobulin staining of the meningitis cases showed distinctive increased deposit of IgM and IgG (IgM > IgG) in arteries as compared to the non-meningitis control cases, suggesting some sort of role of antigen-induced vasculitis in pneumococcal meningitis. However, we observed no difference in immunoglobulin deposition patterns between the control meningitis and delayed cerebral thrombosis cases, suggesting that accumulation of immune complexes is not the key driver of delayed cerebral thrombosis.

We used anti-pneumococcal capsule antibody to demonstrate the presence of pneumococcal cell wall components with circular enhancement in all meningitis cases with considerable differences in density. Groups of intact capsules were present in the cytoplasm of inflammatory cells, and isolated ones seemed to be present extracellularly. We did not observe gross differences in the presence of pneumococcal capsule between patients with and without DCT. In a previous post-mortem study, including 14 patients with pneumococcal meningitis, *S. pneumoniae* has been detected using Gram and silver staining in the subarachnoid, perivascular and ventricular spaces, but not within the brain parenchyma [28]. The presence of pneumococcal capsule in CSF and brain up to 35 days after initiation of antibiotic treatment may be suggested

to be a source for an ongoing (or resurging) inflammatory response. The lack of bacterial growth in repeated CSF cultures in DCT patients argues against ongoing bacterial infection [12]. As the pneumococcal capsules were observed in patients with and without DCT, it cannot be the only mechanism leading to DCT. Previously, we described complement factor 5a to be higher in DCT patients and identified genetic variation in the complement factor 5 gene to influence disease course [12, 29]. Potentially, the pneumococcal capsules only elicit a severe secondary inflammatory response in patients genetically prone to be pro-inflammatory.

DCT is a rare but devastating complication of bacterial meningitis. Adjunctive dexamethasone therapy seems to predispose patients with bacterial meningitis to this complication [12]. Infective intracranial aneurysms may be found in DCT patients although the consequences of this finding is unclear as it may be a marker of a more general cerebral vasculopathy or lead to direct infectious thromboembolisms. No evidence for accumulation of immune complexes or bacteria in blood vessels, or for infectious vasculitis, was found as explanation for the secondary deterioration and massive cerebral infarction of these patients. We observed pneumococcal cell wall components up to 35 days after start of antibiotics treatment that may be a source of ongoing or resurging inflammation. Although speculative, our findings indicate a persistent pro-inflammatory reaction that initially is suppressed by adjunctive dexamethasone treatment. Additional immunosuppressive treatment may therefore be beneficial in DCT patients, as previously suggested.

Authors' contributions
J-YL performed the pathological studies and drafted the manuscript, MCB and DB identified the patients and corrected the manuscript for intellectual content, EA corrected the manuscript for intellectual content, DB supervised the study. All authors read and approved the final manuscript.

Author details
[1] Department of Neurology, Academic Medical Center, University of Amsterdam, Amsterdam Neuroscience, PO Box 22660, 1100 DD Amsterdam, The Netherlands. [2] Department of Neuropathology, Academic Medical Center, University of Amsterdam, Amsterdam Neuroscience, Amsterdam, The Netherlands. [3] Stichting Epilepsie Instellingen Nederland (SEIN), Cruquius, The Netherlands.

Competing interests
Financial disclosure statement: the authors have no financial disclosures to report.

Funding
Study's funding and support: This study was supported by the Netherlands Organization for Health Research and Development (ZonMw; NWO-Veni-Grant [916.13.078], and NWO-Vidi-Grant [917.17.308] to MB, NWO-Vidi grant [016.116.358] to DB), the Academic Medical Center (AMC Fellowship to DB) and the European Research Council (ERC Starting Grant to DB).

References

1. van de Beek D, de Gans J, Spanjaard L, Weisfelt M, Reitsma JB, Vermeulen M. Clinical features and prognostic factors in adults with bacterial meningitis. N Engl J Med. 2004;351:1849–59.
2. Bijlsma MW, Brouwer MC, Kasanmoentalib ES, et al. Community-acquired bacterial meningitis in adults in the Netherlands, 2006–2014: a prospective cohort study. The Lancet Infectious diseases 2015.
3. van de Beek D, Brouwer M, Hasbun R, Koedel U, Whitney CG, Wijdicks E. Community-acquired bacterial meningitis. Nat Rev Dis Primers. 2016;2:16074.
4. Mook-Kanamori BB, Geldhoff M, van der Poll T, van de Beek D. Pathogenesis and pathophysiology of pneumococcal meningitis. Clin Microbiol Rev. 2011;24:557–91.
5. de Gans J, van de Beek D. European dexamethasone in adulthood bacterial meningitis study I. Dexamethasone in adults with bacterial meningitis. N Engl J Med. 2002;347:1549–56.
6. van de Beek D, de Gans J, McIntyre P, Prasad K. Steroids in adults with acute bacterial meningitis: a systematic review. Lancet Infect Dis. 2004;4:139–43.
7. Brouwer MC, Heckenberg SG, de Gans J, Spanjaard L, Reitsma JB, van de Beek D. Nationwide implementation of adjunctive dexamethasone therapy for pneumococcal meningitis. Neurology. 2010;75:1533–9.
8. van de Beek D, Brouwer MC, Thwaites GE, Tunkel AR. Advances in treatment of bacterial meningitis. Lancet. 2012;380:1693–702.
9. Hoogman M, van de Beek D, Weisfelt M, de Gans J, Schmand B. Cognitive outcome in adults after bacterial meningitis. J Neurol Neurosurg Psychiatry. 2007;78:1092–6.
10. Lucas MJ, Brouwer MC, van de Beek D. Neurological sequelae of bacterial meningitis. J Infect. 2016;73:18–27.
11. van de Beek D, de Gans J, Tunkel AR, Wijdicks EF. Community-acquired bacterial meningitis in adults. N Engl J Med. 2006;354:44–53.
12. Lucas MJ, Brouwer MC, van de Beek D. Delayed cerebral thrombosis in bacterial meningitis: a prospective cohort study. Intensive Care Med. 2013;39:866–71.
13. Schut ES, Brouwer MC, de Gans J, Florquin S, Troost D, van de Beek D. Delayed cerebral thrombosis after initial good recovery from pneumococcal meningitis. Neurology. 2009;73:1988–95.
14. Wittebole X, Duprez T, Hantson P. Delayed cerebral ischaemic injury following apparent recovery from Streptococcus pneumoniae meningitis. Acta Clin Belg. 2016;71:343–6.
15. Steiner I. Past as prologue: delayed stroke as a parainfectious process of bacterial meningitis? Neurology. 2009;73:1945–6.
16. Kawaguchi T, Ogawa Y, Inoue T, Tominaga T. Cerebral arteritis with extremely late onset secondary to bacterial meningitis—case report. Neurol Med Chir (Tokyo). 2011;51:302–5.
17. Rice CM, Ramamoorthi M, Renowden SA, Heywood P, Whone AL, Scolding NJ. Cerebral ischaemia in the context of improving, steroid-treated pneumococcal meningitis. QJM Mon J Assoc Physician. 2012;105:473–5.
18. Kato Y, Takeda H, Dembo T, Tanahashi N. Delayed recurrent ischemic stroke after initial good recovery from pneumococcal meningitis. Intern Med. 2012;51:647–50.
19. Engelen-Lee JY, Brouwer MC, Aronica E, van de Beek D. Pneumococcal meningitis: clinical-pathological correlations (meningene-path). Acta Neuropathol Commun. 2016;4:26.
20. Ducruet AF, Hickman ZL, Zacharia BE, et al. Intracranial infectious aneurysms: a comprehensive review. Neurosurg Rev. 2010;33:37–46.
21. Nakahara I, Taha MM, Higashi T, et al. Different modalities of treatment of intracranial mycotic aneurysms: report of 4 cases. Surg Neurol. 2006;66:405–9 **(discussion 9–10)**.
22. Palacios A, Llorente AM, Ordonez O, Martinez de Aragon A. Intracranial mycotic aneurysm in a 5 month-old infant with pneumococcal meningitis. Enferm Infecc Microbiol Clin. 2017;35:267–9.
23. Choi KH, Park MS, Kim JT, et al. Infectious intracranial aneurysm presenting with a series of strokes as a complication of pneumococcal meningitis. Eur Neurol. 2012;68:260.
24. Cohen JE, Itshayek E, Gomori JM, et al. Spontaneous thrombosis of cerebral aneurysms presenting with ischemic stroke. J Neurol Sci. 2007;254:95–8.
25. Emmi G, Silvestri E, Squatrito D, et al. Thrombosis in vasculitis: from pathogenesis to treatment. Thromb J. 2015;13:15.
26. Mook-Kanamori BB, Fritz D, Brouwer MC, van der Ende A, van de Beek D. Intracerebral hemorrhages in adults with community associated bacterial meningitis in adults: should we reconsider anticoagulant therapy? PLoS One. 2012;7:e45271.
27. Kumar V, Aster JC. Robbins & Cotran. Pathologic basis of disease. 9th ed. New York: Elsevier; 2014.
28. Guarner J, Liu L, Bhatnagar J, et al. Neutrophilic bacterial meningitis: pathology and etiologic diagnosis of fatal cases. Mod Pathol. 2013;26:1076–85.
29. Woehrl B, Brouwer MC, Murr C, et al. Complement component 5 contributes to poor disease outcome in humans and mice with pneumococcal meningitis. J Clin Invest. 2011;121:3943–53.

6

Anemia at pediatric intensive care unit discharge: prevalence and risk markers

Pierre Demaret[1,2]* iD, Oliver Karam[3,4] iD, Marisa Tucci[5], Jacques Lacroix[5], Hélène Behal[6], Alain Duhamel[6], Frédéric Lebrun[1], André Mulder[1] and Stéphane Leteurtre[2,7]

Abstract

Background: Anemia is prevalent at pediatric intensive care unit (PICU) admission and incident during PICU stay, but little is known about anemia at PICU discharge. Anemia after critical illness is an important issue because it could impact post-PICU outcome. We aimed to estimate the prevalence of anemia at PICU discharge and to determine its risk markers.

Methods: This is an ancillary study of a prospective observational study on transfusion practices conducted in the PICU of a tertiary care children's hospital. All children consecutively admitted to the PICU during a 1-year period were considered for inclusion. Data were prospectively collected from medical charts, except for hemoglobin (Hb) levels at PICU and hospital discharge that were collected retrospectively. Anemia was defined by an Hb concentration below the lower limit of the normal range for age.

Results: Among the 679 children retained for analysis, 390 (57.4%) were anemic at PICU discharge. After multivariate adjustment, anemia at PICU admission was the strongest risk marker of anemia at PICU discharge. The strength of this association varied according to age (interaction): The odds ratio (OR) (95% CI) of anemia at PICU discharge was 4.85 (1.67–14.11) for 1–5-month-old infants anemic versus not anemic at PICU admission, and it was 73.13 (13.43, 398.19) for adolescents anemic versus not anemic at PICU admission. Children admitted after a non-cardiac surgery had an increased risk of anemia at PICU discharge [OR 2.30 (1.37, 3.88), $p = 0.002$]. The proportion of anemic children differed between age categories, while the median Hb level did not exhibit significant variations according to age.

Conclusions: Anemia is highly prevalent at PICU discharge and is strongly predicted by anemia at PICU admission. The usual age-based definitions of anemia may not be relevant for critically ill children. The consequences of anemia at PICU discharge are unknown and deserve further scrutiny.

Keywords: Child, Anemia, Erythrocyte, Pediatric intensive care unit, Pediatric, Outcome

Background

Anemia, defined as a concentration of hemoglobin (Hb) below the lower limit of the normal range for age (Table 1) [1], is a common issue in critically ill patients: Approximately two-thirds of critically ill adults are anemic at admission to the intensive care unit (ICU) [2, 3] and up to 98% of them have been reported to be anemic by ICU day 8 [4]. Anemia is frequent in pediatric ICU (PICU) as well: In a large North American multicenter study, one-third of the critically ill children with a PICU stay of at least 2 days were anemic at PICU admission and an additional 40% became anemic during their PICU stay [5].

Given the high prevalence and incidence of anemia at admission and during ICU stay and given that red blood cell (RBC) transfusion guidelines recommend a restrictive strategy for most critically ill patients [6, 7], it makes sense to wonder about anemia at ICU discharge.

There are scarce data, suggesting that about 85% of adults are anemic when leaving the ICU [8, 9] and that this anemia persists for weeks, most of the patients still being anemic at hospital discharge [9]. It even seems

*Correspondence: pierre.demaret@chc.be
[1] Pediatric Intensive Care Unit, Department of Pediatrics, CHC, Liège, Belgium
Full list of author information is available at the end of the article

Table 1 Hemoglobin thresholds used to diagnose anemia and anemia prevalence at PICU discharge

Age	Hb threshold to diagnose anemia (g/L)	Proportion of patients anemic at PICU discharge in our study[a]
< 1 month	< 130	39/55 (70.9)
1–5 months	< 95	32/105 (30.5)
6–59 months	< 110	125/231 (54.1)
5–11 years	< 115	70/119 (58.8)
12–14 years	< 120	55/81 (67.9)
≥ 15 years		
Female	< 120	39/46 (84.8)
Male	< 130	30/42 (71.4)
Total		390/679 (57.4)

[a] Number of anemic children/total number of children in the age category (%)

Hb hemoglobin, *PICU* pediatric intensive care unit

that up to half of adults leaving the ICU with a Hb level < 100 g/L are still anemic 6 months after hospital discharge [10].

Data about anemia at PICU discharge are almost non-existent. In a single-center Canadian study with large exclusion criteria and no cases of cardiac surgery, 94/392 (24%) children were discharged from PICU with anemia [11]. No other pediatric study on this topic has been published so far.

Anemia is far from trivial and is associated with worse outcomes even in non-critically ill patients. For example, anemia is associated with mortality in African children and a recent meta-analysis of nearly 12,000 children showed that the risk of death falls by 24% for each 1 g/dL increase in Hb [12]. Anemia is associated with neurological outcome. For example, prenatal iron deficiency anemia is associated with a worse mental development of the child at 12, 18 and 24 months of age [13], and a lower mean Hb after a hypoxic–ischemic brain injury following cardiac arrest is associated with a higher odd of unfavorable neurological outcome at hospital discharge [14]. Anemia is also associated with a decreased quality of life and with an increase in healthcare resource utilization [15, 16].

These associations between anemia and worse outcomes explain why the question of anemia after critical illness is of high importance. If anemia is frequent at PICU discharge, then it could play an important role in the post-PICU course.

Outcome after discharge from intensive care is a real challenge for PICU physicians. Mortality rates in PICU are very low (2.4%) as recently reported [17]. Cognitive impairments and physical impairments are currently recognized as potential post-intensive care morbidities of importance [18], and anemia may have an impact on both of them. Limited adult data indicate that patients

discharged from ICU with anemia may have a reduced health-related quality of life as compared to the normal population and to non-selected ICU survivors [10]. To our knowledge, no pediatric data have been published so far on this issue.

The first step in assessing the role of anemia at PICU discharge is to determine its prevalence, which is currently unknown. We therefore conducted a study aiming to determine the prevalence of anemia at PICU discharge and its risk markers.

Methods

Study design, study site and population

This study is a post hoc analysis of a single-center prospective database aiming to describe transfusion practices in PICU [19, 20].

The PICU of Sainte-Justine University Hospital is a multidisciplinary PICU, serving both medical and surgical specialties. All consecutive admissions to PICU, from April 21, 2009, to April 20, 2010, were prospectively screened for recruitment. A priori defined exclusion criteria were: newborn with gestational age less than 40 weeks at the time of PICU admission, age less than 3 days or more than 18 years at PICU admission, pregnancy or admission just after labor. We excluded a posteriori all children with no Hb level at PICU discharge (as defined below).

Primary outcome

We retrospectively collected the Hb level at discharge from PICU, defined as follows: the Hb level closest to PICU discharge, collected on a complete blood count after PICU admission and not more than 7 days prior to PICU discharge.

Based on the World Health Organization (WHO) criteria for children aged 6 months and older [21] and on the thresholds proposed in a pediatric textbook for infants younger than 6 months of age [22], we defined anemia as a Hb level < 130 g/L for neonates, < 95 g/L for 1–5-month-old infants, < 110 g/L for 6–59-month-old children, < 115 g/L for 5–11-year-old children, < 120 g/L for 12–14-year-old infants, < 120 g/L for female adolescents aged ≥ 15 years and < 130 g/L for male adolescents aged ≥ 15 years (Table 1).

Data collection

Trained research assistants prospectively collected data daily in a validated case report form. All information was abstracted from medical charts.

Patient characteristics and baseline data collected within 24 h after PICU admission included age, gender, medical past and admission diagnoses. (More than one diagnosis could be attributed to each patient.) A predictive score of mortality, the Pediatric Risk of Mortality (PRISM score, first version) [23], and a descriptive score of severity of multiple organ dysfunction, the Pediatric Logistic Organ Dysfunction (PELOD score, first version) [24], were used to describe severity of illness at PICU admission.

Several data were prospectively collected during the entire PICU stay. Organ dysfunctions and multiple organ dysfunction syndrome (MODS) were defined according to Goldstein et al. [25]. New MODS was diagnosed if a patient with no organ dysfunction or one organ dysfunction at the time of PICU admission developed two or more organ dysfunctions during PICU stay or if he/she died; progressive MODS was diagnosed if a patient who already had MODS at PICU admission developed dysfunction of at least one other organ during PICU stay or if he/she died. Infections were recorded as per medical notes in the patient chart and by following up all cultures done during PICU stay. Severe sepsis and septic shock were defined according to the definitions published by an International Pediatric Sepsis Consensus Conference [25]. Use of extracorporeal support techniques as well as mortality (death in PICU and in hospital) and the length of stay in PICU and in hospital were recorded.

The Hb concentration at hospital discharge was collected retrospectively and was defined as the Hb level closest to hospital discharge, collected after PICU discharge, but not more than 7 days prior to hospital discharge.

Institutional review board approval was obtained for the collection of the initial database, waiving the requirement for written informed consent due to the observational nature of the study.

Statistical analysis
Quantitative variables were expressed as mean (standard deviation) if the variable was normally distributed (as assessed graphically and by using the Shapiro–Wilk test) and as median (interquartile range) if not. Qualitative variables were expressed as frequencies and percentages.

Association between anemia at PICU discharge and each patient characteristic at PICU admission or during PICU stay was first studied by bivariate analysis using a logistic regression with a random subject effect (general linear mixed model, GLMM) that allowed us to account for the occurrence of repeated measures per subject (no more than two admissions per subject).

In order to identify independent risk markers of anemia at PICU discharge, we performed multivariable GLMM analysis using the following steps: First, the variables with a p value less than 0.2 in bivariate analysis were introduced in a multivariable GLMM. The PRISM score was forced into the model, as we wanted to adjust for the

severity of disease. Second, a backward selection at level 0.1 was performed to simplify the model by eliminating variables that were useless in the model. Third, considering the subset of variables selected at the previous step, all the possible first-order interactions were tested in bivariate models. The final multivariable GLMM was obtained by considering the variables selected at the second step and the interactions having a significant level less than 0.1.

Results
Over the 1-year study period, there were 913 consecutive PICU admissions; 71 cases were excluded according to a priori criteria and 163 cases were excluded due to a posteriori criteria (Fig. 1). This left 679 cases for analysis. Children excluded a posteriori differed from those included: They were older (median age (IQR) 53 (12–155) *versus* 39 (6–141) months, $p = 0.019$), were less severely ill (median admission PRISM score 4 (0–6) *versus* 5 (2–9), $p < 0.001$), had less congenital heart disease (8.6% *versus* 23.1%, $p < 0.001$) and had a higher median Hb at PICU admission (122 (108–139) *versus* 110 (95–124) g/L, $p < 0.001$).

Hemoglobin and anemia at PICU discharge
Among the 679 cases retained for analysis, 390 (57.4%) were anemic at PICU discharge. The last Hb before PICU discharge was collected on the day of PICU discharge for 543 (80%) children, 1 day before PICU discharge for 85 (12.5%) children and 2, 3, 4, 5, 6 and 7 days before PICU discharge for 25 (3.7%), 11 (1.6%), 5 (0.7%), 6 (0.9%), 3 (0.4%) and 1 (0.1%) children, respectively. The median Hb (IQR) at PICU discharge was 96 g/L (86–106) in anemic children and 122 g/L (113–133) in non-anemic children ($p < 0.001$) (Fig. 2a). The proportion of anemic children was higher in neonates (70.9%) and adolescents (male 71.4%, female 84.8%), while it was lower in infants aged 1–5 months (30.5%) (Table 1, Fig. 3).

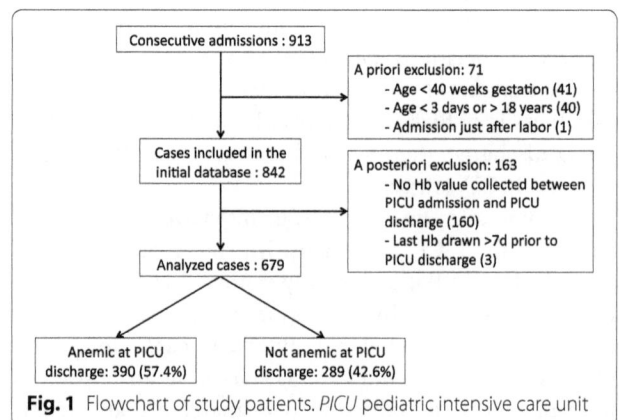

Fig. 1 Flowchart of study patients. *PICU* pediatric intensive care unit

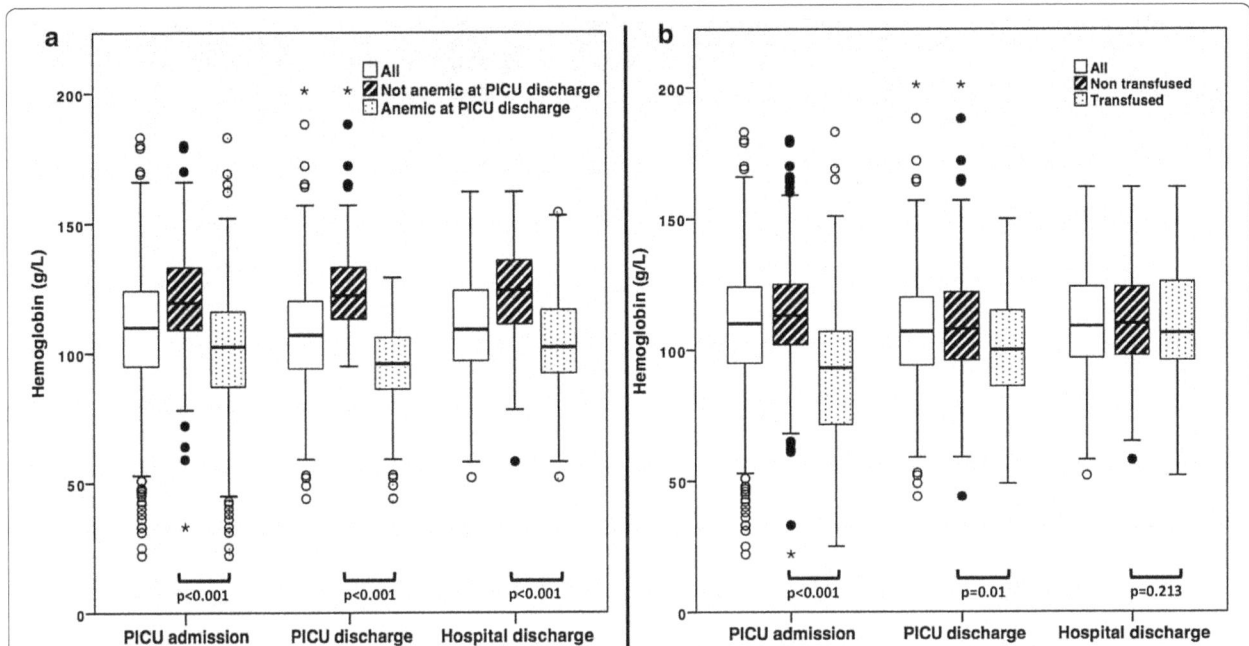

Fig. 2 Whisker plots of the hemoglobin level at PICU admission, PICU discharge and hospital discharge for children anemic and non-anemic at PICU admission (**a**) and for children transfused and non-transfused during their PICU stay (**b**). *PICU* pediatric intensive care unit; points and asterisks represent outliers and extreme outliers, respectively

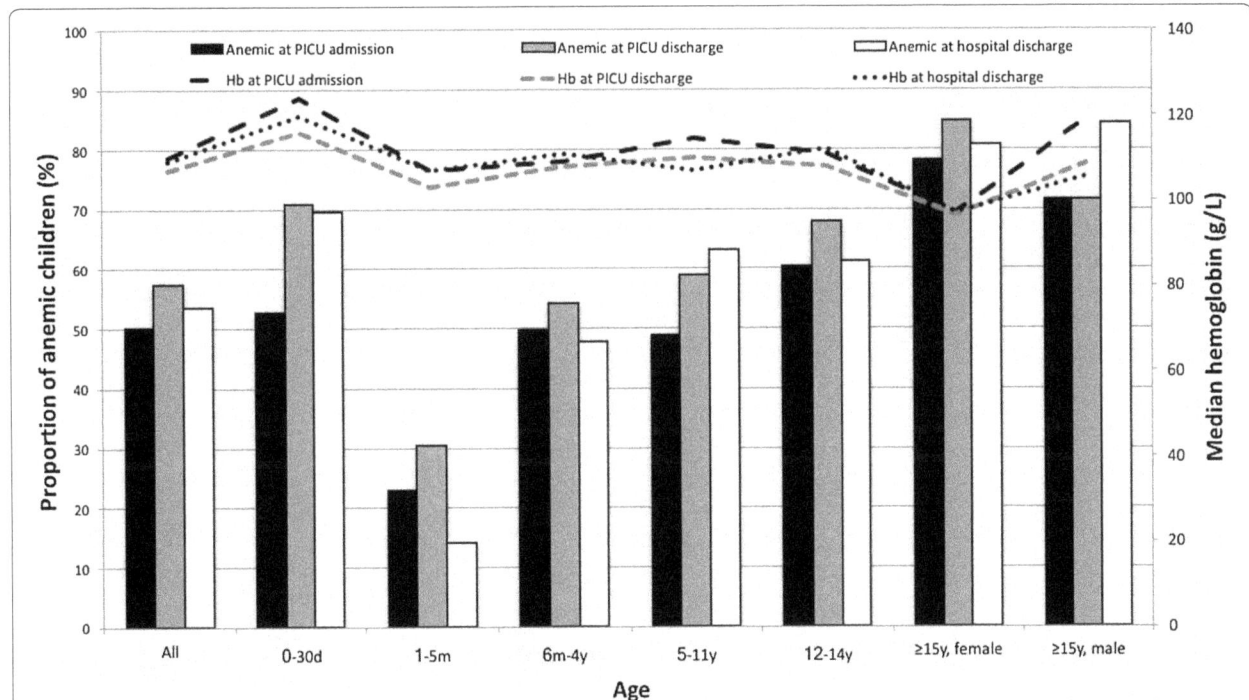

Fig. 3 Double *Y*-axis graph on the proportion of anemic children at PICU admission, PICU discharge and hospital discharge according to age, and median Hb level at PICU admission, PICU discharge and hospital discharge according to age. *Hb* hemoglobin, *PICU* pediatric intensive care unit

Bivariate association between patient, PICU admission or PICU stay characteristics and anemia at PICU discharge
Children anemic at PICU discharge were older than

non-anemic children, and they were more likely to suffer from a cancer and less likely to have cyanotic congenital heart disease (Table 2). Children with a higher admission

Table 2 Bivariate association between patient and PICU stay characteristics and anemia at PICU discharge

	All patients (n = 679)	Not anemic (p = 289)	Anemic (n = 390)	Crude OR (CI$_{95\%}$)	p value
Patient characteristics					
Age (months)	39 (6–141)	20 (4–89)	57.5 (10.8–159.3)		< 0.001
< 1 month	55 (8.1)	16 (5.4)	39 (10.0)	Reference	
1–5 months	105 (15.5)	73 (25.3)	32 (8.2)	0.18 (0.09, 0.38)	
6–59 months	231 (34.0)	106 (36.7)	125 (32.1)	0.48 (0.25, 0.94)	
5–11 years	119 (17.5)	49 (17.0)	70 (17.9)	0.59 (0.29, 1.20)	
12–14 years	81 (11.9)	26 (9.0)	55 (14.1)	0.86 (0.40, 1.88)	
≥ 15 years	88 (13.0)	19 (6.6)	69 (17.7)	1.47 (0.66, 3.30)	
Gender male	353 (52.0)	147 (50.9)	206 (52.8)	1.08 (0.78, 1.50)	0.62
Cancer (n, %)	37 (5.4)	10 (3.5)	27 (6.9)	2.08 (0.99, 4.37)	0.048
Congenital heart disease (n, %)					0.018
Cyanotic	84 (12.4)	49 (17.0)	35 (9.0)	0.49 (0.29, 0.80)	
Non-cyanotic	73 (10.8)	29 (10.0)	44 (11.3)	1.04 (0.61, 1.77)	
No congenital heart disease	522 (76.9)	211 (73.0)	311 (79.7)	Reference	
PICU admission day					
PRISM score					0.35
> 10	125 (18.4)	53 (18.3)	72 (18.5)	0.84 (0.48, 1.46)	
6–10	194 (28.6)	93 (32.2)	101 (25.9)	0.67 (0.40, 1.11)	
1–5	250 (36.8)	101 (34.9)	149 (38.2)	0.91 (0.56, 1.48)	
0	110 (16.2)	42 (14.6)	68 (17.4)	Reference	
PELOD score					0.034
> 20	27 (4.0)	7 (2.4)	20 (5.1)	2.82 (1.09, 7.29)	
11–20	153 (22.5)	56 (19.4)	97 (24.9)	1.71 (1.1, 2.67)	
1–10	271 (39.9)	113 (39.1)	158 (40.5)	1.39 (0.95, 2.03)	
0	228 (33.6)	113 (39.1)	115 (29.5)	Reference	
Lowest Hb (g/L), mean ± SD	108.9 ± 24.3	120.8 ± 20.1	100.4 ± 23.4	0.96 (0.95, 0.96)	< 0.001
Anemia	341 (50.2)	57 (21.1)	284 (75.1)	11.27 (7.63, 16.65)	< 0.001
Lowest platelets count (× 10^9/L), mean ± SD	234.5 ± 133.9	250.2 ± 114.6	223.2 ± 145.2	0.98 (0.97, 0.99)	0.021
Thrombocytopenia[a]	194 (28.6)	63 (23.4)	131 (34.7)	1.72 (1.18, 2.5)	0.005
Admission diagnosis					
Respiratory disease	239 (35.2)	127 (43.9)	112 (28.8)	0.51 (0.36, 0.72)	< 0.001
Infection	254 (37.5)	120 (41.5)	134 (34.4)	0.74 (0.53, 1.04)	0.079
Non-cardiac surgery	165 (24.3)	48 (16.7)	117 (30.2)	2.16 (1.44, 3.21)	< 0.001
Cardiac surgery	106 (15.6)	47 (16.3)	59 (15.1)	0.91 (0.59, 1.42)	0.69
Seizures	49 (7.2)	27 (9.3)	22 (5.6)	0.58 (0.31, 1.07)	0.081
Any shock	46 (6.8)	16 (5.6)	30 (7.7)	1.44 (0.74, 2.79)	0.28
Trauma	23 (3.4)	19 (4.9)	4 (1.4)	3.62 (1.17, 11.26)	0.027
PICU stay					
Transfusion (n, %)					
Any transfusion	176 (25.9)	59 (20.4)	117 (30.0)	1.67 (1.14, 2.45)	0.009
Red blood cells	143 (21.1)	45 (15.6)	98 (25.1)	1.83 (1.21, 2.77)	0.005
Plasma	94 (13.8)	39 (13.5)	55 (14.1)	1.06 (0.66, 1.7)	0.81
Platelets	58 (8.5)	13 (4.5)	45 (11.5)	2.73 (1.4, 5.32)	0.004
Respiratory dysfunction	337 (49.6)	159 (55.0)	178 (45.6)	0.69 (0.5, 0.95)	0.025
Cardiovascular dysfunction	14 (2.1)	4 (1.4)	10 (2.6)	1.91 (0.56, 6.55)	0.30
Hematological dysfunction	115 (16.9)	32 (11.1)	83 (21.3)	2.15 (1.35, 3.42)	0.002
Neurological dysfunction	388 (57.1)	162 (56.1)	226 (57.9)	1.09 (0.79, 1.51)	0.60
Hepatic dysfunction	98 (14.4)	33 (11.4)	65 (16.7)	1.55 (0.97, 2.5)	0.069
Renal dysfunction	24 (3.5)	4 (1.4)	20 (5.1)	3.86 (1.25, 11.95)	0.02

Table 2 continued

	All patients (n = 679)	Not anemic (p = 289)	Anemic (n = 390)	Crude OR (CI$_{95\%}$)	p value
New or progressive MODS	112 (16.5)	43 (14.9)	69 (17.7)	1.22 (0.78, 1.89)	0.38
Death in PICU	25 (3.7)	9 (3.1)	16 (4.1)	1.35 (0.56, 3.24)	0.50
Infection (proven or suspected)	301 (44.3)	137 (47.6)	164 (42.3)	0.81 (0.58, 1.12)	0.20
Severe sepsis/septic shock	63 (9.3)	19 (6.6)	44 (11.3)	1.8 (1.00, 3.26)	0.051
Support techniques (n, %)					
Mechanical ventilation	350 (51.5)	147 (50.9)	203 (52.1)	1.05 (0.76, 1.45)	0.75
Duration (day), median (Q1–Q3)[b]	2 (1–5)	2 (1–5)	3 (1–5)		
ECMO/Berlin heart	8 (1.2)	4 (1.4)	4 (1.0)	0.74 (0.17, 3.24)	0.68
Plasmapheresis	5 (0.7)	1 (0.3)	4 (1.0)	–	–
Renal replacement therapy	13 (1.9)	1 (0.3)	12 (3.1)	9.12 (1.11, 75.09)	0.04
PICU length of stay (day), median (Q1–Q3)[c]	3 (2–6)	3 (2–6)	3 (2–6)		0.70
PICU stay > 48 h (n, %)	450 (66.3)	185 (64.0)	265 (67.9)	1.2 (0.85, 1.68)	0.30

Values are frequencies and percentage unless otherwise specified

OR odds ratio, PICU pediatric intensive care unit, PRISM pediatric risk of mortality, PELOD pediatric logistic organ dysfunction, Hb hemoglobin, SD standard deviation, MODS multiple organ dysfunction syndrome, ECMO extracorporeal membrane oxygenation, CI confidence interval

[a] Odds ratio calculated for an increase of 10×10^9/L

[b] Calculated for patients mechanically ventilated only

[c] Mann–Whitney U test was used for this variable due to its distribution

PELOD score showed an increased risk of anemia at PICU discharge as well as those admitted after non-cardiac surgery or due to trauma.

Anemia and thrombocytopenia at PICU admission were significantly associated with anemia at PICU discharge (OR (95% CI) 11.27 (7.63, 16.65), $p < 0.001$, and 1.72 (1.18, 2.50), $p = 0.005$, respectively). RBC and platelet transfusions during PICU stay were associated with an increased risk of anemia at PICU discharge (OR 1.83 (1.21, 2.77), $p = 0.005$, and 2.73 (1.4, 5.32), $p = 0.004$, respectively), but plasma transfusions were not ($p = 0.81$).

Incidence of anemia after PICU admission

Hb at PICU admission was available for 648 children. Among the 307 (49.8%) children not anemic at PICU admission, 94 (30.6%) were anemic at PICU discharge. These 94 children accounted for one quarter (94/390, 24.1%) of the children anemic at PICU discharge.

Hb levels at PICU admission, PICU discharge and hospital discharge were available in 372 children. Among the 139 (37.4%) children not anemic at PICU admission, 38 (27.3%) became anemic during PICU stay and 19 (13.7%) became anemic during the hospital stay after PICU discharge; 38 (27.3%) were still anemic at hospital discharge.

Multivariable analysis

The adjusted association between anemia at PICU admission and anemia at PICU discharge varied according to age (interaction): The strongest association was for adolescents aged 12–14 years (adjusted OR 33.44 (7.91,

Table 3 Multivariable analysis: risk markers of anemia at PICU discharge

	Adjusted OR (CI$_{95\%}$)	p value
Anemia at PICU admission × age		0.056
Anemia at PICU admission[a]		
< 1 month	9.32 (1.99, 43.75)	
1–5 months	4.85 (1.67, 14.11)	
6 months–4 years	6.79 (3.58, 12.91)	
5–11 years	9.13 (3.57, 23.37)	
12–14 years	33.44 (7.91, 141.33)	
≥ 15 years	73.13 (13.43, 398.19)	
Non-cardiac surgery	2.30 (1.37, 3.88)	0.002
Renal dysfunction	3.19 (0.85, 11.92)	0.083

OR odds ratio, PICU pediatric intensive care unit, CI confidence interval

[a] For each age category, children anemic at PICU admission are compared to non-anemic children (reference group)

141.33)) and ≥ 15 years (adjusted OR 73.13 (13.43, 398.19)), while the lowest association was for infants aged 1–5 months (adjusted OR 4.85 (1.67, 14.11)) (Table 3). Non-cardiac surgery was an independent risk marker of anemia at PICU discharge (OR 2.30 (1.37, 3.88), $p = 0.002$) as well. Renal dysfunction was retained in the final multivariable model, but its association with anemia at PICU discharge was not statistically significant. Admission PRISM score was forced into the multivariate model, but it was not statistically associated with anemia at PICU discharge ($p = 0.62$). All the other variables included in the multivariate analysis were not retained in the final model after backward selection (cancer; congenital heart disease; thrombocytopenia at PICU admission; admission for respiratory disease, infection, seizure or trauma; RBC or platelet transfusion during PICU stay; respiratory, hematological, hepatic or renal dysfunction; severe sepsis/septic shock; renal replacement therapy).

Patient outcomes after PICU discharge

Children anemic at PICU discharge had a longer length of hospital stay after PICU discharge than non-anemic children (Table 4). Hospital mortality after PICU discharge did not differ between the two groups ($p = 0.614$). When analyzing the 386 children for whom an Hb level at hospital discharge was available, we found that a high proportion of children with anemia at PICU discharge were still anemic at hospital discharge (178/247, 72%). Surprisingly 21% (29/139) of children who did not have anemia at PICU discharge developed anemia before hospital discharge.

The mean rate of Hb recovery between PICU and hospital discharge was 14.3 ± 40 g/L/week for the entire cohort; it was 18.5 ± 39.7 g/L/week for children anemic at PICU discharge and 6.7 ± 39.5 g/L/week for non-anemic children ($p < 0.001$)

Hemoglobin, transfusion and anemia at PICU admission, PICU discharge and hospital discharge

Children anemic at PICU discharge already exhibited a lower median Hb at PICU admission as compared with children who were not anemic at PICU discharge, and this difference was still significant at hospital discharge (Fig. 2a). Children transfused with RBCs during their PICU stay had a lower median Hb at PICU admission than non-transfused children, but this difference was reduced (even though still significant) at PICU discharge and was no longer significant at hospital discharge (Fig. 2b).

The proportion of anemic children at PICU admission, PICU discharge and hospital discharge showed the same trend through the age categories: This proportion was highest in female adolescents and lowest in infants aged 1–5 months (Fig. 3). However, such an age-dependant variation is not in phase with the trend of the median Hb level through the age categories: The median Hb level was quite stable from one age category to another and did not significantly decrease in 1–5-month-old infants (Fig. 3).

Discussion

This observational study shows that anemia is frequent at PICU discharge (57% of children included in our study). We identified two independent risk markers of anemia at PICU discharge: anemia at PICU admission (the strongest risk marker, showing an interaction with age) and admission after a non-cardiac surgery. A high proportion (72%) of children discharged from PICU with anemia were still anemic at hospital discharge. Finally, the proportion of anemic children at PICU admission, PICU discharge and hospital discharge varied according to the age categories, while the median Hb level was quite stable through these age categories (Fig. 3).

Anemia of PICU patients: from admission to hospital discharge… and beyond?

Anemia is highly prevalent at PICU admission and incident during PICU stay [5]. Our study shows that this anemia of critical illness is not limited to the acute phase of the disease but is still a significant issue at PICU discharge and maybe even subsequently.

We found that anemia at PICU admission was the stronger predictor of anemia at PICU discharge. We also found that the strength of this association varied according to age. Several hypotheses may be raised to explain such an interaction: Causes of anemia may differ from one age category to another; the erythropoietic response may vary depending on age; nutritional and/or therapeutic supports may change from the neonatal period to adolescence and may be associated with a different course of anemia according to age.

Our data on anemia at hospital discharge are limited since the Hb level at hospital discharge was available for

Table 4 Outcomes after PICU discharge

Outcome	All patients ($n = 679$)	Not anemic ($n = 289$)	Anemic ($n = 390$)	Univariate OR (CI$_{95\%}$)	p value
Hospital length of stay after PICU discharge, median (Q1–Q3)[a]	5 (2–13)	4 (2–9)	6 (3–15)		< 0.001
Death in hospital, n (%)[a]	12 (1.8)	6 (2.2)	6 (1.7)	0.75 (0.24, 2.34)	0.614
Hb at hospital discharge, median (Q1–Q3)[b]	109 (97–124)	124 (111–136)	102 (92–117)		< 0.001
Anemia at hospital discharge (n, %)[b]	207 (54)	29 (21)	178 (72)	9.79 (5.97, 16.1)	< 0.001

Continuous variables are expressed as median (interquartile range)

OR odds ratio, *Hb* hemoglobin, *CI* confidence interval

[a] For children discharged alive from PICU

[b] Available for 386 children

only 386 children. Keeping this limitation in mind, it is nevertheless noteworthy that 72% of children anemic at PICU discharge were still anemic when discharged from hospital. We do not have data on the Hb levels after hospital discharge. In a single-center Canadian cohort, 69% (43/62) of children anemic at PICU discharge were still anemic at hospital discharge, but anemia resolved within 4–6 months in 28 patients who were subsequently followed up [11]. Bateman et al. studied 19 adult patients having left the ICU with an Hb < 100 g/L [10]; only 47% (9/19) recovered from their anemia after 6 months of follow-up, with a median time to recovery of 11 weeks. In our study, the mean rate of Hb recovery between PICU and hospital discharge was 14.3 ± 40 g/L/week for the whole cohort; it was 18.5 ± 39.7 g/L/week for children anemic at PICU discharge and 6.7 ± 39.5 g/L/week for non-anemic children ($p < 0.001$). The rate usually encountered in healthy adults is 10 g/L/week; to our knowledge, the rate of recovery in healthy children has not been established yet [10]. We do not know whether children included in our study received RBCs, iron or erythropoiesis-stimulating agents after PICU discharge: Thus, the rate of Hb recovery we observed cannot be properly interpreted, but it is possible that children anemic at PICU discharge exhibit a better erythropoietic reaction than their adult counterparts.

Our finding that 21% of children without anemia at PICU discharge developed anemia during the subsequent hospital stay is also of importance. Are the causes and consequences of this anemia occurring after PICU discharge the same as those of anemia persisting after PICU discharge? What follow-up strategies should be implemented at PICU discharge, if any? Further studies are clearly required to clarify the epidemiology of this "post-PICU" anemia, to estimate the duration of this anemia and to better understand its mechanisms and its potential impacts.

Is the usual age-based definition of anemia relevant in PICU?

The WHO definition of anemia has been used in many studies. However, this definition has some limitations since it was established more than 40 years ago in a small population sample, without documentation of methodology [29]. Other diagnostic criteria have been proposed but none include pediatric criteria [30].

Studies on the distribution of normal Hb range in a healthy pediatric population are scarce and show quite variable results [31–33]. There is no universal definition of anemia in children. The normal range of Hb depends on several variables including age, race and socioeconomic status. The impact of age is largely explained by the transition from fetal Hb to adult Hb during the first weeks of life. This phenomenon, combined with a down-regulation of EPO production related to the increase in blood oxygen content and tissue oxygenation delivery following birth, leads to the so-called physiologic anemia of infancy [34].

However, according to our results (Fig. 3), children admitted to PICU do not exhibit such an age-based fluctuation of Hb level. The usual age-based definitions of anemia are thus questionable in the PICU setting. We were surprised to find that the proportion of anemic children varied through the age categories (drop in 1–5-month-old infants) while the median Hb level was relatively constant. Our results raise the question of the appropriate Hb level to diagnose anemia in critically ill children: Further research is required to address this question.

Red blood cell transfusions and anemia at PICU and hospital discharge

Children included in our study were transfused according to a restrictive strategy, which recommends transfusion for stable non-cyanotic PICU patients only if their Hb level drops below 70 g/L. In the patients retained for our study, including unstable and cyanotic children, the mean Hb level before the first transfusion was 77.7 ± 22.2 g/L [19]. We do not know to what extent this restrictive RBC transfusion strategy may have impacted the Hb level at PICU discharge. It is plausible that a restrictive strategy increases the risk of anemia at PICU discharge. Indeed, in the Transfusion Requirements in Pediatric Intensive Care Unit study, the overall average lowest Hb concentration from randomization to PICU discharge was 87 ± 4 g/L in the restrictive group and 108 ± 5 g/L in the liberal group ($p < 0.001$), while the Hb levels were similar in these two groups at randomization (80 ± 10 g/L versus 80 ± 9 g/L) [35]. On the other hand, patients transfused with RBCs do not seem to exhibit a greater Hb level than non-transfused patients at (P)ICU discharge. Indeed, it has been shown in a large adult cohort study that the mean Hb difference between transfused and non-transfused patients was high at ICU admission but then decreased over time and becomes nonsignificant [2]. We observed the same trend in our study (Fig. 2b).

All in all, it seems that RBC transfusion during PICU stay is not a reliable tool to distinguish between children who will be anemic at PICU/hospital discharge and those who will not, even when a restrictive transfusion strategy is applied.

Limitations and strengths

Our study has several limitations. First, Hb levels at PICU and hospital discharge were collected retrospectively, which increases the risk of information bias.

Second, the date of occurrence of the variables collected during the PICU stay was not documented, and the Hb we used to characterize anemia at PICU discharge could have been collected within the 7 days prior to discharge. It is thus theoretically possible that a variable considered as a risk marker of anemia at PICU discharge actually occurred after measurement of the discharge Hb. However, we believe that the risk of such protopathic bias is reduced since the discharge Hb was collected the day before or on the day of PICU discharge in 628 out of the 679 included patients (92.5%). Third, the Hb on the day of PICU discharge was not available for all patients, and we considered that a Hb level collected 1 to 7 days before PICU discharge should be a good surrogate of the Hb on the day of PICU discharge. This assertion could not be true and could result in information bias leading to an over- or underestimation of the prevalence of anemia at PICU discharge. However, as stated above, the vast majority of our patients had their last Hb collected the day before or on the day of PICU discharge. The risk of such information bias is thus significantly reduced. Fourth, we excluded 163 cases a posteriori that differed from the included cases; this may have induced a selection bias, which may limit the external validity of our study. Fifth, our study was single center, which also limits its external validity; however, our critical care unit is comparable to most multidisciplinary university-affiliated North American PICUs with regard to case mix and severity of illness. Sixth, our database has been collected in 2009–2010 and some practices may have changed since then, so that our study population may not appropriately reflect children discharged from PICU nowadays.

Our study has also several strengths. This is the first study that evaluates anemia at PICU discharge in a large cohort of critically ill children including neonates and children with congenital heart disease. We enrolled in this study all consecutive PICU admissions over a 1-year period, which resulted in a case mix with a limited risk of selection bias and no influence due to seasonal variation. Finally, all the independent variables were collected prospectively, which is a major asset to minimize information bias.

Conclusions

Anemia is frequent at PICU discharge and is strongly associated with anemia at PICU admission. While previous studies have focused on anemia at PICU admission and during PICU stay, it seems that the anemia of critically ill child is not limited to the acute phase of the critical illness: There seems to be a continuum of anemia from PICU admission to PICU discharge and hospital discharge.

As it is plausible that anemia at PICU discharge is associated with worse outcomes after PICU stay, efforts should be made to better understand its causes and consequences as well as to implement optimal care and follow-up strategies.

Abbreviations
CI: confidence interval; EPO: erythropoietin; Hb: hemoglobin; IL: interleukin; IQR: interquartile range; MODS: multiple organ dysfunction syndrome; OR: odds ratio; PELOD: pediatric logistic organ dysfunction; PICU: pediatric intensive care unit; PRISM: pediatric risk of mortality; RBC: red blood cell; WHO: World Health Organization.

Authors' contributions
PD, SL, JL and MT designed the study; PD, AD and HB conducted data analysis and wrote the tables; PD, SL, JL, MT and OK contributed to data interpretation; PD wrote the manuscript except for "Statistical analysis" section which was written by AD and HB; PD, SL, JL, MT, OK, AM and FL commented on the manuscript. All authors read and approved the final manuscript.

Author details
[1] Pediatric Intensive Care Unit, Department of Pediatrics, CHC, Liège, Belgium. [2] Université de Lille, EA 2694 - Santé Publique: épidémiologie et qualité des soins, 59000 Lille, France. [3] Pediatric Critical Care Unit, Geneva University Hospital, Geneva, Switzerland. [4] Division of Pediatric Critical Care Medicine, Children's Hospital of Richmond at VCU, Richmond, VA, USA. [5] Division of Pediatric Critical Care Medicine, Department of Pediatrics, Sainte-Justine Hospital, Université de Montréal, Montreal, Canada. [6] Université de Lille, EA 2694 - Santé Publique: épidémiologie et qualité des soins, Unité de Biostatistique, 59000 Lille, France. [7] Pediatric Intensive Care Unit, CHU Lille, 59000 Lille, France.

Acknowledgements
The authors thank Nicole Poitras, Mariana Dumitrascu and Christian Dong for their support in the realization of this study.

Competing interests
The authors declare that they have no competing interests.

Funding
This study was supported by the Fonds de la Recherche en Santé du Québec (Grant #24460).

References
1. Kassebaum NJ, Jasrasaria R, Naghavi M, Wulf SK, Johns N, Lozano R, et al. A systematic analysis of global anemia burden from 1990 to 2010. Blood. 2014;123(5):615–24.
2. Corwin HL, Gettinger A, Pearl RG, Fink MP, Levy MM, Abraham E, et al. The CRIT study: anemia and blood transfusion in the critically ill–current clinical practice in the United States. Crit Care Med. 2004;32(1):39–52.
3. Vincent JL, Baron JF, Reinhart K, Gattinoni L, Thijs L, Webb A, et al. Anemia and blood transfusion in critically ill patients. JAMA. 2002;288(12):1499–507.
4. Thomas J, Jensen L, Nahirniak S, Gibney RT. Anemia and blood transfusion practices in the critically ill: a prospective cohort review. Heart Lung J Crit Care. 2010;39(3):217–25.

5. Bateman ST, Lacroix J, Boven K, Forbes P, Barton R, Thomas NJ, et al. Anemia, blood loss, and blood transfusions in North American children in the intensive care unit. Am J Respir Crit Care Med. 2008;178(1):26–33.

6. Lacroix J, Demaret P, Tucci M. Red blood cell transfusion: decision making in pediatric intensive care units. Semin Perinatol. 2012;36(4):225–31.

7. Retter A, Wyncoll D, Pearse R, Carson D, McKechnie S, Stanworth S, et al. Guidelines on the management of anaemia and red cell transfusion in adult critically ill patients. Br J Haematol. 2013;160(4):445–64.

8. Walsh TS, Lee RJ, Maciver CR, Garrioch M, Mackirdy F, Binning AR, et al. Anemia during and at discharge from intensive care: the impact of restrictive blood transfusion practice. Intensive Care Med. 2006;32(1):100–9.

9. Walsh TS, Saleh EE, Lee RJ, McClelland DB. The prevalence and characteristics of anaemia at discharge home after intensive care. Intensive Care Med. 2006;32(8):1206–13.

10. Bateman AP, McArdle F, Walsh TS. Time course of anemia during six months follow up following intensive care discharge and factors associated with impaired recovery of erythropoiesis. Crit Care Med. 2009;37(6):1906–12.

11. Ngo QN, Matsui DM, Singh RN, Zelcer S, Kornecki A. Anemia among pediatric critical care survivors: prevalence and resolution. Crit Care Res Pract. 2013;2013:684361.

12. Scott SP, Chen-Edinboro LP, Caulfield LE, Murray-Kolb LE. The impact of anemia on child mortality: an updated review. Nutrients. 2014;6(12):5915–32.

13. Chang S, Zeng L, Brouwer ID, Kok FJ, Yan H. Effect of iron deficiency anemia in pregnancy on child mental development in rural China. Pediatrics. 2013;131(3):e755–63.

14. Wormsbecker A, Sekhon MS, Griesdale DE, Wiskar K, Rush B. The association between anemia and neurological outcome in hypoxic ischemic brain injury after cardiac arrest. Resuscitation. 2017;112:11–6.

15. Bolge SC, Mody S, Ambegaonkar BM, McDonnell DD, Zilberberg MD. The impact of anemia on quality of life and healthcare resource utilization in patients with HIV/AIDS receiving antiretroviral therapy. Curr Med Res Opin. 2007;23(4):803–10.

16. Yohannes AM, Ershler WB. Anemia in COPD: a systematic review of the prevalence, quality of life, and mortality. Respir Care. 2011;56(5):644–52.

17. Burns JP, Sellers DE, Meyer EC, Lewis-Newby M, Truog RD. Epidemiology of death in the PICU at five U.S. teaching hospitals*. Crit Care Med. 2014;42(9):2101–8.

18. Needham DM, Davidson J, Cohen H, Hopkins RO, Weinert C, Wunsch H, et al. Improving long-term outcomes after discharge from intensive care unit: report from a stakeholders' conference. Crit Care Med. 2012;40(2):502–9.

19. Demaret P, Tucci M, Ducruet T, Trottier H, Lacroix J. Red blood cell transfusion in critically ill children (CME). Transfusion. 2014;54(2):365–75.

20. Karam O, Lacroix J, Robitaille N, Rimensberger PC, Tucci M. Association between plasma transfusions and clinical outcome in critically ill children: a prospective observational study. Vox Sang. 2013;104(4):342–9.

21. World Health Organization: Haemoglobin concentrations for the diagnosis of anaemia and assessment of severity. Vitamin and Mineral Nutrition Information System. Geneva, World Health Organization, 2011 (WHO/NMH/NHD/MNM/11.1) (http://www.who.int/vmnis/indicators/haemoglobin.pdf. Accessed 10 Sept 2015.

22. Behrman RE, Kliegman R, Jenson HB. Nelson textbook of pediatrics. 17th ed. Philadelphia, PA: Saunders; 2004. xlviii, 2618 p.

23. Pollack MM, Ruttimann UE, Getson PR. Pediatric risk of mortality (PRISM) score. Crit Care Med. 1988;16(11):1110–6.

24. Leteurtre S, Martinot A, Duhamel A, Proulx F, Grandbastien B, Cotting J, et al. Validation of the paediatric logistic organ dysfunction (PELOD) score: prospective, observational, multicentre study. Lancet. 2003;362(9379):192–7.

25. Goldstein B, Giroir B, Randolph A. International pediatric sepsis consensus conference: definitions for sepsis and organ dysfunction in pediatrics. Pediatr Crit Care Med. 2005;6(1):2–8.

26. Corwin HL. Anemia and blood transfusion in the critically ill patient: role of erythropoietin. Crit Care. 2004;8(Suppl 2):S42–4.

27. Hayden SJ, Albert TJ, Watkins TR, Swenson ER. Anemia in critical illness: insights into etiology, consequences, and management. Am J Respir Crit Care Med. 2012;185(10):1049–57 **PubMed PMID: 22281832**.

28. Lasocki S, Longrois D, Montravers P, Beaumont C. Hepcidin and anemia of the critically ill patient: bench to bedside. Anesthesiology. 2011;114(3):688–94.

29. Cappellini MD, Motta I. Anemia in clinical practice-definition and classification: does hemoglobin change with aging? Semin Hematol. 2015;52(4):261–9.

30. Beutler E, Waalen J. The definition of anemia: what is the lower limit of normal of the blood hemoglobin concentration? Blood. 2006;107(5):1747–50.

31. Sherriff A, Emond A, Hawkins N, Golding J. Haemoglobin and ferritin concentrations in children aged 12 and 18 months. ALSPAC Children in Focus Study Team. Arch Dis Child. 1999;80(2):153–7.

32. Jopling J, Henry E, Wiedmeier SE, Christensen RD. Reference ranges for hematocrit and blood hemoglobin concentration during the neonatal period: data from a multihospital health care system. Pediatrics. 2009;123(2):e333–7.

33. Stevens GA, Finucane MM, De-Regil LM, Paciorek CJ, Flaxman SR, Branca F, et al. Global, regional, and national trends in haemoglobin concentration and prevalence of total and severe anaemia in children and pregnant and non-pregnant women for 1995–2011: a systematic analysis of population-representative data. Lancet Glob Health. 2013;1(1):e16–25.

34. Widness JA. Pathophysiology of anemia during the neonatal period, including anemia of prematurity. NeoReviews. 2008;9(11):e520.

35. Lacroix J, Hebert PC, Hutchison JS, Hume HA, Tucci M, Ducruet T, et al. Transfusion strategies for patients in pediatric intensive care units. N Engl J Med. 2007;356(16):1609–19.

36. McEvoy MT, Shander A. Anemia, bleeding, and blood transfusion in the intensive care unit: causes, risks, costs, and new strategies. Am J Crit Care Off Publ Am Assoc Crit Care Nurses. 2013;22(6 Suppl):eS1–13.

37. Algarin C, Nelson CA, Peirano P, Westerlund A, Reyes S, Lozoff B. Iron-deficiency anemia in infancy and poorer cognitive inhibitory control at age 10 years. Dev Med Child Neurol. 2013;55(5):453–8.

38. Dlugaj M, Winkler A, Weimar C, Durig J, Broecker-Preuss M, Dragano N, et al. Anemia and mild cognitive impairment in the german general population. J Alzheimer's Dis JAD. 2015;49(4):1031–42.

39. Milman N. Postpartum anemia I: definition, prevalence, causes, and consequences. Ann Hematol. 2011;90(11):1247–53.

40. Farag YM, Keithi-Reddy SR, Mittal BV, Surana SP, Addabbo F, Goligorsky MS, et al. Anemia, inflammation and health-related quality of life in chronic kidney disease patients. Clin Nephrol. 2011;75(6):524–33.

41. Adams KF Jr, Pina IL, Ghali JK, Wagoner LE, Dunlap SH, Schwartz TA, et al. Prospective evaluation of the association between hemoglobin concentration and quality of life in patients with heart failure. Am Heart J. 2009;158(6):965–71.

Removal of totally implanted venous access ports for suspected infection in the intensive care unit: a multicenter observational study

Marie Lecronier[1]* [iD], Sandrine Valade[2], Naike Bigé[3], Nicolas de Prost[4], Damien Roux[5], David Lebeaux[6,7], Eric Maury[3], Elie Azoulay[2], Alexandre Demoule[1,8], Martin Dres[1,8] and on behalf of the GrrrOH (Group for Research in Respiratory Intensive Care Onco-Hematology)

Abstract

Background: While no data support this practice, international guidelines recommend the removal of totally implanted venous access ports (TIVAPs) in patients with suspicion of TIVAP-related bloodstream infection admitted in the intensive care unit (ICU) for a life-threatening sepsis.

Methods: During this multicenter, retrospective and observational study, we included all patients admitted in five ICU for a life-threatening sepsis in whom a TIVAP was removed between January 2012 and December 2014. We aimed (1) at determining the proportion of confirmed TIVAP-related infections and (2) at assessing short- and long-term survival of patients with and without TIVAP-related infections.

Results: One hundred and fifty-one patients (58 ± 14 years, 62% males) were included between 2012 and 2014. TIVAP-related infections were confirmed in 68 patients (45%). Demographic characteristics were similar between patients with and without TIVAP-related infections. SOFA score on admission per point increase [odd ratio (OR), 0.86 interval confidence (IC) 95% (0.8–0.9), $p < 0.01$] and local signs of infection [OR 4.0, IC 95% (1.1–15.6), $p = 0.04$] were significantly associated with TIVAP-related infection. Patients with TIVAP-related infection had lower ICU and 6-month mortality as compared to their counterparts (9 vs. 40%, respectively, $p < 0.01$; and 50 vs. 66%, respectively, $p = 0.04$). TIVAP-related infection was significantly associated with ICU survival [OR 0.2, IC 95% (0.05–0.5), $p < 0.01$].

Conclusions: TIVAP-related infection was confirmed in nearly one out of two cases of life-threatening sepsis in patients in whom it has been removed. TIVAP-related infection was associated with a good prognosis, as compared to patients with other causes of infection.

Keywords: Sepsis, Intensive care unit, Totally implantable venous access ports

Background

Totally implanted venous access ports (TIVAPs) are commonly used for patients requiring long-term or iterative treatments such as antineoplastic chemotherapy, parenteral nutrition and transfusion [1–3]. Even if TIVAPs are associated with a low risk of infection, they still remain a source of infections potentially leading to life-threatening sepsis and subsequent admission in the intensive care unit (ICU) [4, 5].

In case of tunnel or port-pocket infection, TIVAP-related bloodstream infection is obviously strongly suspected and the device should be promptly removed [6]. However, local signs of infection are frequently lacking [7–10]. International guidelines support the removal

*Correspondence: marie.lecronier@aphp.fr
[1] Service de Pneumologie et Réanimation Médicale (Département "R3S"), Groupe Hospitalier Pitié-Salpêtrière Charles Foix, Assistance Publique-Hôpitaux de Paris, 75013 Paris, France
Full list of author information is available at the end of the article

of TIVAP in case of TIVAP-related bloodstream infection, with complication like severe sepsis or/and septic shock (use of vasopressors) [6, 11], although no data support this practice. Removal of TIVAP may have deleterious consequences in critically ill patients. First, patients with TIVAP are frequently frail and exposed to uncontrolled bleeding (low platelets and coagulation disorders). Second, removal of TIVAP is a surgical procedure that may interfere with the management of the ongoing sepsis [12–15]. Eventually, removing TIVAP may defer administration of chemotherapy or specific treatments once patients are discharged from the ICU. Therefore, removal of TIVAP is an important decision that should be supported by clinical evidences, but predictive factors of TIVAP-related infections are lacking in ICU patients. Likewise, no study regarding the prognosis of TIVAP-related infections has been conducted outside the ICU [16–20]. In light with this, the present study was designed to address three main objectives: (1) to determine the proportion of confirmed TIVAP-related infections in a population of patients admitted in the ICU in whom a TIVAP was removed for life-threatening sepsis, (2) to identify predictive factors of confirmed TIVAP infection in patients admitted to the ICU and (3) to assess short- and long-term outcome of patients with TIVAP-related infection and compare them with their counterparts in whom TIVAP was removed without confirmation of infection.

Patients and methods

This retrospective, multicenter, observational study was conducted in five ICU located in academic hospitals. The study period extended from January 2012 through December 2014. The Institutional Review Board of the French Intensive Care Society approved the study (CE SRLF15-52).

Selection of patients

Using clinical microbiology laboratory databases, we identified retrospectively all the patients admitted in participating ICU in whom a TIVAP was removed during the ICU stay and sent to the microbiology laboratory. Each patient's record was analyzed by two investigators (ML and MD) and those patients who fulfilled the following criteria were entered into the study: (1) age > 18 years, (2) sepsis, severe sepsis or septic shock, defined according to criteria of the Surviving Sepsis Campaign's definition [21], as the main reason for TIVAP removal. Of notice, peripherally inserted central catheters and surgically inserted long-term central venous catheters others than TIVAP were not considered for the study. In addition, patients with TIVAP removed before ICU admission or

for another reason than sepsis (thrombosis, uselessness) were also not included in the study.

Data collection

The following data were extracted from each patient's medical record: age, gender, clinical and biological variables on admission. Simplified Acute Physiology Score (SAPS) 2 [22] and Sequential Organ Failure Assessment (SOFA) [23] were calculated upon ICU admission. Predisposing risk factors for TIVAP-related infections were also collected: immunosuppression status (i.e., hematological malignancies, solid organ transplant, recent antineoplastic chemotherapy for cancer or HIV infection), time since TIVAP insertion, main indication of the TIVAP (antineoplastic chemotherapy, parenteral nutrition), date of last antineoplastic chemotherapy and delay between ICU admission and removal of the device. We also looked through each patient's record for local signs of infection (induration or erythema, warmth and pain or tenderness along the tract of a catheterized vein) whenever it was described and general sign of infection (fever defined as temperature $\geq 38°3$, hypothermia defined as temperature $< 36°$, hypotension defined as systolic blood pressure < 90 mmHg or mean blood pressure < 65 mmHg). Advanced life support measures taken during the ICU stay (mechanical ventilation and vasopressors) and antibiotics regimens were recorded for each patient. Microbiological data were collected as follows: positive culture of TIVAP catheter tip or port reservoir, positive blood culture from the TIVAP and from a peripheral vein with the differential time to positivity. We also collected information regarding use of appropriate antibiotic in initial regimen (antibiotics with in vitro activity against the infecting agent). Finally, we recorded length of ICU stay, time spent under invasive mechanical ventilation and vasopressors. Mortality was determined in the ICU, at 28 days and 6 months after ICU admission.

Definitions

Culture of TIVAP was considered as positive if the tip or port reservoir (indoor or outdoor) was positive. Positivity of TIVAP tip culture was defined according to the same modality across all the microbiological laboratories of participating centers. It was defined on blood agar plate by quantitative method after vortexing or sonication (taking into account pathogens present in their inner or outer surfaces) with a cutoff of ≥ 1000 colony-forming units (CFU)/mL [24–26]. Growth of < 1000 CFU/mL from a catheter by quantitative method was considered as catheter contamination. TIVAP box culture was performed according to each clinical microbiology laboratory-own protocol, such as immersion of the case in broth and then sowing on blood agar plate or chocolate plate, needle puncture and aspiration of the case contents then sowing, or swab from outside the case then sowing. In all these techniques, a qualitative culture was performed.

Definition of TIVAP-related infection was adapted from the Infectious Diseases Society of America (IDSA) guidelines [6] as one of the following conditions:

1. TIVAP-related bloodstream infection, defined as (1) a positive culture of the TIVAP (catheter tip or reservoir's port) associated with a positive peripheral blood culture with the same microorganism (same species and same antibiotic susceptibility testing) or (2) a differential time to positivity of a blood culture drawn from the catheter versus from a peripheral vein (positivity of the catheter blood sample at least 2 h before the peripheral blood sample) [27, 28];
2. Local or general (fever $\geq 38°3$ or $< 36°$ and chills) signs of infection, positive culture of TIVAP (catheter tip or the reservoir's port) and regression of clinical signs of infection after TIVAP removal despite a negative peripheral blood culture.

We also included patients who did not meet the two above conditions but who had positive blood culture without other suspected infection and regression of clinical signs of infection after TIVAP removal despite negative culture of TIVAP (catheter tip or the reservoir's port).

Exclusive TIVAP-related infection was defined by TIVAP-related infection that was not associated with any other documented source of infection among lower respiratory, digestive or urinary tract infection.

Statistical analysis

Continuous variables are expressed as mean ± standard deviation or median (interquartile range). Categorical variables are expressed as number and relative frequencies. Patients were categorized a posteriori into two groups according to microbiologic findings: patients with or without TIVAP-related infection. Continuous variables were tested for normality using the Shapiro–Wilk test. Gaussian variables were compared using a t test and non-normally distributed variables using a Mann–Whitney test. Categorical variables were compared with Chi-square test. The primary endpoint was the prevalence of TIVAP-related infection. A stepwise logistic regression analysis was performed to identify variables associated with TIVAP-related infection and with ICU and 28-day mortality. Variables found to have univariate association ($p < 0.05$) with the outcome of interest were considered in the final model. Kaplan–Meier survival curves for patients with and without TIVAP-related infections were computed for 6-month mortality. For all final

comparisons, a two-tailed p value less than or equal to 0.05 was considered statistically significant. The statistical analysis was performed with SAS statistical V9.3 software (SAS Institute Inc., Cary, NC, USA).

Results
Characteristics upon ICU admission

Over the study period, 151 patients met the inclusion criteria and were retained in the analysis (see flowchart, Additional file 1: Figure S1). Main characteristics of the patients are presented in Table 1. One hundred and forty-eight (98%) patients were immunosuppressed, and 50 patients (33%) had neutropenia. Antineoplastic chemotherapy was administrated in 131 patients (87%) in the last 6 months, and 18 (12%) of the patients were receiving parenteral nutrition. Severe sepsis was present in 48 patients (32%) and septic shock in 93 (62%).

Proportion and features of TIVAP-related infection

TIVAP-related infection was found in 68 patients (45%). Among these 68 patients, the diagnosis of TIVAP-related infection was retained because of (1) TIVAP-related bloodstream infection with the association of a positive peripheral blood culture with a positive culture of the TIVAP (tip or reservoir) in 33 patients (48%) or a differential time to positivity of a blood culture drawn from the catheter versus from a peripheral vein in 11 patients (16%); (2) a positive culture of the TIVAP and the regression of clinical signs of infection after TIVAP removal in 12 (18%) patients (negative peripheral blood culture) or (3) a positive blood culture associated with favorable outcome after TIVAP removal in 12 (18%) patients (negative tip or reservoir culture of the TIVAP). A growth of 100 CFU/mL of *Staphylococcus epidermidis* was found in two patients who were classified as catheter contamination (without TIVAP-related infection).

Regarding microbiological findings, TIVAP-related infections were associated with 53% (36/68) of Gram-negative rods, 44% (30/68) of Gram-positive cocci and 7% (5/68) of *Candida* sp. (see Table 2). Sixty-nine percent of patients with TIVAP-related infection had no other focus of infection and were subsequently classified as exclusive TIVAP-related infection (see Additional file 1: Table S1). Among patients with infectious other than TIVAP-related infections, 65% had positive microbiological samples (see Table 3; Additional file 1: Table S2).

Characteristics of the patients according to the presence or absence of TIVAP-related infections

Demographic characteristics of patients with and without TIVAP-related infections were not different (Table 1). Parenteral nutrition was more frequent in patients with TIVAP-related infections. In addition, SAPS2 and SOFA

Table 1 Clinical characteristics and laboratory features upon intensive care unit admission

Characteristic	All $n = 151$	TIVAP-related infection $n = 68$	No TIVAP-related infection $n = 83$	p value
Age, year	58 ± 14	57 ± 14	58 ± 14	0.58
Female gender, n (%)	58 (38)	30 (44)	28 (34)	0.19
Transfer from the emergency room, n (%)	47 (31)	21 (31)	26 (31)	1.00
Transfer from the ward, n (%)	104 (69)	47 (69)	57 (69)	1.00
SAPS2	52 ± 17	47 ± 15	56 ± 17	<0.01
SOFA	9 ± 4	7 ± 4	10 ± 4	<0.01
TIVAP-related infection risk factors, n (%)				
Immunosuppression	148 (98)	66 (97)	82 (99)	0.44
Hematological malignancies	72 (48)	28 (41)	44 (53)	0.14
Solid organ cancer	71 (47)	35 (51)	36 (43)	0.32
Metastatic cancer	44 (29)	24 (35)	20 (24)	0.13
Recent chemotherapy (< 6 months)	131 (87)	58 (85)	73 (88)	0.63
Parenteral nutrition	18 (12)	14 (21)	4 (5)	<0.01
Clinical signs				
Temperature < 36 or ≥ 38.3 °C, n (%)	111 (74)	55 (81)	56 (67)	0.08
Systolic blood pressure, mmHg	98 ± 27	97 ± 29	99 ± 25	0.54
Mean blood pressure, mmHg	69 ± 20	69 ± 23	70 ± 18	0.77
Glasgow Score Scale	13 ± 3	14 ± 3	13 ± 4	0.04
Local sign of infection, n (%)	15 (10)	12 (18)	3 (4)	<0.01
Biological signs				
White blood cells < 1 Giga/l, n (%)	50 (33)	19 (28)	31 (37)	0.22
Platelet counts, Giga/l	116 ± 113	124 ± 99	110 ± 123	0.45
Prothrombin time, %	64 ± 17	69 ± 17	60 ± 17	<0.01
Serum creatinine, µmol/l	142 ± 119	126 ± 113	155 ± 123	0.13
Bicarbonate, mmol/l	20 ± 5	21 ± 5	20 ± 6	0.05
Arterial lactate, mmol/l	3.4 ± 3.2	3.3 ± 3.0	3.6 ± 3.3	0.61

Categorical variables are expressed as no. (%) and continuous variables as mean ± SD

SAPS2 Simplified Acute Physiology Score, *SOFA* Sepsis-Related Organ Failure Assessment, *TIVAP* totally implanted venous access port

score were higher in patients with infectious other than TIVAP-related infections as compared to their counterparts. Local signs of infection were present in 18% of the patients with a TIVAP-related infection versus 4% for their counterparts ($p < 0.01$). There was no difference regarding the presence of neutropenia upon admission between patients with TIVAP-related infection and patients without.

By multivariate logistic regression analysis, two factors were independently associated with TIVAP-related infection: SOFA score upon admission per point increase [odd ratio (OR) 0.86 interval confidence (IC) 95% (0.80–0.90), $p < 0.01$] and local signs of infection [OR 4.0 IC 95% (1.1–15.6), $p = 0.04$].

Therapeutic management and outcome

Patients with infections other than TIVAP-related infections received more vasopressors and were more likely to require mechanical ventilation than their counterparts (Table 4). There was no significant difference in

terms of antibiotics management between both groups. The duration of ICU stay was similar between patients with and without TIVAP-related infections. Overall ICU mortality was 26%. Patients with TIVAP-related infection had lower ICU, 28-day and 6-month mortality as compared to their counterparts (Table 4; Fig. 1). In addition, patients with exclusive TIVAP-related infection had a lower ICU mortality as compared to patients who had TIVAP-related infection and another focus of infection: 2% (1/47) versus 24% (5/21), respectively ($p < 0.01$).

Table 5 displays the variables associated with 28-day mortality, and Tables 2 and 3 show microbiological findings associated with 28-day mortality among patients with and without TIVAP-related infections, respectively. By multivariate logistic regression analysis, three factors were independently associated with higher 28-day mortality: SOFA at admission per point increase [OR 1.3 IC 95% (1.1–1.6), $p < 0.01$], the use of mechanical ventilation [OR 11 IC 95% (2.8–41.2), $p < 0.01$] and hematological malignancies [OR 3.2 IC 95% (1.1–9.1), $p = 0.03$].

Table 2 Microbiological findings in patients with totally implanted venous access ports-related infections and association with 28-day mortality (univariate analysis)

	All n = 68	Alive n = 54	Dead n = 14	p value
Gram-negative bacilli, n (%)	36 (53)	32 (59)	4 (29)	0.07
Enterobacteriaceae	27 (40)	25 (46)	2 (14)	0.03
Escherichia coli	8 (12)	8 (15)	0 (0)	0.19
Klebsiella pneumoniae	7 (10)	6 (11)	1 (7)	0.99
Enterobacter cloacae	7 (10)	7 (13)	0 (0)	0.33
Other Enterobacteriaceae	6 (9)	5 (9)	1 (7)	0.99
Pseudomonas aeruginosa	8 (12)	6 (11)	2 (14)	0.99
Stenotrophomonas maltophilia	1 (2)	1 (2)	0 (0)	0.99
Acinetobacter sp.	1 (2)	1 (2)	0 (0)	0.99
Gram-positive cocci, n (%)	30 (44)	21 (39)	9 (64)	0.13
Staphylococcus aureus	9 (13)	5 (9)	4 (29)	0.09
Coagulase-negative staphylococci	19 (28)	15 (28)	4 (29)	0.99
Enterococcus sp.	2 (3)	1 (2)	1 (7)	0.37
Other Gram-positive cocci	1 (2)	1 (2)	0 (0)	0.99
Candida sp., n (%)	5 (7)	2 (4)	3 (21)	0.06
Polymicrobial, n (%)	6 (9)	4 (7)	2 (14)	0.59

Data are expressed as n (%)

Table 3 Microbiological findings in patients without TIVAP (totally implanted venous access port)-related infections and association with 28-day mortality (univariate analysis)

	All n = 83	Alive n = 43	Dead n = 40	p value
Gram-negative bacilli, n (%)	34 (41)	17 (40)	17 (43)	0.83
Enterobacteriaceae	26 (31)	15 (35)	11 (28)	0.49
Escherichia coli	14 (17)	7 (16)	7 (18)	0.99
Klebsiella pneumoniae	7 (9)	4 (9)	3 (8)	0.99
Enterobacter cloacae	3 (4)	2 (5)	1 (3)	0.99
Other Enterobacteriaceae	9 (11)	7 (16)	2 (5)	0.16
Pseudomonas aeruginosa	6 (7)	1 (2)	5 (13)	0.10
Acinetobacter sp.	2 (3)	1 (2)	1 (3)	0.99
Gram-positive cocci, n (%)	22 (27)	8 (19)	14 (35)	0.13
Staphylococcus aureus	4 (5)	2 (5)	2 (5)	0.99
Coagulase-negative staphylococci	4 (5)	0 (0)	4 (10)	0.05
Enterococcus sp.	10 (12)	3 (7)	7 (18)	0.18
Other Gram-positive cocci	5 (6)	3 (7)	2 (5)	0.99
Other bacteria, n (%)	4 (5)	4 (9)	0 (0)	0.12
Candida sp., n (%)	8 (10)	4 (9)	4 (10)	0.99
Polymicrobial, n (%)	16 (19)	7 (16)	9 (23)	0.58

Data are expressed as n (%)

One factor, TIVAP-related infection, was independently associated with lower 28-day mortality [OR 0.2 IC 95% (0.1–0.7), $p = 0.02$].

Additional file 1: Table S3 displays the variables associated with ICU mortality. By multivariate logistic regression analysis, two factors were independently associated with higher ICU mortality: SOFA at admission per point increase [OR 1.4 IC 95% (1.2–1.7), $p < 0.01$] and the use of mechanical ventilation [OR 14.0 IC 95% (3.6–56.0), $p < 0.01$]. One factor, TIVAP-related infection, was independently associated with lower ICU mortality [OR 0.16 IC 95% (0.05–0.5), $p < 0.01$].

Discussion

This study is seemingly the first reporting characteristics and outcome of patients admitted for a life-threatening sepsis in the ICU whose TIVAP has been removed. Our findings can be summarized as follows: (1) TIVAP-related infection was confirmed in almost half of the patients; (2) except for a low value of SOFA score and local signs of infection, no other variable was found to be independently associated with TIVAP-related infection upon admission; and (3) patients with TIVAP-related infection had a better prognosis than patients with other source of infection.

Proportion of TIVAP-related infection

The proportion of patients in whom a TIVAP-related infection was confirmed was 45%. Being the first study addressing this issue in the ICU, our results are hardly comparable. Indeed, most of previous studies were conducted outside the ICU [4, 5, 10, 17, 19, 20, 29]. For instance, in two studies [8, 9], among patient whose TIVAP was removed because of a suspected infection, TIVAP-related infection was confirmed in two thirds of the patients (19/29 and 15/23, respectively). Based on our findings, the remaining key question is whether this 45% rate is high enough to justify TIVAP removal as supported by international guidelines [6] or whether these recommendations should be questioned. A higher rate (> 80%) would have made clearly acceptable the TIVAP removal (and all its consequences), whereas a lower rate (< 20%) would have discouraged current practices in term of potential harmful effects. While this 45% rate of TIVAP-related infection could be considered disappointing, it might represent the lower bounder of the proportion of patients with TIVAP-related infection. Indeed, all our patients received antibiotics prior ICU admission, a condition that could easily lead to false-negative microbiological findings [30]. As a matter of fact, this could have artificially underestimated the rate of patients with confirmed TIVAP-related infections. A randomized controlled trial might be necessary to definitively support the removal of TIVAP in case of severe sepsis or septic shock.

Another important finding is that a concomitant infection focus was evidenced in approximately one-third of

Table 4 Therapeutic management and outcome of patients with and without TIVAP (totally implanted venous access port)-related infection

Characteristic	All patients $n = 151$	TIVAP-related infections $n = 68$	No TIVAP-related infections $n = 83$	p value
Time between ICU admission and TIVAP withdrawal, days	1 (0–2)	1 (0–1)	1 (0–2)	0.09
Antibiotics				
Beta lactam antibiotic, n (%)	143 (95)	63 (93)	80 (96)	0.49
Glycopeptide/linezolid, n (%)	78 (52)	38 (57)	40 (48)	0.29
Use of MV, n (%)	74 (49)	24 (35)	50 (60)	< 0.01
MV duration, days	0 (0–5)	0 (0–3)	2 (0–7)	0.26
Vasopressors, n (%)	103 (68)	37 (55)	66 (80)	< 0.01
Vasopressors, days	2 (0–3)	1 (0–2)	2 (1–4)	0.04
ICU length of stay, days	5 (3–10)	4 (3–6)	6 (3–12)	0.40
ICU mortality, n (%)	39 (26)	6 (9)	33 (40)	< 0.01
28-day mortality, n (%)	54 (36)	14 (20.5)	40 (48)	< 0.01
6-Month mortality, n (%)	89 (59)	34 (50)	55 (66)	0.04

Categorical variables are expressed as no. (%) and continuous variables as median (interquartile range)

TIVAP totally implanted venous access port, *ICU* intensive care unit, *MV* mechanical ventilation

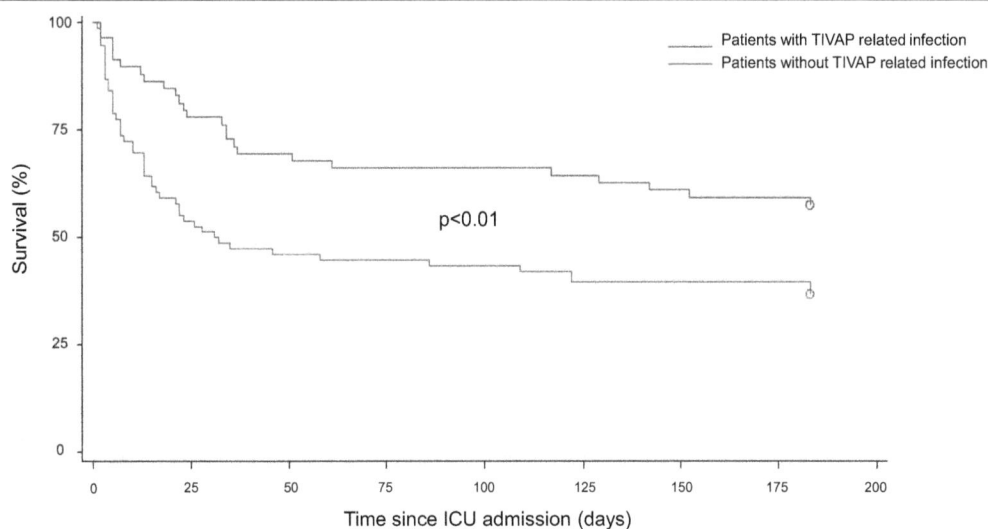

Fig. 1 Kaplan–Meier survival curve with 6-month mortality in patients with and without totally implanted venous access port (TIVAP)-related infections

patients with TIVAP-related infection. In half of these cases, the same pathogen was responsible (Additional file 1: Table S1). Whether this focus was the primary source or an hematogenous seeding from the TIVAP-related infection is unknown. This finding points out the importance of an extensive investigation even though a TIVAP infection is identified.

Factors associated with TIVAP-related infection
While a 45% rate of confirmed TIVAP-related infection may be acceptable, identifying associated factors of

TIVAP-related infection upon admission would be helpful to prevent patients from undue procedures. Unfortunately, our study failed at providing new insightful clues in this purpose. Immunosuppression, a known risk factor for infection [4, 31–33], was equally present in both groups. By contrast, the use of parenteral nutrition, another recognized risk factor for TIVAP-related infection [34–36], was used more frequently in patients with TIVAP-related infection, but this finding remained infrequent and was not confirmed in multivariate analysis. While local signs of infection have been reported to be

Table 5 Variables associated with 28-day mortality

	All $n = 151$	Alive $n = 97$	Dead $n = 54$	p value
Age, year	58 ± 14	57 ± 15	59 ± 13	0.40
Female gender, n (%)	58 (38)	41 (43)	17 (32)	0.71
SAPS2	52 ± 17	47 ± 13	62 ± 19	<0.01
SOFA	9 ± 4	7 ± 3.5	11 ± 4.5	<0.01
TIVAP-related infection	68 (45)	55 (57)	13 (24)	<0.05
TIVAP-related infection risk factors, n (%)				
Immunosuppression	148 (98)	97 (100)	51 (95)	0.99
Hematological malignancies	72 (48)	43 (44)	29 (54)	<0.05
Solid organ cancer	71 (47)	52 (54)	19 (35)	0.12
Metastatic cancer	44 (29)	31 (32)	13 (24)	0.55
Recent chemotherapy (<6 months)	131 (87)	88 (91)	43 (80)	0.85
Parenteral nutrition	18 (12)	13 (14)	5 (9)	0.34
Initial presentation				
Systolic blood pressure, mmHg	98 ± 27	98 ± 27	101 ± 28	0.55
Mean blood pressure, mmHg	69 ± 20	69 ± 19	72 ± 24	0.44
Glasgow Score Scale	13 ± 3	14 ± 3	13 ± 3	0.20
White blood cells, Giga/l	7.6 ± 13.2	7.6 ± 15.6	7.6 ± 10.2	0.98
Platelet counts, Giga/l	116 ± 113	128 ± 110	91 ± 114	<0.05
Prothrombin time, %	64 ± 17	68 ± 15	55 ± 19	<0.01
Serum creatinine, μmol/l	142 ± 119	125 ± 106	176 ± 137	0.01
Bicarbonate, mmol/l	20 ± 5	21 ± 6	19 ± 5	<0.01
Arterial blood lactate, mmol/l	3.4 ± 3.2	2.7 ± 2.2	5 ± 4	<0.01
Treatments				
Time between ICU admission and device withdrawal, days	1.8 ± 3.5	1.6 ± 2.8	2.2 ± 4.5	0.35
Use of MV, n (%)	74 (49)	37 (38)	37 (69)	<0.01
MV duration, days	4 ± 7	4 ± 7	5 ± 5	0.32
Use of vasopressors, n (%)	103 (68)	62 (64)	41 (76)	<0.01
Vasopressors duration, days	3 ± 4	2 ± 3	4 ± 5	<0.01
ICU stay, days	8 ± 9	9 ± 10	8 ± 7	0.53

Categorical variables are expressed as no. (%) and continuous variables as mean $\pm$ SD

ICU intensive care unit, *SOFA* Sepsis-Related Organ Failure Assessment, *SAPS2* Simplified Acute Physiology Score, *TIVAP* totally implanted venous access port, *MV* mechanical ventilation

present from 7 to 33% of the cases [8–10, 17, 20], in our patient series, only few had local sign of infection (18%). But it's important to specify that information about local signs of infection is difficult to collect in a retrospective study. They are not systematically looked for and their identification may vary between healthcare providers when clear definitions are not used. Interestingly, it was independently associated with TIVAP-related infection in our study.

TIVAP-related infections: impact on prognosis

While ICU mortality of sepsis is still high, up to 20% in latest publications [37–39], it reaches even higher rates in immunocompromised patients, between 40 and 60% [40]. In the present study, we report a lower mortality: 26%

for ICU mortality and 36% at 28 days. While expected mortality (predicted by SAPS2 score) was around 40%, patients with TIVAP-related infections had a much lower mortality (9%). Moreover, ICU mortality was 2% in patients with exclusive TIVAP-related infection (no other infection focus). TIVAP-related infection was significantly associated with highest ICU and 28-day survival, whereas high SOFA score upon admission and the need for mechanical ventilation were significantly associated with ICU mortality and at 28 days. The low mortality observed in patients with exclusive TIVAP-related infections may be explained by the strong experience in the management of immunocompromised patients of participating ICUs. As a matter of fact, the precociousness of source control was probably a major driver of such a favorable outcome. In agreement with other studies, neutropenia was not significantly related to mortality [41–44]. Interestingly, patients who had both TIVAP-related infections and another focus had a worst prognosis than patients who had only TIVAP-related infection. In light with this, our study provides an important message for physicians managing immunosuppressed patients with severe presentation (septic shock, need for mechanical ventilation). While admission in the ICU of such patients is sometimes questioned, our findings suggest that in case of TIVAP-related infection, those patients have a short ICU stay and good prognosis. Likewise, our findings suggest that in patients admitted for a suspected TIVAP-related infection who do not recover shortly, this diagnosis should be questioned.

Limits

While reporting the first cohort of TIVAP-related infections in the ICU, this retrospective study has some limitations. As we obtained data from patient's medical charts, we cannot pretend to be exhaustive in data collection. Important information such as presence of thrombosis or endocarditis associated with TIVAP-related infection would have been interesting, but not all patients had a Doppler ultrasonography at time of admission. Then, it is likely that all patients with TIVAP admitted in participating ICU were not enrolled in the study since the main inclusion criteria was TIVAP removal. As a matter of fact, our inclusion criteria could have biased the true incidence of TIVAP-related infection toward overestimation. Due to the retrospective nature of the study, it was not possible to systematically identify patients who may have been admitted in our ICUs with a TIVAP in place that was not removed. The fact that positive blood cultures were available prior TIVAP removal may have also influenced clinicians' decision. However, ICUs participating in the study had homogeneous practices regarding admission policy of immunocompromised patients and the decision to remove TIVAP in case of life-threatening sepsis. Last, the definition of TIVAP-related infection was extended to patients with positive blood culture without other suspected infection ($n = 12$) and regression of clinical signs of infection after TIVAP removal despite negative culture of TIVAP (catheter tip or the reservoir's port). Since all our patients received antibiotics prior TIVAP removal, a condition that could fairly lead to misclassification, we estimated legitimate to consider these twelve patients as having TIVAP-related infection.

Conclusion

In almost one out of two cases, TIVAP-related infection was evidenced in immunosuppressed patients admitted in the ICU for sepsis and in whom the device has been removed. With the exception of local signs of infection, no other associated factor could have been identified. TIVAP-related infection was associated with a good prognosis, as compared to patients with other causes of infection.

Abbreviations

TIVAP: totally implanted venous access port; ICU: intensive care unit; SAPS II: Simplified Acute Physiology Score II; SOFA: Sequential Organ Failure Assessment; HIV: human immunodeficiency virus; IDSA: Infectious Diseases Society of America; CFU: colony-forming unit; OR: odd ratio; CI: confidence interval.

Authors' contributions

ML participated in the conception and design of the study, performed the literature search, performed the data analysis and drafted the manuscript. SV helped to collect data. NB helped to collect data. NdeP helped to collect data and helped to revise the manuscript. DR helped to collect data and helped to revise the manuscript. DL, EM, EA and AD helped to revise the manuscript. MD designed the study, helped to draft the manuscript and helped to revise the manuscript. All authors read and approved the final manuscript.

Author details

[1] Service de Pneumologie et Réanimation Médicale (Département "R3S"), Groupe Hospitalier Pitié-Salpêtrière Charles Foix, Assistance Publique-Hôpitaux de Paris, 75013 Paris, France. [2] Service de Réanimation médicale, Groupe Hospitalier Saint-Louis – Lariboisière – Fernand-Widal, Assistance Publique-Hôpitaux de Paris, Paris, France. [3] Service de Réanimation médicale, Groupe Hospitalier Est Parisien, Hôpital Saint-Antoine Paris, Assistance Publique-Hôpitaux de Paris, Paris, France. [4] Service de Réanimation médicale, Groupe Hospitalier Henri Mondor, Assistance Publique-Hôpitaux de Paris, Créteil, France. [5] Service de Réanimation médico-chirurgicale, Groupe Hospitalier Paris Nord, Hôpital Louis-Mourier, Assistance Publique-Hôpitaux de Paris, Colombes, France. [6] Service de Microbiologie, Unité Mobile de Microbiologie Clinique, Hôpital Européen Georges Pompidou, Assistance Publique-Hôpitaux de Paris, Paris, France. [7] Université Paris Descartes, Sorbonne Paris Cité, Paris, France. [8] INSERM, UMRS1158 Neurophysiologie respiratoire expérimentale et clinique, Sorbonne Universités, UPMC Univ Paris 06, Paris, France.

Acknowledgements

The authors would like to thank all the microbiologist from each center, for providing the clinical microbiology laboratory data to identify and include the patients.

Competing interests

Alexandre Demoule has signed research contracts with Medtronic (Dublin, Ireland), Maquet (Solna, Sweden) and Philips (Carlsbad, CA); he has also received personal fees from Medtronic (Dublin, Ireland), Maquet (Solna, Sweden), Fisher&Paykel (Kingston, Milton Keynes, UK), Resmed, Hamilton and MSD (Courbevoie, France). Martin Dres received personal fees from Pulsion Medical System (Feldkirchen, Germany) and Astra Zeneca (Cambridge, UK). Jean-Damien Ricard received travel expenses from Fisher&Paykel (Kingston, Milton Keynes, UK) to attend scientific meetings. Damien Roux received personal fees from Astellas (Levallois-Perret, France). The other authors declare that they have no competing interests.

Funding

MD was supported by the French Intensive Care Society, Paris, France (bourse de mobilité 2015); The 2015 Short Term Fellowship Program of the European Respiratory Society, Lausanne, Switzerland; The 2015 Bernhard Dräger Award for advanced treatment of acute respiratory failure of the European Society of Intensive Care Medicine, Brussels, Belgium; the Assistance Publique-Hôpitaux de Paris, Paris, France; and the Fondation pour la Recherche Médicale, Paris, France (FDM 20150734498).

References

1. Niederhuber JE, Ensminger W, Gyves JW, Liepman M, Doan K, Cozzi E. Totally implanted venous and arterial access system to replace external catheters in cancer treatment. Surgery. 1982;92:706–12.
2. Biffi R, Toro A, Pozzi S, Di Carlo I. Totally implantable vascular access devices 30 years after the first procedure. What has changed and what is still unsolved? Support Care Cancer. 2014;22:1705–14.
3. Barbetakis N, Asteriou C, Kleontas A, Tsilikas C. Totally implantable central venous access ports. Analysis of 700 cases. J Surg Oncol. 2011;104:654–6.
4. Groeger JS, Lucas AB, Thaler HT, Friedlander-Klar H, Brown AE, Kiehn TE, et al. Infectious morbidity associated with long-term use of venous access devices in patients with cancer. Ann Intern Med. 1993;119:1168–74.
5. Chang L, Tsai J-S, Huang S-J, Shih C-C. Evaluation of infectious complications of the implantable venous access system in a general oncologic population. Am J Infect Control. 2003;31:34–9.
6. Mermel LA, Allon M, Bouza E, Craven DE, Flynn P, O'Grady NP, et al. Clinical practice guidelines for the diagnosis and management of intravascular catheter-related infection: 2009 Update by the Infectious Diseases Society of America. Clin Infect Dis. 2009;49:1–45.
7. Safdar N, Maki DG. Inflammation at the insertion site is not predictive of catheter-related bloodstream infection with short-term, noncuffed central venous catheters. Crit Care Med. 2002;30:2632–5.
8. Whitman ED, Boatman AM. Comparison of diagnostic specimens and methods to evaluate infected venous access ports. Am J Surg. 1995;170:665–9.
9. Douard MC, Arlet G, Longuet P, Troje C, Rouveau M, Ponscarme D, et al. Diagnosis of venous access port-related infections. Clin Infect Dis. 1999;29:1197–202.
10. Hsu J-F, Chang H-L, Tsai M-J, Tsai Y-M, Lee Y-L, Chen P-H, et al. Port type is a possible risk factor for implantable venous access port-related bloodstream infections and no sign of local infection predicts the growth of gram-negative bacilli. World J Surg Oncol. 2015;13:288.
11. Timsit J-F. Updating of the 12th consensus conference of the Société de Réanimation de langue française (SRLF): catheter related infections in the intensive care unit. Ann Fr Anesth Réanim. 2005;24:315–22.
12. Seymour CW, Kahn JM, Martin-Gill C, Callaway CW, Yealy DM, Scales D, et al. Delays from first medical contact to antibiotic administration for sepsis. Crit Care Med. 2017;45:759–65.
13. Bagshaw SM, Lapinsky S, Dial S, Arabi Y, Dodek P, Wood G, et al. Acute kidney injury in septic shock: clinical outcomes and impact of duration of hypotension prior to initiation of antimicrobial therapy. Intensive Care Med. 2009;35:871–81.
14. Kumar A, Roberts D, Wood KE, Light B, Parrillo JE, Sharma S, et al. Duration of hypotension before initiation of effective antimicrobial therapy is the critical determinant of survival in human septic shock. Crit Care Med. 2006;34:1589–96.
15. Lundberg JS, Perl TM, Wiblin T, Costigan MD, Dawson J, Nettleman MD, et al. Septic shock: an analysis of outcomes for patients with onset on hospital wards versus intensive care units. Crit Care Med. 1998;26:1020–4.
16. Lebeaux D, Fernández-Hidalgo N, Chauhan A, Lee S, Ghigo J-M, Almirante B, et al. Management of infections related to totally implantable venous-access ports: challenges and perspectives. Lancet Infect Dis. 2014;14:146–59.
17. Lebeaux D, Larroque B, Gellen-Dautremer J, Leflon-Guibout V, Dreyer C, Bialek S, et al. Clinical outcome after a totally implantable venous access port-related infection in cancer patients: a prospective study and review of the literature. Medicine (Baltimore). 2012;91:309–18.
18. Raad I, Hanna H, Maki D. Intravascular catheter-related infections: advances in diagnosis, prevention, and management. Lancet Infect Dis. 2007;7:645–57.
19. Sotir MJ, Lewis C, Bisher EW, Ray SM, Soucie JM, Blumberg HM. Epidemiology of device-associated infections related to a long-term implantable vascular access device. Infect Control Hosp Epidemiol. 1999;20:187–91.
20. Vidal M, Genillon JP, Forestier E, Trouiller S, Pereira B, Mrozek N, et al. Outcome of totally implantable venous-access port-related infections. Méd Mal Infect. 2016;46:32–8.
21. Dellinger RP, Levy MM, Rhodes A, Annane D, Gerlach H, Opal SM, et al. Surviving sepsis campaign: international guidelines for management of severe sepsis and septic shock: 2012. Crit Care Med. 2013;41:580–637.
22. Le Gall JR, Lemeshow S, Saulnier F. A new Simplified Acute Physiology Score (SAPS II) based on a European/North American multicenter study. JAMA. 1993;270:2957–63.
23. Vincent JL, Moreno R, Takala J, Willatts S, De Mendonça A, Bruining H, et al. The SOFA (Sepsis-related Organ Failure Assessment) score to describe organ dysfunction/failure. On behalf of the Working Group on Sepsis-Related Problems of the European Society of Intensive Care Medicine. Intensive Care Med. 1996;22:707–10.
24. Brun-Buisson C, Abrouk F, Legrand P, Huet Y, Larabi S, Rapin M. Diagnosis of central venous catheter-related sepsis. Critical level of quantitative tip cultures. Arch Intern Med. 1987;147:873–7.
25. Cleri DJ, Corrado ML, Seligman SJ. Quantitative culture of intravenous catheters and other intravascular inserts. J Infect Dis. 1980;141:781–6.
26. Safdar N, Fine JP, Maki DG. Meta-analysis: methods for diagnosing intravascular device-related bloodstream infection. Ann Intern Med. 2005;142:451–66.
27. Blot F, Nitenberg G, Chachaty E, Raynard B, Germann N, Antoun S, et al. Diagnosis of catheter-related bacteraemia: a prospective comparison of the time to positivity of hub-blood versus peripheral-blood cultures. Lancet. 1999;354:1071–7.
28. Blot F, Schmidt E, Nitenberg G, Tancrède C, Leclercq B, Laplanche A, et al. Earlier positivity of central-venous-versus peripheral-blood cultures is highly predictive of catheter-related sepsis. J Clin Microbiol. 1998;36:105–9.
29. Pegues D, Axelrod P, McClarren C, Eisenberg BL, Hoffman JP, Ottery FD, et al. Comparison of infections in Hickman and implanted port catheters in adult solid tumor patients. J Surg Oncol. 1992;49:156–62.
30. Rijnders BJ, Van Wijngaerden E, Vandecasteele SJ, Stas M, Peetermans WE. Treatment of long-term intravascular catheter-related bacteraemia with antibiotic lock: randomized, placebo-controlled trial. J Antimicrob Chemother. 2005;55:90–4.
31. Howell PB, Walters PE, Donowitz GR, Farr BM. Risk factors for infection of adult patients with cancer who have tunnelled central venous catheters. Cancer. 1995;75:1367–75.
32. Adler A, Yaniv I, Steinberg R, Solter E, Samra Z, Stein J, et al. Infectious complications of implantable ports and Hickman catheters in paediatric haematology-oncology patients. J Hosp Infect. 2006;62:358–65.
33. Lebeaux D, Zarrouk V, Leflon-Guibout V, Lefort A, Fantin B. Totally implanted access port-related infections: features and management. Rev Méd Interne. 2010;31:819–27.
34. Penel N, Neu J-C, Clisant S, Hoppe H, Devos P, Yazdanpanah Y. Risk factors for early catheter-related infections in cancer patients. Cancer. 2007;110:1586–92.
35. Santarpia L, Pasanisi F, Alfonsi L, Violante G, Tiseo D, De Simone G, et al. Prevention and treatment of implanted central venous catheter (CVC)—related sepsis: a report after six years of home parenteral nutrition (HPN). Clin Nutr Edinb Scotl. 2002;21:207–11.
36. Touré A, Chambrier C, Vanhems P, Lombard-Bohas C, Souquet J-C, Ecochard R. Propensity score analysis confirms the independent effect of parenteral nutrition on the risk of central venous catheter-related bloodstream infection in oncological patients. Clin Nutr Edinb Scotl. 2013;32:1050–4.
37. Damiani E, Donati A, Serafini G, Rinaldi L, Adrario E, Pelaia P, et al. Effect of performance improvement programs on compliance with sepsis bundles and mortality: a systematic review and meta-analysis of observational studies. PLoS ONE. 2015;10:e0125827.
38. Kaukonen K-M, Bailey M, Suzuki S, Pilcher D, Bellomo R. Mortality related to severe sepsis and septic shock among critically ill patients in Australia and New Zealand, 2000–2012. JAMA. 2014;311:1308–16.
39. Stevenson EK, Rubenstein AR, Radin GT, Wiener RS, Walkey AJ. Two decades of mortality trends among patients with severe sepsis: a comparative meta-analysis. Crit Care Med. 2014;42:625–31.
40. Pène F, Percheron S, Lemiale V, Viallon V, Claessens Y-E, Marqué S, et al. Temporal changes in management and outcome of septic shock in patients with malignancies in the intensive care unit. Crit Care Med. 2008;36:690–6.

41. Azoulay E, Mokart D, Pène F, Lambert J, Kouatchet A, Mayaux J, et al. Outcomes of critically ill patients with hematologic malignancies: prospective multicenter data from France and Belgium—A Groupe de Recherche Respiratoire en Réanimation Onco-Hématologique Study. J Clin Oncol. 2013;31:2810–8.

42. Darmon M, Azoulay E, Alberti C, Fieux F, Moreau D, Le Gall J-R, et al. Impact of neutropenia duration on short-term mortality in neutropenic critically ill cancer patients. Intensive Care Med. 2002;28:1775–80.

43. Mokart D, Darmon M, Resche-Rigon M, Lemiale V, Pène F, Mayaux J, et al. Prognosis of neutropenic patients admitted to the intensive care unit. Intensive Care Med. 2015;41:296–303.

44. Vandijck DM, Benoit DD, Depuydt PO, Offner FC, Blot SI, Van Tilborgh AK, et al. Impact of recent intravenous chemotherapy on outcome in severe sepsis and septic shock patients with hematological malignancies. Intensive Care Med. 2008;34:847–55.

8

Reliability of respiratory pressure measurements in ventilated and non-ventilated patients in ICU: an observational study

Clément Medrinal[1,2,3*], Guillaume Prieur[4], Yann Combret[5,6], Aurora Robledo Quesada[3], Tristan Bonnevie[1,2,7], Francis Edouard Gravier[7], Eric Frenoy[8], Olivier Contal[9] and Bouchra Lamia[1,2,4,10]

Abstract

Background: Assessment of maximum respiratory pressures is a common practice in intensive care because it can predict the success of weaning from ventilation. However, the reliability of measurements through an intubation catheter has not been compared with standard measurements. The aim of this study was to compare maximum respiratory pressures measured through an intubation catheter with the same measurements using a standard mouthpiece in extubated patients.

Methods: A prospective observational study was carried out in adults who had been under ventilation for at least 24 h and for whom extubation was planned. Maximal respiratory pressure measurements were carried out before and 24 h following extubation.

Results: Ninety patients were included in the analyses (median age: 61.5 years, median SAPS2 score: 42.5 and median duration of ventilation: 7 days). Maximum respiratory pressures measured through the intubation catheter were as reliable as measurements through a standard mouthpiece (difference in maximal inspiratory pressure: mean bias $= -2.43 \pm 14.43$ cmH$_2$O and difference in maximal expiratory pressure: mean bias $= 1.54 \pm 23.2$ cmH$_2$O).

Conclusion: Maximum respiratory pressures measured through an intubation catheter were reliable and similar to standard measures.

Keywords: Intensive care unit, Mechanical ventilation, Respiratory muscles

Background

Mechanical ventilation generally results in a loss of respiratory muscle strength [1, 2]. The prevalence of respiratory muscle weakness is high, and the causes are multifactorial [3–5]. Assessment of respiratory muscle strength is becoming common practice in intensive care. Assessment techniques range from diaphragm ultrasound to measurement of maximum respiratory pressures. Respiratory muscle strength has been established as prognostic of successful weaning and mortality [6–8].

Measurement of maximum respiratory pressures is a simple, non-invasive method to quantify the global strength of the inspiratory and expiratory muscles. Pressures can be measured using a manometer with a unidirectional valve or the "Negative Inspiratory Force" (NIF) function available on most ventilators. However, these methods require full patient cooperation. Several protocols have thus been developed for use in intensive care to ensure accurate measurements with or without cooperation from the patient [9]. Several studies have attempted to determine optimal methods to ensure quality measurements that are reliable [10–12].

Respiratory pressure measurements are commonly carried out, while the patient is intubated as part of the evaluation to determine the likely success of extubation [5,

*Correspondence: medrinal.clement.mk@gmail.com
[3] Intensive Care Unit Department, Groupe Hospitalier du Havre, Avenue Pierre Mendes France, 76290 Montivilliers, France
Full list of author information is available at the end of the article

7]. It is important to carry out longitudinal evaluations of respiratory muscle strength after mechanical ventilation in order to increase understanding of the relationship between strength and long-term rates of mortality [7]. However, the methods used to measure respiratory pressures differ between intubation and extubation and, along with other factors such as lack of patient cooperation and discomfort, this could lead to different values being recorded. To our knowledge, no, or few, studies have evaluated respiratory pressure measurements in non-ventilated patients in ICU, and the reliability of these measurements has not been compared between intubation and extubation.

The aim of this study was to compare maximum respiratory pressures measured through an intubation catheter (intubated patients) with the same measurement using a standard mouthpiece (extubated patients). The secondary aims were to analyse correlations between the two measurements.

Method

Study design and participants

This study was part of a larger, prospective observational cohort study conducted in an 18-bed intensive care unit (ICU) between January 2014 and December 2014 [7]. The study was approved by our Institutional Review Board (Comité de Protection des Personnes Nord-Ouest 3); NCT02363231 www.clinicaltrials.gov. In conformity with the Declaration of Helsinki, all patients participated voluntarily.

Patients were included if they were over 18 years of age and had undergone a minimum of 24 h of MV. They were not included if they had chronic loss of autonomy (a KATZ score below 6/6 [13], a degenerative neurological pathology with disabling muscle weakness, were agitated prior to the evaluation (Ramsay score of 1 or Richmond Agitation-Sedation Scale (RASS) greater than 1) or a decision to withhold life sustaining treatment had been made. Patients who were included but had to be re-intubated during the first 24 h of extubation were excluded from the analysis.

Study protocol

In our ICU, patients are assessed daily (without sedation) to determine whether they are ready to wean from MV. If a patient fulfils extubation criteria and level of cooperation is satisfactory, a weaning trial is carried out under pressure support (inspiratory positive airway pressure of 7 cmH_2O with no expiratory positive airway pressure for 30–120 min) [14]. For the purpose of the study, if the trial was successful and extubation was planned, the patient underwent maximum inspiratory and expiratory pressure

measurements (MIPs and MEPs) (intubation condition). Twenty-four hours following extubation, MIPs and MEPs were re-measured, this time using a mouthpiece (mouthpiece condition).

Demographic data, reasons for admission to ICU and comorbidities were collected at the time of inclusion, prior to carrying out the MIP and MEP measurements under MV.

In both conditions, the MIP and MEP measurements were carried out with the patient lying in bed with the backrest inclined to 45°. Respiratory physiotherapy was carried out first to ensure that secretions were evacuated, and endotracheal aspiration was carried out for intubated patients.

An electronic manometer, micro-RPM® (Eolys, PAYS), with a unidirectional valve was used to measure respiratory pressures. In both conditions, MIP was measured at the residual volume and patients were instructed accordingly.

In the intubation condition, the manometer was connected to the endotracheal tube using a catheter mount. The patient was disconnected from the ventilator for a minimum of 20 s [11].

In the mouthpiece condition, it was not possible to leave the manometer in position for 20 s. MIP was measured after a maximal exhalation (at the residual volume).

MEP was measured after a maximal inspiration in both conditions. Three MIP and three MEP measurements were carried out for each patient, and the best result was used for the analysis.

Statistical analysis

Descriptive statistics are reported as counts and percentages for categorical data, and means and standard deviations or medians and 25th–75th percentiles for continuous variables, depending on the normality of the distribution. Differences between values were evaluated using a Wilcoxon matched-pairs signed rank test. Univariate linear regression analysis was performed using the least squares method. The Bland–Altman limits of agreement method was used to calculate bias and precision.

Statistical analyses were performed using GraphPad Prism 5. A two-tailed p value of 0.05 was considered significant for all analyses.

Results

One hundred and twenty-four patients were included in the larger study. Of these, 101 accepted to carry out additional measurements. Eleven patients required re-intubation within 24 h of extubation and were excluded from the analysis. Ninety patients thus underwent MIP and MEP measurements in both conditions.

Patient characteristics are described in Table 1. Briefly, 43% of the patients were women, median age was 61.5 years, median BMI was 28.6 kg/m^2, median SAPS2 score was 42.5 and median duration of MV was 7 days.

Median MIP value was 28 (21.7–40.2) cmH$_2$O in the intubation condition and 27 (19–38) cmH$_2$O in the mouthpiece condition ($p = 0.02$). Linear regression showed a significant correlation between the values in each condition ($r = 0.64$ 95% CI [0.5–0.75]; $p < 0.0001$).

The Bland–Altman analysis showed that the MIP values between intubation and extubation were clinically comparable (mean bias (ΔMIP) $= -2.43 \pm 14.43$ cmH$_2$O). (See Fig. 1).

There was no statistically significant difference in MEP values between conditions [47 (30–74) vs. 53.5 (34–76.2) cmH$_2$O; $p = 0.2$]. There was a strong significant correlation between the MEP values in each condition ($r = 0.71$ 95% CI [0.6–0.8]; $p < 0.0001$).

There was no clinical difference between the values in the two conditions as shown by the Bland–Altman analysis (mean bias (ΔMEP) $= 1.54 \pm 23.2$ cmH$_2$O) (See Fig. 2).

No patient-related factors were found to be associated with the measurement bias (age, BMI, SAPS2, number of days under mechanical ventilation, extubation failure). However, there was a correlation between the ΔMIP and the ΔMEP ($r = 0.49$ 95% CI [0.31–0.64]; $p < 0.0001$).

There was a significant correlation between MIP and MEP values in each condition (respectively $r = 0.61$ 95% CI [0.45–0.72]; $p < 0.0001$ and $r = 0.66$ 95% CI [0.52–0.77]; $p < 0.0001$).

Discussion

This study found [1] that the methods of measuring respiratory pressures in intubated and extubated patients produced clinically similar results for both MIP and MEP, and [2] there were strong correlations between the MIP and MEP values in both conditions.

Assessment of respiratory pressures is common practice in ICU [4, 5, 7, 9–12]. Although other tools may more accurately assess muscle strength, measures of respiratory pressure are used to determine if a patient is ready to wean from MV, as well as the prognosis [7, 15]. For this reason, we believed it was important to evaluate the validity of measurements in intubated patients compared with post-extubation measurements using a mouthpiece in order to longitudinally evaluate changes in respiratory muscle strength.

Measurement of maximal respiratory pressures requires patient cooperation, which can be difficult when patients are intubated; however, similar pressures were recorded during intubation and extubation, with slightly higher pressures during intubation. This could

Table 1 Cohort characteristics

	N = 90
Female, n (%)	39 (43)
Age, mean (SD)	61.5 (14)
Body mass index (Kg/m^2), median (25th–75th percentile)	28.6 (24.4–32)
SAPS II at ICU admission, median (25th–75th percentile)	42.5 (31–57)
No. of admissions to ICU within the last year, n (%)	4 (4.4)
Main diagnosis	
Pneumonia, n (%)	32 (35)
Sepsis, n (%)	8 (9)
COPD/asthma exacerbation, n (%)	12 (13)
Cardiac failure, n (%)	12 (13)
Drug overdose/acute mental status change, n (%)	11 (12)
Intra-abdominal sepsis with surgery, n (%)	14 (15)
Trauma, n (%)	1 (4)
Co-morbidity	
Chronic pulmonary disease, n (%)	23 (25)
Obesity, n (%)	27 (30)
Chronic cardiac insufficiency, n (%)	13 (14)
Cancer, n (%)	15 (17)
Chronic kidney disease, n (%)	14 (15)
Diabetes mellitus, n (%)	17 (19)
Between admission and awakening	
Septic shock, n (%)	45 (50)
ARDS, n (%)	13 (14)
Renal failure, n (%)	30 (33)
Use of catecholamines, n (%)	58 (64)
Use of neuromuscular blockers, n (%)	58 (64)
No. of days of neuromuscular blockers, median (25–75th percentile)	1 (0–3)
Use of corticosteroids, n (%)	21 (78)
Ventilator use (days), median (25th–75th percentile)	7 (4–9)

SAPS simplified acute physiology score, *ICU* intensive care unit, *No.* number, *COPD* chronic obstructive pulmonary disease, *ARDS* acute respiratory distress syndrome

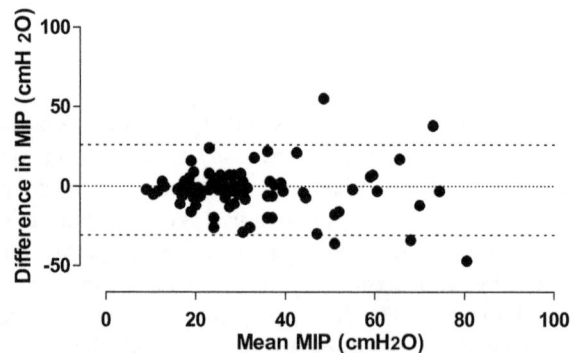

Fig. 1 Bland–Altman analysis of maximal inspiratory pressure correlations: difference versus mean

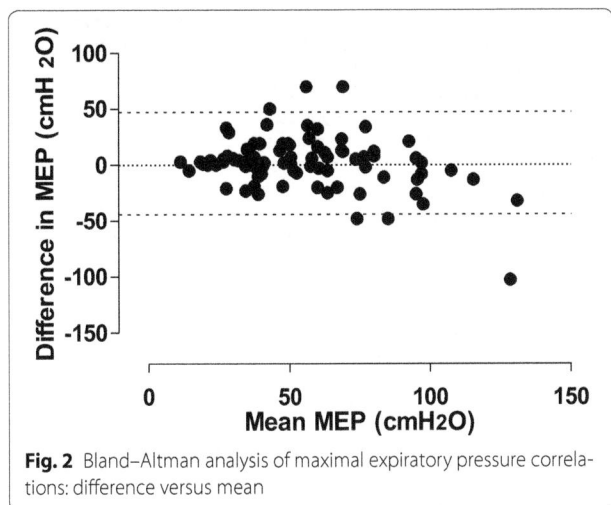

Fig. 2 Bland–Altman analysis of maximal expiratory pressure correlations: difference versus mean

be explained by the fact that mouth leak cannot occur when the patient is intubated with the balloon inflated or because the measurement was carried out over 20 s when the patients were intubated [11]. One study compared the conventional method (values taken at the maximum pressure plateau maintained for at least 1 s) with Marini's method [10] (measurement of inspiratory pressure with a unidirectional valve over 20 s) in 54 patients. MIP was 28% higher using Marini's method with a coefficient of variation of around 10%, indicating good reliability. This procedure can be used for intubated patients but is not reliable in extubated patients. Nevertheless, in the present study, mean MIP variation between the two conditions was $- 2.43$ cmH_2O $(- 8.4\%)$ and for MEP was 1.54 cmH_2O (7%), confirming good reliability across conditions and measurements.

The results of this study showed a relationship between MIP and MEP. MEP reflects the patient's capacity to cough, and a low MEP is associated with delayed weaning [15]; however, studies tend to focus on inspiratory muscle strength, neglecting expiratory muscle strength. MIP is reported to be predictive of successful extubation, and we recently showed that low MIP before extubation (MIP $\leq$ 30 cmH_2O) was an independent predictor of an increase in mortality risk 1 year following extubation [7]. However, several authors have stated that values obtained in intubated patients may be underestimated [9, 12, 15]. In the current study, we found that Marini's method (occlusion for 20 s) produced clinically similar values to measurements carried out with a mouthpiece following recommendations [16]. This indicates that if the patient is sufficiently alert, the values are not underestimated and are therefore reliable across different conditions, allowing accurate follow-up of respiratory capacity.

This study has several limitations. Firstly, the observational design comprises several types of inherent bias and we did not perform a sample size calculation. Secondly, it was not possible to evaluate patients who were re-intubated within 24 h. Thirdly, the pressure measurements were not taken in exactly the same conditions. The second measurement 24 h following extubation may have been affected by respiratory muscle fatigue. Finally, we evaluated peak pressure, not pressure maintained over 1 s as recommended [16]. However, the recommendations are more relevant out of ICU where measurements of respiratory pressure differ considerably from the bedside measurements used in ICU [11].

This study has several strengths. The sample size was large and representative of the population of patients in ICU. The test evaluated is simple and easy to carry out at the patient's bedside. Moreover, we showed that the measurements were reliable across two common conditions in ICU (intubated and extubated patients).

Conclusion

Respiratory pressure measurements are reliable in both intubated and non-intubated patients. These results corroborate those of previous studies. Measurements of respiratory pressure can thus be carried out reliably when the patient is intubated and repeated following weaning from MV to carry out longitudinal evaluations of respiratory muscle recovery.

Abbreviations
BMI: body mass index; CI: confidence intervals; ICU: intensive care unit; MIP: maximal inspiratory pressure; MEP: maximal expiratory pressure; MV: mechanical ventilation; NIF: negative inspiratory force; RASS: Richmond Agitation-Sedation Scale; SAPS: simplified acute physiology score.

Author's contributions
C.M., G.P., Y.C., O.C and B.L. designed the study. C.M., B.L. and O.C. coordinated the study. C.M., G.P., E.F., A.R.Q., T.B and F.G. were responsible for patient screening, enrolment, diaphragm assessment, and follow-up. C.M., E.F. O.C. and B.L. analysed the data and wrote the manuscript. All authors contributed to the interpretation of the data and provided comments on the report at various stages of development. All authors approved this manuscript in its final form.

Author details
[1] Normandie Univ, UNIROUEN, EA3830 - GRHV, 76000 Rouen, France. [2] Institute for Research and Innovation in Biomedicine (IRIB), 76000 Rouen, France. [3] Intensive Care Unit Department, Groupe Hospitalier du Havre, Avenue Pierre Mendes France, 76290 Montivilliers, France. [4] Pulmonology Department, Groupe Hospitalier du Havre, Avenue Pierre Mendes France, 76290 Montivilliers, France. [5] Institut de Recherche Expérimentale et Clinique (IREC), Pôle de Pneumologie, ORL and Dermatologie, Université Catholique de Louvain, Brussels 1200, Belgium. [6] Physiotherapy Department, Groupe Hospitalier du Havre, Avenue Pierre Mendes France, 76290 Montivilliers, France. [7] ADIR Association, Bois Guillaume, France. [8] Intensive Care Unit Department, Hôpital Jacques Monod, 76290 Montivilliers, France. [9] University of Applied Sciences and Arts Western Switzerland (HES-SO), Avenue de Beaumont, 1011 Lausanne, Switzerland. [10] Intensive Care Unit, Respiratory Department, Rouen University Hospital, Rouen, France.

Competing interests
The authors declare that they have no competing interests.

Funding
This study was supported by grants from ADIR Association. The funder had no direct influence on the design of the study, the analysis of the data, the data collection, drafting of the manuscript or the decision to publish.

References
1. Levine S, Nguyen T, Taylor N, Friscia ME, Budak MT, Rothenberg P, et al. Rapid disuse atrophy of diaphragm fibers in mechanically ventilated humans. N Engl J Med. 2008;358(13):1327–35.
2. Demoule A, Molinari N, Jung B, Prodanovic H, Chanques G, Matecki S, et al. Patterns of diaphragm function in critically ill patients receiving prolonged mechanical ventilation: a prospective longitudinal study. Ann Intensive Care. 2016;6(1):75.
3. Dres M, Dube BP, Mayaux J, Delemazure J, Reuter D, Brochard L, et al. coexistence and impact of limb muscle and diaphragm weakness at time of liberation from mechanical ventilation in medical intensive care unit patients. Am J Respir Crit Care Med. 2017;195(1):57–66.
4. Medrinal C, Prieur G, Frenoy E, Combret Y, Gravier FE, Bonnevie T, et al. Is overlap of respiratory and limb muscle weakness at weaning from mechanical ventilation associated with poorer outcomes? Intensive Care Med. 2017;43(2):282–3.
5. Jung B, Moury PH, Mahul M, de Jong A, Galia F, Prades A, et al. Diaphragmatic dysfunction in patients with ICU-acquired weakness and its impact on extubation failure. Intensive Care Med. 2016;42(5):853–61.
6. Demoule A, Jung B, Prodanovic H, Molinari N, Chanques G, Coirault C, et al. Diaphragm dysfunction on admission to the intensive care unit. Prevalence, risk factors, and prognostic impact-a prospective study. Am J Respir Crit Care Med. 2013;188(2):213–9.
7. Medrinal C, Prieur G, Frenoy E, Robledo Quesada A, Poncet A, Bonnevie T, et al. Respiratory weakness after mechanical ventilation is associated with one-year mortality—a prospective study. Crit Care. 2016;20(1):231.
8. Zambon M, Greco M, Bocchino S, Cabrini L, Beccaria PF, Zangrillo A. Assessment of diaphragmatic dysfunction in the critically ill patient with ultrasound: a systematic review. Intensive Care Med. 2017;43(1):29–38.
9. Moxham J, Goldstone J. Assessment of respiratory muscle strength in the intensive care unit. Eur Respir J. 1994;7(11):2057–61.
10. Marini JJ, Smith TC, Lamb V. Estimation of inspiratory muscle strength in mechanically ventilated patients: the measurement of maximum inspiratory pressure. J Crit Care. 1986;1(1):32–8.
11. Caruso P, Friedrich C, Denari SD, Ruiz SA, Deheinzelin D. The unidirectional valve is the best method to determine maximum inspiratory pressure during weaning. Chest. 1999;115(4):1096–101.
12. Spadaro S, Marangoni E, Ragazzi R, Mojoli F, Verri M, Longo L, et al. A methodological approach for determination of maximum inspiratory pressure in patients undergoing invasive mechanical ventilation. Minerva Anestesiol. 2015;81(1):33–8.
13. Katz S, Akpom CA. A measure of primary sociobiological functions. Int J Health Serv. 1976;6(3):493–508.
14. Boles JM, Bion J, Connors A, Herridge M, Marsh B, Melot C, et al. Weaning from mechanical ventilation. Eur Respir J. 2007;29(5):1033–56.
15. De Jonghe B, Bastuji-Garin S, Durand MC, Malissin I, Rodrigues P, Cerf C, et al. Respiratory weakness is associated with limb weakness and delayed weaning in critical illness. Crit Care Med. 2007;35(9):2007–15.
16. ATS/ERS Statement on respiratory muscle testing. Am J Respir Crit Care Med. 2002;166(4):518–624.

9

Skin microcirculatory reactivity assessed using a thermal challenge is decreased in patients with circulatory shock and associated with outcome

Diego Orbegozo, Wasineenart Mongkolpun, Gianni Stringari, Nikolaos Markou, Jacques Creteur, Jean-Louis Vincent* and Daniel De Backer*

Abstract

Background: Shock states are characterized by impaired tissue perfusion and microcirculatory alterations, which are directly related to outcome. Skin perfusion can be noninvasively evaluated using skin laser Doppler (SLD), which, when coupled with a local thermal challenge, may provide a measure of microcirculatory reactivity. We hypothesized that this microvascular reactivity would be impaired in patients with circulatory shock and would be a marker of severity.

Methods: We first evaluated skin blood flow (SBF) using SLD on the forearm and on the palm in 18 healthy volunteers to select the site with maximal response. Measurements were taken at 37 °C (baseline) and repeated at 43 °C. The 43 °C/37 °C SBF ratio was calculated as a measure of microvascular reactivity. We then evaluated the SBF in 29 patients with circulatory shock admitted to a 35-bed department of intensive care and in a confirmatory cohort of 35 patients with circulatory shock.

Results: In the volunteers, baseline SBF was higher in the hand than in the forearm, but the SBF ratio was lower (11.2 [9.4–13.4] vs. 2.0 [1.7–2.6], $p < 0.01$) so we used the forearm for our patients. Baseline forearm SBF was similar in patients with shock and healthy volunteers, but the SBF ratio was markedly lower in the patients (2.6 [2.0–3.6] vs. 11.2 [9.4–13.4], $p < 0.01$). Shock survivors had a higher SBF ratio than non-survivors (3.2 [2.2–6.2] vs. 2.3 [1.7–2.8], $p < 0.01$). These results were confirmed in the second cohort of 35 patients. In multivariable analysis, the APACHE II score and the SBF ratio were independently associated with mortality.

Conclusions: Microcirculatory reactivity is decreased in patients with circulatory shock and has prognostic value. This simple, noninvasive test could help in monitoring the peripheral microcirculation in acutely ill patients.

Keywords: Skin blood flow, Skin laser Doppler, Capillary blood flow, Perfusion, Nitric oxide, Peripheral circulation, Laser Doppler flowmetry

Background

Circulatory shock is a life-threatening condition affecting about one-third of patients admitted to the intensive care unit (ICU) [1, 2]. Regardless of the underlying pathophysiological mechanisms, the hallmark of shock states is altered tissue perfusion, which if not rapidly corrected leads to organ dysfunction and death [3, 4]. Recent data have highlighted the prognostic importance of microcirculatory abnormalities in patients with shock using noninvasive bedside techniques, such as sublingual video-microscopy [5–8]. The hallmark of these alterations is decreased capillary density, and microvascular blood flow with increased heterogeneity of perfusion [9, 10]. Interestingly, these microcirculatory abnormalities

*Correspondence: jlvincent@intensive.org; ddebacke@ulb.ac.be
Department of Intensive Care, Erasme University Hospital, Université Libre de Bruxelles, Route de Lennik 808, 1070 Brussels, Belgium

are not explained by routinely measured global macro-hemodynamic variables, making it attractive to assess them directly [11, 12].

The microcirculation can also be studied by evaluating the response generated by a hypoxic stress event, such as during a transient vascular occlusion test (VOT) [7, 8]. Near-infrared spectroscopy (NIRS) or laser Doppler techniques can be used to indirectly or directly evaluate a transient increase in flow after a VOT [13–15]. Studies using these techniques have shown that endothelial reactivity is impaired in sepsis and is associated with organ dysfunction and outcome [16, 17]. However, VOTs are not easily standardized (duration of occlusion and/or tissue oxygen saturation [StO_2] reached) [16, 18]. In addition, VOTs may alter local metabolism [19]. Alternative methods to evaluate microvascular recruitment are, therefore, of interest.

Local heating of the skin may represent an alternative means of evaluating microvascular reactivity. Skin laser Doppler (SLD) (also known as laser Doppler flowmetry) can be used to assess skin blood flow (SBF) during a thermal challenge [14]. This technique uses an optical fiber to direct light from a low-power laser source to the skin and to collect the back-scattered light. The shift in light wavelength is proportional to the red blood cell velocity in the studied skin area, providing a noninvasive measurement of SBF expressed as arbitrary perfusion units (PUs) [20]. New SLD flow probes can heat the explored tissue in a controlled way, making it possible to perform a dynamic test of capillary reactivity by increasing local temperature [14]. However, there are no published data evaluating this test in patients with circulatory shock.

We hypothesized that reactivity of the skin microcirculation, evaluated as the skin blood flow ratio, during a thermal challenge would be impaired in patients with circulatory shock. We also assessed whether these alterations could be explained by other hemodynamic parameters and were correlated with patient outcome.

Methods
This prospective, observational study was conducted in our 35-bed Department of Intensive Care. Institutional Ethical Committee approval was obtained, and informed consent was obtained from each participant or the next of kin.

Protocol
To assess the most appropriate probe position for an SLD thermal challenge, we first studied 18 healthy volunteers. They were comfortably seated in a quiet, temperature-controlled room for at least 15 min before each experiment. Heart rate, respiratory rate and hemoglobin saturation were evaluated noninvasively by pulse oximetry using a Siemens SC 9000 monitor (Siemens, Erlangen, Germany). Noninvasive measurements of mean arterial pressure (MAP) were taken in the opposite arm to that used for the SLD blood flow measurements.

We then studied, in 2013, a cohort of 29 critically ill adult patients admitted with a diagnosis of circulatory shock, defined as the need for norepinephrine infusion to maintain a MAP of at least 65 mmHg, associated with an altered mental status, acute oliguria defined as a urine output < 0.5 ml/Kg/h or an arterial lactate level > 2 mmol/L [4]. Screening of ICU admissions, collection of data and SLD measurements were performed by doctors not involved in patient management. All SLD measurements were taken as soon as possible after completion of initial resuscitation, i.e., when an adequate arterial pressure for that patient had been reached (determined by the treating physician), and norepinephrine doses had been stable for 1 h. A second SLD measurement was taken, when possible, 48 h after the first measurement.

Having analyzed the results from our first patient cohort, we repeated the study in a second, confirmatory cohort of critically ill patients with circulatory shock (using the same definition) admitted in 2015. Patients were evaluated by an investigator who had not been involved in the initial study and at just one time point during the first day of hospitalization after initial resuscitation.

We collected demographic and clinical data on admission and classified patients as having sepsis or not, based on standard criteria [21]. At the time of each SLD measurement, we collected all available hemodynamic and respiratory data from ongoing patient monitors and recorded the central body temperature. We also collected biochemical and laboratory data from clinical records, including the most recent blood gas analysis. The APACHE II score [22] was calculated using the worst data during the first 24 h in the ICU. The sequential organ failure assessment (SOFA) score [23] was calculated from the data present at the time of the SLD measurements. Patients were grouped according to ICU outcome (dead or alive) for further analysis.

Skin laser Doppler measurements
All SLD measurements were taken using the PeriFlux System 5000 monitor (Perimed, Jarfalla, Sweden), and data were continuously collected (PeriSoft software 2.5.5; Perimed) for further analysis. For the thermal challenge, a small angled thermostatic SLD probe 457 (Perimed) with 0.25 mm fiber separation was used. This probe also allows skin temperature measurement at site of application. The SLD machine emits a beam of laser light with a wavelength of 780 nm that allows skin evaluation at a

depth of 0.5–1 mm. The initial skin temperature was measured with the thermostatic probe prior to each measurement. In the healthy volunteers, the probe was placed on the skin of the volar face of the proximal forearm and on the palm of the same arm. In the patients, the SLD probe was placed on the forearm without the arterial line. The probe was kept in position using the double-sided tape provided with the SLD monitor. All participants were asked to abstain from any activity during the study period to prevent any possible artifacts in the recorded signals [13].

To limit differences between subjects in the basal temperature, SBF was recorded at a local skin temperature of 37 °C allowing for at least three minutes of stabilization. Thereafter, a thermal challenge was performed by increasing the probe temperature abruptly (0.1 °C/s) from 37 to 43 °C. After 9 min at 43 °C, the SBF was recorded (Additional file 1: Figure S1). We chose to increase the temperature to 43 °C, because our preliminary experience indicated that using lower thresholds (39 °C or 41 °C) reduced the amplitude of the response, making it more difficult to detect potential differences. We calculated the SBF ratio (SBF obtained at 43 °C/SBF obtained at 37 °C) as a simple measure of microvascular reactivity in the explored area.

Statistical analysis

Statistical analyses were performed using SPSS 22.0 (IBM, New York, NY) software. Variables were assessed for normality of distribution using skewness and kurtosis tests and Q–Q plots. Continuous variables are presented as means ± standard deviations or median values with percentiles (25–75%) depending on the presence or absence of normality. Categorical data are presented as numbers of events and percentages. Repeated measurements were compared using a paired Student's t test or Wilcoxon signed rank test, as appropriate. Comparisons between different cohorts were made using an unpaired t test or Mann–Whitney U test as appropriate. Proportions were compared with a Chi-square test or Fisher's exact test as appropriate. We plotted the sensitivity and specificity using a receiving operating characteristics (ROC) graph, and the area under the curve (AUC) was calculated for the different variables as a measure of their ability to predict mortality. To assess possible explanatory variables correlated with the SBF ratio, we plotted individual data on graphs and calculated the Pearson or Spearman correlation coefficient (r) as appropriate. Univariate and multivariate analyses (binary logistic regressions) were performed to identify the ability of different variables to predict ICU mortality, calculating the odds ratios and their respective 95% confidence intervals.

In a post hoc analysis considering that the APACHE II score was directly correlated and the SBF ratio inversely correlated with mortality, we calculated the ratio between the two factors (APACHE II score/SBF ratio) in an attempt to improve their prognostic value.

A two-sided p value less than 0.05 was considered as significant for all analyses.

Results
Healthy volunteers
The main characteristics of the volunteers are listed in Additional file 1: Table S1. Comparisons of measurements taken in the hand and the forearm are shown in Fig. 1 and Additional file 1: Table S2. Baseline values of SBF at 37 °C were lower in the forearm than in the hand, but the SBF ratio was higher in the forearm.

Patients: initial cohort
The main demographic and baseline characteristics of the 29 patients are listed in Table 1: 16 (55%) had septic and 13 (45%) cardiogenic shock. Eleven patients died in the ICU (44%). Times from ICU admission until the first measurement were similar in survivors and non-survivors: 6 (4–17) versus 7 (5–14) h ($p = 0.59$). The patients had a similar baseline SBF to the healthy volunteers, but a lower SBF at 43 °C, which resulted in a lower SBF ratio (Table 2). SBF values at baseline and at 43 °C were similar in survivors and non-survivors, but survivors had significantly higher SBF ratios (Table 2). A comparison of the SBF ratios in volunteers, survivors and non-survivors is shown in Fig. 2.

SLD measurements were repeated at 48 h in 20 of the patients. At that time point, the survivors had a somewhat higher SBF ratio than the non-survivors although the differences were not statistically significant [3.1 (2.4–4.3) vs. 2.3 (1.5–3.1), $p = 0.08$] (Additional file 1: Figure S2). The difference in the SBF ratio between T0 and T48 was not significant in survivors or non-survivors (Additional file 1: Figure S3).

There were no significant correlations between the SBF ratio and any hemodynamic or blood gas-derived variable, administration of vasoactive drugs (Additional file 1: Figure S4), presence of sepsis (Additional file 1: Table S3), degree/severity of organ dysfunction (SOFA score), initial forearm temperature or the difference between the central to forearm temperature (Additional file 1: Figure S5).

The SBF ratio and the APACHE II score had similar ROC AUCs to predict survival (0.73 [0.55–0.91] vs. 0.74 [0.56–0.92], respectively) (Fig. 3). There was no significant correlation between the SBF ratio and the APACHE II score ($r = 0.047$, $p > 0.05$), so that we calculated their combined ratio, which resulted in a larger ROC AUC to

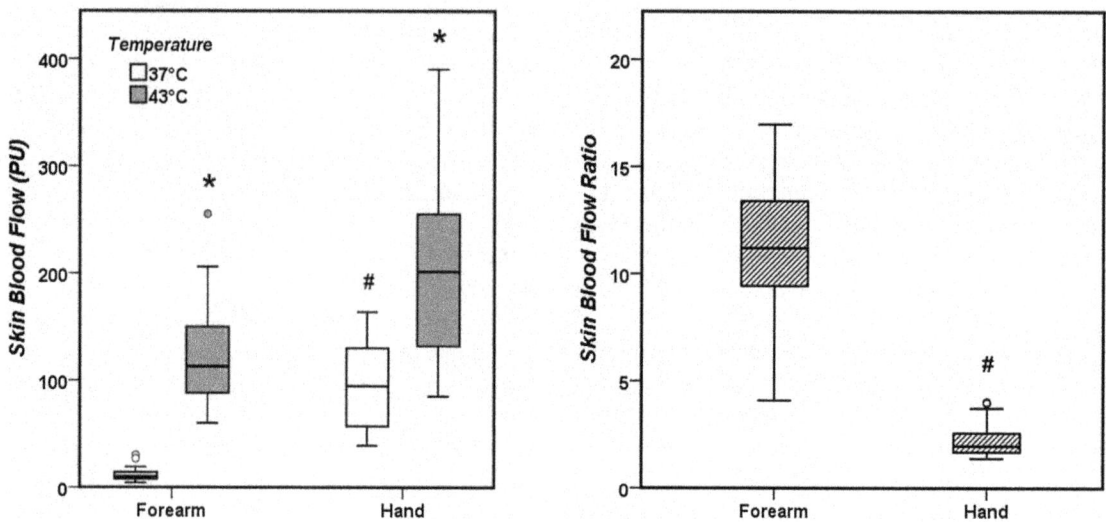

Fig. 1 Comparison of skin blood flow measurements at different temperatures on the forearm and the hand in healthy volunteers. In the right panel, the ratio of skin blood flow obtained between 43 and 37 °C is presented. *$p < 0.05$ compared with measurements at 37 °C; #$p < 0.05$ compared with forearm measurements

predict survival than that for either measure alone (0.90 [0.79–1.00], Fig. 3).

Considering a cutoff ratio of 3 for the SBF ratio, the specificity and sensitivity were 91 and 56%, respectively, to predict survival. Considering a cutoff value of 2 for the SBF ratio, the specificity and sensitivity were 36 and 83%, respectively.

In multivariable analysis, taking into consideration the SOFA score, the blood lactate concentration, the mean arterial pressure, the norepinephrine dose and the presence of sepsis, only the APACHE II score and the SBF ratio were independently correlated with mortality (Additional file 1: Table S4).

Patients: confirmatory cohort

The demographic and baseline characteristics of the 35 patients in the confirmatory cohort are listed in Table 1: 28 had septic (80%) and 7 cardiogenic (20%) shock. Eighteen patients died in the ICU (51%). SBF values at baseline were similar in survivors and non-survivors, but survivors had significantly higher SBF values at 43 °C and larger SBF ratios (Table 2).

There were no significant correlations between the SBF ratio and any hemodynamic or blood gas-derived variable, dose of vasoactive drugs, presence of sepsis (Additional file 1: Table S3), degree/severity of organ dysfunction (SOFA score), initial forearm temperature or the difference between the central to forearm temperature (all p values > 0.05).

The ROC AUCs to predict survival were 0.85 (0.73–0.98) and 0.77 (0.60–0.94) for the SBF ratio and the APACHE II score, respectively. The ratio between the

APACHE II score and the SBF ratio resulted in an ROC AUC to predict survival of 0.91 (0.82–1.00) (Fig. 3).

Considering a cutoff ratio of 3 for the SBF ratio, the specificity and sensitivity to predict survival were 83 and 71%, respectively. Considering a cutoff value of 2 for the SBF ratio, the specificity and sensitivity for prediction of survival were 50 and 88%, respectively.

Discussion

In this study, reactivity of the skin microcirculation during a thermal challenge was compromised in patients with circulatory shock, and this impairment was related to outcome. This phenomenon could not be explained by other hemodynamic variables and was independent of regularly used scoring systems, such as the SOFA and the APACHE II score.

As far as we know, this is the first report to assess the skin microvascular reactivity (or vasodilatation) during a thermal challenge in shock patients. Several previous reports have used an ischemic challenge to assess microcirculatory reactivity [7] and shown that post-occlusive reactive hyperemia is impaired in patients with sepsis and septic shock, and this has been correlated with poor outcomes [15–17, 24]. However, this condition is not pathognomonic of sepsis and is also present in hemorrhagic [25] and cardiogenic [19, 26] shock. Our data also show that the degree of impairment in microvascular reactivity during a thermal challenge was similar in septic and cardiogenic shock. Nevertheless, studies in patients with just cardiogenic, septic or hemorrhagic shock may be of interest to further investigate whether the effects of a thermal

Table 1   Main baseline characteristics of patients with circulatory shock

Variable	Initial cohort				Confirmatory cohort			
	Total (n = 29)	Survivors (n = 18)	Non-survivors (n = 11)	P	Total (n = 35)	Survivors (n = 17)	Non-survivors (n = 18)	P
Age (years)	67 ± 11	64 ± 12	71 ± 8	0.11	64 ± 16	61 ± 16	67 ± 16	0.30
Body mass index (kg/m²)	26 ± 6	25 ± 5	27 ± 8	0.66	28 ± 5	27 ± 5	28 ± 5	0.29
Septic shock [n (%)]	16 (55)	9 (50)	7 (64)	0.82	28 (80)	13 (77)	15 (83)	0.61
Cardiogenic shock [n (%)]	13 (45)	9 (50)	4 (36)	0.82	7 (20)	4 (23)	3 (17)	0.61
Chronic kidney disease [n (%)]	8 (28)	7 (39)	1 (9)	0.11	8 (23)	4 (24)	4 (22)	1.00
Chronic arterial hypertension [n (%)]	20 (69)	11 (61)	9 (82)	0.41	11 (31)	5 (29)	6 (33)	0.80
Diabetes mellitus [n (%)]	12 (41)	7 (39)	5 (46)	0.73	11 (31)	5 (29)	6 (33)	0.80
Coronary artery disease [n (%)]	9 (31)	5 (28)	4 (36)	0.69	8 (23)	3 (18)	5 (28)	0.69
Mean arterial pressure (mmHg)	75 ± 13	73 ± 9	77 ± 17	0.52	73 ± 9	72 ± 7	75 ± 10	0.28
Heart rate (bpm)	97 ± 25	99 ± 25	95 ± 27	0.67	99 ± 22	101 ± 22	98 ± 22	0.71
Central venous pressure (mmHg)	11 (8–12)	11 (7–12)	11 (9–13)	0.28	9 (7–12)	8 (6–11)	10 (8–12)	0.23
Cardiac output (L/min)	4.0 (3.4–5.7) n = 18	3.8 (3.2–4.7) n = 11	4.1 (3.5–6.8) n = 7	0.44	4.8 (3.5–6.3) n = 32	4.8 (3.4–6.7) n = 16	4.6 (3.6–5.6) n = 16	0.68
Central temperature (°C)	36.8 (36.0–37.5)	37.1 (36.2–37.8)	36.5 (35.9–37.3)	0.19	36.9 (36.6–37.5)	36.8 (36.6–37.2)	37.0 (36.6–37.6)	0.71
Basal forearm temperature (°C)	32.0 (31.1–32.7)	32.1 (31.1–32.7)	31.4 (30.7–32.7)	0.58	30.6 (29.1–31.6)	30.5 (28.9–31.6)	30.7 (30.0–31.8)	0.55
Central to basal forearm temperature (°C)	5.1 (4.2–6.1)	5.0 (4.5–6.4)	5.0 (4.2–5.6)	0.44	6.5 (5.6–7.6)	7.4 (5.2–7.9)	6.4 (5.8–7.1)	0.54
pH	7.35 ± 0.07	7.36 ± 0.06	7.33 ± 0.09	0.29	7.35 ± 0.12	7.33 ± 0.13	7.36 ± 0.11	0.42
PCO₂ (mmHg)	38 ± 8	39 ± 9	35 ± 8	0.22	37 ± 11	40 ± 14	35 ± 8	0.22
Lactate (mmol/L)	2.4 (1.6–4.8)	1.9 (1.5–2.9)	3.2 (1.6–6.3)	0.35	1.7 (1.2–2.6)	1.6 (1.1–2.7)	1.8 (1.3–2.4)	0.78
Mechanical ventilation [n (%)]	25 (86)	15 (83)	10 (91)	1.00	25 (71)	10 (59)	15 (84)	0.11
PaO₂/FiO₂ ratio	192 (132–293)	196 (128–310)	192 (145–250)	0.93	166 (124–244)	189 (124–247)	146 (120–211)	0.24
Creatinine (mg/dL)	1.4 (1.0–1.7)	1.4 (0.9–1.6)	1.6 (1.0–2.2)	0.44	1.3 (0.8–2.0)	1.3 (0.8–1.9)	1.2 (0.8–2.1)	0.82
Total bilirubin (mg/dL)	0.9 (0.5–2.1)	0.9 (0.5–1.8)	1.6 (0.6–2.8)	0.30	0.8 (0.5–2.7)	0.8 (0.5–2.7)	0.9 (0.5–2.6)	0.58
Platelets (× 10³/μL)	163 (92–243)	160 (92–243)	163 (65–307)	0.93	52 (13–79)	58 (25–108)	22 (7–67)	0.06
Leukocytes (cells × 10³/μL)	12.4 (8.5–17.7)	11.7 (8.2–17.7)	12.4 (8.5–17.7)	0.95	12.0 (8.5–19.9)	12.5 (10.4–21.9)	10.8 (4.7–17.0)	0.16
Number of patients receiving sedatives [n (%)]	17 (59)	10 (56)	7 (64)	0.67	8 (23)	4 (24)	4 (22)	1.00
Number of patients receiving opiates [n (%)]	22 (76)	14 (78)	8 (73)	1.00	7 (20)	4 (24)	3 (17)	0.69
APACHE II score	26 ± 8	23 ± 7	30 ± 8	0.03	26 ± 8	22 ± 8	29 ± 6	< 0.01
SOFA score	10 ± 3	10 ± 3	12 ± 3	0.04	10 ± 5	9 ± 5	11 ± 4	0.13

Table 1 (continued)

Variable	Initial cohort				Confirmatory cohort			
	Total ($n = 29$)	Survivors ($n = 18$)	Non-survivors ($n = 11$)	P	Total ($n = 35$)	Survivors ($n = 17$)	Non-survivors ($n = 18$)	P
Number of patients receiving dobutamine [n (%)]	13 (45)	7 (39)	6 (54)	0.41	6 (17)	2 (24)	2 (11)	0.40
Dobutamine dose at moment of thermal challenge (mcg/Kg/min)	0 (0–10)	0 (0–5)	10 (0–15)	0.24	0 (0–0)	0 (0–0)	0 (0–0)	0.42
Norepinephrine dose at moment of thermal challenge (mcg/Kg/min)	0.32 (0.11–0.50)	0.28 (0.11–0.41)	0.43 (0.11–0.84)	0.43	0.12 (0.08–0.55)	0.12 (0.07–0.41)	0.20 (0.08–0.62)	0.36
ICU length of stay (days)	8.0 (3.5–16.0)	8.6 (4.4–16.0)	6.5 (2.1–19.6)	0.44	5.3 (3.2–9.0)	4.7 (4.0–9.0)	6.0 (3.2–8.0)	0.70

Table 2 Comparison of skin laser Doppler (SLD) variables between volunteers and patients and between survivors and non-survivors

SLD variable	Healthy volunteers and initial cohort			Initial cohort			Confirmatory cohort		
	Volunteers ($n = 18$)	Patients ($n = 29$)	P	Survivors ($n = 18$)	Non-survivors ($n = 11$)	P	Survivors ($n = 17$)	Non-survivors ($n = 18$)	P
Skin blood flow 37 °C (PU)	10.3 (8.0–14.2)	13.0 (10.1–19.5)	0.16	13.4 (10.0–21.6)	13.0 (10.1–19.5)	0.44	12.4 (8.0–17.3)	15.0 (10.2–19.3)	0.44
Skin blood flow 43 °C (PU)	112.8 (88.0–150.0)	36.4 (25.6–76.9)	<0.01	51.8 (25.6–77.2)	33.7 (16.5–39.0)	0.76	57.4 (41.5–71.5)	33.1 (21.8–41.6)	<0.01
Skin blood flow ratio	11.2 (9.4–13.4)	2.6 (2.0–3.6)	<0.01	3.2 (2.2–6.2)	2.3 (1.7–2.8)	<0.01	3.7 (2.9–6.2)	2.1 (1.6–2.5)	<0.01

PU perfusion units

challenge are indeed similar across different shock etiologies. Our results were not correlated with other regularly used parameters, but this is not surprising considering the considerable previous literature showing dissociation between the macro- and microcirculations [11, 12].

Importantly, an ischemic challenge can significantly alter local metabolism. Hence, some NIRS-derived variables, such as the descending slope (the rate of decrease in tissue oxygen saturation during a VOT and correlated with tissue oxygen consumption), may be affected by some degree of ischemic preconditioning in the studied tissue, limiting the reproducibility of results over a short time period [19]. The thermal challenge that we propose allows the SBF to return to baseline within minutes, enabling the test to be repeated in the same area. If there are concerns about alterations in local metabolism, the challenged area is very small (compared to the complete extremity involved during a VOT), so that the test can be repeated in an adjacent area.

The mechanisms underlying a thermal challenge are different to those of an ischemic challenge. As the skin temperature increases, the SBF increases until a maximum plateau value is reached [27–29]. More specifically, an initial short-lived phase of rapid vasodilation, which is neurally driven, is followed by a more gradual but protracted increase in SBF that is dependent on local nitric oxide (NO) production stimulated by endothelial NO synthase [27–31]. Thus, the use of this very simple and noninvasive test may provide an indirect assessment of the local NO pathway. NO plays a major role in the local control of the microcirculation and in its interaction with red blood cells [32, 33]. It also plays an important role in the pathophysiology of sepsis and septic shock [34, 35] and of cardiogenic shock [36, 37]. Interestingly, during endotoxin infusion in healthy volunteers, recruitment of the skin microcirculation through a thermal challenge that involves NO-dependent pathways was impaired, whereas post-occlusive reactive vasodilation was not [38]. Thus,

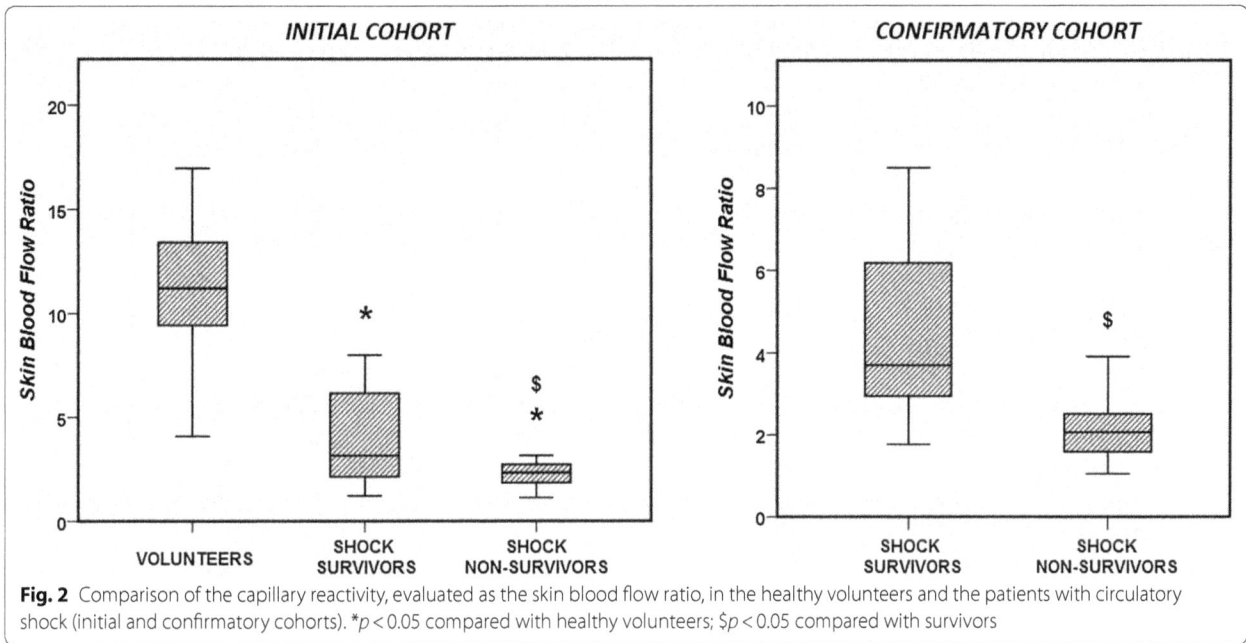

Fig. 2 Comparison of the capillary reactivity, evaluated as the skin blood flow ratio, in the healthy volunteers and the patients with circulatory shock (initial and confirmatory cohorts). *$p < 0.05$ compared with healthy volunteers; $p < 0.05$ compared with survivors

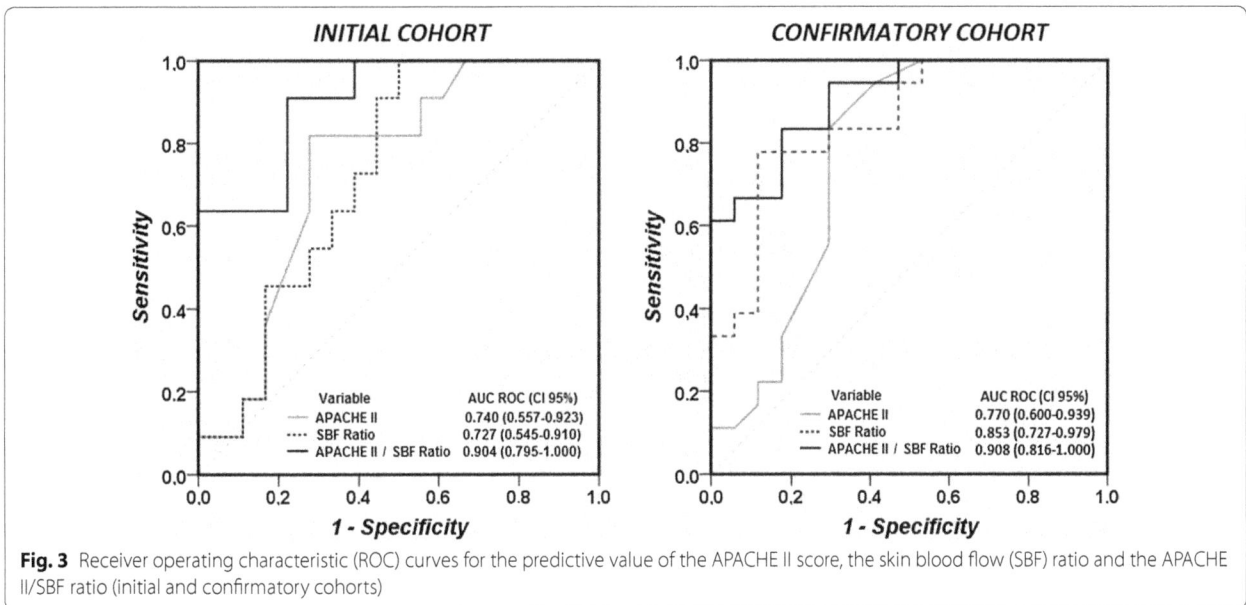

Fig. 3 Receiver operating characteristic (ROC) curves for the predictive value of the APACHE II score, the skin blood flow (SBF) ratio and the APACHE II/SBF ratio (initial and confirmatory cohorts)

the worse outcome in patients with shock who had compromised skin microvascular reactivity after the thermal challenge may reflect altered NO pathways. Nevertheless, physiological or basic science studies need to be conducted to verify the role of the NO pathway in our observations.

Two important technical aspects should be discussed further: the position of the probe on the forearm and the duration of the thermal challenge. Intuitively, the skin area used to perform SLD with a thermal challenge should have the highest potential recruitment even if the baseline SBF is relatively low. SLD studies have shown that the cutaneous microcirculation in healthy volunteers is very heterogeneous with lower blood flow values in the forearm than in the palm and lower values in the metacarpal spaces than in the fingertips [14, 39]. Similar observations have been made for other areas of the body, such as the torso, feet and face, and this heterogeneity has been confirmed by other techniques evaluating skin perfusion [40–44]. When performing a thermal challenge in different cutaneous regions, Metzler-Wilson et al. [40] showed that recruitment was higher in the forearm than in the palm. We confirmed this finding in our healthy volunteers.

Different temperature thresholds and heating times have been proposed when performing a thermal challenge [28, 29, 38, 40, 41]. However, 30 min may be needed to reach the maximal SBF during the test [28, 29], a period that is too long in critically ill patients who often need rapid changes in therapy. During pilot studies (data not shown), we observed that the best temperature to demonstrate a response was 43 °C. We also observed that we were not able to identify the initial short-lived phase of rapid vasodilation in all patients (this does not mean that the neural stimulus was absent, but just difficult to track with this technology), but when present it had already disappeared at 9 min and its analysis was difficult to standardize (time to peak versus maximum peak versus slope). For these practical reasons, we arbitrarily chose to limit the duration of the thermal challenge to 9 min. Hence, we did not evaluate the maximal recruitment of the skin microcirculation, but a surrogate value (the slope or speed of the microcirculation recruitment) within a reasonable observation period.

Other limitations should also be acknowledged. First, we included a relatively small number of patients, potentially limiting the statistical power of our analyses and possibly accounting for the lack of significant difference in microvascular reactivity between survivors and non-survivors, particularly at 48 h. Moreover, although we found similar results in our two cohorts, external validation of our data is still necessary. Second, although the forearm is a very accessible area in most critically ill patients and has the additional benefit of high potential recruitability with a thermal challenge, studies using different skin locations may also be informative. Further studies are also required to describe the evolution of these alterations over time and their changes with specific therapies (fluid bolus, transfusions, change in vasopressor dose, etc.). Although we focused on mortality as an outcome measure, future studies could also specifically assess relationships with other clinical outcomes, including changes in SOFA scores over time. Third, the presence of fever may represent a confounding factor that should be taken into account; however, the local temperature on the forearm was always less than 37 °C and there was no apparent correlation with the resulting SBF ratio. Fourth, we did not collect data from a control cohort of elderly patients (a factor that can influence the vascular response); however, our control group was designed to provide a picture of the normal physiological response and, more importantly, our main findings are related to the differences between survivors and non-survivors. Fifth, we did not compare the results of the thermal challenge to results from other concomitant measures of

the microcirculation. However, our recent observations indicate that VOTs can induce ischemic preconditioning and alter local metabolism [19], which would need to be taken into account if a skin thermal challenge was performed in the same area. Finally, although it is impossible to extrapolate our skin measurements to other microvascular networks in different organs, the strong association we found with outcomes and the simplicity of this technique makes it attractive for future research.

Conclusion

SLD with a thermal challenge is a technique that allows simple, noninvasive evaluation of skin microcirculatory reactivity. Using this technique, we have demonstrated that reactivity of skin microcirculation during a thermal challenge is compromised in patients with circulatory shock, is related to outcome and combination with the APACHE II score can improve its prognostic value.

Abbreviations
AUC: area under the curve; ICU: intensive care unit; MAP: mean arterial pressure; NIRS: near-infrared spectroscopy; NO: nitric oxide; PU: perfusion units; ROC: receiver operating characteristic; SBF: skin blood flow; SLD: skin laser Doppler; SOFA: sequential organ failure assessment; StO_2: tissue oxygen saturation; VOT: vascular occlusion test.

Authors' contributions
DO, NM, JC, JLV, DDB conceived and designed the study; DO, WM, GS and NM performed and analyzed the measurements; DO wrote the first draft of the manuscript. DO, WM, GS, NM, JC, JLV and DDB revised the text for intellectual content. All the authors read and approved the final manuscript.

Acknowledgements
None.

Competing interests
The authors have no competing interests to declare related to this manuscript.

Funding
No external funding.

References
1. Sakr Y, Reinhart K, Vincent JL, Sprung CL, Moreno R, Ranieri VM, et al. Does dopamine administration in shock influence outcome? results of the sepsis occurrence in acutely Ill patients (SOAP) study. Crit Care Med. 2006;34:589–97.
2. De Backer D, Biston P, Devriendt J, Madl C, Chochrad D, Aldecoa C, et al. Comparison of dopamine and norepinephrine in the treatment of shock. N Engl J Med. 2010;362:779–89.
3. Weil MH, Shubin H. Proposed reclassification of shock states with special reference to distributive defects. Adv Exp Med Biol. 1971;23:13–23.
4. Vincent JL, De Backer D. Circulatory shock. N Engl J Med. 2013;369:1726–34.
5. Edul VS, Enrico C, Laviolle B, Vazquez AR, Ince C, Dubin A. Quantitative assessment of the microcirculation in healthy volunteers and in patients with septic shock. Crit Care Med. 2012;40:1443–8.
6. den Uil CA, Lagrand WK, van der Ent M, Jewbali LS, Cheng JM, Spronk PE, et al. Impaired microcirculation predicts poor outcome of patients with

acute myocardial infarction complicated by cardiogenic shock. Eur Heart J. 2010;31:3032–9.

7. De Backer D, Donadello K, Cortes DO. Monitoring the microcirculation. J Clin Monit Comput. 2012;26:361–6.

8. Lima A, Bakker J. Noninvasive monitoring of peripheral perfusion. Intensive Care Med. 2005;31:1316–26.

9. De Backer D, Creteur J, Preiser JC, Dubois MJ, Vincent JL. Microvascular blood flow is altered in patients with sepsis. Am J Respir Crit Care Med. 2002;166:98–104.

10. Trzeciak S, Dellinger RP, Parrillo JE, Guglielmi M, Bajaj J, Abate NL, et al. Early microcirculatory perfusion derangements in patients with severe sepsis and septic shock: relationship to hemodynamics, oxygen transport, and survival. Ann Emerg Med. 2007;49(88–98):98.

11. De Backer D, Donadello K, Sakr Y, Ospina-Tascon G, Salgado D, Scolletta S, et al. Microcirculatory alterations in patients with severe sepsis: impact of time of assessment and relationship with outcome. Crit Care Med. 2013;41:791–9.

12. De Backer D, Orbegozo CD, Donadello K, Vincent JL. Pathophysiology of microcirculatory dysfunction and the pathogenesis of septic shock. Virulence. 2014;5:73–9.

13. Wright CI, Kroner CI, Draijer R. Non-invasive methods and stimuli for evaluating the skin's microcirculation. J Pharmacol Toxicol Methods. 2006;54:1–25.

14. Roustit M, Blaise S, Millet C, Cracowski JL. Reproducibility and methodological issues of skin post-occlusive and thermal hyperemia assessed by single-point laser Doppler flowmetry. Microvasc Res. 2010;79:102–8.

15. Doerschug KC, Delsing AS, Schmidt GA, Haynes WG. Impairments in microvascular reactivity are related to organ failure in human sepsis. Am J Physiol Heart Circ Physiol. 2007;293:H1065–71.

16. Creteur J, Carollo T, Soldati G, Buchele G, De Backer D, Vincent JL. The prognostic value of muscle StO$_2$ in septic patients. Intensive Care Med. 2007;33:1549–56.

17. Payen D, Luengo C, Heyer L, Resche-Rigon M, Kerever S, Damoisel C, et al. Is thenar tissue hemoglobin oxygen saturation in septic shock related to macrohemodynamic variables and outcome? Crit Care. 2009;13(Suppl 5):S6.

18. Gomez H, Torres A, Polanco P, Kim HK, Zenker S, Puyana JC, et al. Use of non-invasive NIRS during a vascular occlusion test to assess dynamic tissue O(2) saturation response. Intensive Care Med. 2008;34:1600–7.

19. Orbegozo Cortes D, Puflea F, De Backer D, Creteur J, Vincent JL. Near infrared spectroscopy (NIRS) to assess the effects of local ischemic preconditioning in the muscle of healthy volunteers and critically ill patients. Microvasc Res. 2015;102:25–32.

20. Vongsavan N, Matthews B. Some aspects of the use of laser Doppler flow meters for recording tissue blood flow. Exp Physiol. 1993;78:1–14.

21. Levy MM, Fink MP, Marshall JC, Abraham E, Angus D, Cook D, et al. 2001 SCCM/ESICM/ACCP/ATS/SIS international sepsis definitions conference. Crit Care Med. 2003;31:1250–6.

22. Knaus WA, Draper EA, Wagner DP, Zimmerman JE. APACHE II: a severity of disease classification system. Crit Care Med. 1985;13:818–29.

23. Vincent JL, Moreno R, Takala J, Willatts S, De Mendonca A, Bruining H, et al. The SOFA (sepsis-related organ failure assessment) score to describe organ dysfunction/failure. On behalf of the working group on sepsis-related problems of the European society of intensive care medicine. Intensive Care Med. 1996;22:707–10.

24. Shapiro NI, Arnold R, Sherwin R, O'Connor J, Najarro G, Singh S, et al. The association of near-infrared spectroscopy-derived tissue oxygenation measurements with sepsis syndromes, organ dysfunction and mortality in emergency department patients with sepsis. Crit Care. 2011;15:R223.

25. Duret J, Pottecher J, Bouzat P, Brun J, Harrois A, Payen JF, et al. Skeletal muscle oxygenation in severe trauma patients during haemorrhagic shock resuscitation. Crit Care. 2015;19:141.

26. Petroni T, Harrois A, Amour J, Lebreton G, Brechot N, Tanaka S, et al. Intra-aortic balloon pump effects on macrocirculation and microcirculation in cardiogenic shock patients supported by venoarterial extracorporeal membrane oxygenation. Crit Care Med. 2014;42:2075–82.

27. Taylor WF, Johnson JM, O'Leary D, Park MK. Effect of high local temperature on reflex cutaneous vasodilation. J Appl Physiol Respir Environ Exerc Physiol. 1984;57:191–6.

28. Minson CT, Berry LT, Joyner MJ. Nitric oxide and neurally mediated regulation of skin blood flow during local heating. J Appl Physiol. 1985;2001(91):1619–26.

29. Kellogg DL Jr. In vivo mechanisms of cutaneous vasodilation and vasoconstriction in humans during thermoregulatory challenges. J Appl Physiol. 1985;2006(100):1709–18.

30. Kellogg DL Jr, Liu Y, Kosiba IF, O'Donnell D. Role of nitric oxide in the vascular effects of local warming of the skin in humans. J Appl Physiol. 1985;1999(86):1185–90.

31. Kellogg DL Jr, Zhao JL, Wu Y. Roles of nitric oxide synthase isoforms in cutaneous vasodilation induced by local warming of the skin and whole body heat stress in humans. J Appl Physiol. 1985;2009(107):1438–44.

32. Vaughn MW, Kuo L, Liao JC. Effective diffusion distance of nitric oxide in the microcirculation. Am J Physiol. 1998;274:H1705–14.

33. Kim-Shapiro DB, Schechter AN, Gladwin MT. Unraveling the reactions of nitric oxide, nitrite, and hemoglobin in physiology and therapeutics. Arterioscler Thromb Vasc Biol. 2006;26:697–705.

34. Lupp C, Baasner S, Ince C, Nocken F, Stover JF, Westphal M. Differentiated control of deranged nitric oxide metabolism: a therapeutic option in sepsis? Crit Care. 2013;17:311.

35. Cauwels A. Nitric oxide in shock. Kidney Int. 2007;72:557–65.

36. Hollenberg SM, Cinel I. Bench-to-bedside review: nitric oxide in critical illness—update 2008. Crit Care. 2009;13:218.

37. Alexander JH, Reynolds HR, Stebbins AL, Dzavik V, Harrington RA, Van de Werf F, et al. Effect of tilarginine acetate in patients with acute myocardial infarction and cardiogenic shock: the TRIUMPH randomized controlled trial. JAMA. 2007;297:1657–66.

38. Engelberger RP, Pittet YK, Henry H, Delodder F, Hayoz D, Chiolero RL, et al. Acute endotoxemia inhibits microvascular nitric oxide-dependent vasodilation in humans. Shock. 2011;35:28–34.

39. Ninet J, Fronek A. Cutaneous postocclusive reactive hyperemia monitored by laser Doppler flux metering and skin temperature. Microvasc Res. 1985;30:125–32.

40. Metzler-Wilson K, Kellie LA, Tomc C, Simpson C, Sammons D, Wilson TE. Differential vasodilatory responses to local heating in facial, glabrous and hairy skin. Clin Physiol Funct Imaging. 2012;32:361–6.

41. Del Pozzi AT, Hodges GJ. To reheat, or to not reheat: that is the question: the efficacy of a local reheating protocol on mechanisms of cutaneous vasodilatation. Microvasc Res. 2015;97:47–54.

42. Roustit M, Millet C, Blaise S, Dufournet B, Cracowski JL. Excellent reproducibility of laser speckle contrast imaging to assess skin microvascular reactivity. Microvasc Res. 2010;80:505–11.

43. Bezemer R, Klijn E, Khalilzada M, Lima A, Heger M, van Bommel J, et al. Validation of near-infrared laser speckle imaging for assessing microvascular (re)perfusion. Microvasc Res. 2010;79:139–43.

44. Pauling JD, Shipley JA, Raper S, Watson ML, Ward SG, Harris ND, et al. Comparison of infrared thermography and laser speckle contrast imaging for the dynamic assessment of digital microvascular function. Microvasc Res. 2012;83:162–7.

10

Oleic acid chlorohydrin, a new early biomarker for the prediction of acute pancreatitis severity in humans

Enrique de-Madaria[1], Xavier Molero[2], Laia Bonjoch[3], Josefina Casas[4], Karina Cárdenas-Jaén[1], Andrea Montenegro[2] and Daniel Closa[3*] (iD)

Abstract

Background: The early prediction of the severity of acute pancreatitis still represents a challenge for clinicians. Experimental studies have revealed the generation of specific halogenated lipids, in particular oleic acid chlorohydrin, in the early stages of acute pancreatitis. We hypothesized that the levels of circulating oleic acid chlorohydrin might be a useful early prognostic biomarker in acute pancreatitis in humans.

Methods: In a prospective, multicenter cohort study, plasma samples collected within 24 h after presentation in the emergency room from 59 patients with acute pancreatitis and from 9 healthy subjects were assessed for oleic acid chlorohydrin levels.

Results: Pancreatitis was mild in 30 patients, moderately severe in 16 and severe in 13. Oleic acid chlorohydrin levels within 24 h after presentation were significantly higher in patients that later progressed to moderate and severe acute pancreatitis. Using 7.49 nM as the cutoff point, oleic acid chlorohydrin distinguished mild from moderately severe-to-severe pancreatitis with high sensitivity/specificity (96.6/90.0%) and positive/negative predictive values (90.3/96.4%). Using 32.40 nM as the cutoff value sensitivity, specificity, positive and negative predictive values were all 100% for severe acute pancreatitis. It was found to be a better prognostic marker than BISAP score, hematocrit at 48 h, SIRS at admission, persistent SIRS or C-reactive protein at 48 h.

Conclusions: Oleic acid chlorohydrin concentration in plasma is elevated in patients with acute pancreatitis on admission and correlates with a high degree with the final severity of the disease, indicating that it has potential to serve as an early prognostic marker for acute pancreatitis severity.

Keywords: Acute pancreatitis, Chlorohydrins, Inflammation, Fatty acids, SIRS

Background

Acute pancreatitis (AP) is an abrupt inflammatory process of the pancreas that often involves peripancreatic tissues and distant organs [1] and is one of the most common causes of hospital admission due to gastrointestinal disease [2]. The severity of the disease is highly variable, ranging from a mild and self-limited form to a severe disease with local and systemic complications that may lead to multiorgan failure and death [3].

The early prediction of severity becomes a critical issue in the management of AP. When the prediction is accurate, it allows for proper patient stratification with clinical management implications: Patients predicted at risk of developing severe AP will get enhanced hemodynamic support and close monitoring aimed at prompt recognition of local or systemic complications that may require specific treatment. Unfortunately, our ability to identify with high accuracy those severe cases early in the course of the disease is still unsatisfactory. The current prediction of severity is mainly based on multifactorial scores

*Correspondence: daniel.closa@iibb.csic.es
[3] Department of Experimental Pathology, IIBB-CSIC, IDIBAPS, c/Rosselló 161, 7°, 08036 Barcelona, Spain
Full list of author information is available at the end of the article

(Ranson, Imrie, APACHE-II, BISAP, etc.) [4, 5]. However, some of them are cumbersome to calculate (APACHE-II, Ranson, Imrie) and, most importantly, these scoring systems have a limited accuracy for mortality or persistent organ failure (> 48 h) [5–8]. In addition, some reports indicate that these scoring systems are not superior to easier-to-determine biomarkers, such as blood urea nitrogen, C-reactive protein (CRP), hematocrit or creatinine [6]. In this scenario, a blood biomarker with improved accuracy in predicting severe AP (as compared to previously described predictors) would be a step forward toward better early management of patients with severe AP.

In previous studies using an experimental model of taurocholate-induced acute pancreatitis in rats, we observed the generation and release to the bloodstream of specific halogenated lipids [9]. The infiltration and activation of polymorphonuclear neutrophils in the pancreas, but also in surrounding areas of adipose tissue, result in the generation of hypochlorous acid (HOCl) from hydrogen peroxide (H_2O_2) and chloride ions, in a reaction catalyzed by myeloperoxidase (MPO) [10]. The combination of high MPO and pancreatic lipase activity results in the generation and release of fatty acid chlorohydrins (Fig. 1), being the oleic acid chlorohydrin (OAC) the most abundant of them.

It is important to note that the generation of these halogenated fatty acids requires a combination of processes that are triggered during the development of pancreatitis, particularly when the enhanced inflammatory response acquires such characteristics that herald the progression to severe AP. This inflammatory response involves the recruitment of macrophages and neutrophils to the damaged pancreas and to the surrounding adipose tissue. These cells release active MPO in the areas where large amounts of pancreatic lipase catalyze the hydrolysis of triacylglycerols from adipocytes [11]. Therefore, fatty acid chlorohydrins (and in particular OAC) generation is fostered by the combined action of two enzymatic systems (myeloperoxidase and lipase) that are overactive in severe AP. Furthermore, OAC can be released to the bloodstream and its blood levels quantitated.

Experimental studies pointed to an interesting correlation between the levels of circulating OAC and the severity of acute pancreatitis [12]. However, the potential use of plasma OAC concentration as an early biomarker

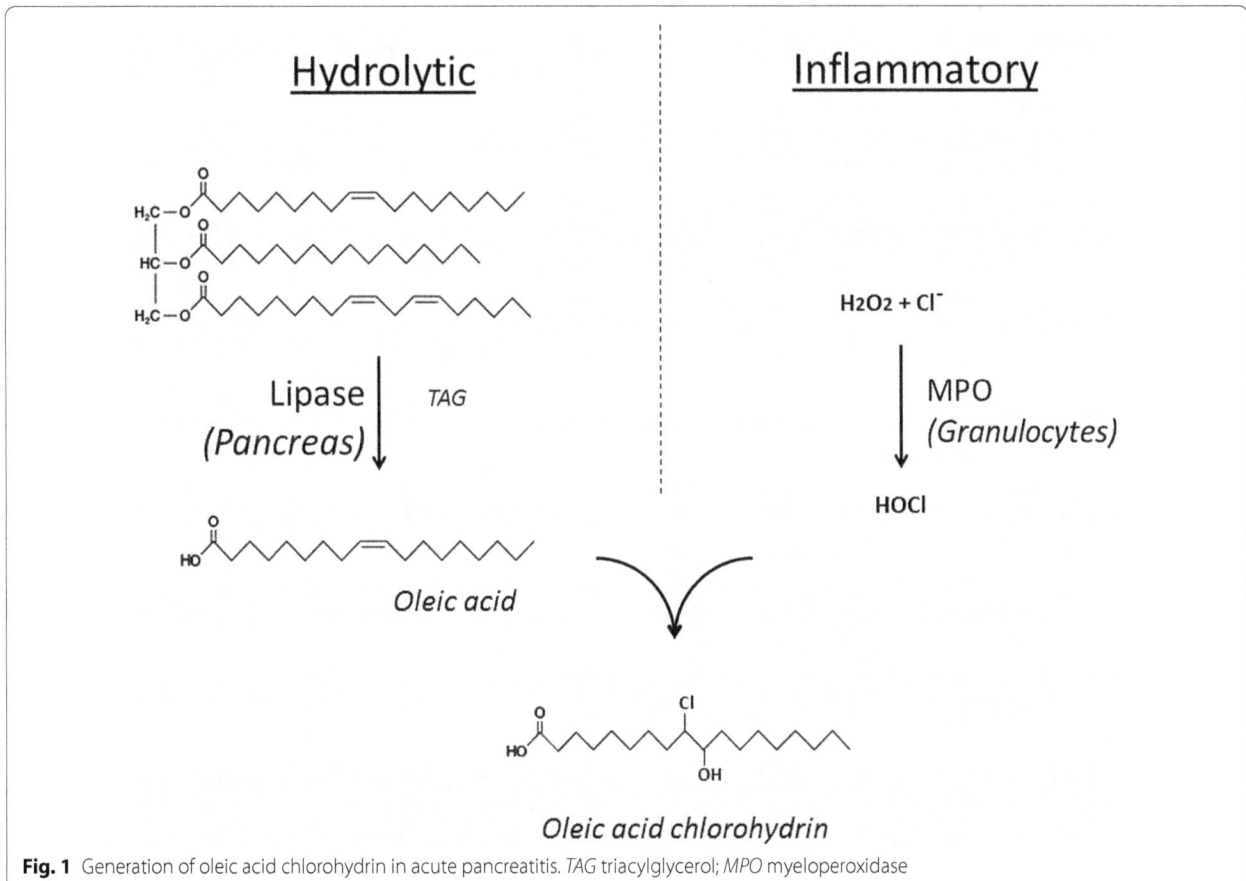

Fig. 1 Generation of oleic acid chlorohydrin in acute pancreatitis. *TAG* triacylglycerol; *MPO* myeloperoxidase

for severe AP in humans has not been evaluated yet. In this study, we assessed the effectiveness and feasibility of OAC in the early prediction of severity of acute pancreatitis in humans.

Methods

The relationship between OAC plasma levels and outcome of AP was studied in a prospective cohort of consecutive patients from two medical centers: Hospital General Universitario de Alicante (Alicante, Spain) and Hospital Universitari Vall d'Hebron (Barcelona, Spain). The study protocol was approved by the ethic committee of both centers and followed the Declaration of Helsinki Ethical Principles for Medical Research Involving Human Subjects. The patients signed an informed consent before entering the study.

Study population

Adult ($\geq$ 18 years) patients with AP were prospectively recruited for 6 months. AP was defined according to the revised Atlanta classification. At least two of the following three features should be presented: (1) abdominal pain consistent with acute pancreatitis (acute onset of a persistent, severe, epigastric pain often radiating to the back); (2) serum lipase activity (or amylase activity) at least three times greater than the upper limit of normal; and (3) characteristic findings of acute pancreatitis on contrast-enhanced computed tomography (CECT) and less commonly on magnetic resonance imaging (MRI) or on transabdominal ultrasonography [13]. We excluded patients with recurrent acute pancreatitis, chronic pancreatitis, pancreatitis due to malignancy, pregnant patients, patients with time from onset of disease to presentation in the emergency room greater than 24 h and patients being hospitalized for more than 24 h at the time of recruitment.

Variables

Local and systemic complications were defined according to the revised Atlanta classification [13], and systemic inflammatory response syndrome (SIRS) was defined according to usual criteria [14]. We compared the prognostic accuracy of OAC with other commonly used prognostic markers and scores: BISAP score [15], C-reactive protein at 48 h from presentation [16], presence of SIRS criteria at emergency room and presence of persistent SIRS (> 48 h) [17, 18] and hematocrit at emergency room higher than 44% [19]. Charlson comorbidity index was used to describe comorbidity [20].

Outcome variables were defined according to the revised Atlanta classification [13]: moderately severe-to-severe disease (presence of local or systemic complications in general), severe disease (presence of persistent organ failure) and in-hospital mortality.

Blood samples

Blood samples were collected from each patient within 24 h after presentation in the emergency room, drawn into 5-ml heparin-treated tubes and centrifuged for 10 min at 1500×g. The plasma was then collected and stored at − 40 °C until analysis. Healthy controls were recruited from hospital staff. Assessment of OAC concentration was done blindly.

Oleic acid chlorohydrin analysis by mass spectrometry

Samples were fortified with 18,18,18-d3-octadecanoic acid (20 nmol) and extracted with hexane (four volumes). The organic extract was evaporated and lipid extracts were derivatized with bis-trimethylsilyltrifluoroacetamide and injected the GC–MS system [21]. Endogenous levels of fatty acid chlorohydrins were thus quantified by selected ion monitoring (SIM).

Gas chromatography coupled to electron impact (70 eV) mass spectrometry was carried out as described [21] with minor modifications. Selected ions were those at m/z 344 and m/z 359 ([(M-CH3)$^+$ and (M)$^+$, trimethylsilyl (TMS) derivative of internal standard]; m/z 215 (TMS derivative of oleic acid chlorohydrin) and m/z 317 (common to the TMS derivatives of both the chlorohydrins of oleic and linoleic acids).

Statistical methods

Results are expressed in mean (SD), median (Q1, Q3) or n (%). Normality was assessed by means of the Shapiro–Wilk test. Quantitative variables were compared with qualitative variables by means of the Student t/Mann–Whitney tests (2 categories) or ANOVA/Kruskal–Wallis tests (> 2 categories). Qualitative variables were compared by means of the Chi-square test, with Fisher's correction when necessary. Receiver operating characteristics (ROC) curves were calculated for assessing the prognostic accuracy and for determining the best cutoff points. Sensitivity (Se), specificity (Sp) and positive/negative predictive values (PPV and NPV, respectively) were calculated. A P value less than 0.05 indicated statistical significance, but we applied the Bonferroni correction when multiple comparisons were performed. Statistical analyses were performed using SPSS 19.0 (SPSS, Inc., Chicago, Illinois, USA).

Results

Demographic, clinical and biochemical characteristics of patients

Fifty-nine patients and nine healthy subjects entered the study. Based on the revised Atlanta classification [13], 30 patients had mild AP, 16 developed moderately severe AP and 13 severe AP. As the two hospitals are transferal centers where they derived the most serious cases, the percentage of severe pancreatitis is relatively high. Patient's basal clinical characteristics as well as outcomes according to severity are shown in Table 1. Gallstones were the main etiological factor, followed by alcohol abuse and endoscopic retrograde cholangiopancreatography (ERCP). Eight patients with severe AP died (5 of them with infected pancreatic necrosis). No significant differences were observed in age, gender or BMI > 30 between groups.

Oleic acid chlorohydrin levels in plasma

Median OAC plasma concentration raised as the severity of AP increased. Significant differences in plasma OAC levels were detected among the different group categories of AP studied: mild, moderately severe and severe (Fig. 2), with lower levels in the mild acute pancreatitis group (median 2.6 nM; 1.3–5) as compared with moderate (14.7 nM; 9.1–22.65) and severe (65.2 nM; 42–71.4) groups. OAC was significantly different in all the possible comparisons between controls, mild, moderately severe and severe categories (Fig. 2). In control samples, OAC was only detected in a few samples (0.0 nM; 0–3.1).

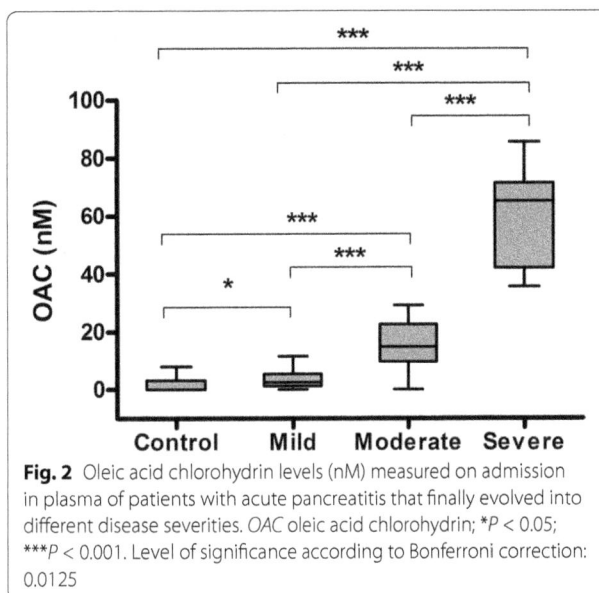

Fig. 2 Oleic acid chlorohydrin levels (nM) measured on admission in plasma of patients with acute pancreatitis that finally evolved into different disease severities. *OAC* oleic acid chlorohydrin; *P < 0.05; ***P < 0.001. Level of significance according to Bonferroni correction: 0.0125

Prognostic accuracy of OAC and other predictors

Regarding the prediction of moderately severe-to-severe AP, the ROC curves for OAC, BISAP score and CRP are shown in Fig. 3. OAC levels had a higher ROC AUC

Table 1 Demographic characteristics and outcomes of the study patients according to severity

	Global sample (n = 59)	Mild (n = 30)	Moderately severe (n = 16)	Severe (n = 13)	P
Age (years)	64 (50.5–77)	62.5 (49.5, 72.3)	66.5 (53.5, 77.8)	77 (42, 81.5)	0.5
Female sex	33 (55.9%)	19 (63.3%)	9 (56.3%)	5 (38.5%)	0.3
Etiology					0.065
Biliary	24 (40.7%)	13 (43.3%)	7 (43.8%)	4 (30.8%)	
Alcohol	8 (13.6%)	1 (3.3%)	4 (25%)	3 (23.1%)	
Post-ERCP	7 (11.9%)	3 (10%)	2 (12.5%)	2 (15.4%)	
BMI > 30 kg/m^2	14 (23.7%)	7 (23.3%)	3 (18.8%)	4 (30.8%)	0.749
BISAP score	1 (1, 2)	1 (0, 1.3)	2 (1, 3)	2 (1, 3)	0.005
Charlson index	0 (0, 1)	0 (0, 1)	1 (0, 2)	1 (2.5)	0.035
CRP at 48 h (mg/dL)	10.9 (3–24.2)	4.3 (1.8, 12.7)	19.8 (9.6, 28.4)	30.4 (23.2, 39.3)	<0.001
OAC (nM)	7 (2.3–22.6)	2.6 (1.3, 5)	14.7 (9.1, 22.6)	65.2 (42, 71.4)	<0.001
SIRS at ER	29 (49.2%)	9 (30%)	11 (68.8%)	9 (75%)	0.007
SIRS > 48 h	14 (23.7%)	0	3 (18.8%)	11 (84.6%)	<0.001
Pancreatic necrosis	9 (15.3%)	0	3 (18.8%)	6 (46.2%)	0.001
Peripancreatic necrosis	15 (25.4%)	0	9 (56.3%)	6 (46.2%)	<0.001
Infected necrosis	5 (8.5%)	0	0	5 (38.5%)	<0.001
Persistent organ failure	13 (22%)	0	0	13 (100%)	<0.001
Hospital stay (days)	12 (7–18.5)	8.5 (6, 12.3)	14 (11, 20)	32.5 (3.8, 52.3)	0.014
Mortality		0	0	8 (61.5%)	<0.001

Results in median (p25, p75) or n (%)

BISAP Bedside index of severity in acute pancreatitis, *SIRS* systemic inflammatory response syndrome, *OAC* oleic acid chlorohydrin, *CRP* C-reactive protein, *ERCP* endoscopic retrograde cholangiopancreatography, *ER* emergency room. Please note that persistent organ failure defines the severe category on the revised Atlanta classification

P statistical significance for the comparison between the mild, moderately severe and severe categories

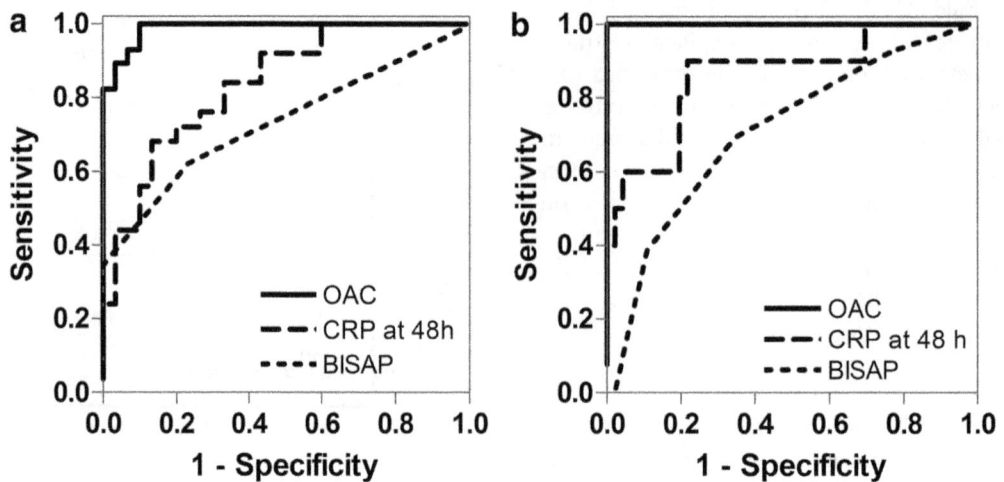

Fig. 3 ROC curves of oleic acid chlorohydrin (OAC), C-reactive protein (CRP) and BISAP score for the prediction of acute pancreatitis severity. **a** ROC curve for the prediction of moderately severe-to-severe disease. **b** ROC curve for the prediction of severe disease. *OAC* oleic acid chlorohydrin. *CRP at 48 h* C-reactive protein at 48 h from admission. *BISAP* bedside index of severity in acute pancreatitis

Table 2 Area under the receiver operating characteristics curve for the prediction of moderately severe-to-severe disease, severe disease (persistent organ failure) and mortality for oleic acid chlorohydrin, BISAP score and C-reactive protein

Outcome to predict	Predictor	AUC (95% CI)
Moderately severe-to-severe disease	OAC	0.954 (0.886–1)
	BISAP score	0.732 (0.601–0.863)
	CRP 48 h	0.837 (0.734–0.941)
Severe disease (persistent organ failure)	OAC	1
	BISAP score	0.709 (0.547–0.871)
	CRP 48 h	0.860 (0.720–1)
Mortality	OAC	0.931 (0.866–0.997)
	BISAP score	0.808 (0.668–0.948)
	CRP 48 h	0.772 (0.529–1)

AUC Area under the receiver operating characteristics curve, *CI* confidence intervals, *OAC* oleic acid chlorohydrin, *BISAP* Bedside index of severity in acute pancreatitis, *CRP 48 h* C-reactive protein at 48 h from admission

than BISAP score and CRP (Table 2). Using 7.49 nM as the cutoff point, OAC plasma concentration at admission could readily predict moderately severe or severe AP with a sensitivity of 96.6%, specificity of 90.0%, positive predictive value (PPV) of 90.3% and negative predictive value (NPV) of 96.4%. Sensitivity and NPV for OAC were higher than for other commonly used predictors (Table 3).

OAC was an excellent predictor of severe disease (and persistent organ failure), again associated with higher AUC (1) than BISAP score and CRP (Table 2; Fig. 3). Using 32.40 nM as the cutoff value, OAC predicted

severe disease with 100% sensitivity, specificity, PPV and NPV. This accuracy was higher than any other predictor evaluated in this study (Table 4).

It is interesting to note that all of the above results did not change significantly when data from patients recruited at each participating hospital were processed independently, indicating that the test performed equally well at the two hospitals.

Discussion

Early identification of severe forms of AP is essential for successful management of affected patients. Unfortunately, early reliable and sensitive predictive markers of severity are not at hand for application in clinical practice beyond popular multifactorial scores [22–24]. Moderately severe-to severe acute pancreatitis is believed to be the result of a multifactorial process that involves tissue necrosis, hydrolytic enzyme activation, release of inflammatory cytokines, generation of reactive oxygen species and synthesis of bioactive lipid mediators. In addition, some of these events take place in extra-pancreatic organs and none of them, by its own, is directly linked to the severity of the disease. Of note, pancreas-derived mediators that proved valuable for severity prediction in experimental animals have failed to predict the future course of pancreatitis when applied to human disease. The concomitant activation of different local and systemic processes explains the need for multifactorial scoring systems developed to predict the severity of AP, including Ranson criteria, APACHE-II or BISAP [5].

Fatty acid chlorohydrins are halogenated lipids generated by the action of hypochlorous acid on unsaturated

Table 3 Prognostic accuracy of OAC for moderately severe-to-severe disease compared to other widely used predictors

Variable	Se	Sp	PPV	NPV
OAC ≥ 7.49 nM	96.6	90	90.3	96.4
SIRS at ER	71.4	70	69	72.4
Persistent SIRS	48.3	100	100	65.9
HTC at ER > 44%	44.8	66.7	56.5	55.6
BISAP ≥ 3	34.5	100	100	61.2
CRP ≥ 15 mg/dL at 48 h	68	80	73.9	75

Se Sensitivity, *SP* specificity, *PPV/NPV* positive/negative predictive values, *POF* persistent organ failure, *OAC* oleic acid chlorohydrin, *SIRS* systemic inflammatory response syndrome, *HTC* hematocrit, *BISAP* bedside index of severity in acute pancreatitis, *CRP* C-reactive protein

Table 4 Prognostic accuracy of OAC for severe disease (persistent organ failure) and mortality compared to other widely used predictors

Variable	Outcome to predict	Se	Sp	PPV	NPV
OAC ≥ 32.4 nM	Severe disease	100	100	100	100
	Mortality	100	90.2	61.5	100
SIRS at ER	Severe disease	75	56.5	31	89.7
	Mortality	85.7	54.9	20.7	96.6
Persistent SIRS	Severe disease	84.6	93.3	78.6	95.5
	Mortality	75	84	42.9	95.5
HTC at ER > 44%	Severe disease	38.5	60.9	21.7	77.8
	Mortality	25	58.8	8.7	83.3
BISAP ≥ 3	Severe disease	38.5	89.1	50	83.7
	Mortality	50	88.2	40	91.8
CRP ≥ 15 mg/dL at 48 h	Severe disease	90	68.9	39.1	96.9
	Mortality	80	62	17.4	96.9

Se Sensitivity, *SP* specificity, *PPV/NPV* positive/negative predictive values, *POF* persistent organ failure, *OAC* oleic acid chlorohydrin, *SIRS* systemic inflammatory response syndrome, *HTC* hematocrit, *BISAP* bedside index of severity in acute pancreatitis, *CRP* C-reactive protein

fatty acids [10]. Although absent in control conditions, they can be released to the bloodstream during AP due to the combined effect of high lipase and MPO activities. Since this combination is characteristic of severe pancreatic/peripancreatic damage and enhanced systemic response, the presence of fatty acid chlorohydrins could only be expected to occur under the simultaneous activation of both hydrolytic and inflammatory processes that, when combined, are associated with the progression from mild to severe AP. Importantly, a number of pro-inflammatory activities have also been reported for fatty acid chlorohydrins, including the induction of P-selectin and the activation of macrophages [9, 25].

The value of lipid metabolites as indicators of increased severity of AP has been progressively recognized. There are also some clues that point to an active role of lipid

mediators in the progression of mild to severe AP, in particular on the systemic effects that may lead to organ failure. Obesity or increased intra-abdominal fat is associated with severe AP, possibly through a mechanism related to the lipotoxic action of unsaturated fatty acids released by the effect of lipase on triglycerides of visceral adipocytes. In a series of elegant experiments, Navina et al. [26] demonstrated the pathogenic role of unsaturated fatty acids released during pancreatitis on inflammation, necrosis, multisystem organ failure and mortality. The measurement of chlorohydrins of fatty acids is a further step on this direction since the presence of these molecules indicates that, in addition to the effects of hydrolytic enzymes released by the pancreas, the inflammatory microenvironment required for the halogenation of fatty acids becomes relevant in distant organs. Even when these reactions are only relevant in local scenarios, the plasma levels of OAC are ultimately related to increased severity of AP and to multiorgan failure. The experimental study in rats indicates that release of OAC depends on the action of lipase following a kinetic similar to that observed for oleic acid, whereas its final course seems to be related to the hepatic uptake of free fatty acids [9]. Chlorinated fatty acids have been reported to be catabolized by hepatocytes through ω-oxidation and subsequent β-oxidation and their final products are rapidly excreted in urine [27]. Altogether it suggests that OAC could be a useful prognostic parameter but only in the initial stages of acute pancreatitis.

Our results in human patients confirm the expectations generated in experimental studies and show the value of OAC in predicting the course and outcome of AP. OAC was particularly accurate in predicting persistent organ failure and mortality, the most important outcome variables in AP. Our data reveal that levels of OAC measured on admission allow for discriminating the different degrees of severity to be developed on the progression of the disease in the long run, which should have a direct impact on the clinical management of these patients. According to our data, OAC concentrations higher than 32.4 nM are associated with severe AP, while a cutoff value of 7.5 distinguishes mild from moderate and severe disease.

Like many other studies focusing on research of prognostic biochemical markers, our study also has a number of methodological and technical limitations. The study includes patients from two hospitals, but, as expected, the number of patients in moderate and severe groups was significantly lower than in mild group. Therefore, out of 59 patients with AP only 13 had severe pancreatitis and 16 moderately severe. Although the results obtained allow to discriminate between these three groups with a good statistical level, there is no doubt that more studies with a much higher number of patients need to be done. Anyway, OAC was very accurate to detect severity and was compared with preexisting predictors of severity that were applied to the same sample showing a lower accuracy. On the other hand, the generation of OAC through the incorporation of the HOCl to the 9,10 double bond of oleic acid results in the formation of two isomeric chlorohydrins (the 9-chloro, 10-OTMS 18:0 chlorohydrin and the 9-OTMS, 10-chloro 18:0 chlorohydrin). These compounds are not separated by the GC column and, although this limitation may have little impact on the overall results of our study, we have to acknowledge that our data indicate the sum of the two isomers. In addition, it must be taken into account that, although the measure of OAC by gas chromatography/mass spectrometry is too complex and slow to be applied to clinical practice, ELISA tests similar to those for prostaglandins and other lipid metabolites can be easily developed allowing for much faster measurements of OAC. Availability of faster and easier assays methods will make easier to confirm our results in larger samples of patients. In this line, although these encouraging results have been obtained from two independent cohorts of patients from two different and geographically remote hospital centers, they should be validated in larger cohort studies performed by other groups. In case of similar results, OAC would be, by far, the most accurate early predictor of severe acute pancreatitis ever described.

Conclusions

In summary, this study demonstrates that OAC is generated during AP, it can be measured in plasma, and its levels correlate with pancreatitis severity. Our findings indicate that oleic acid chlorohydrin is an accurate early prognostic biomarker to be used in patients with acute pancreatitis.

Abbreviations
AP: acute pancreatitis; OAC: oleic acid chlorohydrin; CRP: C-reactive protein; ROC: receiver operating characteristics; BISAP: bedside index for severity in acute pancreatitis; SIRS: systemic inflammatory response syndrome; POF: persistent organ failure.

Authors' contributions
DC, E-dM and XM conceived of the study, designed the experiments, analyzed data and wrote the manuscript. JC, LB, KC and AM obtained and processed samples and analyzed data. All authors read and approved the final manuscript.

Author details
[1] Pancreatic Unit, Department of Gastroenterology, Hospital General Universitario de Alicante, Instituto de Investigación Sanitaria y Biomédica de Alicante (ISABIAL - Fundación FISABIO), Alicante, Spain. [2] Exocrine Pancreatic Diseases Research Group, Hospital Universitari Vall d'Hebron, Institut de Recerca (VHIR), Universitat Autònoma de Barcelona, CIBEREHD, Barcelona, Spain. [3] Department of Experimental Pathology, IIBB-CSIC, IDIBAPS, c/Rosselló 161, 7°, 08036 Barcelona, Spain. [4] RUBAM, Department of Biomedicinal Chemistry, IQAC-CSIC, Barcelona, Spain.

Acknowledgements
The authors thank Alexandre Garcia for excellent technical assistance.

Competing interests
The authors declare that they have no competing interests.

Funding
This work was supported by a research grant from the Carlos III Institute of Health with reference FIS PI13/00019 and co-funded with European Union ERDF funds (European Regional Development Fund). L. Bonjoch is supported by a predoctoral fellowship from Generalitat de Catalunya (AGAUR, FI DGR 2013).

References
1. Beger HG, Rau BM. Severe acute pancreatitis: clinical course and management. World J Gastroenterol WJG. 2007;13:5043–51.
2. Peery AF, Crockett SD, Barritt AS, et al. Burden of gastrointestinal, liver, and pancreatic diseases in the United States. Gastroenterology. 2015;149(1731–41):e3.
3. Frossard J-L, Steer ML, Pastor CM. Acute pancreatitis. Lancet. 2008;371:143–52.
4. Gao W, Yang H-X, Ma C-E. The value of BISAP Score for predicting mortality and severity in acute pancreatitis: a systematic review and meta-analysis. PLoS ONE. 2015;10:e0130412.
5. Papachristou GI, Muddana V, Yadav D, et al. Comparison of BISAP, Ranson's, APACHE-II, and CTSI scores in predicting organ failure, complications, and mortality in acute pancreatitis. Am J Gastroenterol. 2010;105:435–41.
6. Mounzer R, Langmead CJ, Wu BU, et al. Comparison of existing clinical scoring systems to predict persistent organ failure in patients with acute pancreatitis. Gastroenterology. 2012;142:1476–82 (quiz e15–6).
7. Chauhan S, Forsmark CE. The difficulty in predicting outcome in acute pancreatitis. Am J Gastroenterol. 2010;105:443–5.
8. Bollen TL, Singh VK, Maurer R, et al. A comparative evaluation of radiologic and clinical scoring systems in the early prediction of severity in acute pancreatitis. Am J Gastroenterol. 2012;107:612–9.
9. Franco-Pons N, Casas J, Fabriàs G, et al. Fat necrosis generates proinflammatory halogenated lipids during acute pancreatitis. Ann Surg. 2013;257:943–51.
10. Spickett CM. Chlorinated lipids and fatty acids: an emerging role in pathology. Pharmacol Ther. 2007;115:400–9.
11. Gea-Sorlí S, Bonjoch L, Closa D. Differences in the inflammatory response induced by acute pancreatitis in different white adipose tissue sites in the rat. PLoS ONE. 2012;7:e41933.
12. Aho HJ, Suonpää K, Ahola RA, et al. Experimental pancreatitis in the rat. Ductal factors in sodium taurocholate-induced acute pancreatitis. Exp Pathol. 1984;25:73–9.
13. Banks PA, Bollen TL, Dervenis C, et al. Classification of acute pancreatitis—2012: revision of the Atlanta classification and definitions by international consensus. Gut. 2013;62:102–11.
14. Rangel-Frausto MS, Pittet D, Costigan M, et al. The natural history of the systemic inflammatory response syndrome (SIRS). A prospective study. JAMA. 1995;273:117–23.
15. Wu BU, Johannes RS, Sun X, et al. The early prediction of mortality in acute pancreatitis: a large population-based study. Gut. 2008;57:1698–703.
16. Leese T, Shaw D, Holliday M. Prognostic markers in acute pancreatitis: Can pancreatic necrosis be predicted? Ann R Coll Surg Engl. 1988;70:227–32.
17. Buter A, Imrie CW, Carter CR, et al. Dynamic nature of early organ dysfunction determines outcome in acute pancreatitis. Br J Surg. 2002;89:298–302.
18. Johnson CD, Abu-Hilal M. Persistent organ failure during the first week as a marker of fatal outcome in acute pancreatitis. Gut. 2004;53:1340–4.
19. Brown A, Orav J, Banks PA. Hemoconcentration is an early marker for organ failure and necrotizing pancreatitis. Pancreas. 2000;20:367–72.

20. Charlson ME, Pompei P, Ales KL, et al. A new method of classifying prognostic comorbidity in longitudinal studies: development and validation. J Chronic Dis. 1987;40:373–83.

21. Winterbourn CC, van den Berg JJ, Roitman E, et al. Chlorohydrin formation from unsaturated fatty acids reacted with hypochlorous acid. Arch Biochem Biophys. 1992;296:547–55.

22. Karpavicius A, Dambrauskas Z, Gradauskas A, et al. The clinical value of adipokines in predicting the severity and outcome of acute pancreatitis. BMC Gastroenterol. 2016;16:99.

23. Staubli SM, Oertli D, Nebiker CA. Laboratory markers predicting severity of acute pancreatitis. Crit Rev Clin Lab Sci. 2015;52:273–83.

24. Di M-Y, Liu H, Yang Z-Y, et al. Prediction models of mortality in acute pancreatitis in adults: a systematic review. Ann Intern Med. 2016;165:482–90.

25. Dever G, Wainwright CL, Kennedy S, et al. Fatty acid and phospholipid chlorohydrins cause cell stress and endothelial adhesion. Acta Biochim Pol. 2006;53:761–8.

26. Navina S, Acharya C, DeLany JP, et al. Lipotoxicity causes multisystem organ failure and exacerbates acute pancreatitis in obesity. Sci Transl Med. 2011;3:107.

27. Brahmbhatt VV, Albert CJ, Anbukumar DS, et al. {Omega}-oxidation of {alpha}-chlorinated fatty acids: identification of {alpha}-chlorinated dicarboxylic acids. J Biol Chem. 2010;285:41255–69.

Interstitial pneumonia with autoimmune features: an additional risk factor for ARDS?

Giacomo Grasselli[1][*] [ID], Beatrice Vergnano[2], Maria Rosa Pozzi[3], Vittoria Sala[2], Gabriele D'Andrea[4], Vittorio Scaravilli[1], Marco Mantero[5], Alberto Pesci[6,7] and Antonio Pesenti[1,5]

Abstract

Background: Interstitial pneumonia with autoimmune features (IPAF) identifies a recently recognized autoimmune syndrome characterized by interstitial lung disease and autoantibodies positivity, but absence of a specific connective tissue disease diagnosis or alternative etiology. We retrospectively reviewed the clinical presentation, diagnostic workup and management of seven critically ill patients who met diagnostic criteria for IPAF. We compared baseline characteristics and clinical outcome of IPAF patients with those of the population of ARDS patients admitted in the same period.

Results: Seven consecutive patients with IPAF admitted to intensive care unit for acute respiratory distress syndrome (ARDS) were compared with 78 patients with ARDS secondary to a known risk factor and with eight ARDS patients without recognized risk factors. Five IPAF patients (71%) survived and were discharged alive from ICU: Their survival rate was equal to that of patients with a known risk factor (71%), while the subgroup of patients without risk factors had a markedly lower survival (38%). According to the Berlin definition criteria, ARDS was severe in four IPAF patients and moderate in the remaining three. All had multiple organ dysfunction at presentation. The most frequent autoantibody detected was anti-SSA/Ro52. All patients required prolonged mechanical ventilation (median duration 49 days, range 10–88); four received extracorporeal membrane oxygenation and one received low-flow extracorporeal CO_2 removal. All patients received immunosuppressive therapy.

Conclusions: This is the first description of a cohort of critical patients meeting the diagnostic criteria for IPAF presenting with ARDS. This diagnosis should be considered in any critically ill patient with interstitial lung disease of unknown origin. While management is challenging and level of support high, survival appears to be good and comparable to that of patients with ARDS associated with a known clinical insult

Keywords: Interstitial pneumonia with autoimmune features, Lung-dominant connective tissue disease, ARDS, ECMO

Background

The term "connective tissue disease" (CTD) refers to a heterogeneous group of disease that targets the connective tissues of the body. The autoimmune CTDs are caused by overactivity of the immune system, resulting in the production of autoantibodies. Their diagnosis is based on the combination of clinical history, physical examination and laboratory and radiologic findings, according to the established diagnostic criteria [1, 2].

Clinical presentation ranges from mild symptoms to life-threatening manifestations. Up to 30% of patients with CTD require intensive care unit (ICU) admission, and the CTD is frequently diagnosed during the ICU stay [3, 4]. The main reason for ICU admission is acute respiratory failure (ARF): type and frequency of lung involvement vary among the different CTDs [5], but a typical presentation is represented by interstitial lung disease (ILD) [6, 7].

*Correspondence: giacomo.grasselli@unimi.it
[1] Dipartimento di Anestesia, Rianimazione ed Emergenza-Urgenza, Fondazione IRCCS Ca' Granda, Ospedale Maggiore Policlinico, Via Francesco Sforza 35, 20122 Milan, Italy
Full list of author information is available at the end of the article

The early recognition of the etiology of ILD (CTD, environmental exposures, drugs or idiopathic conditions) is crucial to choose the appropriate therapeutic strategy but can be really challenging. Nonetheless, a significant number of patients with ILD have clinical and/or serologic features suggesting an autoimmune etiology but do not fulfill established diagnostic criteria for a definite CTD: In these cases, different definitions have been proposed like undifferentiated CTD (UCTD) [8, 9], lung-dominant CTD (LD-CTD) [10, 11] and autoimmune-featured ILD (AIF-ILD) [12], but none of these is universally accepted. Recently, a consensus on the term "interstitial pneumonia with autoimmune features" (IPAF) has been reached by a joint European Respiratory Society (ERS)–American Thoracic Society (ATS) task force [13].

We present here for the first time a series of seven patients meeting the diagnostic criteria for IPAF requiring ICU admission for acute respiratory distress syndrome (ARDS) and multiple organ failure. Baseline characteristics and clinical outcome of IPAF patients were compared with those of the population of ARDS patients admitted in the same period.

Methods

Patient population

We retrospectively reviewed the electronic files of patients with a diagnosis of ARDS (according to the Berlin definition criteria) [14] admitted to the tertiary level ICUs of San Gerardo Hospital in Monza and of Fondazione IRCCS Ca' Granda Ospedale Maggiore Policlinico in Milan (Italy) from May 2012 to October 2016. Based on the presence or absence of a recognized risk factor for ARDS among those listed in the Berlin definition criteria [14], patients were subdivided into two groups: (1) patients with a known risk factor; (2) patients without a known risk factor. The latter group was further subdivided into two subgroups according to the presence of diagnostic criteria for IPAF [13]: a. patients with IPAF (study group); b. patients without both a recognized risk factor and not fulfilling the criteria for IPAF.

The following data at ICU admission were recorded: demographics (sex, age), comorbidities, severity scores (SAPSII and SOFA), risk factors for ARDS, PaO_2/FiO_2 (P/F) ratio, intrapulmonary shunt (Qs/Qt), ventilator and respiratory mechanics parameters [positive end-expiratory pressure (PEEP), tidal volume (Vt), plateau pressure (P_{plat}), driving pressure (ΔP), respiratory rate (RR), static respiratory system compliance (C_{rs})].

P_{plat} was measured during an end-inspiratory pause of at least 2 s ; ΔP was defined as $P_{plat} - PEEP_{tot}$; static C_{rs} was calculated as Vt/ΔP.

The following outcome data were collected: use of prone positioning, need for extracorporeal membrane oxygenation (ECMO) support, duration of invasive mechanical ventilation (IMV) and ECMO (if applicable), ICU length of stay (ICU-LOS) and ICU mortality.

IPAF was diagnosed according to the criteria described by the joint ATS–ERS task force (Table S1) [13].

In all patients with IPAF (study group) and with ARDS without known risk factors, computed tomography (CT) of the chest and bronchoalveolar lavage (BAL) were performed within 2 days from ICU admission, and their findings were reviewed according to the ATS Guidelines [15, 16]. Timing, dose and schedule of administration of steroid therapy and other eventual immunosuppressive treatments were recorded. Episodes of ventilator-associated pneumonia (VAP) occurring in IPAF patients were analyzed. Finally, in patients with IPAF we obtained long-term follow-up data on lung morphology (by CT scan), respiratory function (by spirometry) and immunological status.

Statistical analysis

Data are presented as absolute frequency (% of the included patients) or as median and interquartile range. To evaluate differences between patients' groups, the Kruskal–Wallis test and Pearson's Chi-squared test were utilized to compare continuous and nominal variables, respectively. Two-tailed values of p below 0.05 were considered statistically significant. The JMP 11 statistical program (SAS Institute Inc, Cary, NC) was used for statistical analysis.

Results

Data from 93 patients with ARDS were reviewed. As previously described, patient population was subdivided into three groups (Fig. 1): (1) patients with a known risk factor for ARDS ($n = 78$); (2) patients without risk factors but fulfilling the diagnostic criteria for IPAF ($n = 7$); (3) patients without risk factors and not meeting the criteria for IPAF ($n = 8$).

Among the 78 patients with ARDS secondary to a known clinical insult, pneumonia was the most frequent risk factor (47 cases, 13 of viral origin), as shown in Fig. 1.

Description of IPAF patients

Seven patients (four males and three females) with ARF due to a newly diagnosed ILD meeting the diagnostic criteria for IPAF were identified. Median age was 61 years (IQR 55–64); median SAPS II and SOFA scores at admission were 32 (32–36) and 11 (11–12.5), respectively. Five patients (71%) survived: Their median ICU stay was 54 (23–78) days and they were all discharged alive from the hospital. Two patients died 72 and 23 days after ICU admission, respectively (Table 1).

All patients were admitted to the hospital for acute dyspnoea and hypoxemia. Extrathoracic symptoms were

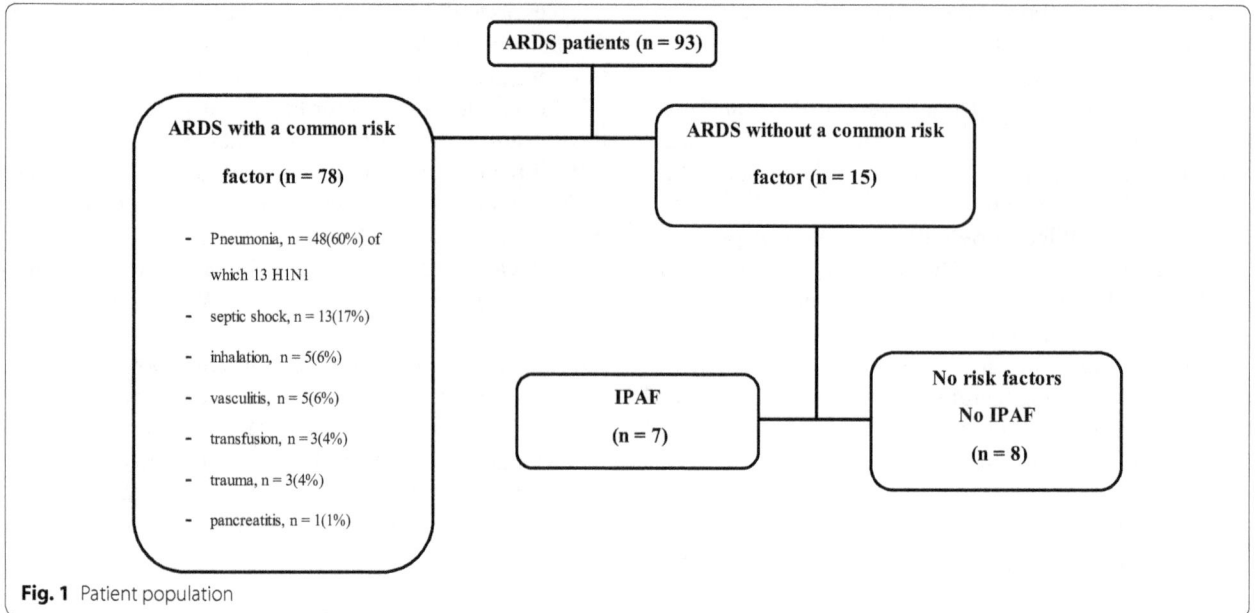

Fig. 1 Patient population

few and nonspecific (fatigue, weight loss, fever), and none had skin lesions or arthritis. No patient had previous history of ILD and/or CTD, and detailed medication and occupational history were negative.

According to the oxygenation criteria established by the Berlin definition [14], three patients had moderate and four had severe acute respiratory distress syndrome (ARDS); however, in none of them a "known clinical insult" [14] could be identified as the cause of ARDS. At admission, median P/F ratio was 120 mmHg (range 80–163) and median respiratory system compliance 26 ml/cmH$_2$O. All patients required intubation and invasive mechanical ventilation (MV). At first day of MV, median positive end-expiratory pressure (PEEP) was 12 cmH$_2$O, plateau airway pressure 26 cmH$_2$O and tidal volume 380 mL (Table 1). The time course of selected parameters during the ICU stay is depicted in Additional file 1: Figure S1. The following rescue therapies were applied: recruitment maneuvers (all patients), inhaled nitric oxide (three patients) and prone positioning (four patients). The median duration of MV was 49 days (21–81) and six subjects (85%) were tracheostomized. Five patients (71%) required an extracorporeal respiratory support with venovenous extracorporeal membrane oxygenation (ECMO) in four cases and with low-flow extracorporeal CO$_2$ removal (ECCO$_2$R) with a dedicated device (Prolung™, Estor) in one case. Three of these patients survived and the median ECMO duration was 53 days (17–63).

All patients needed vasopressor support during the ICU stay and two presented with shock at admission. One patient required continuous renal replacement therapy.

Bacterial, viral or fungal infections were excluded in all patients by means of a complete microbiological workup, consisting of cultural, serological and molecular biology tests on blood, urine and BAL samples.

Other potentially reversible causes, such as pneumothorax, pulmonary embolism, left heart failure, acute eosinophilic pneumonia and hypersensitivity pneumonia, were ruled out.

Findings of BAL samples and CT scans are detailed in Table 2. Briefly, cytomorphological analysis of BAL showed mixed alveolitis with significant lymphocytosis (>30%) in three cases and significant neutrophilia (>50%) in two other patients, without signs of viral inclusion or diffuse alveolar hemorrhage.

At CT scans, consolidations were present in all cases and mainly found in subpleural caudal areas, often associated with perilobular opacities (Fig. 2a; Additional file 1: Figure S2). Ground-glass opacities, in some cases with subpleural sparing, were also quite common but more diffuse and predominant at follow-up scans (Fig. 2b; Additional file 1: Figure S2). In four patients, mediastinal or hilar lymphadenopathies (with a diameter greater than 10 mm) were observed, while pleural effusion was present in only one case. Of the five patients who survived, two had limited or widespread organizing pneumonia (OP) consolidations; one had typical features of AIP/DAD with ground-glass opacities, patchy consolidations and fibrotic changes; one had extensive ground-glass opacities in lower lobes with some cysts suggestive of lymphocytic interstitial pneumonia (LIP) but with atypical extensive superimposition of "crazy-paving" pattern; the last one had and OP/nonspecific

Table 1 Patient characteristics, ventilator and respiratory mechanics parameters (at admission) severity scores (at admission) and clinical outcomes of the seven IPAF patients included in the study

PT	Age (years)	Sex	PEEP (cmH$_2$O)	P$_{plat}$ (cmH$_2$O)	ΔP (cmH$_2$O)	C$_{rs}$ (mL/cmH$_2$O)	P/F (mmHg)	Qs/Qt	SAPS II score	SOFA score	ICU stay (days)	MV duration (days)	ECMO duration (days)	Outcome
PT1	62	M	16	25	9	42	80	51	37	11	84	81	64	Alive
PT2	45	M	12	30	18	22	97	54	37	10	72	72	63	Dead
PT3	50	M	14	26	12	30	141	35	24	11	95	88	53	Alive
PT4	66	F	10	31	21	12	120	NA	36	13	23	21	0	Alive
PT5	61	M	14	29	15	26	163	NA	32	14	10	10	0	Alive
PT6	74	F	12	26	14	27	77	25	32	12	23	23	0 (ECCO$_2$R)	Dead
PT7	61	F	12	24	14	14	122	26	32	11	54	49	17	Alive

P$_{plat}$: end-inspiratory plateau pressure; ΔP: driving pressure; C$_{rs}$: respiratory system compliance; P/F: PaO$_2$/FiO$_2$ ratio; Qs/Qt: intrapulmonary shunt; SAPS Simplified Acute Physiology Score; SOFA Sequential Organ Failure Assessment, ICU intensive care unit, MV mechanical ventilation, ECMO extracorporeal membrane oxygenation; ECCO$_2$R: extracorporeal CO$_2$ removal; NA not available

Table 2 Autoantibodies pattern, BAL and CT scan findings of IPAF patients

PT	Autoantibodies	BAL	CT findings at presentation	ILD pattern at CT	CT findings at follow-up
PT 1	ANA; SSA/Ro52; anti-centromere	Lymphocytic cellular pattern (MA 42%; L 35%; PMN 14%; E 2%)	Extensive GGO with crazy-paving mainly in dependent zones and with subpleural sparing; consolidations in costophrenic sulci; some cystic lesions mainly in lower areas	LIP	Minimal diffuse GGO and subpleural reticulations; rare traction bronchiolectasis; enlarged cystic lesions (20 months)
PT 2	SSA/Ro52	Neutrophilic cellular pattern (MA 9%; L 0%; PMN 91%; E 0%); Foam cells +++	Focal subpleural and peribroncovascular consolidations in upper lobes and extensive consolidations of RLL, with air bronchogram	OP	Extensive parenchymal fibrosis with large bilateral pleural effusions (after 2 months of ICU stay)
PT3	SSA/Ro52	Physiological cellular pattern (MA 93%; L 2%; PMN 5%, E 0%); Foam cells +++	Subpleural consolidations with air bronchogram, mainly in lower lobes, with peribrobular consolidations in RUL	OP	Diffuse reticulations with architectural distortion and subpleural curvilinear lines; limited traction bronchiectasis (17 months)
PT 4	ANA; SSA/Ro52	Neutrophilic cellular pattern (MA 9%; L 9%; PMN 83%; E 5%)	Limited gravity-dependent consolidations with air bronchogram and GGO; some areas of perilobular consolidations	OP	Gradual development of extensive GGO with reticulations, mainly in lower lobes with traction bronchiectasis (24 months)
PT 5	Anti-Jo1; SSA/Ro52	Lymphocytic cellular pattern (MA 27%; L 57%; PMN 14%; E 2%)	Diffuse GGO with subpleural sparing and crazy paving; subpleural consolidations mainly dorsal; initial signs of fibrosis with corkscrew-like traction bronchiectasis in RUL consolidated areas	AIP/DAD	Minimal subpleural GGO with reticulations; traction bronchiolectasis in RUL (23 months)
PT 6	ANA; SSA/Ro52	Lymphocytic cellular pattern (MA 60%; L 30%; PMN 10%; E 0%)	Bilateral consolidations with air bronchogram in lower lobes and dorsal segments of upper lobes. Some GGO in lower lobes and anterior segments of upper lobes. Limited reticulations anteriorly	OP	NA
PT 7	ANA (nucleolar pattern)	Physiological cellular pattern (MA 95%; L 1%; PMN 3%, E 1%)	Bilateral quite extensive GGO in upper and lower lobes, with subpleural and peribronchovascular distribution, associated with minimal reticulations in upper lobes and limited consolidations in lower lobes	OP/NSIP overlap	NA

ANA antinuclear antibodies, RUL right upper lobe, GGO ground-glass opacities, RLL right lower lobe, MA macrophages, L lymphocytes, PMN polymorphonuclear cells, E eosinophils, LIP lymphocytic interstitial pneumonia, OP organizing pneumonia, AIP acute interstitial pneumonia, DAD diffuse alveolar damage, NA not available

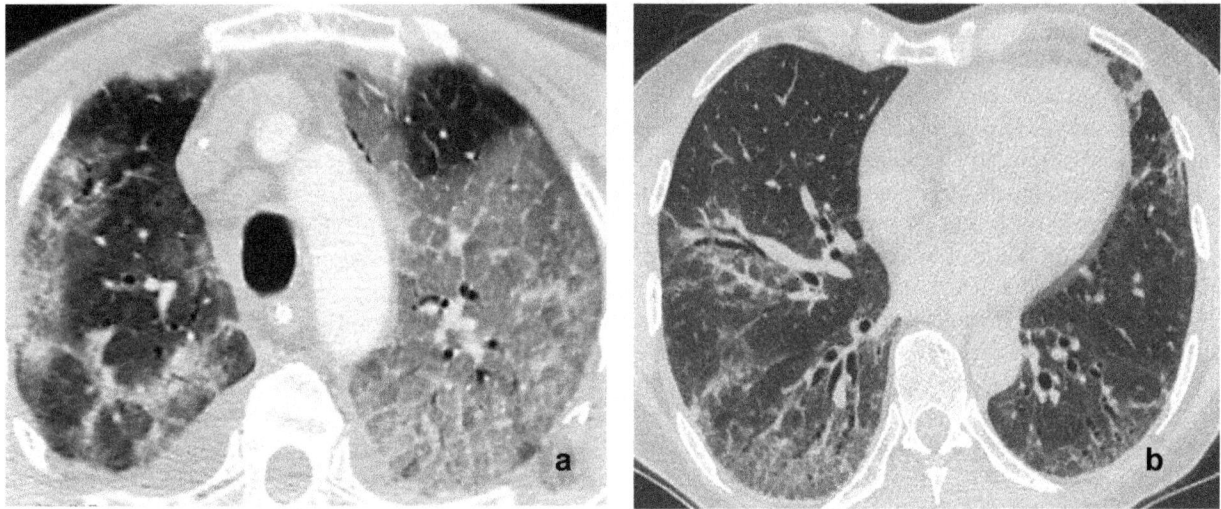

Fig. 2 a Contrast-enhanced computed tomography scan of the thorax of Patient 5 at the level of the carina at ICU admission (slice thickness 2 mm). The picture shows bilateral, diffuse ground-glass opacities with partial subpleural sparing and crazy-paving pattern. **b** Follow-up high-resolution computed tomography scan of the thorax of Patient 4 at the level of the middle lobe (slice thickness 1 mm). The picture shows bilateral, mainly dorsal ground-glass opacities with reticulations and traction bronchiectasis

interstitial pneumonia (NSIP) overlap pattern. Both patients who died had an OP pattern at presentation, but in one of them the initial OP pattern rapidly progressed to acute interstitial pneumonia/diffuse alveolar damage (AIP/DAD) pattern and he subsequently developed striking extensive fibrotic parenchymal involvement. Follow-up scans were obtained in the first four surviving patients after a median interval from hospital discharge of 20 months. Patients with OP pattern at presentation developed ground-glass opacities both in new parenchymal territories and in previously consolidated areas. Three patients developed mild to moderate signs of fibrosis (traction bronchiectasis and mild parenchymal distortion), but no patient developed honeycombing. Representative images from baseline and follow-up CT scans of the first five patients are presented in Additional file 1: Figure S2.

A complete autoantibody panel was obtained, consisting of antinuclear antibodies (ANA), anti-SSA/Ro52, anti-SSB/LA, anti-ribonucleoprotein, anti-Scl70, anti-Smith, anti-Jo1, anti-centromere, anti-double-stranded DNA, anti-neutrophil cytoplasmic antibody (ANCA), cyclic anti-citrullinated peptide and rheumatoid factor (RF). All patients had anti-SSA/Ro52; one patient had high titer ANA and anti-centromere autoantibodies and one was positive for anti-Jo1. Since no other causes of ILD were identified, extrathoracic symptoms were nonspecific and pulmonary manifestations were by far the most important, all patients met the criteria for IPAF.

All patients received immunosuppressive therapy while in ICU, after a median interval of 10 days from admission. Five of them received high doses of methylprednisolone (1000 mg/day for 3 days and then 1 mg/kg/day), followed by cyclophosphamide (10–15 mg/kg every 2–3 weeks); they also received iv immunoglobulin infusion, and two were treated with cyclosporine for inadequate response to cyclophosphamide. The remaining two patients were treated with methylprednisolone (1 mg/kg/day) without loading dose.

Five patients (71%) developed a ventilator-associated pneumonia, after a median time interval of 19 (10–31) days from admission: Pneumonia was caused by multidrug-resistant Gram-negative bacteria in three cases and by Aspergillus fumigatus in one case.

The median follow-up of the first four surviving patients was 21 months. At the last visit, forced vital capacity range was 77–112% and diffusing lung capacity for carbon monoxide 39–95% of predicted and no patient requires oxygen supplementation. Immunological follow-up examinations showed that anti-SSA/Ro52 became negative in three out of four patients. Maintenance immunosuppressive therapy with low-dose prednisone, azathioprine and mycophenolate is ongoing in three patients.

All IPAF patients, except from the two who died, gave their written informed consent to publication. Due to the retrospective nature of the study and since written consent was obtained from the study patients, ethics committee approval was waived according to local regulations.

Comparison between IPAF patients and control population

Table 3 shows the comparison of baseline characteristics and clinical outcome among the three patient groups. We did not find significant differences in regard to demographics, severity of hypoxemia (P/F ratio and Qs/Qt) and ventilator and respiratory mechanics parameters. IPAF patients tended to have a higher median SOFA score compared to both control groups (11 vs 8 vs 8.5; $p = 0.068$) and a higher frequency of use of prone positioning (86 vs 53 vs 43%; $p = 0.197$) and ECMO (71 vs 41 vs 25%; $p = 0.176$). ICU survival of IPAF patients was exactly equal to that of patients with a known risk factor (71%), while it was markedly higher than that of the patients without risk factors (38%); however, due to the small number of patients, this difference was not statistically significant. Compared to the other subgroups, IPAF patients had significantly longer median ICU-LOS (54 vs 19 vs 15.5 days; $p = 0.0045$) and duration of IMV (49 vs 17 vs 15.5 days; $p = 0.031$) and ECMO (53 vs 9.5 vs 28; $p = 0.006$).

In all the eight control patients without risk factors, microbiological and immunological screening resulted negative. Revision of chest CT scans and BAL performed in these patients did not allow the identification of a typical radiologic or cytomorphologic pattern, similarly to what observed IPAF patients. Of note, in all these patients a course of corticosteroid therapy was performed, mainly for "nonresolving ARDS."

Discussion

In this paper, we reviewed the clinical presentation, diagnostic workup and management of seven critically ill patients with IPAF. Our patients had an extremely severe clinical picture, with ARDS and multiple organ failure; they required prolonged mechanical ventilation and, in three cases, prolonged ECMO support. To the best of our knowledge, this is the first description of a cohort of patients with IPAF requiring ICU admission and invasive ventilation. Compared to the control population of ARDS patients admitted in the same period, ICU survival of patients with IPAF was equal to that of patients with ARDS associated with a known risk factor, while it was markedly higher than that of the subgroup of patients without risk factors (71 vs 38%). Hence, in our case series, IPAF patients had similar baseline characteristics and outcome to patients with ARDS associated with a recognized clinical insult, while patients without a known risk factor had a worse outcome. Of note, despite similar severity of hypoxemia and impairment of respiratory mechanics, IPAF patients had a significantly higher ICU-LOS and duration of IMV and required more frequently prone positioning and ECMO. Our findings confirm the data of Gibelin et al. [17] on a large series of ARDS patients: they observed that patients lacking exposure to common risk factors had a significantly higher mortality (66%) than other ARDS patients and found that the

Table 3 Patient characteristics, severity scores at admission, ventilator and respiratory mechanics parameters at admission and clinical outcome data in the three groups of patients included in the study

	ARDS with known risk factors	No risk factors	IPAF	p
Gender (male)	54 (69%)	1 (25%)	4 (57%)	0.763
Age (years)	55 (45–67.25)	58.5 (38.5–72.25)	61 (50–66)	0.726
SAPS II	41.5 (31–50.5)	42 (35–59)	32 (32–37)	0.133
SOFA	8 (5.75–12)	8.5 (8–11)	11 (11–13)	0.068
PaO_2/FiO_2 (mmHg)	93 (67.75–125.25)	103 (62.75–150.75)	120 (80–141)	0.515
PEEP (mmHg)	12.5 (10–15)	10 (7.25–14.75)	12 (10–14)	0.303
Compliance (mL/cmH$_2$O)	29.4 (24–37)	26.5 (16.25–43.5)	26 (14–30)	0.336
Intrapulmonary shunt (%)	35 (25–46.5)	33 (14.5–40.5)	35 (25.5–52.5)	0.588
Plateau pressure (cmH$_2$O)	28 (26–30)	27.5 (22.5–29.75)	26 (25–30)	0.796
Driving pressure (cmH$_2$O)	14 (11–18)	15.5 (10.25–21.25)	14 (12–18)	0.977
ECMO	32 (41%)	2 (25%)	5 (71%)	0.176
Tracheostomy	45 (58%)	3 (43%)	5 (71%)	0.557
Pronation	41 (53%)	3 (43%)	6 (86%)	0.197
Survival	55 (71%)	3 (38%)	5 (71%)	0.159
ICU length of stay (days)	19 (8.75–32.25)*	15.5 (5.5–35.75)*	54 (23–84)	0.045
ECMO duration (days)	9.5 (6–13)*	28 (8–48)	53 (17–63)	0.006
IMV duration (days)	17 (6–28.5)*	15.5 (5.5–34.25)*	49 (21–81)	0.031

Data are presented as absolute frequency (% of the included patients) or as median and interquartile range

IPAF interstitial pneumonia with autoimmune features, *SAPS II* Simplified Acute Physiology Score, *SOFA* Sequential Organ Failure Assessment, *PEEP* positive end-expiratory pressure, *ECMO* extracorporeal membrane oxygenation, *ICU* intensive care unit, *IMV* invasive mechanical ventilation

* $p < 0.05$ versus IPAF group

absence of known risk factors was independently associated with mortality (adjusted OR 2.06). Of note, De Prost et al. [18] recently published a secondary analysis on the cohort of ARDS patients without risk factors included in the LUNG SAFE study: ARDS without risk factors accounted for 8.3% of all ARDS cases and in 80% of these patients the etiology of ARDS was not identified.

Identification of the etiology of ILDs and their management remain a clinical challenge. The low incidence of ILD-associated ARF requiring ICU admission is a major obstacle to the assessment of outcome predictors and treatment optimization. Moreover, available studies report a high mortality among patients requiring invasive MV [7, 19, 20], ranging from 47 to 89.7%. For these reasons, ICU physicians tend to be reluctant to admit patients with ILD of uncertain etiology and are even more reluctant to administer immunosuppressive drugs in the absence of a definite diagnosis of an autoimmune disease.

Many authors have underlined the need to categorize patients with prevalent pulmonary involvement in probable autoimmune origin but with insufficient diagnostic criteria for a definite CTD. The rheumatologist would classify these patients as UCTD [8]; however, UCTD usually identifies patients with milder disease, nonspecific clinical features and low incidence of pulmonary involvement [2, 9].

Thus, Vij proposed the definition AIF-ILD [12]: Diagnostic criteria are the presence of ILD associated with at least one symptom/sign and one abnormal serologic test. In Vij's retrospective review of 200 patients with ILD, 63 were classified as AIF-ILD and had significantly lower survival rates than patients with ILD associated with a definite CTD.

An alternative classification has been presented by Fischer, who proposed the definition of LD-CTD for "cases where ILD has a rheumatologic flavor as supported by specific autoantibodies and yet does not meet criteria for a defined CTD based on the lack of adequate extrathoracic features" [11]. However, ICU physicians are still not familiar with these diagnostic categories: Neither AIF-LD nor LD-CTD was considered in the large survey published by Dumas on 363 critically ill patients with systemic rheumatic diseases [21].

In the attempt to create consensus, an ERS-ATS task force recently proposed the definition of IPAF [13], based on the combination of at least one feature from at least two of three diagnostic domains: clinical (specific extrathoracic manifestations), serologic (specific circulating autoantibodies) and morphologic (suggestive radiologic or histopathologic pattern). The main characteristics of the classification are summarized in Additional file 1: Table S1.

All our patients but one were positive for anti-SSA/Ro52: Ro52 is a protein implicated in the process of ubiquitination and is upregulated at sites of autoimmune inflammation [22]. Several studies have demonstrated that anti-Ro52 is associated with ILD in patients with CTD, particularly in anti-synthetases syndromes [23]. Anti-tRNA synthetases were detected only in one of our patients, who had anti-Jo1 positivity but did not meet the diagnostic criteria for the anti-synthetase syndrome. However, diagnostic assays for anti-tRNA synthetases other than anti-Jo1 were not routinely available in our hospitals before 2015, and this might have reduced our ability to diagnose the disease.

As noted above, the definition of IPAF requires the presence of morphologic features, namely nonspecific interstitial pneumonia (NSIP), organizing pneumonia (OP) or lymphoid interstitial pneumonia (LIP) patterns at HRTC or lung biopsy [13]. Histologic and radiologic presentation in these patients is unspecific and variable, as recently demonstrated by Omote in a series of 44 patients with LD-CTD who underwent open lung biopsy [24]: the major histologic patterns were usual interstitial pneumonia (UIP) followed by NSIP, and UIP pattern was associated with worse prognosis. Similar findings were described in two recent studies on larger cohorts of patients meeting the diagnostic criteria for IPAF: More than half of the patients had a high-confidence diagnosis of UIP pattern on CT that was associated with worse prognosis particularly when associated with honeycombing or pulmonary artery enlargement [25–27]. We did not identify any specific radiologic (CT scan) or cytologic (BAL) findings in IPAF patients; a significant lymphocytosis in BAL, which strongly suggests an autoimmune etiology, was indeed observed only in three patients. Interestingly, none of these patients had a UIP pattern on CT scan, and this may explain the good clinical outcome of our cohort. Interestingly, lack of a typical CT scan and BAL findings was observed also in control patients without common risk factors. However, we acknowledge that the correlation between lung histology and radiologic pattern at CT scan may be quite poor, especially in critically ill patients undergoing mechanical ventilation.

One important limitation of our study is the lack of histologic data, due to the high risk of serious complications when a lung biopsy is performed during mechanical ventilation and ECMO. We acknowledge that lung histology is extremely helpful in patients with ARDS of unknown origin or in cases of nonresolving ARDS, since it can provide important diagnostic and prognostic information and guide patient management [28, 29]. Another limitation resides in the very small number of patients, which limits statistical power of the analysis even in case of large differences among the subgroups; moreover, the limited sample size precluded the possibility of performing a multivariate analysis of risk factors associated with mortality.

To the best of our knowledge, this is the first report of a series of critical patients fulfilling the diagnostic criteria for IPAF requiring ICU admission for ARDS. The number of patients is small, but the patient population is very well characterized and the clinical condition is rare. We think that our patient series demonstrates that the possibility of an autoimmune etiology and in particular the diagnosis of IPAF must be considered in any critically ill patient with "ARDS" according to the Berlin definition criteria but without a known risk factor. Once the diagnosis is established, these patients should receive a "full code" treatment, including ECMO if necessary, especially if the CT scan does not show a UIP pattern with associated signs of fibrosis or pulmonary hypertension. Management of IPAF patients is really challenging, but they can have a very good outcome if the appropriate therapy is instituted: immunosuppressive treatment can lead to a significant improvement in pulmonary manifestations and should be initiated as soon as an infectious cause has been excluded.

However, selecting the appropriate diagnostic and therapeutic strategy is extremely complex and requires a multidisciplinary approach: the intensivist should become part of a team together with the rheumatologist, the pulmonologist, the radiologist and the pathologist.

Conclusions

Interstitial pneumonia with autoimmune features (IPAF) is a rare autoimmune form of interstitial lung disease that can present acutely with ARDS and multiple organ failure, requiring ICU admission and advanced life support measures (included ECMO, if needed). This diagnosis should be considered in any patient presenting with interstitial pneumonia and ARDS lacking exposure to common risk factors for ARDS. In our small cohort of patients, the clinical response to immunosuppressive therapy was good, with a survival rate equal to that of patients with ARDS associated with a known clinical insult. Findings of the present study need to be confirmed prospectively on larger patient series.

Abbreviations

AIF-ILD: Autoimmune-featured interstitial lung disease; ANA: Antinuclear antibodies; ARDS: Acute respiratory distress syndrome; ARF: Acute respiratory Failure; ATS: American Thoracic Society; BAL: Bronchoalveolar lavage; CT: Computed tomography; CTD: Connective tissue disease; ECMO: Extracorporeal membrane oxygenation; ERS: European Respiratory Society; ICU: Intensive care unit; ILD: Interstitial lung disease; IPAF: Interstitial pneumonia with autoimmune features; LD-CTD: Lung-dominant connective tissue disease; LIP: Lymphocytic interstitial pneumonia; MV: Mechanical ventilation; NSIP: Non-specific interstitial pneumonia; OP: Organizing pneumonia; RF: Rheumatoid factor; UCTD: Undifferentiated connective tissue disease; UIP: Usual interstitial pneumonia.

Authors' contributions

GG takes responsibility for the content of the manuscript and contributed substantially to the study design, data analysis and interpretation, preparation, writing and submission of this manuscript. BV, VS, MM and VS contributed to data collection and interpretation, preparation and writing of this manuscript. MRP, AP contributed to study design, data interpretation, review and final approval of the manuscript. GD analyzed all the radiologic studies and contributed to writing, review and submission of the manuscript. AP contributed to study design, review and final approval of the manuscript. All authors read and approved the final manuscript.

Author details

[1] Dipartimento di Anestesia, Rianimazione ed Emergenza-Urgenza, Fondazione IRCCS Ca' Granda, Ospedale Maggiore Policlinico, Via Francesco Sforza 35, 20122 Milan, Italy. [2] Dipartimento di Emergenza-Urgenza, Ospedale San Gerardo, Monza, Italy. [3] Dipartimento di Medicina, Unità Operativa di Reumatologia, Ospedale San Gerardo, Monza, Italy. [4] Unità Operativa di Radiodiagnostica, Ospedale San Gerardo, Monza, Italy. [5] Dipartimento di Fisiopatologia Medico Chirurgica e dei Trapianti, Università degli Studi di Milano, Milan, Italy. [6] Dipartimento di Medicina e Chirurgia, Università Milano Bicocca, Monza, Italy. [7] Clinica Pneumologica, Ospedale San Gerardo, Monza, Italy.

Acknowledgements

We are indebted to Prof. Giacomo Bellani and Prof. Francesco Blasi for their critical reading of the manuscript and for their helpful comments and suggestions.

Competing interests

Giacomo Grasselli received payment for lectures from Thermo-Fisher and Pfizer Pharmaceuticals and travel–accommodation–congress registration support from Biotest. (All these relationships are unrelated with the present work) No conflict of interest has been declared by co-authors.

Funding

No financial support was received for the study, including funding from NIH or HHMI and departmental or institutional funding

References

1. Goldblatt F, O'Neill SG. Clinical aspects of autoimmune rheumatic diseases. Lancet. 2013;382:797–808.
2. Vij R, Strek ME. Diagnosis and treatment of connective tissue disease-associated interstitial lung disease. Chest. 2013;143:814–24.
3. Janssen NM, Karnad DR, Guntupalli KK. Rheumatologic diseases in the intensive care unit: epidemiology, clinical approach, management and outcome. Crit Care Clin. 2002;18:729–48.
4. Quintero OL, Rojas-Villarraga A, Mantilla RD, Anaya JM. Autoimmune diseases in the intensive care unit. An update. Autoimmun Rev. 2013;12:380–95.
5. Cottin V. Idiopathic interstitial pneumonias with connective tissue diseases features: a review. Respirology. 2016;21:245–58.
6. Corte TJ, Copley SJ, Desai SR, Zappala CJ, Hansell DM, Nicholson AG, et al. Significance of connective tissue disease features in idiopathic interstitial pneumonia. Eur Respir J. 2012;39:661–8.
7. Zafrani L, Lemiale V, Lapidus N, Lorillon G, Schlemmer B, Azoulay E. Acute respiratory failure in critically ill patients with interstitial lung disease. PLoS ONE. 2014;9(8):e104897.
8. Mosca M, Neri R, Bombardieri S. Undifferentiated connective tissue diseases (UCTD): a review of the literature and a proposal for preliminary classification criteria. Clin Exp Rheumatol. 1999;17:615–20.

9. Kinder BW, Collard HR, Koth L, Daikh DI, Wolters PJ, Elicker B. Idiopathic nonspecific interstitial pneumonia: lung manifestation of undifferentiated connective tissue disease? Am J Respir Crit Care Med. 2007;176:691–7.

10. Fischer A, du Bois RM. Interstitial lung disease in connective tissue disorders. Lancet. 2012;380:689–98.

11. Fischer A, West SG, Swigris JJ, Brown KK, du Bois RM. Connective tissue disease-associated interstitial lung disease: a call for clarification. Chest. 2010;138:251–6.

12. Vij R, Noth I, Strek ME. Autoimmune-featured interstitial lung disease: a distinct entity. Chest. 2011;140:1292–9.

13. Fischer A, Antoniou KM, Brown KK, Cadranel J, Corte TJ, du Bois RM, et al. ERS/ATS Task Force on Undifferentiated Forms of CTD-ILD: an official European Respiratory Society/American Thoracic Society research statement: interstitial pneumonia with autoimmune features. Eur Respir J. 2015;46:976–87.

14. ARDS Definition Task Force. Acute respiratory distress syndrome: the Berlin Definition. JAMA. 2012;307:2526–33.

15. Travis WD, Costabel U, Hansell DM, King TE Jr, Lynch DA, Nicholson AG, et al. ATS/ERS Committee on Idiopathic Interstitial Pneumonias: an official American Thoracic Society/European Respiratory Society statement: update of the international multidisciplinary classification of the idiopathic interstitial pneumonias. Am J Respir Crit Care Med. 2013;188:733–48.

16. Meyer KC, Raghu G, Baughman RP, Brown KK, Costabel U, Du Bois RM, et al. American Thoracic Society Committee on BAL in Interstitial Lung Disease: an official American Thoracic Society clinical practice guideline: the clinical utility of bronchoalveolar lavage cellular analysis in interstitial lung disease. Am J Respir Crit Care Med. 2012;185:1004–14.

17. Gibelin A, Parrot A, Maitre B, Brun-Buisson C, Mekontso Dessap A, Fartoukh M, et al. Acute respiratory distress syndrome mimickers lacking common risk factors of the Berlin definition. Intensive Care Med. 2016;42:164–72.

18. De Prost N, Pham T, Carteaux G, Mekontso Dessap A, Brun-Buisson C, Fan E, Bellani G, et al. Etiologies, diagnostic work-up and outcomes of acute respiratory distress syndrome with no common risk factor: a prospective multicenter study. Ann Intensive Care. 2017;7:69.

19. Fernandez-Perez ER, Yilmaz M, Jenad H, Daniels CE, Ryu JH, Hubmayr RD, et al. Ventilator settings and outcome of respiratory failure in chronic interstitial lung disease. Chest. 2008;133:1113–9.

20. Gungor G, Tatar D, Salturk C, Cimen P, Karakurt Z, Kirakli C, et al. Why do patients with interstitial lung diseases fail in the ICU? A two-center cohort study. Respir Care. 2013;58:525–31.

21. Dumas G, Géri G, Montlahuc C, Chemam S, Dangers L, Pichereau C, et al. Outcomes in critically ill patients with systemic rheumatic disease: a multicenter study. Chest. 2015;148(4):927–35.

22. Oke V, Wahren-Herlenius M. The immunobiology of Ro52 (TRIM21) in autoimmunity: a critical review. J Autoimmun. 2012;39:77–82.

23. La Corte R, Lo Monaco A, Locaputo A, Dolzani F, Trotta F. In patients with antisynthetase syndrome the occurrence of anti-Ro/SSA antibodies causes a more severe interstitial lung disease. Autoimmunity. 2006;39:249–53.

24. Omote N, Taniguchi H, Kondoh Y, Watanabe N, Sakamoto K, Kimura T, et al. Lung-dominant connective tissue disease. Clinical, radiologic and histologic features. Chest. 2015;148:1438–46.

25. Oldham JM, Adegunsoye A, Valenzi E, Lee C, Witt L, Chen L, et al. Characterisation of patients with interstitial pneumonia with autoimmune features. Eur Respir J. 2016;47:1767–75.

26. Luppi F, Wells AU. Interstitial Pneumonia with Autoimmune Features (IPAF): a work in progress. Eur Respir J. 2016;47:1622–4.

27. Chung JH, Montner SM, Adegunsoye A, Lee C, Oldham JM, Husain AN, et al. CT findings, radiologic-pathologic correlation, and imaging predictors of survival for patients with interstitial pneumonia with autoimmune features. Am J Roentgenol. 2017;208:1229–36.

28. Guerin C, Bayle F, Leray V, Debord S, Stoian A, Yonis H, et al. Open lung biopsy in nonresolving ARDS frequently identifies diffuse alveolar damage regardless of the severity stage and may have implications for patient management. Intensive Care Med. 2015;41:222–30.

29. Aublanc M, Perinel S, Guerin C. Acute respiratory distress syndrome: the role of lung biopsy. Curr Opin Crit Care. 2017;23:24–9.

12

Point-of-care ultrasonography in Brazilian intensive care units: a national survey

José Augusto Santos Pellegrini[1], Ricardo Luiz Cordioli[2,3,7*], Ana Cristina Burigo Grumann[4], Patrícia Klarmann Ziegelmann[5] and Leandro Utino Taniguchi[6]

Abstract

Background: Point-of-care ultrasonography (POCUS) has recently become a useful tool that intensivists are incorporating into clinical practice. However, the incorporation of ultrasonography in critical care in developing countries is not straightforward.

Methods: Our objective was to investigate current practice and education regarding POCUS among Brazilian intensivists. A national survey was administered to Brazilian intensivists using an electronic questionnaire. Questions were selected by the Delphi method and assessed topics included organizational issues, POCUS technique and training patterns, machine availability, and main applications of POCUS in daily practice.

Results: Of 1533 intensivists who received the questionnaire, 322 responded from all of Brazil's regions. Two hundred and five (63.8%) reported having access to an ultrasound machine dedicated to the intensive care unit (ICU); however, this was more likely in university hospitals than in non-university hospitals (80.6 vs. 59.6%; risk ratio [RR] = 1.35 [1.16–1.58], $p = 0.002$). The main applications of POCUS were ultrasound-guided central vein catheterization (49.4%) and bedside echocardiographic assessment (33.9%). Two hundred and fifty-eight (80.0%) reported having at least one POCUS-trained intensivist in their staff (trained units). Trained units were more likely to perform routine ultrasound-guided jugular vein catheterization than non-trained units (38.6 vs. 16.4%; RR = 2.35 [1.31–4.23], $p = 0.001$). The proportion of POCUS-trained intensivists and availability of a dedicated ultrasound machine were both independently associated with performing ultrasound-guided jugular vein catheterization (RR = 1.91 [1.32–2.77], $p = 0.001$) and (RR = 2.20 [1.26–3.29], $p = 0.005$), respectively.

Conclusions: A significant proportion of Brazilian ICUs had at least one intensivist with POCUS capability in their staff. Although ultrasound-guided central vein catheterization constitutes the main application of POCUS, adherence to guideline recommendations is still suboptimal.

Keywords: Ultrasonography, Critical care, Survey

Background

Point-of-care ultrasonography (POCUS) has recently become a useful and widely disseminated tool that intensivists are incorporating into clinical practice. Assimilation timeframe varies according to the geographic, economic, and structural characteristics in which the practitioner is working. POCUS assists physicians to diagnose different causes of clinical deterioration and respiratory and/or hemodynamic failure, to tailor medical interventions (e.g., fluid therapy and mechanical ventilation adjustments), and to guide invasive procedures [1–3].

Despite guidelines that recommend the use of POCUS in different scenarios of critical care [3, 4], the incorporation of ultrasonography into clinical practice is not

*Correspondence: rlcordioli@gmail.com
[7] Department of Intensive Care Unit, Hospital Israelita Albert Einstein, 627, Albert Einstein St., São Paulo 05652-900, Brazil
Full list of author information is available at the end of the article

straightforward. For central venous catheterization (CVC), recent data showed that 18% of French intensivists reported that they routinely use ultrasonography [5], while 44% and 37% of emergency medicine specialists [6] and anesthesiologists [7], respectively, reported never using ultrasonography for CVC guidance.

Previous studies assessed the implementation of POCUS in critical care [5, 8–10]. Methodologies for collecting data were varied: while some authors applied electronic mailing and waited for spontaneous return, or based their findings on self-reported previous experience, others adopted cross-sectional epidemiological sampling consisting of punctual observations [9]. Similar studies revealing ultrasonographic patterns of use in intensive care units (ICUs) in developing regions are still lacking.

Brazil's large territory and policies of public health system organization lead to challenges in access of health care personnel to the population, access to medical education, and the incorporation of new technologies into clinical practice. Therefore, precise information about regionalization, training methods, and preferential applications could help guide national entities in achieving more efficient dissemination of ultrasonography across Brazilian ICUs, potentially improving the quality of delivered care.

Surveys are standard tools that are increasingly used for assessing various aspects of health care, including educational, technological, and organizational aspects [11], as well as for investigating translation from scientific research to clinical practice [12]. Consisting of descriptive or explanatory questions, surveys can support the incorporation of medical evidence in current patient care.

Therefore, the purpose of our study was to utilize a survey to assess current practice and education of POCUS by Brazilian intensivists, as well as to assess the dissemination of ultrasonography and main applications in ICUs across Brazil. By evaluating the frequency of use and barriers of implementing ultrasonography, we can identify gaps in medical education and incorporate recommended clinical practices to critical care.

Methods

This study was conducted with the logistic support of AMIBNet (the Brazilian network of research in intensive care) and *Ecografia em Terapia Intensiva* (ECOTIN), the national training program of POCUS for intensivists. No financial support was received from any source.

The ECOTIN program is an initiative of the Brazilian Intensivists Medical Association (AMIB), which was conceived in 2010. It consists of a board of POCUS experts who developed a teaching method and conduct short duration courses throughout Brazil. The ECOTIN course encompasses physical principles of ultrasound, knobology, echocardiographic and lung ultrasound basic techniques, as well as incorporating supervised, practical activities to allow participants to demonstrate expertise acquisition.

Questions were selected using the Delphi method. Four of the authors developed a set of questions of interest, which were then subjected to three rounds of appreciation. One author served as a facilitator, assessing agreement among the other three authors and providing feedback between rounds. Rounds were stopped when consensus was reached for all questions in the set. No physical meetings occurred. All of the panel members are formally certified intensivists and well-known experts in POCUS techniques and teaching. Three of the panel members are from the board of the ECOTIN group.

The survey consisted of 32 questions (Additional file 1) assessing the geographic location, type of hospital and type of ICU, availability of an ultrasound (US) machine, training in POCUS techniques, use and daily practice of US-guided CVC and other applications of POCUS (e.g., echocardiography, measuring the optic nerve sheath diameter, lung and abdominal studies), medical residents' education in POCUS, and perceived barriers to the implementation of ultrasonography. All questions focused on POCUS performed by intensivists, not on complementary exams done by other physicians (e.g., radiologist or cardiologist). Skip logic was used when appropriate to ease the burden on respondents.

A web-based platform (SurveyMonkey®, www.surveymonkey.com) was used for the survey according to recent recommendations [12]. Initially, a group of 12 ICU physicians tested the questionnaire. After an interval of 3 weeks, a retest was performed by the same 12 physicians to verify reliability. The survey was physician-centered and was directly sent to intensivists subscribed to the AMIBnet mailing list. The questionnaire was available for 6 months (from September 2016 to March 2017). Reminders were sent via e-mail to potential participants on three occasions, every 2 months.

Survey respondents were stratified according to the training status of POCUS: trained versus non-trained. Trained status was dependent on having at least one intensivist with formal POCUS training working in the ICU staff. Additionally, questions gathered data on the proportion of staff that were trained in POCUS.

Statistical analysis

Categorical variables were presented as absolute numbers and percentages and compared using the Chi-square test with standardized adjusted residuals analysis (for tables larger than 2×2) and the Fisher exact test (for 2×2 comparisons). A two-sided p value < 0.05 was considered statistically significant. Risk ratios (RRs) and 95% confidence intervals were calculated for associated measurements.

Multivariate analysis through Poisson linear models with robust estimation were constructed to identify variables that are independently associated with an important quality-of-care marker: US-guided internal jugular vein (IJV) puncture, in compliance with international guidelines [13–15]. A priori interest factors were those plausibly associated: the type of institution (university vs. non-university), presence of an intensivist on a daily basis, availability of a dedicated US machine, intensivists' formal certification in critical care, proportion of POCUS-trained intensivists (low vs. high level), and payoff. For the construction of the multivariate model, we used forced simultaneous entry—all candidate variables remained in the model regardless of statistical significance. Outputs from this analysis are summarized as RRs.

All analyses were performed using Statistical Package for Social Science (SPSS), version 21.0 (IBM Corp., Armonk, NY, USA).

Results
Characteristics of the study population
From September 2016 to March 2017, 1533 intensivists were contacted by electronic mail. Of these, 322 responded (20.7% response rate) from all Brazilian regions. Of the units where respondents were working, private hospitals represented 46% while clinical-surgical units represented 72%. Three hundred and three units (94%) had a certified ICU physician attending daily rounds (Table 1).

Two hundred and five (63.8%) of the respondents stated that they had access to a US machine dedicated to the ICU (Table 2). There were disparities throughout Brazil's territory in this subject ($p=0.017$). Availability of a dedicated US machine was more likely in university than in non-university hospitals (80.6 vs. 59.6%, respectively; RR = 1.35 [1.16–1.58], $p=0.002$).

US-guided CVC was the main indication of POCUS, representing 49.4% of indications, followed by bedside echocardiography (33.9%). Pleuropulmonary and abdominal ultrasonographic examinations were infrequently reported (8.5 and 8.2%, respectively). According to 59% of the respondents, chest x-rays are performed on a daily basis in more than 50% of the patients. This was negatively associated with the frequency of lung ultrasound examination ($p=0.028$).

Sixteen respondents (5.1%) stated that they use a prespecified form for summarizing data concerning examinations. The exam results images and clips) were electronically recorded 14.6% of the time.

Table 1 Baseline characteristics of the study population

Characteristic	n (322)
Region within Brazil	
Southwest	191 (59.7)
South	58 (18.1)
Northeast	43 (13.4)
Central-West	19 (5.9)
North	9 (2.8)
Hospital's type	
Private	148 (46)
Public	107 (33.2)
University	67 (20.8)
ICU type	
Mixed, clinico-surgical	231 (72)
Clinical	43 (13.4)
Pediatrics	22 (6.8)
Surgical	13 (4.0)
Trauma	12 (3.7)
Number of beds	
< 10	130 (40.5)
11–20	107 (33.2)
21–40	47 (14.6)
> 41	37 (11.5)
Attendance of a certified intensivist during daily rounds	
Full-time (morning and afternoon)	151 (46.9)
Part time (morning or afternoon)	152 (47.2)
None	19 (5.9)

ICU intensive care unit

Competence and training of POCUS
Two hundred fifty-eight (80.0%) respondents reported to have at least one intensivist with formal POCUS training working in their staff (Table 3). We designated these as trained units for the following comparisons. We did not identify significant differences across Brazil's territory according to training. The most frequently reported training structure was one- to two-day courses (65%).

ECOTIN trained 53% of the participants. The implementation of the ECOTIN training method was associated with the type of hospital: 67 and 49% of university and non-university hospital workers reported ECOTIN training, respectively (RR = 1.35 [1.1–1.67], $p=0.013$). ECOTIN training prevalence was heterogeneous among Brazil's regions ($p=0.001$).

Medical residents were present in 69% of the units, including critical care medicine residents in 44%. There were no structured training modules for US-guided CVC in 54% of cases. Twenty-six respondents (8.1%) said that their residents use simulation techniques to learn how to perform US-guided CVC.

Table 2 POCUS characteristics

Characteristic	n (322)
Dedicated ultrasound machine availability	
No	116 (36.1)
Yes, without Doppler imaging	35 (10.9)
Yes, with Continuous and Pulsatile Doppler	63 (19.6)
Yes, with Continuous, Pulsatile and Tissue Doppler	107 (33.3)
Proportion of patients assessed by POCUS on a regular basis	
<10%	124 (39)
11–25%	100 (31.4)
26–50%	55 (17.3)
51–75%	22 (6.9)
>75%	17 (5.3)
POCUS type	
US-guided CVC insertion	156 (49.4)
Cardiac assessment	107 (33.9)
Lung	27 (8.5)
Abdominal	26 (8.2)
POCUS recording	
No recording	170 (54.5)
Registered on patient's records	102 (32.7)
Electronically stored and registered on patient's records	47 (14.6)
Medical report formally provided	16 (5.1)
Payoffs	
None	278 (90.3)
Only for the institution	13 (4.2)
Only for the physician	4 (1.3)
For both the institution and the physician	13 (4.2)

POCUS point-of-care ultrasound, *US* ultrasound, *CVC* central vein catheterization

Table 3 Medical trainment in POCUS

Characteristic	n (322)
Trainment status	
Yes—ECOTIN	60 (18.7)
Yes—ECOTIN and other courses	111 (34.6)
Yes—only other courses	87 (27.1)
None	63 (19.6)
Trainment modality	
1–2 days courses	163 (65.2)
2 days–1 week	46 (18.4)
1 week–1 month	8 (3.2)
>1 month	33 (13.2)
Proportion of medical staff trained in POCUS	
<10%	125 (50)
11–25%	68 (27.2)
26–50%	38 (15.2)
51–75%	11 (4.4)
>76%	8 (3.2)
Medical residents	
Yes—Critical care medicine	138 (44.1)
Yes—Other specialties	76 (24.3)
None	99 (31.6)
Medical residents POCUS training modality	
Practice-based only	118 (54.1)
Lecture-based trainment available	44 (20.2)
Simulation-based	26 (11.9)
No trainment	30 (13.8)

POCUS point-of-care ultrasound, *ECOTIN* ecografia em terapia intensiva

As aforementioned, we stratified respondents and their respective units into trained versus non-trained units based on self-reporting of training. We observed that the training status in POCUS affected the pattern of some answers (Table 4), such as availability of a dedicated US machine, proportion of patients assessed by POCUS and the density of certified intensivists.

The most frequent POCUS applications were distinct according to individual capability ($p < 0.001$; Fig. 1a): US-guided CVC and pulmonary ultrasonography was positively associated with trained individuals.

The status of POCUS training was negatively associated with exam payoff: fourteen (5.6%) of the trained units reported payoffs, compared to 27.6% of the non-trained units (RR = 0.20 [0.11–0.39], $p < 0.001$).

US-guided CVC

According to the study participants, 58.5% of the units dealt with a monthly incidence density of less than 200 catheter-days and, in 54.5% of the cases, a catheter-related bloodstream infection of less than 2 events per 1000 catheter-days. The two most common approaches for CVC were the US-guided IJV (36.2%) and landmark-guided subclavian vein approaches (35.6%).

Respondents were questioned about the frequency with which CVC is US-guided in their units. In 22.8% of cases, IJV catheterization was "always" guided (in line with international guidelines). The most frequent answer was "only in specific situations" (45%). One hundred thirty-one (40.7%) of the participants classified the recommendations for routine use of ultrasonography when catheterizing the IJV as "weak". For subclavian access, 78% of the respondents reported "rarely" using US, while 5% reported routinely using it; two hundred twenty-seven (70.5%) physicians classified the recommendation supporting US for subclavian puncture as "weak".

Patterns of preferences for CVC according to training status are represented in Fig. 1b. US-guided IJV was the first choice for trained individuals (41%), in contrast to the landmark-guided subclavian approach (48.4%) for those not trained. Overall, eighty-five percent of non-trained individuals preferred landmark-guided CVC.

Table 4 Competence and POCUS

Characteristic	Trained (258)	Not trained (63)	Risk Ratio (95% CI)	p value
Dedicated ultrasound machine	184 (71.3)	22 (34.9)	2.04 (1.44–2.89)	<0.001
High intensity of certified intensivists	160 (62)	21 (33.3)	1.86 (1.29–2.67)	<0.001
>10% of patients assessed by POCUS on daily basis	165 (64.7)	29 (46.8)	1.38 (1.04–1.83)	0.013
Routine US-guided IJV catheterization	96 (38.6)	10 (16.4)	2.35 (1.31–4.23)	0.001
Payoff	14 (5.6)	16 (27.6)	0.20 (0.11–0.39)	<0.001

POCUS point-of-care ultrasound, *CI* confidence interval, *US* ultrasound, *IJV* internal jugular vein

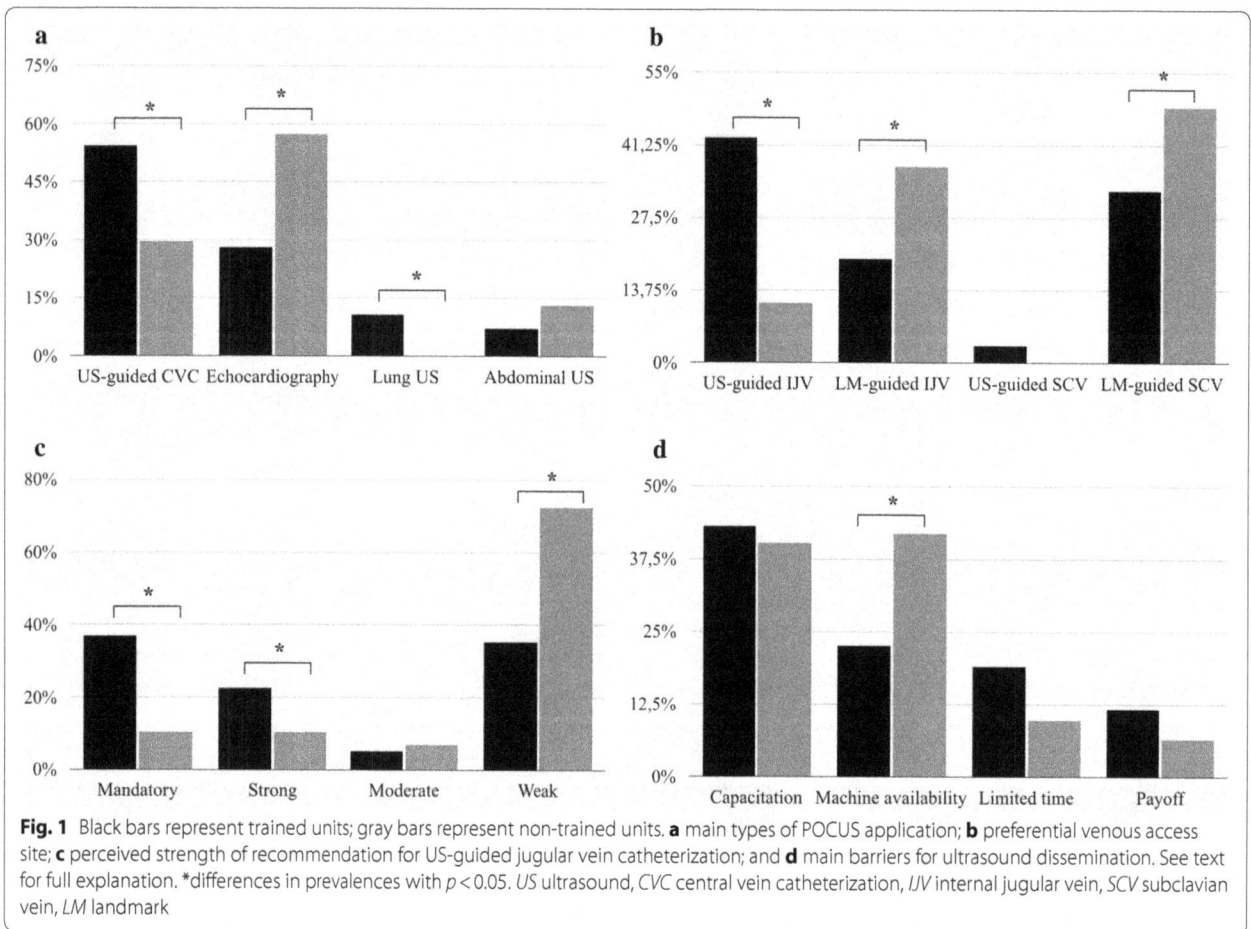

Fig. 1 Black bars represent trained units; gray bars represent non-trained units. **a** main types of POCUS application; **b** preferential venous access site; **c** perceived strength of recommendation for US-guided jugular vein catheterization; and **d** main barriers for ultrasound dissemination. See text for full explanation. *differences in prevalences with p < 0.05. *US* ultrasound, *CVC* central vein catheterization, *IJV* internal jugular vein, *SCV* subclavian vein, *LM* landmark

Physicians' perception about strength of recommendation for US-guided IJV catheterization appears to be affected by their training status. While answers of "routine use" or "strong recommendation" were associated with trained units, "weak recommendation" was associated with non-trained units (p < 0.001; Fig. 1c). For the subclavian route, the same pattern was identified (p < 0.001).

Other invasive procedures that were reported to be "usually" US-guided included thoracentesis (49%), paracentesis (31.5%), and arterial line insertion (27%).

Routine US-guided IJV puncture

Routine US (defined as more than two-thirds of the time) was used by 38.6% of the trained individuals compared to 16.4% of the non-trained ones (RR = 2.35 [1.31–4.23], p = 0.001).

Most of the factors plausibly associated with routine US-guided IJV puncture (as defined above) were statistically associated in univariate analysis (all factors except payoff). Considering multivariate analysis, two factors maintained independent association: dedicated ultrasound machine availability (RR = 2.20 [1.26–3.29],

$p=0.005$) and proportion of POCUS-trained intensivists (RR $=1.91$ [1.32 - 2.77], $p=0.001$) (Additional file 2: Table S1).

Barriers for nationwide dissemination of POCUS

One hundred thirty-three (41.3%) of the respondents answered that physicians' training was the greatest barrier in the dissemination of ultrasonography across the Brazilian territory. When comparing the types of institutions, private hospitals responded differently ($p=0.012$); in these institutions, limited intensivist time when considering other tasks was more relevant than medical capability or other limitations.

Main barriers to the dissemination of ultrasonography according to the training status are represented in Fig. 1d. Non-trained respondents were more likely to classify the availability of a dedicated US machine as the most relevant barrier (not training itself) ($p=0.021$).

Discussion

The main findings of this survey can be summarized as follows: (1) availability of a dedicated US machine in Brazilian ICUs is still suboptimal; (2) US-guided CVC insertion is the main application of POCUS, followed by echocardiography, and lung ultrasonography is rarely performed; (3) a large proportion of assessed intensivists are trained in POCUS, but as there is a predominance of courses with a short duration and workshop structure, medical residents are being trained in POCUS in an unstructured fashion); and 4) training is associated with several aspects of POCUS application, including US-guided IJV catheterization, an important marker of quality of care regarding ultrasonography in critical care medicine.

Availability of a dedicated US machine is obviously a fundamental aspect for the dissemination of POCUS. While two-thirds of the respondents in this study reported having this machine in their units, authors in other countries [8, 16] have reported higher rates. Some specific regions in Brazil and non-university hospitals were less likely to have a dedicated US machine. Our results indicated that a dedicated US machine is independently associated with adherence to US-guided IJV catheterization.

Similar rates of training in POCUS were reported from 70 to 81% in Europe and the United States [6, 8, 9], although precise information concerning the training structure and specific curriculum is scarce. Other authors [5] have reported even higher rates. Our results on this subject, however, are unique: although previous studies [5, 6, 8] have focused on specific areas within POCUS education (e.g., US-guided venous catheterization or echocardiography), we assessed general aspects

of ultrasonography of the critically ill. Additionally, we aimed to directly assess the intensivists and their self-perception of training, in contrast to previous studies [9] that designed questionnaires for ICU coordinators regarding their medical staff's capability. Medical residents in Brazil are beginning to learn ultrasonography in their education, although this is done in an unstructured and potentially heterogeneous way.

POCUS training issues are one of the major challenges of ultrasound dissemination in Brazil and other low- and middle-income countries. When heterogeneous training modalities coexist, it is difficult to ensure that all kinds of training provide comparable efficacy and competence acquisition. Standardization of training structures, both for medical residents and for those already working as intensivists, is needed, as those training structures influence intensivists' perceptions and use of evidence-based practices.

Reaching a balance between uniform accessibility to US machines and achieving minimum requirements of quality in care delivery remains an important future objective for Brazil. Realistic simulation should be provided in a method that is scalable and replicable. Medical associations of developing countries should contextualize international recommendations on POCUS training [17, 18] for specific guidelines in Brazilian (and other developing country) contexts.

Zielezkiewicz et al. [9] demonstrated in a 1-day prevalence study in Europe that 13% of the POCUS examinations performed were for central venous puncture, and that nearly half of the CVCs were US-guided. In the present survey, we assessed physicians' self-reporting practice, not real procedures; nevertheless, US-guided CVC insertion was identified as the major indication for POCUS by Brazilian intensivists. This behavior was also more pronounced in environments with a high level of training: the proportion of trained staff was identified as independently associated with adherence to US-guided IJV puncture. Overall adherence to routine US-guided IJV catheterization recommendations was relatively low (22.8%), compared to other critical care scenarios [19–21].

Lung ultrasonography, although infrequently reported, also showed a positive association with educational status. Lung ultrasound prevalence was negatively associated with routine chest x-ray, indicating a potential role of POCUS in reducing radiation exposure. This finding, however, is exploratory due to low adherence to lung ultrasound examination in this study. Other authors have previously reported similar data [22, 23].

Our results contrast with other studies, as US-guided CVC insertion represents the major indication for POCUS in Brazil. This could be explained by several reasons: the evidence concerning CVC guidance is solid, reducing adverse event rates and improving procedural success; the learning curve for US-guided IJV catheterization appears to be smoother than, for example, cardiac assessment and hemodynamic monitoring; some of the US machines available in Brazilian ICUs are relatively basic technology, and do not offer Doppler techniques or cardiac assessment software.

Our study has several limitations. First, inherent self-selection bias can influence our results. Physicians who already use ultrasonography were more likely to complete the survey; however, we obtained answers from a wide range of respondents from all Brazilian regions, representing private and public institutions, as well as clinical, surgical, and mixed units. Second, self-reporting, while providing direct answers from the practitioner, risks data precision. Instead of obtaining objective real-time measures, our study was based on physicians' impressions, which could be a distorted representation of actual practices. This limitation has been previously recognized [24]. Third, as we obtained direct responses from the intensivists, large ICUs could be redundantly represented, which could also bias our results. Nevertheless, our sample consisted of intensivists working in small units (40.5% had less than 10 beds) with part time intensivist presence (47.2%), indicating that although some degree of redundancy may have occurred, it was likely of minor influence to our results. Finally, we aimed to construct direct, objective questions that could reduce misunderstanding as much as possible. Our intention was to minimize the survey burden effect [25] that could potentially minimize our return rate. Nevertheless, our questionnaire was validated in a standard way, as previously described [12].

Conclusions

The rate of dissemination of POCUS in Brazilian ICUs is nearing rates reported in other countries. Although US-guided CVC insertion constitutes the main application of POCUS, adherence to international recommendations remains suboptimal. POCUS training, although including various relevant aspects of care, is heterogeneous, as is medical resident education regarding POCUS. Future research could address these gaps and help to better achieve POCUS dissemination in developing countries.

Abbreviations

CVC: central venous catheterization; ECOTIN: Ecografia em Terapia Intensiva (ultrasonography in intensive care); ICU: intensive care unit; IJV: internal jugular vein; POCUS: point-of-care ultrasonography; RR: risk ratio; US: ultrasound.

Authors' contributions
Drs. JASP and LUT had full access to all data and take responsibility for the writing of the manuscript, the integrity of the data and the accuracy of the final analysis. Dr. Ziegelmann was responsible for biostatistical consultation and data interpretation. Dr. Cordioli and Grumann contributed substantially to the study design, data acquisition, and analysis and interpretation of the results. All authors read and approved the final manuscript.

Author details
[1] Department of Critical Care Medicine, Hospital de Clínicas de Porto Alegre, Universidade Federal do Rio Grande do Sul, Porto Alegre, Brazil. [2] Department of Critical Care Medicine, Hospital Israelita Albert Einstein, São Paulo, Brazil. [3] Department of Critical Care Medicine, Alemão Oswaldo Cruz Hospital, São Paulo, Brazil. [4] Department of Critical Care Medicine, Nereu Ramos Hospital, Florianópolis, Brazil. [5] Statistics Department and Post-Graduation Program in Epidemiology, Universidade Federal do Rio Grande do Sul, Porto Alegre, Brazil. [6] Department of Critical Care Medicine, Hospital das Clínicas de São Paulo, FMUSP, São Paulo, Brazil. [7] Department of Intensive Care Unit, Hospital Israelita Albert Einstein, 627, Albert Einstein St., São Paulo 05652-900, Brazil.

Acknowledgements
The authors would like to thank the FIPE-HCPA (Fundo de Incentivo à Pesquisa of Hospital de Clínicas de Porto Alegre) for their support in manuscript publication.

Competing interests
The authors declare that they have no competing interests.

References
1. Lichtenstein D, van Hooland S, Elbers P, Malbrain ML. Ten good reasons to practice ultrasound in critical care. Anaesthesiol Intensive Ther. 2014;46(5):323–35.
2. Cardenas-Garcia J, Mayo PH. Bedside ultrasonography for the intensivist. Crit Care Clin. 2015;31(1):43–66.
3. Frankel HL, Kirkpatrick AW, Elbarbary M, Blaivas M, Desai H, Evans D, et al. Guidelines for the appropriate use of bedside general and cardiac ultrasonography in the evaluation of critically ill patients—part I: general ultrasonography. Crit Care Med. 2015;43(11):2479–502.
4. Levitov A, Frankel HL, Blaivas M, Kirkpatrick AW, Su E, Evans D, et al. Guidelines for the appropriate use of bedside general and cardiac ultrasonography in the evaluation of critically ill patients—part II: cardiac ultrasonography. Crit Care Med. 2016;44(6):1206–27.
5. Maizel J, Bastide MA, Richecoeur J, Frenoy E, Lemaire C, Sauneuf B, et al. Practice of ultrasound-guided central venous catheter technique by the French intensivists: a survey from the BoReal study group. Ann Intensive Care. 2016;6(1):76.
6. Soni NJ, Reyes LF, Keyt H, Arango A, Gelfond JA, Peters JI, et al. Use of ultrasound guidance for central venous catheterization: a national survey of intensivists and hospitalists. J Crit Care. 2016;36:277–83.
7. Bailey PL, Glance LG, Eaton MP, Parshall B, McIntosh S. A survey of the use of ultrasound during central venous catheterization. Anesth Analg. 2007;104(3):491–7.
8. Quintard H, Philip I, Ichai C. French survey on current use of ultrasound in the critical care unit: ECHOREA. Ann Fr Anesth Reanim. 2011;30(11):e69–73.
9. Zieleskiewicz L, Muller L, Lakhal K, Meresse Z, Arbelot C, Bertrand PM, et al. Point-of-care ultrasound in intensive care units: assessment of 1073 procedures in a multicentric, prospective, observational study. Intensive Care Med. 2015;41(9):1638–47.
10. Berlet T, Fehr T, Merz TM. Current practice of lung ultrasonography (LUS) in the diagnosis of pneumothorax: a survey of physician sonographers in Germany. Crit Ultrasound J. 2014;6(1):16.

11. Estenssoro E, Alegria L, Murias G, Friedman G, Castro R, Nin Vaeza N, et al. Organizational issues, structure, and processes of care in 257 ICUs in Latin America: a study from the Latin America intensive care network. Crit Care Med. 2017;45(8):1325–36.

12. Burns KE, Duffett M, Kho ME, Meade MO, Adhikari NK, Sinuff T, et al. A guide for the design and conduct of self-administered surveys of clinicians. CMAJ. 2008;179(3):245–52.

13. Lamperti M, Bodenham AR, Pittiruti M, Blaivas M, Augoustides JG, Elbarbary M, et al. International evidence-based recommendations on ultrasound-guided vascular access. Intensive Care Med. 2012;38(7):1105–17.

14. American Society of Anesthesiologists Task Force on Central Venous A, Rupp SM, Apfelbaum JL, Blitt C, Caplan RA, Connis RT, et al. Practice guidelines for central venous access: a report by the American Society of Anesthesiologists Task Force on Central Venous Access. Anesthesiology. 2012;116(3):539–73.

15. Troianos CA, Hartman GS, Glas KE, Skubas NJ, Eberhardt RT, Walker JD, et al. Special articles: guidelines for performing ultrasound guided vascular cannulation: recommendations of the American Society of Echocardiography and the Society of Cardiovascular Anesthesiologists. Anesth Analg. 2012;114(1):46–72.

16. Eisen LA, Leung S, Gallagher AE, Kvetan V. Barriers to ultrasound training in critical care medicine fellowships: a survey of program directors. Crit Care Med. 2010;38(10):1978–83.

17. Mayo PH, Beaulieu Y, Doelken P, Feller-Kopman D, Harrod C, Kaplan A, et al. American College of Chest Physicians/La Societe de Reanimation de Langue Francaise statement on competence in critical care ultrasonography. Chest. 2009;135(4):1050–60.

18. Expert Round Table on Echocardiography in ICU. International consensus statement on training standards for advanced critical care echocardiography. Intensive Care Med. 2014;40(5):654–66.

19. Jain MK, Heyland D, Dhaliwal R, Day AG, Drover J, Keefe L, et al. Dissemination of the Canadian clinical practice guidelines for nutrition support: results of a cluster randomized controlled trial. Crit Care Med. 2006;34(9):2362–9.

20. Reschreiter H, Maiden M, Kapila A. Sedation practice in the intensive care unit: a UK national survey. Crit Care. 2008;12(6):R152.

21. Safdar N, Musuuza JS, Xie A, Hundt AS, Hall M, Wood K, et al. Management of ventilator-associated pneumonia in intensive care units: a mixed methods study assessing barriers and facilitators to guideline adherence. BMC Infect Dis. 2016;16:349.

22. Peris A, Tutino L, Zagli G, Batacchi S, Cianchi G, Spina R, et al. The use of point-of-care bedside lung ultrasound significantly reduces the number of radiographs and computed tomography scans in critically ill patients. Anesth Analg. 2010;111(3):687–92.

23. Oks M, Cleven KL, Cardenas-Garcia J, Schaub JA, Koenig S, Cohen RI, et al. The effect of point-of-care ultrasonography on imaging studies in the medical ICU: a comparative study. Chest. 2014;146(6):1574–7.

24. Brunkhorst FM, Engel C, Ragaller M, Welte T, Rossaint R, Gerlach H, et al. Practice and perception—a nationwide survey of therapy habits in sepsis. Crit Care Med. 2008;36(10):2719–22.

25. Crawford SDCM, Lamias MJ. Web surveys: perceptions of burden. Soc Sci Comput Rev. 2001;19:146–62.

13

Extracorporeal membrane oxygenation for severe Middle East respiratory syndrome coronavirus

Mohammed S. Alshahrani[1][*], Anees Sindi[2], Fayez Alshamsi[5], Awad Al-Omari[6], Mohamed El Tahan[7], Bayan Alahmadi[3], Ahmed Zein[8], Naif Khatani[3], Fahad Al-Hameed[4,9], Sultan Alamri[10], Mohammed Abdelzaher[11], Amenah Alghamdi[12], Faisal Alfousan[12], Adel Tash[13], Wail Tashkandi[14], Rajaa Alraddadi[15], Kim Lewis[16], Mohammed Badawee[17], Yaseen M. Arabi[18], Eddy Fan[19] and Waleed Alhazzani[20]

Abstract

Background: Middle East respiratory syndrome (MERS) is caused by a coronavirus (MERS-CoV) and is characterized by hypoxemic respiratory failure. The objective of this study is to compare the outcomes of MERS-CoV patients before and after the availability of extracorporeal membrane oxygenation (ECMO) as a rescue therapy in severely hypoxemic patients who failed conventional strategies.

Methods: We collected data retrospectively on MERS-CoV patients with refractory respiratory failure from April 2014 to December 2015 in 5 intensive care units (ICUs) in Saudi Arabia. Patients were classified into two groups: ECMO versus conventional therapy. Our primary outcome was in-hospital mortality; secondary outcomes included ICU and hospital length of stay.

Results: Thirty-five patients were included; 17 received ECMO and 18 received conventional therapy. Both groups had similar baseline characteristics. The ECMO group had lower in-hospital mortality (65 vs. 100%, $P = 0.02$), longer ICU stay (median 25 vs. 8 days, respectively, $P < 0.01$), and similar hospital stay (median 41 vs. 31 days, $P = 0.421$). In addition, patients in the ECMO group had better PaO2/FiO2 at days 7 and 14 of admission to the ICU (124 vs. 63, and 138 vs. 36, $P < 0.05$), and less use of norepinephrine at days 1 and 14 (29 vs. 80%; and 36 vs. 93%, $P < 0.05$).

Conclusions: ECMO use, as a rescue therapy, was associated with lower mortality in MERS patients with refractory hypoxemia. The results of this, largest to date, support the use of ECMO as a rescue therapy in patients with severe MERS-CoV.

Keywords: Coronavirus infection, Extracorporeal membrane oxygenation, Rescue therapy, Signs and symptoms respiratory

Background

Middle East respiratory syndrome (MERS), which was first described in 2012, is caused by a novel coronavirus (MERS-CoV). The World Health Organization (WHO) as of 5 December 2016 reported 1917 confirmed cases of the MERS-CoV infection globally with an overall mortality rate of 35% [1]. The majority of cases were reported in Saudi Arabia, wherein 1567 were confirmed cases, and of which 649 (41%) died [2]. Human coronaviruses were first identified in the mid-1960s and usually cause mild upper-respiratory tract illness. In 2012, the first confirmed case of MERS-CoV was reported from Saudi Arabia [3].

MERS-CoV infection is associated with significant mortality related to the virulence of the virus, nature of the disease, and the lack of effective therapy. Patients

*Correspondence: msshahrani@uod.edu.sa; mohammadalshahrani@hotmail.com
[1] Department of Emergency and Critical Care, King Fahad Hospital of the University-Dammam University, PO Box 40236, Al Khobar 31952, Saudi Arabia
Full list of author information is available at the end of the article

with MERS-CoV who develop acute respiratory distress syndrome (ARDS) are at a high risk of dying from refractory hypoxemia, multiorgan failure, and septic shock [4].

Current interventions such as lung protective ventilation, prone ventilation, and neuromuscular blocking agents have been shown in randomized trials to improve mortality in patients with ARDS [5–7]. However, in some patients, these conventional measures fail to maintain adequate oxygenation; therefore, other rescue therapies are considered, such as different modes of ventilation, inhaled pulmonary vasodilators, and extracorporeal membrane oxygenation (ECMO). Anticipated difficulties in patient recruitment, study design, and ethical concerns affect the feasibility of conducting randomized clinical trials that examine the efficacy of ECMO in this population. Therefore, observational studies are a reasonable alternative. In this study, we aim to describe the effect of ECMO rescue therapy on patient-important outcomes in patients with severe MERS-CoV.

Methods

ECMO program

In response to the large MERS-CoV outbreak, the Saudi Ministry of Health implemented a national ECMO program in April 2014. The Saudi ECMO program provided a rapid transportation chain system (Medevac system), isolated intensive care unit (ICU) beds, and venovenous (V-V) ECMO machines in selected centers across the country. An ECMO team was created that was available 24 h a day/7 days a week. The team included an intensivist trained in ECMO, a cardiac surgeon, a perfusionist, and ECMO-trained nurses. The intensivist on the ECMO team triaged all calls from other centers based on predefined criteria, wherein patients were predetermined to be candidates to receive ECMO or not. Criteria for eligibility to receive ECMO were based on the Extracorporeal Life Support Organization (ELSO) [8] guidelines and are listed below.

Study design and settings

We retrospectively identified patients who would have been eligible for ECMO but did not receive it because the ECMO program was not available at that time (prior to April 2014). The intervention (ECMO) group was included from five main ECMO centers in three major cities in Saudi Arabia after the program initiation (April 2014 to December 2015). All participating hospitals were accredited by the Joint Commission International and had closed ICUs with 24-h coverage by trained intensivists. We obtained ethics approval from the Saudi Ministry of Health ethics review board and from individual centers' ethics boards.

Case definition and ECMO eligibility

Patients were candidates to receive ECMO if they have met the following criteria:

1. Laboratory-confirmed MERS-CoV according to the WHO criteria, which use real-time RT-PCR, assays targeting the up, Orf1a, or Orf1b regions of the MERS-CoV genome from nasopharyngeal swab, tracheal aspirates, or bronchoalveolar lavage (BAL) [9].
2. Were admitted to the ICU and on invasive mechanical ventilation.
3. Met ECMO initiation criteria:

   a. Severe respiratory failure defined as a $PaO2/FiO2 < 100$ on $FiO2 > 0.9$ and/or
   b. Murray score 3–4 despite optimal care for 6 h or more and/or
   c. CO_2 retention on mechanical ventilation despite high P-plat (> 30 cm H_2O)

4. None of the following contraindications to ECMO:

   a. mechanical ventilation at high settings (FiO2 > 0.9, P-plat > 30) for ≥ 7 days
   b. recent central nervous system hemorrhage
   c. existence of non-recoverable terminal disease

The ECMO group included patients who met the above criteria and received ECMO after implementing the ECMO program from April 2014 to December 2015. We included all patients with MERS-CoV who received ECMO during that period. The control group were patients who met the above criteria but did not receive ECMO in the period prior to the introduction of ECMO program (prior to April 2014). Weaning from ECMO was primarily based on clinical improvement demonstrated by adequate oxygenation and gas exchange shown in vital signs, blood gases, and chest X-ray. The decision for readiness of a patient to be weaned from ECMO was left to the judgment of treating clinician and the ECMO team. The weaning process followed the ELSO criteria as follow: weaning starts by decreasing the flow to 1L/min while keeping the sweep of 100% (to maintain SPO2 > 95%). If SPO2 remains within target, a trial of clamping the catheters and keeping the patient on the ventilator at appropriate settings was attempted.

Data collection

We designed an electronic pretested data abstraction forms; the forms were pilot tested prior to data collection to ensure accuracy and reproducibility. Trained personnel collected the data at each participating center under the supervision of the local principal investigators. Research personnel collected data on patients' demographics, comorbidities, Acute Physiology and Chronic Health Evaluation II (APACHE II) score, laboratory results (hemoglobin concentration, white blood and platelets counts, kidney function, blood gases), ventilator modes and settings, interventions used to treat refractory hypoxemia (prone ventilation, use of neuromuscular blocking drugs, and pulmonary vasodilators), vasoactive support, antimicrobial and antiviral therapy, steroid use, and primary and secondary outcome data.

Statistical analysis

Data were tested for normality using the Kolmogorov–Smirnov test. A repeated-measures analysis of variance was performed. Fischer's exact test was used for the categorical data. Independent t test was used to compare the continuous variables in the two groups. The Mann–Whitney U test was performed to compare the nonparametric values of the two groups. Data were expressed as median (interquartile range (IQR) [range]), number (proportion), or mean (SD) as appropriate. The volume of cases was not enough to allow a priori power analysis. However, a post hoc power analysis indicated that the current sample size of 35 patients is powered to detect 35% absolute difference in mortality rate, with a type I error of 0.05 and a power of 80%. A value of $P < 0.05$ was considered statistically significant.

Results

Baseline characteristics

Eighty patients with confirmed MERS-CoV infection were admitted to the ICUs of participating centers from April 2014 to December 2015. Thirty-five patients met our eligibility criteria and were included in the analysis, 17 in the ECMO group and 18 in the control group. As shown in Table 1, the baseline characteristics were similar in both groups; the median ages were (46 vs. 50 years), and mean APACHE II score (28 vs. 31) were not statistically different. ($P = 0.48$ and $P = 0.12$; respectively).

Adjunctive therapies were used in both groups. Ribavirin was used significantly more often in the ECMO group compared to the control group (82 vs. 24%, $P = 0.001$), interferon was also used more in the ECMO cohort compared to controls (65 vs. 24%, $P = 0.016$), and the use of steroids was similar in both groups (53 vs. 72%, $P = 0.24$). At day one of eligibility to ECMO, more patients in the control group required hemodynamic support with norepinephrine compared to ECMO group; however, both groups had similar use of epinephrine and dobutamine, continuous renal replacement therapy (CRRT), modes of ventilation, positive end-expiratory pressure (PEEP), and neuromuscular blocking agents (Tables 2 and 3).

Table 1 Patients characteristics

Variable	Group 1 ECMO (n = 17)[a]	Group 2 Control (n = 18)	P value
Age median [IQR]	45.5 [28.5–58.5]	50 [33–63.5]	0.484
Gender (male) n (%)	12 (70.6%)	11 (61.1%)	0.556
Weight (kg)	87.4 (25.4)	87.5 (21.4)	0.989
Height (cm)	167.4 (10.1)	161.6 (6.1)	0.100
Body surface area (kg/m^{-2})	1.95 (0.31)	1.90 (0.26)	0.712
APACHE II median [IQR][b]	27.8 [23–29.8]	31 [24–29.5]	0.120
Pregnancy n (%)	1 (5.9%)	1 (5.6%)	0.493
Comorbidities n (%)			
Diabetes	8 (47.1%)	10 (55.6%)	0.616
Hypertension	5 (29.1%)	7 (38.9%)	0.725
Coronary artery disease	1 (5.9%)	1 (5.6%)	0.493
Heart failure	0 (0%)	1 (5.6%)	0.975
Bronchial asthma	2 (11.8%)	2 (11.1%)	0.638
COPD[c]	2 (11.8%)	0 (0%)	0.442
Acute kidney injury	2 (11.8%)	1 (5.6%)	0.975
Chronic kidney disease	1 (5.9%)	4 (22.2%)	0.371
Liver disease	0 (0%)	2 (11.1%)	0.493
Immunocompromised	0 (0%)	1 (5.6%)	0.975
Preexisting risk factors for ARDS n (%)[d]	0 (0%)	0 (0%)	
Bacterial co-infection n (%)	7 (41.2%)	4 (22.2%)	0.401

Data are presented as median [minimum–maximum], number (%), or mean (SD)

[a] *ECMO* extracorporeal membrane oxygenation

[b] *APACHE II* Acute Physiology and Chronic Health Evaluation score II

[c] *COPD* chronic obstructive pulmonary disease

[d] *ARDS* acute respiratory distress syndrome

Alveolar recruitment maneuver was used in one patient in the ECMO group. None of the patients received prone ventilation. Throughout days 1–14, more patients in the control group developed renal impairment and had significantly lower PaO2/FiO2 ratio (Table 3). Other laboratory values were similar between both groups (Table 4). However, due to the small sample size, it was not feasible to adjust for all confounding factors.

The intervention

In the ECMO group, the V-V mode was used in all patients via the percutaneous cannulation approach for vascular access. Femoral–femoral access was used in 65% of patients, while femoral–jugular access was used in 35% of cases. ECMO access was inserted by a cardiac surgeon in 70% of cases and by a cardiac intensivist in the remaining 30%. Chest X-ray was used to confirm successful cannulation in 16 patients and transesophageal echocardiography (TEE) in one patient. Blood flow (L min^{-1}), revolutions per minute, and sweep gas among ECMO patients had a mean (SD) of 3.8 (0.77), 3148.7

Table 2 Circulatory and renal support during the study period

	Day 1		Day 3		Day 7		Day 10		Day 14	
	ECMO (n = 17)	Non-ECMO (n = 18)	ECMO (n = 14)	Non-ECMO (n = 15)	ECMO (n = 14)	Non-ECMO (n = 15)	ECMO (n = 14)	Non-ECMO (n = 15)	ECMO (n = 14)	Non-ECMO (n = 14)
Use of norepinephrine n (%)	5 (29.4%)	12 (80%)*	8 (57.1%)	11 (73.3%)	7 (50%)	13 (86.7%)	7 (50%)	12 (80%)	5 (35.7%)	13 (92.9%)*
Max. dose ($\mu g\,kg^{-1}\,min^{-1}$)	0.08 (0.16)	0.13 (0.25)	0.04 (0.55)	0.15 (0.17)*	0.04 (0.58)	0.43 (0.69)*	0.15 (0.30)	0.06 (0.09)	0.44 (0.58)	0.5 (0.71)
Use of dobutamine n (%)	2 (11.8%)	2 (11.1%)	0 (0%)	0 (0%)	0 (0%)	0 (0%)	0 (0%)	0 (0%)	0 (0%)	0 (0%)
Max. dose ($\mu g\,kg^{-1}\,min^{-1}$)	1.5 (2.21)	5.0 (8.66)	NA	NA	NA	NA	NA	NA	NA	NA
Use of epinephrine n (%)	0 (0%)	NA	0 (0%)	NA	0 (0%)	1 (6.7%)	1 (7.1%)	NA	1 (5.9%)	NA
Max. dose ($\mu g\,kg^{-1}\,min^{-1}$)	NA	NA	NA	NA	NA	1.1 (0.90)	0.10 (0.14)	NA	1.5 (0.00)	NA
Use of CRRT n (%)[a]	3 (17.6%)	4 (22.2%)	7 (50%)	6 (40%)	8 (57.1%)	6 (46.7%)	5 (35.7%)	3 (20%)	2 (14.3%)	1 (7.10%)

Results are presented as number (%) or mean (SD)

*P < 0.05 vs. ECMO group

[a] CRRT continuous renal replacement therapy

Table 3 Ventilatory support data during the study period; data are presented as number (%) or mean (SD)

	Day 1		Day 3		Day 7		Day 10		Day 14	
	ECMO (n = 17)	Non-ECMO (n = 18)	ECMO (n = 14)	Non-ECMO (n = 15)	ECMO (n = 14)	Non-ECMO (n = 15)	ECMO (n = 14)	Non-ECMO (n = 15)	ECMO (n = 14)	Non-ECMO (n = 14)
Invasive ventilation n (%)	17 (100%)	18 (100%)	14 (100%)	16 (100%)	14 (100%)	15 (100%)	11 (78.6%)	14 (93.3%)	5 (35.7%)	13 (92.9%)*
Mode of ventilation										
CMV	6 (35.3%)	10 (55.6%)	7 (50%)	11 (68.8%)	6 (42.8%)	8 (53.3%)	4 (36.4%)	6 (42.9%)	1 (20%)	11 (84.6%)*
PCV	3 (17.6%)	2 (11.1%)	4 (28.6%)	1 (6.3%)	4 (28.5%)	3 (20%)	3 (27.3%)	5 (35.7%)	3 (60%)	0 (0%)*
VCV	4 (23.5%)	4 (22.2%)	1 (7.1%)	2 (12.5%)	1 (7.1%)	1 (6.7%)	1 (9.1%)	2 (14.3%)	1 (20%)	0 (0%)
PRVC	2 (11.8%)	1 (5.6%)	3 (21.4%)	0 (0%)	1 (7.1%)	2 (13.3%)	0 (0%)	1 (7.1%)	0 (0%)	1 (7.7%)
APRV	1 (6.7%)	1 (5.6%)	1 (7.1%)	0 (0%)	1 (7.1%)	1 (6.7%)	0 (0%)	0 (0%)	0 (0%)	1 (7.7%)
SIMV	1 (5.9%)	0 (0%)	0 (0%)	0 (0%)	0 (0%)	0 (0%)	1 (9.1%)	0 (0%)	0 (0%)	0 (0%)
PSV	0 (0%)	0 (0%)	0 (0%)	0 (0%)	0 (0%)	0 (0%)	1 (9.1%)	0 (0%)	0 (0%)	0 (0%)
CPAP	0 (0%)	0 (0%)	0 (0%)	0 (0%)	0 (0%)	0 (0%)	1 (9.1%)	0 (0%)	0 (0%)	0 (0%)
HFOV	0 (0%)	0 (0%)	0 (0%)	1 (6.3%)	1 (7.1%)	0 (0%)	0 (0%)	0 (0%)	0 (0%)	0 (0%)
FiO_2 (%)	0.67 (0.29)	0.80 (0.24)	0.59 (0.24)	0.79 (0.25)*	0.50 (0.21)	0.73 (0.24)*	0.50 (0.25)	0.66 (0.27)	0.33 (0.17)	0.72 (0.38)*
PaO_2/FiO_2 ratio (%)	115 (110.2)	109 (93.9)	109 (81.51)	63 (62.7)	124 (106.9)	63 (66.1)*	138 (139.5)	36 (66.4)*	237 (42.11)	85 (31.95)*
PEEP (cm H_2O)	12 (3.97)	12 (6.4)	13 (3.94)	14 (4.8)	11 (3.61)	14 (5.6)	11 (4.04)	11 (5.7)	10 (7.20)	13 (7.0)
Use of NMBs n (%)	8 (53.3%)	12 (66.7%)	10 (76.9%)	12 (80%)	10 (71.4)	8 (53.3%)	4 (36.4%)	3 (20%)	2 (40%)	0 (0%)

CMV continuous mandatory ventilation, PCV pressure-controlled ventilation, VCV volume-controlled ventilation, PRVC pressure-regulatory volume control ventilation, APRV airway pressure release ventilation, SIMV synchronised intermittent mandatory ventilation, PSV pressure-support ventilation, CPAP continuous positive airway pressure, HFOV high-frequency oscillatory ventilation, FiO_2 inspired oxygen fraction, PaO_2/FiO_2 arterial oxygen tension to FiO_2 ratio, PEEP positive end-expiratory pressure, ARM alveolar recruitment maneuver, NMBs neuromuscular blocking drugs

*$P < 0.05$ versus ECMO group

Table 4 Laboratory data

	Day 1 ECMO	Day 1 Non-ECMO	Day 3 ECMO	Day 3 Non-ECMO	Day 7 ECMO	Day 7 Non-ECMO	Day 10 ECMO	Day 10 Non-ECMO	Day 14 ECMO	Day 14 Non-ECMO
Hemoglobin (g dL⁻¹)	10.9 (2.44)	10.6 (2.93)	10.3 (1.37)	10.9 (2.31)	9.6 (1.31)	9.9 (1.51)	9.7 (1.29)	8.8 (1.10)	9.3 (0.83)	9.4 (1.10)
WBCs × 10⁻⁹ L	9.9 (4.05)	12.5 (7.64)	13.9 (7.08)	9.6 (5.42)	15.5 (9.09)	16.7 (14.04)	16.0 (7.23)	28.3 (19.30)	13.3 (10.51)	12.6 (1.10)
Platelets × 10⁻⁹ L	180 (127.5)	210 (124.9)	149 (87.32)	206 (103.5)	144 (113.7)	195 (101.5)	157 (142.3)	197 (80.1)	183 (158.9)	185 (107.5)
BUN (mg dL⁻¹)	36 (25.6)	27 (24.12)	42 (29.1)	29 (23.32)	33 (30.7)	35 (27.69)	43 (34.3)	58 (53.61)	13 (7.2)	37 (32.35)
Creatinine (μmol L⁻¹)	205 (149.90)	201 (166.61)	210 (145.69)	254 (153.75)	140 (88.0)	223 (132.83)	160 (100.9)	295 (182.23)	74 (34.40)	289 (133.75)*
Arterial blood gases										
pH	7.39 (0.07)	7.24 (0.19)*	7.35 (0.11)	7.28 (0.13)	7.35 (0.06)	7.24 (0.15)*	7.34 (0.09)	7.27 (0.14)	7.29 (0.22)	7.32 (0.01)
PaCO₂ (mmHg)	38.8 (8.88)	44.5 (14.71)	41.5 (8.94)	53.2 (19.21)*	41.7 (5.77)	57.8 (20.51)*	44.5 (17.91)	48.1 (11.81)	60.7 (45.08)	53.7 (20.93)
HCO₃ (mEq L⁻¹)	23.2 (4.11)	21.5 (7.01)	23.3 (5.16)	23.4 (2.61)	24.2 (4.71)	22.9 (6.12)	22.0 (4.36)	22.1 (4.41)	23.6 (6.98)	26.0 (3.31)
PaO₂ (mmHg)	83.7 (42.48)	92.7 (76.02)	71.1 (16.61)	58.7 (18.00)	81.9 (44.52)	66.1 (20.81)	92.1 (37.13)	79.1 (24.71)	78.2 (41.21)	61.0 (32.16)

Data are presented as mean (SD)

ECMO extracorporeal membrane oxygenation, WBCs white blood cells, BUN blood urea nitrogen, PaCO₂ arterial carbon dioxide tension, HCO₃ bicarbonate, PaO₂ arterial oxygen tension

* P < 0.05 versus ECMO group

(933.8), and 21.6 (63.2), respectively. Patients who were in the same city, where ECMO centers were situated, were transported via ground ambulances; otherwise, patients were transported via fixed wing medical evacuation airplane. No complication was reported during patients' transportation.

ECMO-related mechanical complications occurred in 3 (18%) patients; one patient developed pneumothorax that was treated with chest tube insertion, and two patients had major bleeding immediately after the initiation of ECMO.

Outcome

Compared to the control group, the ECMO group had significantly lower in-hospital mortality (65 vs. 100%; $P = 0.02$), longer ICU stay (25 vs. 8 days; $P = 0.001$) (Table 5 and Fig. 1). Less use of norepinephrine at days 1 and 14 ($P < 0.05$), and better oxygenation (higher PaO_2/FiO_2 ratio) throughout days 7–14 (Table 2).

Table 5 Outcomes of patients treated with ECMO compared to patients managed without ECMO

Variable	ECMO (n = 17)	Control (n = 18)	P value
In-hospital mortality n (%)	11 (64.7%)	18 (100%)	0.020
ICU length of stay (days)[a]	22.5 [12.5–28.3]	7 [4.3–11.5]	0.001
Hospital length of stay (days)	25 [6.3–56.5]	47 [5–76.5]	0.421
Time to death (days)	32 [1–68]	47 [1-93]	0.422
Cause of death n (%)			
Septic shock/infection	7 (41.2%)	4 (22.2%)	0.401
Refractory hypoxemia	3 (17.6%)	2 (11.1%)	0.975
Others (undetermined)	1 (5.9%)	12 (66.7%)	0.042

Data are presented as number (%), mean (SD), or median [minimum–maximum]

[a] *ICU* intensive care unit

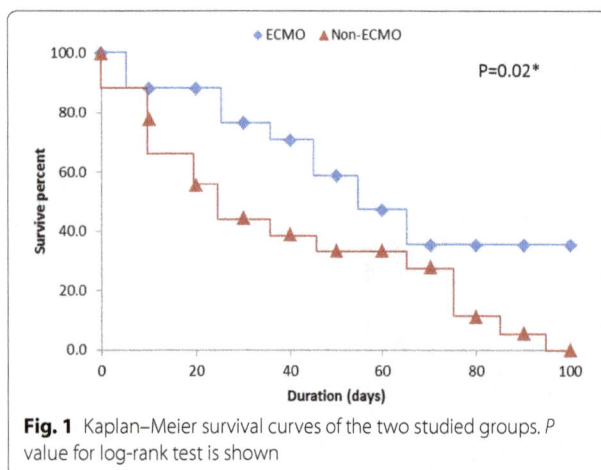

Fig. 1 Kaplan–Meier survival curves of the two studied groups. *P* value for log-rank test is shown

Discussion

In this retrospective cohort study, we found that ECMO rescue therapy was associated with lower in-hospital mortality, better oxygenation, and fewer organ failures compared to historical control (usual care) in patients with severe MERS-CoV. However, the length of hospital stay was the same and a possible explanation is that during the crisis phase, patients were mechanically ventilated in the ward when ICU beds are full, and it is possible that this could have contributed to similar stay in hospital in both groups.

Although ELSO issued guidelines on the use of ECMO in patients with ARDS, these guidelines do not address specific disease context, and are difficult to generalize to the heterogeneous ARDS population. Therefore, we conducted this observational study to report on the efficacy and safety of ECMO in patients with severe MERS-CoV infection.

There is a single case report in the literature looking at ECMO in MERS-CoV patients. Guery et al. described the use of ECMO in two patients with acute respiratory failure secondary to MERS-CoV infection in France, where both patients developed severe hypoxia and increasing oxygen requirements, leading to mechanical ventilation and ECMO use. One patient died, and the other survived after approximately 2 months in hospital [10].

ECMO use in respiratory failure has been reported with variable survival rates. The first 2 randomized clinical trials (RCTs) failed to prove superiority of ECMO over conventional management [11, 12]. However, the severe adult respiratory failure (CESAR) trial showed improved 6-month survival in patients who were referred early to an ECMO center [13]. This was the largest clinical trial to investigate the efficacy of early use ECMO in patients with ARDS. Despite concerns about the trial design and possible differences in steroid use and ventilator strategies, these results contributed to the increasing use of ECMO worldwide.

In this study, we observed no significant differences in the use of adjunctive therapies except for ribavirin use in the ECMO group. The benefit of antiviral therapy in MERS-CoV infection remains unclear. Recent Korean guidelines published during the 2015 MERS-CoV outbreak in South Korea suggested the use of antiviral therapy in patients with severe MERS-CoV [14].

In patients with respiratory failure from H1N1 infection who required the use of ECMO, the survival rate varied considerably between studies ranging from 35 to 90% [15–28]. There was a large variation in survival rates, which could be explained by differences in patients' baseline characteristics and severity of illness. In one study, older, obese, diabetic, or immunocompromised patients were found to be at a higher risk of developing severe

MERS-CoV infection [28–31]. In this study, the two groups were comparable at baseline, and there were no significant differences between groups in any of these variables. Another large observational study examined the predictors of death in H1N1 patients who underwent V–V ECMO and found that creatinine and bilirubin levels, systemic arterial pressure, hematocrit, and pre-ECMO hospital length of stay were associated with higher mortality [32].

Another important factor is the center experience and volume of cases; this could have contributed to the variability in survival rates with ECMO use. A recent study by Barbaro et al. [33] demonstrated that centers with > 30 ECMO cases/year had better survival rates than centers with less than 6 cases per year. In Saudi Arabia, ECMO was not available except in one center until the MERS-CoV crisis; thereafter, the ECMO program was implemented as a therapeutic option for patients with refractory hypoxemia. ECMO interventions were run in tertiary centers with equipped ICUs by most experienced intensivists and perfusionists who received training in ECMO prior to the start of the program.

Although more ECMO patients received ribavirin and interferon therapy, we do not believe that this difference has an impact to our findings. Published reports on this therapy are limited, but none showed significant improvement with this combination [34–36]. The largest study to date published in abstract format [37] showed no reduction in mortality. Therefore, we believe that the imbalance of co-interventions between the two groups is unlikely to affect the estimation of treatment effect.

In regard to infection control issues, caregivers safety of ECMO patients was organized and maintained by aggressive measures which were applied strictly and monitored closely with all admissions were taken to airborne isolated rooms which impacted the containment of the virus plus applying the universal protective personal measures all the time during the patients encounter. Because of these stringent measures, there were no reports by or about any caregiver of any ECMO patient being affected.

To our knowledge, this is the largest study to describe outcomes in patients with MERS-CoV who received ECMO. There are several strengths to our study: the "before and after" design allowed us to compare ECMO cases to a control group with similar demographics and within the same institutions. We also collected data on important variables and confounders, and conducted adjusted analyses to assess the impact on the results. We adhered to the Strengthening the Reporting of Observational studies in Epidemiology (STROBE) guidelines [38].

Despite the strengths of our study, it has several important limitations. First, the retrospective nature of this study renders it at risk of bias. All patients in the control group died, which may be explained by the severity of illness, as these were patients who had ARDS and were eligible otherwise. We cannot rule out the possibility of selection bias, as we were unable to track all transfer requests due to the outbreak and crisis at the time, leaving us with limited information. In addition, some patients were transferred from non-participating ECMO centers; therefore, baseline pre-ECMO data such as blood gases and ventilator settings could not be obtained. Furthermore, due to insufficient documentation during the outbreak and crisis circumstances, we were not able to track the ECMO requests to the referral call center.

There were differences in some co-interventions (e.g., antiviral therapy), and the influence of unmeasured confounders cannot be excluded. Such concerns can only be addressed in RCTs; however, conducting RCT is likely to be challenging in the context of epidemics. This study was not designed to compare the cost of 2 interventions; although it is an important outcome that could help the clinicians and stakeholders to make decisions. Lastly, the small sample size limited our ability to perform an adequate multivariate analysis. Similar to other ECMO studies, it is difficult to determine if the mortality was the result of refractory respiratory failure or other causes like septic shock or other organs failure.

In summary, the use of ECMO was associated with lower mortality in patients with severe MERS-CoV infection and refractory hypoxia. Future randomized trials, although challenging to conduct, are highly needed to confirm or dispute these observations. Until more data are available, ECMO could be considered as a rescue therapy in selected MERS-CoV patients with refractory hypoxemia.

Abbreviations
APACHE II: Acute Physiology and Chronic Health Evaluation II; ARDS: acute respiratory distress syndrome; CRRT: continuous renal replacement therapy; ECMO: extracorporeal membrane oxygenation; ELSO: Extracorporeal Life Support Organization; ICU: intensive care units; MERS: Middle East respiratory syndrome; MERS-CoV: Middle East respiratory syndrome coronavirus; PEEP: positive end-expiratory pressure; RCT: randomized clinical trials; TEE: transesophageal echocardiography; WHO: World Health Organization.

Authors' contributions
MS, AS, BA, WH was involved in conception and design. MS, FS, AO, BA, AZ, NK, FH, SA, MA, AG, FF, AT, WT, RR, MB, YA, WH helped in acquisition, analysis, and interpretation. MS, WH, AS, MT, BA, AT, WT, KL, YA, EF contributed to drafting the manuscript for important intellectual content. MS, WH, AS, MT, BA, AT, WT, KL, YA, EF helped in final approval of the version to be published. All authors read and approved the final manuscript.

Author details
[1] Department of Emergency and Critical Care, King Fahad Hospital of the University-Dammam University, PO Box 40236, Al Khobar 31952, Saudi Arabia. [2] Department of Medicine/Intensive Care, King Abdulaziz University, Jeddah, Saudi Arabia. [3] King Abdulaziz University, Jeddah, Saudi Arabia. [4] King Abdulaziz Medical City, NGHA, Jeddah, Saudi Arabia. [5] Department of Internal Medicine, College of Medicine and Health Sciences, United Arab Emirates

University, Al Ain, UAE. [6] Medical Director of Critical Care, Dr. Suliman Al-Habib Group, AlFaisal University, Riyadh, Saudi Arabia. [7] Department of Anesthesiology, Dammam University, Dammam, Saudi Arabia. [8] Department of ICU, King Fahad Hospital, Jeddah, Saudi Arabia. [9] Intensive Care Department, King Saud bin Abdulaziz University for Health Sciences, Jeddah, Saudi Arabia. [10] Department of ICU National Hospital, Internal Medicine and Critical Care, Riyadh, Saudi Arabia. [11] Critical Care Medicine Department, Cairo University Hospitals, Cairo, Egypt. [12] Department of Internal Medicine, King Abdulaziz University, Jeddah, Saudi Arabia. [13] Department of Cardiac Surgery, King Abdullah Medical City, Makkah, Saudi Arabia. [14] Department of Surgery/Intensive Care, King Abdulaziz University, Jeddah, Saudi Arabia. [15] Community Medicine Department, Ministry of Health, Jeddah, Saudi Arabia. [16] Department of Medicine, Division of Critical Care, McMaster University, Hamilton, Canada. [17] Department of Critical Care, Prince Sultan Military Medical City, Riyadh, Saudi Arabia. [18] King Abdullah International Medical Research Center, King Saud bin Abdulaziz University for Health Sciences, Riyadh, Saudi Arabia. [19] Interdepartmental Division of Critical Care Medicine, University of Toronto, Toronto, Canada. [20] Department of Clinical Epidemiology and Biostatistics, McMaster University, Hamilton, Canada.

Acknowledgements
We wish to acknowledge the Saudi Ministry of Health for implementing a national ECMO program in April 2014 who assisted us throughout the course of this research. We thank our colleagues from all participating ICUs throughout Saudi Arabia who provided insight and expertise that greatly assisted the research, and for their comments on an earlier version of the manuscript.

Competing interests
The authors declare that they have no competing interests.

Funding
All authors declare that they receive no support from any commercial organization or company.

References
1. http://www.who.int/emergencies/mers-cov/mers-summary-2016.pdf. Assessed 12 March 2017.
2. http://www.moh.gov.sa/en/CCC/PressReleases/Pages/default.aspx. Assessed 12 March 2017.
3. Zaki AM, van Boheemen S, Bestebroer TM, Osterhaus AD, Fouchier RA. Isolation of a novel coronavirus from a man with pneumonia in Saudi Arabia. N Engl J Med. 2012;367(19):1814–20.
4. Who Mers-Cov Research Group. State of knowledge and data gaps of middle East respiratory syndrome coronavirus (MERS-CoV) in humans. PLoS Curr. 2013;5(1):1–32.
5. Brower R, Matthay M, Morris A, Schoenfeld D, Thompson BT, Wheeler A. Ventilation with lower tidal volumes as compared with traditional tidal volumes for acute lung injury and the acute respiratory distress syndrome. The acute respiratory distress syndrome network. N Engl J Med. 2000;342(18):1301–8.
6. Guerin C, Reignier J, Richard JC, Beuret P, Gacouin A, Boulain T, et al. Prone positioning in severe acute respiratory distress syndrome. N Engl J Med. 2013;368(23):2159–68.
7. Papazian L, Forel JM, Gacouin A, Penot-Ragon C, Perrin G, Loundou A, et al. Neuromuscular blockers in early acute respiratory distress syndrome. N Engl J Med. 2010;363(12):1107–16.
8. https://www.elso.org/Portals/0/IGD/Archive/FileManager/929122ae88cu sersshyerdocumentselsoguidelinesgeneralalleclsversion1.3.pdf.
9. Corman VM, Muller MA, Costabel U, Timm J, Binger T, Meyer B, et al. Assays for laboratory confirmation of novel human coronavirus (hCoV-EMC) infections. Euro Surveill. 2012;17:49.
10. Guery B, Poissy J, el Mansouf L, Sejourne C, Ettahar N, Lemaire X, et al. Clinical features and viral diagnosis of two cases of infection with Middle East respiratory syndrome coronavirus: a report of nosocomial transmission. Lancet. 2013;381(9885):2265–72.
11. Morris AH, Wallace CJ, Menlove RL, Clemmer TP, Orme JF Jr, Weaver LK, et al. Randomized clinical trial of pressure-controlled inverse ratio ventilation and extracorporeal CO2 removal for adult respiratory distress syndrome. Am J Respir Crit Care Med. 1994;149(2 Pt 1):295–305.
12. Zapol WM, Snider MT, Hill JD, Fallat RJ, Bartlett RH, Edmunds LH, et al. Extracorporeal membrane oxygenation in severe acute respiratory failure. A randomized prospective study. JAMA. 1979;242(20):2193–6.
13. Peek GJ, Mugford M, Tiruvoipati R, Wilson A, Allen E, Thalanany MM, et al. Efficacy and economic assessment of conventional ventilatory support versus extracorporeal membrane oxygenation for severe adult respiratory failure (CESAR): a multicentre randomised controlled trial. Lancet. 2009;374(9698):1351–63.
14. Chong YP, Song JY, Seo YB, Choi JP, Shin HS, Rapid RT. Antiviral treatment guidelines for middle East respiratory syndrome. Infect Chemother. 2015;47(3):212–22.
15. Holzgraefe B, Broome M, Kalzen H, Konrad D, Palmer K, Frenckner B. Extracorporeal membrane oxygenation for pandemic H1N1 2009 respiratory failure. Minerva Anestesiol. 2010;76(12):1043–51.
16. Noah MA, Peek GJ, Finney SJ, Griffiths MJ, Harrison DA, Grieve R, et al. Referral to an extracorporeal membrane oxygenation center and mortality among patients with severe 2009 influenza A(H1N1). JAMA. 2011;306(15):1659–68.
17. Takeda S, Kotani T, Nakagawa S, Ichiba S, Aokage T, Ochiai R, et al. Extracorporeal membrane oxygenation for 2009 influenza A(H1N1) severe respiratory failure in Japan. J Anesth. 2012;26(5):650–7.
18. Davies A, Jones D, Bailey M, Beca J, et al. Extracorporeal membrane oxygenation for 2009 influenza A(H1N1) acute respiratory distress syndrome. JAMA. 2009;302(17):188–95.
19. Cianchi G, Bonizzoli M, Pasquini A, Bonacchi M, Zagli G, Ciapetti M, et al. Ventilatory and ECMO treatment of H1N1-induced severe respiratory failure: results of an Italian referral ECMO center. BMC Pulm Med. 2011;11:2.
20. Zangrillo A, Biondi-Zoccai G, Landoni G, Frati G, Patroniti N, Pesenti A, et al. Extracorporeal membrane oxygenation (ECMO) in patients with H1N1 influenza infection: a systematic review and meta-analysis including 8 studies and 266 patients receiving ECMO. Crit Care. 2013;17(1):R30.
21. Pham T, Combes A, Roze H, Chevret S, Mercat A, Roch A, et al. Extracorporeal membrane oxygenation for pandemic influenza A(H1N1)-induced acute respiratory distress syndrome: a cohort study and propensity-matched analysis. Am J Respir Crit Care Med. 2013;187(3):276–85.
22. Hodgson CL, Hayes K, Everard T, Nichol A, Davies AR, Bailey MJ, et al. Long-term quality of life in patients with acute respiratory distress syndrome requiring extracorporeal membrane oxygenation for refractory hypoxaemia. Crit Care. 2012;16(5):R202.
23. Beurtheret S, Mastroianni C, Pozzi M, D'Alessandro C, Luyt CE, Combes A, et al. Extracorporeal membrane oxygenation for 2009 influenza A (H1N1) acute respiratory distress syndrome: single-centre experience with 1-year follow-up. Eur J Cardiothorac Surg. 2012;41(3):691–5.
24. Hou X, Guo L, Zhan Q, Jia X, Mi Y, Li B, et al. Extracorporeal membrane oxygenation for critically ill patients with 2009 influenza A (H1N1)-related acute respiratory distress syndrome: preliminary experience from a single center. Artif Organs. 2012;36(9):780–6.
25. Roch A, Lepaul-Ercole R, Grisoli D, Bessereau J, Brissy O, Castanier M, et al. Extracorporeal membrane oxygenation for severe influenza A (H1N1) acute respiratory distress syndrome: a prospective observational comparative study. Intensive Care Med. 2010;36(11):1899–905.
26. Bonastre J, Suberviola B, Pozo JC, Guerrero JE, Torres A, Rodriguez A, et al. Extracorporeal lung support in patients with severe respiratory failure secondary to the 2010–2011 winter seasonal outbreak of influenza A (H1N1) in Spain. Med Intensiva. 2012;36(3):193–9.
27. Patroniti N, Zangrillo A, Pappalardo F, Peris A, Cianchi G, Braschi A, et al. The Italian ECMO network experience during the 2009 influenza A(H1N1) pandemic: preparation for severe respiratory emergency outbreaks. Intensive Care Med. 2011;37(9):1447–57.
28. Al-Tawfiq JA, Hinedi K, Ghandour J, Khairalla H, Musleh S, Ujayli A, et al. Middle East respiratory syndrome coronavirus: a case-control study of hospitalized patients. Clin Infect Dis. 2014;59(2):160–5.
29. Arabi YM, Arifi AA, Balkhy HH, Najm H, Aldawood AS, Ghabashi A, et al. Clinical course and outcomes of critically ill patients with middle East respiratory syndrome coronavirus infection. Ann Intern Med. 2014;160(6):389–97.

30. Assiri A, Al-Tawfiq JA, Al-Rabeeah AA, Al-Rabiah FA, Al-Hajjar S, Al-Barrak A, et al. Epidemiological, demographic, and clinical characteristics of 47 cases of middle East respiratory syndrome coronavirus disease from Saudi Arabia: a descriptive study. Lancet Infect Dis. 2013;13(9):752–61.

31. Assiri A, McGeer A, Perl TM, Price CS, Al Rabeeah AA, Cummings DA, et al. Hospital outbreak of middle East respiratory syndrome coronavirus. N Engl J Med. 2013;369(5):407–16.

32. Pappalardo F, Pieri M, Greco T, Patroniti N, Pesenti A, Arcadipane A, et al. Predicting mortality risk in patients undergoing venovenous ECMO for ARDS due to influenza A (H1N1) pneumonia: the ECMOnet score. Intensive Care Med. 2013;39(2):275–81.

33. Barbaro RP, Odetola FO, Kidwell KM, Paden ML, Bartlett RH, Davis MM, et al. Association of hospital-level volume of extracorporeal membrane oxygenation cases and mortality. Analysis of the Extracorporeal Life Support Organization registry. Am J Respir Crit Care Med. 2015;191(8):894–901.

34. Al-Tawfiq JA, Momattin H, Dib J, Memish ZA. Ribavirin and interferon therapy in patients infected with the middle East respiratory syndrome oronavirus:an observational study. Int J Infect Dis. 2014;20:42–6. https://doi.org/10.1016/j.ijid.2013.12.003.

35. Omrani AS, et al. Ribavirin and interferon alfa-2a for severe middle East respiratory syndrome coronavirus infection: a retrospective cohort study. Lancet Inf Dis. 2014;14(11):1090–5.

36. Shalboub S, et al. IFN-α2a or IFN-β1a in combination with ribavirin to treat middle East respiratory syndrome coronavirus pneumonia: a retrospective study. J Antimicrob Chemother. 2015;70(7):2129–32.

37. Arabi YM et al. Effect of Ribavirin and Interferon on the Outcome of Critically III patients with MERS. http://www.atsjournals.org/doi/abs/10.1164/ajrccm-conference.2017.195.1_MeetingAbstracts.A6067.

38. Von Elm E, Altman DG, Egger M, Pocock SJ, Gotzsche PC, Vandenbroucke JP, et al. The Strengthening the Reporting of Observational Studies in Epidemiology (STROBE) statement: guidelines for reporting observational studies. J Clin Epidemiol. 2008;61(4):344–9.

14

Heparin-binding protein (HBP) improves prediction of sepsis-related acute kidney injury

Jonas Tverring[1]*⊙, Suvi T. Vaara[2,3], Jane Fisher[1], Meri Poukkanen[4], Ville Pettilä[2], Adam Linder[1] and the FINNAKI Study Group

Abstract

Background: Sepsis-related acute kidney injury (AKI) accounts for major morbidity and mortality among the critically ill. Heparin-binding protein (HBP) is a promising biomarker in predicting development and prognosis of severe sepsis and septic shock that has recently been proposed to be involved in the pathophysiology of AKI. The objective of this study was to investigate the added predictive value of measuring plasma HBP on admission to the intensive care unit (ICU) regarding the development of septic AKI.

Methods: We included 601 patients with severe sepsis or septic shock from the prospective, observational FINNAKI study conducted in seventeen Finnish ICUs during a 5-month period (1 September 2011–1 February 2012). The main outcome measure was the development of KDIGO AKI stages 2–3 from 12 h after admission up to 5 days. Statistical analysis for the primary endpoint included construction of a clinical risk model, area under the receiver operating curve (ROC area), category-free net reclassification index (cfNRI) and integrated discrimination improvement (IDI) with 95% confidence intervals (95% CI).

Results: Out of 511 eligible patients, 101 (20%) reached the primary endpoint. The addition of plasma HBP to a clinical risk model significantly increased ROC area (0.82 vs. 0.78, $p = 0.03$) and risk classification scores: cfNRI 62.0% (95% CI 40.5–82.4%) and IDI 0.053 (95% CI 0.029–0.075).

Conclusions: Plasma HBP adds predictive value to known clinical risk factors in septic AKI. Further studies are warranted to compare the predictive performance of plasma HBP to other novel AKI biomarkers.

Keywords: Acute kidney injury, Sepsis, Biomarker, Heparin-binding protein, Risk model

Background

Acute kidney injury (AKI) accounts for major morbidity and mortality among the critically ill, and septic shock is a leading cause for AKI [1]. Current AKI diagnosis is defined by a decrease in urine output (UOP) or an increase in serum creatinine (SCr) [2]. Unfortunately, SCr is a late marker of declined kidney function and does not adequately reflect damage to kidney cells. There is a broad consensus that more sensitive and specific biomarkers are needed [3]. Despite considerable research efforts, no novel biomarkers of AKI are currently in widespread clinical use. Heparin-binding protein (HBP), also known as azurocidin or cationic antimicrobial protein of 37 kDa, is a mediator of inflammation and vascular permeability that is released from activated neutrophils and has been shown to correlate with sepsis development, severity and prognosis [4–6]. HBP has recently been suggested to be involved in the pathophysiology of AKI with data from a murine model and a human cell line [7]. In two recent papers, plasma HBP performed well in predicting septic AKI, first among 296 patients with septic shock and second among 59 patients with severe sepsis, respectively [7, 8]. However, neither of those studies presented any statistical analysis on added predictive value to clinical risk factors. Accordingly, we aimed to investigate whether plasma HBP would add predictive value to known clinical risk factors regarding development of septic AKI.

*Correspondence: jonas.tverring@med.lu.se
[1] Division of Infection Medicine, Department of Clinical Sciences, Lund University, BMC B14, 221 84 Lund, Sweden
Full list of author information is available at the end of the article

Methods

Patients

This was a post hoc study of the prospective, observational, multicentre FINNAKI study. Patients with severe sepsis or septic shock diagnosed on day one and who had plasma samples available from admission to the ICU were included in the current study. The FINNAKI study consecutively included all emergency ICU admission and the elective admissions with an ICU stay of above 24 h from seventeen Finnish ICUs during a 5-month period (1 September 2011–1 February 2012) and reported the incidence, risk factors and 90-day mortality of patients with AKI. In brief, exclusion criteria for the FINNAKI study were patients who (1) had end-stage renal disease requiring maintenance dialysis, (2) were organ donors, (3) received intermediate care, (4) had received renal replacement therapy (RRT) while enrolled in the study during a previous ICU admission, (5) were transferred from another ICU where the data collection for the study was fulfilled or (6) were not permanently living in Finland or were unable to give consent due to insufficient language skills. Further details for the FINNAKI study have been published in detail previously [9].

Definitions

AKI was defined and staged using the kidney disease: improving global outcomes (KDIGO) guidelines using both daily serum creatinine and hourly urine output measurements [2]. Baseline SCr was defined as the latest value from the previous year excluding the last week preceding admission. If baseline SCr was not available, SCr was estimated by the modification in diet in renal disease (MDRD) [10] equation assuming a glomerular filtration rate of 75 ml/1.73 m^2. Severe sepsis and septic shock were defined using American College of Chest Physicians/Society of Critical Care Medicine guidelines [11].

Data and sample collection

The Ethics Committee of the Department of Surgery, Helsinki and Uusimaa Hospital District approved the study protocol, and each participant or his/her proxy gave written informed consent. Patient demographics, medical history, severity scores, length of stay, physiologic data and hospital mortality were collected from the Finnish Intensive Care Consortium prospective database (Tieto Ltd, Helsinki, Finland) and with a study-specific case report form. AKI status was screened at admission and during the first 5 days of ICU stay. All data collection was blinded to the index test results. Plasma samples were collected immediately at ICU admission or after 2 h at the latest and directly centrifuged, aliquoted and frozen to − 80 °C. Plasma samples were sent on dry ice between Helsinki, Finland, and Lund, Sweden, for plasma HBP analyses.

HBP test analyses

Plasma HBP concentration was measured in duplicate using a commercial HBP ELISA (Axis-Shield Diagnostics, Dundee, UK) according to the manufacturer's directions. Intra-test variability was controlled through repeated analyses when the coefficient of variation (%CV) was above 10%. Analyses were performed with positive and negative controls, by the same laboratory personnel and blinded to clinical outcomes.

Clinical endpoints

The primary endpoint was the development of new AKI stages 2–3 from 12 h after admission up to 5 days. The endpoint also included patients who developed AKI stage 2 within 12 h and then worsened to stage 3 within the 5 days. Secondary endpoints assessed all patients from admission to the ICU and included fluid balance within 24 h, maximum sequential organ failure assessment (SOFA) score within 5 days, initiation of RRT within 5 days and 28-day mortality, respectively.

Sample size

The primary endpoint analysis ($n = 511$) and the secondary endpoint analyses ($n = 601$) were performed on available patients, samples and data.

Statistical analyses

We constructed a risk model using multivariable logistic regression and compared its predictive performance for the primary endpoint with and without addition of plasma HBP using area under the receiver operating curve (ROC area) and category-free net reclassification index (cfNRI) and integrated discrimination improvement (IDI). CfNRI and IDI are presented for events, non-events and totals with bootstrapped 95% confidence intervals (95% CI) based on 10,000 replications. Testing for the equality of the ROC area was done using an algorithm suggested by DeLong [12]. We also present positive likelihood ratio (LR+) for categorised plasma HBP and ROC area for continuous plasma HBP to predict the primary endpoint. Two-by-two contingency tables were used to calculate sensitivity, specificity, positive predictive value (PPV) and negative predictive value (NPV) for plasma HBP at a binary cut-off. Sensitivity analyses were performed with changes to the primary endpoint regarding outcome definition, missing data, competing risks and baseline imbalance, respectively, and tested for ROC area with 95% CI. Univariable logistic regression was used to calculate the odds ratio (OR) presented in the baseline characteristics. The secondary endpoints were evaluated using independent-sample *t* tests, Mann–Whitney *U* test, ROC area, Kaplan–Meier survival curve and log rank (Mantel–Cox) test, as appropriate. We used missing at random assumptions and performed complete case analysis, in all cases except for baseline creatinine, which was required for AKI diagnosis, and was estimated using the MDRD equation [10]. Results are presented with 95% CI whenever applicable. Medians are presented together with interquartile ranges (IQRs). For all analyses, except when constructing the risk model, two-sided p values less than 0.05 were considered statistically significant. The software used for statistical analysis was SPSS (SPSS version 24.0, IBM Corp., Chicago, USA) and STATA (STATA MP 14.2, StataCorp, Texas, USA).

Results

Patient characteristics

We included a total of 601 patients with severe sepsis or septic shock from the FINNAKI cohort and analysed HBP concentration on plasma samples from admission to the ICU. One patient was excluded due to missing identification number on target sample. Ninety patients were excluded from the primary endpoint analysis because they had already developed AKI stages 2–3 within 12 h, resulting in 511 evaluable patients in the primary analysis (Fig. 1). Baseline characteristics did not differ significantly regarding age, gender, baseline creatinine, source of admission, presence of hypertension, diabetes and medication pre-ICU admission except for use of colloid starch. However, patients developing stages 2–3 AKI had more often chronic kidney disease and positive blood cultures, as well as having a greater disease severity in terms of SAPS II score, vasopressor use on day one, development of septic shock, need for mechanical ventilation and higher creatinine and lactate levels pre-ICU admission, as compared to patients who did not develop stages 2–3 AKI (Table 1). For further data on infection characteristics, see Additional file 1; Table S1.

Patient outcomes

Out of 511 patients, 101 (20%) reached the primary endpoint of KDIGO AKI stages 2–3 from 12 h after admission up to 5 days. Thirty-one (6%) patients developed at highest AKI stage 2, and 70 (14%) patients developed at AKI stage 3, out of which 48 (9%) received renal replacement therapy (RRT). Four hundred and ten patients (80%) did not develop stages 2–3 AKI; 283 patients never developed AKI (55%); and 127 patients developed stage 1 (25%), as shown in Fig. 1. Data on fluid balance were available for 550 patients (8.5% missing) and were collected on the first day from ICU admission with a median time to measurement of 17 h (IQR 11–22 h). Median fluid balance in absolute volume was positive 1209 ml

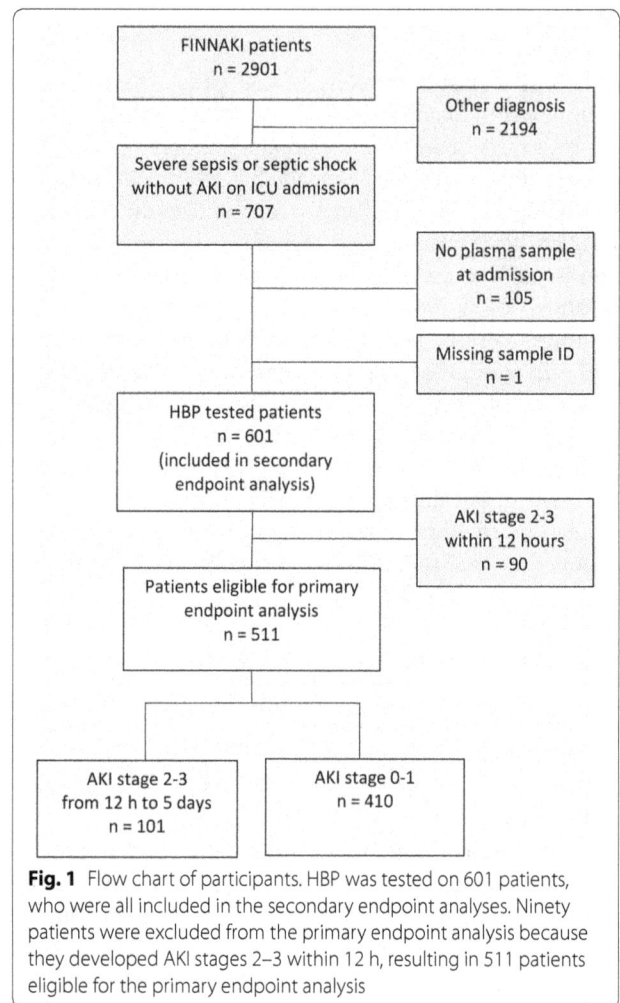

Fig. 1 Flow chart of participants. HBP was tested on 601 patients, who were all included in the secondary endpoint analyses. Ninety patients were excluded from the primary endpoint analysis because they developed AKI stages 2–3 within 12 h, resulting in 511 patients eligible for the primary endpoint analysis

(IQR − 18 to + 3085 ml) and in fluid balance (kg) per weight was + 1.6% (IQR 0.0–4.1%). Median of maximum SOFA score during the first 5 days was 8 points (IQR 6–11) for all 601 patients. A total of 145 patients (24.1%) died within 28 days from ICU admission.

HBP test results

Mean plasma HBP concentration on ICU admission for all patients was 40 ng/ml, and standard deviation was 65 ng/ml. Median plasma HBP was 19 ng/ml, and IQR was 9.1–39 ng/ml. The distribution of plasma HBP was left-shifted as compared to the normal curve. We set the binary cut-off for a high versus a low plasma HBP at 20 ng/ml, which is comparable to that of other studies (15 ng/ml in Linder et al. [5] and 30 ng/ml in Linder et al. [6]). Categorised plasma HBP based on quartiles resulted the following groups: HBP $\leq$ 10 ng/ml, HBP $> 10 \leq 20$ ng/ml, HBP $> 20 \leq 40$ ng/ml and HBP > 40 ng/ml, respectively. Among primary endpoint positive patients, plasma HBP was significantly elevated

Table 1 Patient characteristics

	AKI stages 0–1 (n = 410, where of 127 stage 1)	AKI stages 2–3 (n = 101, where of 70 stage 3)	No data (n)	Odds ratio (95% CI) univariable	p value univariable	Odds ratio (95% CI) multivariable risk model
Age (years)	65 (54–74)	69 (56–79)	0	1.02 (1.00–1.03)	0.02	1.01 (1.00–1.03)
Gender (female)	153 (37.3%)	39 (38.6%)	0	1.06 (0.68–1.65)	> 0.3	*
Weight (kg)	80 (68–90)	79 (68–91)	0	1.01 (1.00–1.02)	> 0.3	*
Baseline SCr (μmol/l)	75 (60–89)	83 (66–119)	118	1.01 (1.01–1.02)	< 0.001	‡
Severity of disease						
SAPS II score (points)	38 (30–46)	54 (40–64)	0	1.06 (1.05–1.08)	< 0.001	§
SAPS II without points for renal or age	23 (17–29)	26 (19–36)	0	1.03 (1.02–1.05)	< 0.001	1.04 (1.02–1.06)
Vasopressor on day one	265 (65%)	80 (79%)	0	2.08 (1.24–3.51)	< 0.01	†
Mechanical ventilation	253 (62%)	77 (76%)	0	1.99 (1.21–3.28)	< 0.01	†
Septic shock	289 (71%)	89 (88%)	0	3.11 (1.64–5.88)	< 0.01	†
Comorbidity						
Chronic kidney disease	24 (5.9%)	13 (13%)	0	2.38 (1.16–4.85)	0.02	‡
Renal transplant	5 (1.2%)	1 (1.2%)	2	0.81 (0.09–7.00)	> 0.3	*
Diabetes	93 (23%)	27 (27%)	0	1.24 (0.76–2.05)	> 0.3	*
Hypertension	211 (52%)	48 (48%)	2	0.85 (0.55–1.31)	> 0.3	*
Systolic heart failure	48 (12%)	9 (8.9%)	4	0.76 (0.36–1.61)	> 0.3	*
COPD	63 (15%)	12 (12%)	6	0.74 (0.38–1.43)	> 0.3	*
Any malignancy	53 (13%)	18 (18%)	0	1.46 (0.81–2.62)	0.21	‡
Chronic liver failure	17 (4.1%)	4 (4.0%)	7	0.96 (0.32–2.92)	> 0.3	*
Source of admission						
Emergency department	142 (35%)	34 (34%)	2	0.95 (0.60–1.51)	> 0.3	*
Hospital ward	136 (33%)	35 (35%)	2	1.06 (0.67–1.68)	> 0.3	*
Operating room	87 (21%)	27 (27%)	2	1.35 (0.82–2.22)	0.24	‡
High-dependency unit	28 (6.8%)	5 (5.0%)	2	0.71 (0.27–1.88)	> 0.3	*
Other	15 (3.7%)	0	2	0.00 (0.00–0.00)	> 0.3	*
Laboratory results max pre-ICU						
SCr (μmol/l) 48 h	85 (62–122)	156 (92–248)	21	1.01 (1.01–1.02)	< 0.001	1.01 (1.01–1.02)
Lactate (mmol/L) 24 h	2.0 (1.2–3.4)	3.3 (1.9–6.1)	184	1.14 (1.06–1.22)	< 0.001	#
Leucocyte (10^9/L) 24 h	12 (8–17)	14 (8–18)	50	1.01 (0.99–10.3)	> 0.3	*
CRP (mg/L) 24 h	157 (64–270)	176 (52–257)	17	1.00 (1.00–1.00)	> 0.3	*
Treatment 48 h pre-ICU						
Immunosuppressive	36 (8.8%)	10 (9.9%)	5	1.13 (.054–2.35)	> 0.3	*
ACE inhibitor or ARB	107 (26%)	22 (22%)	9	0.82 (0.48–1.38)	> 0.3	*
NSAID	66 (16%)	15 (15%)	30	0.87 (0.47–1.60)	> 0.3	*
Diuretic	168 (41%)	44 (44%)	22	1.13 (0.72–1.78)	> 0.3	*
Colloid starch	48 (12%)	23 (23%)	17	2.19 (1.26–3.81)	< 0.01	‡
Radiocontrast	88 (22%)	21 (21%)	2	0.96 (0.56–1.63)	> 0.3	*
Source of infection						
Pulmonary	224 (55%)	34 (34%)	0	0.42 (0.27–0.67)	< 0.001	†
Abdominal	94 (23%)	32 (32%)	0	1.56 (0.97–2.52)	0.07	†
Urinary tract	20 (5%)	16 (16%)	0	3.67 (1.83–7.38)	< 0.001	†
Skin and soft tissue	33 (8%)	8 (8%)	0	0.98 (0.44–2.20)	> 0.3	*
Microbiology						
Blood culture positive	83 (20%)	31 (31%)	133	1.97 (1.16–3.35)	0.01	†
E. coli	11 (2.7%)	9 (8.9%)	133	3.76 (1.50–9.44)	< 0.01	†

Table 1 continued

	AKI stages 0–1 (n = 410, where of 127 stage 1)	AKI stages 2–3 (n = 101, where of 70 stage 3)	No data (n)	Odds ratio (95% CI) univariable	p value univariable	Odds ratio (95% CI) multivariable risk model
Other gram negative	23 (5.6%)	8 (7.9%)	133	1.51 (0.65–3.53)	> 0.3	*
Strep. pneumoniae	14 (3.4%)	5 (5.0%)	133	1.53 (0.53–4.39)	> 0.3	*

Binary variables are shown as absolute number (percentage), and continuous variables are shown as median (interquartile range). Odds ratio, 95% CI and p values are calculated using univariable logistic regression towards the primary endpoint for the purpose of constructing a clinical risk model. Explanation for variable exclusion from the risk model follows

SAPS Simplified Acute Physiology Score; *COPD* chronic obstructive pulmonary disease; *CRP* C-reactive protein; *ACE* angiotensin-converting-enzyme inhibitor; *ARB* angiotensin II receptor blockers; *NSAID* non-steroidal anti-inflammatory drugs

* Excluded from the risk model due to p value above 0.3 in univariable logistic regression

[†] Excluded because the variable was not indisputably available to treating clinician at admission

[‡] Excluded due to p value above 0.1 in multivariable logistic regression

[§] Excluded because the risk model already contains SAPS without renal or age points

[#] Excluded due to too many missing values

compared to endpoint negative patients' plasma HBP (mean 59 ng/ml and median 33 ng/ml (IQR 15–73 ng/ml) versus mean 28 ng/ml and median 15 ng/ml (IQR 8–29 ng/ml), $p < 0.001$, $n = 511$). Among all patients ($n = 601$) reaching at highest AKI stages 0, 1, 2 and 3, median plasma HBP was 14 ng/ml (IQR 7–28 ng/ml), 19 ng/ml (IQR 9–37 ng/ml), 26 ng/ml (IQR 11–70 ng/ml) and 30 ng/ml (IQR 15–76 ng/ml), respectively. The plasma HBP levels for these groups differed significantly in individual comparison between groups in all cases except between AKI stage 2 versus 3, as shown in Additional file 2; Figure S1.

Risk model construction

Only variables presented in Table 1 that were considered indisputably available to the treating physician at ICU admission were eligible for inclusion in the risk model. Variables that had a p value below 0.3 in a univariate logistic regression were included into a multivariable logistic regression and excluded one variable at a time, starting with the highest p value, until only variables with a p value below 0.1 remained. Established AKI risk factors with a p value above 0.3 (CKD, hypertension, diabetes and urinary tract infection) were not included in the risk model because their addition did not affect the ROC area or 95% CI at three decimal places. The final risk model included 489 patients and contained three variables with positive coefficients for the primary endpoint: age, SAPS II without renal and age points and maximum SCr 48 h pre-ICU admission. See Table 1 for further details. Plasma HBP was added to the risk model as a categorical variable based on quartiles because it produced a slightly higher ROC area (0.01 absolute difference) compared to adding plasma HBP as a continuous variable.

Primary endpoint

The ROC area for the risk model including categorical plasma HBP to predict the primary endpoint was 0.82 (95% CI 0.77–0.87) compared to 0.78 (95% CI 0.73–0.84) for the risk model alone ($p = 0.03$, $n = 489$). The total cfNRI was positive 62% (95% CI 41–82%) and total IDI positive 0.053 (95% CI 0.03–0.08). LR+ was 2.73 (95% CI 2.00–3.71) for patients with a plasma HBP above 40 ng/ml and 0.43 (95% CI 0.26–0.71) for patients with a plasma HBP below 10 ng/ml, respectively. Continuous plasma HBP alone had a ROC area of 0.70 (95% CI 0.64–0.76) to predict the primary endpoint. We performed six sensitivity analyses based on ROC area and continuous plasma HBP. See Table 2 and Additional file 1; Tables S2–S5 for further results.

Secondary endpoints

Mean fluid balance within 24 h from ICU admission was significantly higher in patients with a high plasma HBP ($\geq$ 20 ng/ml) compared to patients with a low plasma HBP on ICU admission (+ 2452 ml vs. + 1031 ml, $p < 0.001$). Mean difference in fluid balance per weight was 1.9% (95% CI 1.3–2.5%), and the mean difference in total volume was 1422 ml (95% CI 985–1859 ml). Median fluid balance for each defined plasma HBP quartile ($\leq$ 10, > 10 $\leq$ 20, > 20 $\leq$ 40 and > 40 ng/ml) was 779 ml (IQR − 423 to 2337 ml), 612 ml (IQR − 246 to 2391 ml), 1978 ml (IQR 312–4086 ml) and 2146 ml (IQR 461–3995 ml), respectively, as shown in Fig. 2 and Additional file 3; Figure S2. Maximum SOFA score within 5 days from ICU admission was significantly higher in patients with a high plasma HBP compared to patients with a low plasma HBP on ICU admission (mean points 9.1 vs. 7.4, $p < 0.001$, $n = 601$) with a mean difference of 1.7 points

Table 2 Risk model comparison with and without plasma HBP ($n = 489$)

	Value	95% CI
ROC area: risk model only	0.784*	0.734–0.835
ROC area: risk model + plasma HBP	0.819*	0.770–0.868
cfNRI event	37.4%	18.6–55.1
cfNRI non-event	24.6%	15.2–34.0
cfNRI total	62.0%	40.5–82.4
IDI event	0.042	0.02–0.63
IDI non-event	0.011	0.003–0.019
IDI total	0.053	0.029–0.075

Events refer to the development of the primary endpoint. Categorised plasma HBP based on quartiles was used in the analysis

cfNRI category-free net reclassification index, IDI integrated discrimination improvement

* The difference in ROC area between the risk model with and without plasma HBP was statistically significant ($p = 0.03$)

(95% CI 1.2–2.2). Continuous plasma HBP alone had a ROC area of 0.69 (95% CI 0.63–0.75) to predict initiation of RRT for AKI within 5 days ($n = 91$ out of 601). Patients with a plasma HBP above 20 ng/ml on ICU admission had a significantly higher unadjusted 28-day mortality than patients with a low plasma HBP (28 vs. 21%, $p = 0.03$), as shown in Fig. 2.

Discussion

Key findings

We have found that plasma HBP measured on ICU admission improves prediction of sepsis-related AKI stages 2–3 among mixed general ICU patients. Furthermore, we found that patients with an increased plasma HBP (≥ 20 ng/ml) on ICU admission had a significantly higher fluid balance within 24 h from ICU admission, a higher maximum SOFA score within 5 days and an increased risk of dying within 28 days, respectively, as compared to patients with a low plasma HBP on ICU admission.

Pathophysiological mechanism

HBP's plausibility as a marker of septic organ dysfunction can be supported by its early release in response to an infection and its powerful effects on immune cells and endothelial cells, which may act as causative factors in sepsis [13]. Prefabricated HBP is rapidly released from secretory vesicles of activated neutrophils [14–16]. HBP act as a chemoattractant for neutrophils, T cells and monocytes and enhances monocyte cytokine release, phagocytosis and adhesion to the endothelium [17–20]. HBP also induces cytoskeletal rearrangement and cell contraction, forming gaps in the endothelium, leading to vascular leakage and neutrophil extravasation, which leads to more HBP release from azurophilic granules [21–23]. HBP also induces inflammation and capillary leakage in the kidney, as is supported by findings from Fisher et al. [7], which correspond to two out of three mechanisms in the proposed unifying theory of AKI pathophysiology presented by Gomez et al. [24]. On this background, we present a proposed mechanism to explain the findings from the primary endpoint analysis, as shown in Fig. 3.

Primary endpoint interpretation and performance compared

Translating measures of diagnostic accuracy into clinical use is always a challenge. In this paper, we constructed a

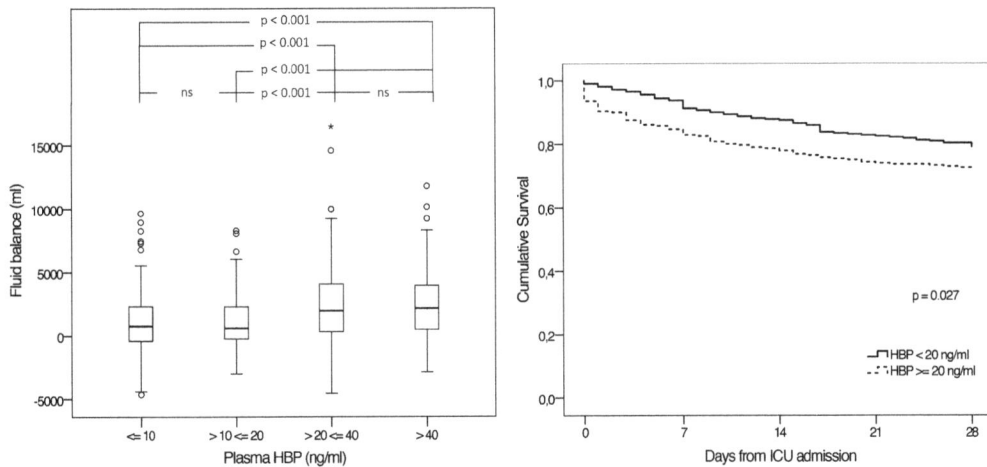

Fig. 2 Fluid balance and 28-day survival. The left boxplot describes patients' fluid balance within 24 h from ICU admission separated by plasma HBP quartiles and includes testing for significant difference between plasma HBP levels of each individual group ($n = 601$, ns: not significant). The right Kaplan–Meier survival curve pictures survival within 28 days from ICU admission among patients with a high versus low plasma HBP on ICU admission ($n = 601$)

risk model to simulate the clinical information available to the treating clinician and then statistically measured the predictive benefit of adding the information from plasma HBP through cfNRI, IDI and improvement in ROC area. The cfNRI was 62%, indicating that about one-third of all patients will benefit from a more correct risk classification (cfNRI max is 200%) when adding plasma HBP to known clinical risk factors. The added predictive value is supported by a significant increase in ROC area of the risk model when adding plasma HBP. The risk model's ROC area is comparable to that of previous studies (0.80 in Kashani et al. [25] and 0.86 in Honore et al. [26]).

We choose only to include patients who developed AKI beyond 12 h from admission in our primary analysis because we considered it most relevant to the treating clinician. AKI diagnosed within 12 h from sampling provides little time for possible clinical intervention.

Furthermore, AKI diagnosed within 12 h will probably reflect kidney cell damage that was already present at biomarker sampling, due to the delayed nature of the current AKI definition based on SCr and UOP, arguably negating the predictive performance of the biomarker. This is probably also true in markers of cell cycle arrest, which are reasonably expressed when kidney cells are already distressed [25]. Conversely, there is evidence to suggest that plasma HBP may have a causative role in septic AKI [7], as shown in Fig. 3.

So far, only two previous studies have examined plasma HBP's performance in predicting AKI. Fisher et al. [7] reported, first, a ROC area of 0.85 to discriminate patients with KDIGO AKI stage 0 versus 2 within 5 days from ICU admission, and second, a ROC area of 0.80 for discriminating AKI stage 0 versus 1–3 after 48 h up to 5 days from ICU admission among 296 patients with septic shock from the Vasopressin and

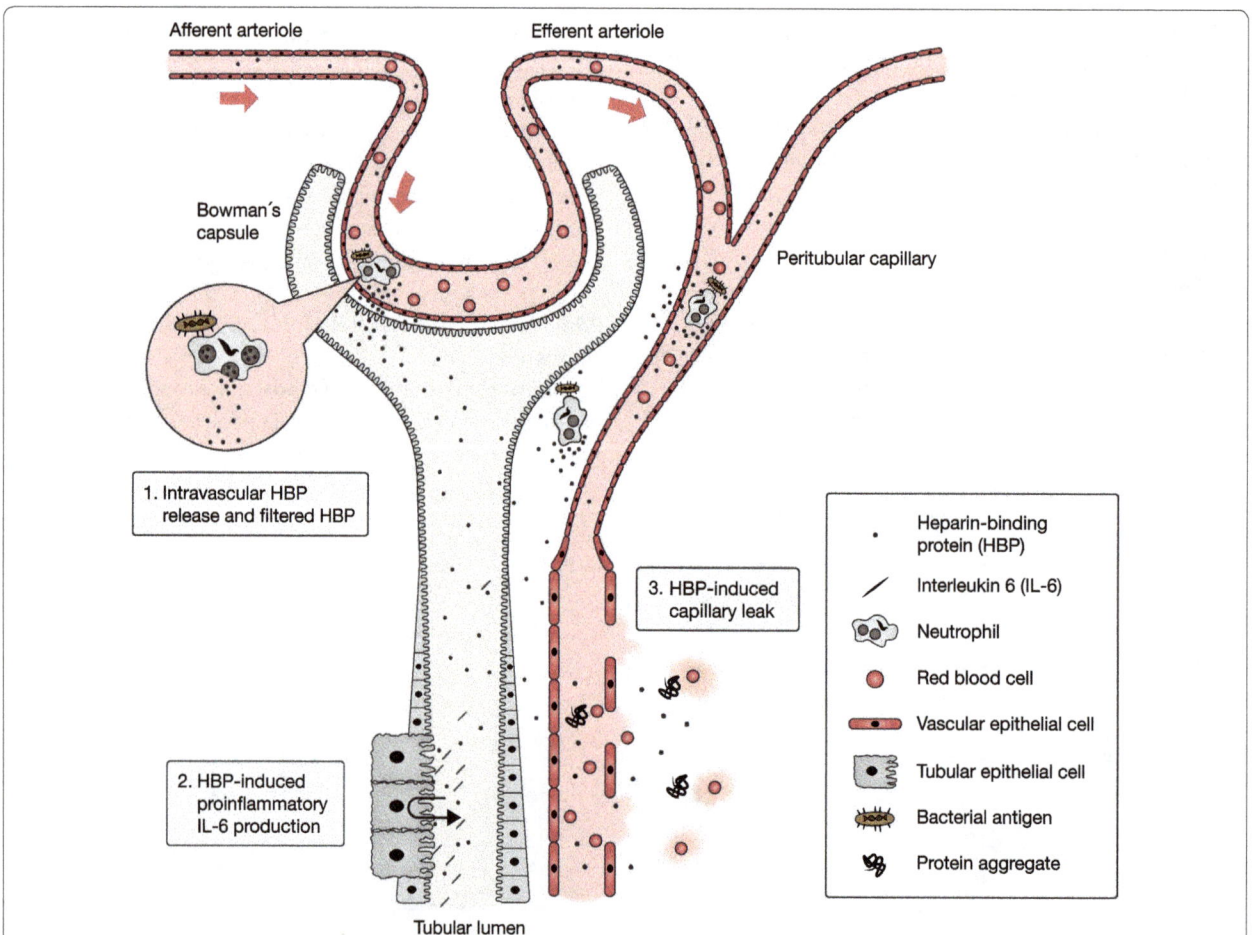

Fig. 3 Proposed mechanism for HBP's involvement in sepsis-related AKI pathophysiology. *1* Neutrophils activated by bacterial antigen release pre-produced HBP from secretory vesicles into peripheral tissue and blood vessels. HBP is filtered through the glomeruli, and the Bowman's capsule into the tubular lumen *2* HBP induces inflammation in tubular epithelial cells, supported by evidence of IL-6 production [7]. *3* HBP act on peritubular vascular cells inducing capillary leakage through loosened tight junctions, supported by evidence of interstitial haemorrhage and protein aggregates in extracellular matrix [7]

Septic Shock Trial (VASST) cohort [27]. Tyden et al. [8] reported a ROC area of 0.70 for plasma HBP measured on ICU admission to predict the development of KDIGO AKI stages 2–3 within 7 days from ICU admission among 245 mixed ICU patients, and a ROC area of 0.88 for the same endpoint in a small subgroup analysis of 59 patients with severe sepsis. However, these results are not directly comparable to our results due to differences in primary endpoint definition, and there were no data on added benefit to clinical risk factors presented in either study.

Our results may be assessed in comparison with the cell cycle arrest biomarkers, namely urine tissue inhibitor of metalloproteinases-2 (TIMP-2) and insulin-like growth factor-binding protein 7 (IGFBP7). Honore et al. [26] present impressive results for the combined biomarker of urine [TIMP-2] * [IGFBP7] to predict KDIGO AKI stages 2–3 within 12 h in 232 ICU patients with severe sepsis and septic shock. However, these results do not clearly translate to our interest of AKI prediction beyond 12 h from admission. The original cohort of the above-mentioned study was published with a supplementary appendix [25] with results for the prediction of AKI (RIFLE Injury or Failure) diagnosed 12–36 h from sample collection in 522 septic and non-septic ICU patients. Here, the ROC area for urine [TIMP-2] * [IGFBP7] was 0.77, cfNRI was 70%, IDI was 0.098 and improvement in risk model ROC area just failed to be statistically significant (0.87 vs. 0.80, $p = 0.06$).

Secondary endpoints interpretation

Patients with an increased plasma HBP on admission had a mean fluid balance that was 1422 ml higher than patients with a low plasma HBP within 24 h from ICU admission. This finding could arguably support HBP's role as a marker of AKI since fluid overload is closely related to AKI and administration of RRT [28]. It also supports the biological role for HBP as a primary mediator of vascular leakage, an important pathophysiological mechanism in septic shock. A high plasma HBP was also associated with a higher maximum SOFA score within 5 days and an increased 28-day mortality, which is in line with earlier research correlating a high plasma HBP to greater sepsis severity and death [5].

Limitations and strengths

First, the study was limited by being designed after sample and data collection. Second, samples had been stored at − 80 °C for over 1 year and shipped on dry ice from Finland to Sweden prior to being analysed. Third, we lacked baseline SCr for 30% of patients, where we had to back-calculate using the recommended MDRD formula. Fourth, no comparison to other biomarkers was made

on the same patients and data, and there was no external validation performed. Strengths of this study include a biologically plausible biomarker, a generally accepted and clinically relevant endpoint, a large sample size from a well-characterised population and results that are robust to several types of statistical analyses.

Conclusion

Plasma HBP is a biologically plausible novel biomarker of sepsis-related AKI that adds predictive value to known clinical risk factors. Further studies are warranted to compare the performance of plasma HBP to other novel AKI biomarkers.

Abbreviations

ACE: angiotensin-converting-enzyme inhibitor; AKI: acute kidney injury; ARB: angiotensin II receptor blockers; cfNRI: category-free net reclassification index; COPD: chronic obstructive pulmonary disease; CRP: C-reactive protein; %CV: coefficient of variation; ELISA: enzyme-linked immunosorbent assay; HBP: heparin-binding protein; ICU: intensive care unit; IDI: integrated discrimination improvement; IGFBP7: insulin-like growth factor-binding protein 7; IL-6: interleukin 6; LR+: positive likelihood ratio; MDRD: modification in diet in renal disease; ng/ml: nanograms per millilitre; NPV: negative predictive value; NSAID: non-steroidal anti-inflammatory drugs; OR: odds ratio; PASS: power analysis and sample size; PPV: positive predictive value; ROC area: area under the receiver operating curve; RRT: renal replacement therapy; SAPS: Simplified Acute Physiology Score; SCr: serum creatinine; SOFA score: sequential organ failure assessment; TIMP-2: tissue inhibitor of metalloproteinases-2; KDIGO: kidney disease: improving global outcomes; UOP: urine output; VASST: vasopressin and septic shock trial.

Authors' contributions

JT performed the laboratory analyses and the statistical analyses, interpreted the data and drafted and finalised the manuscript. STV participated in the design and data gathering of the study and assisted with data interpretation. JF coordinated the laboratory analyses and revised the manuscript critically. MP was an investigator of the FINNAKI study focusing on septic AKI. VP was a major contributor in the design of this study and was the principal investigator of the FINNAKI study. AL is the archival author and coordinator of the study. All the FINNAKI investigators (The FINNAKI study group) participated in the design and data collection of FINNAKI. All authors read and approved the final manuscript.

Author details

[1] Division of Infection Medicine, Department of Clinical Sciences, Lund University, BMC B14, 221 84 Lund, Sweden. [2] Division of Intensive Care Medicine, Department of Anesthesiology, Intensive Care and Pain Medicine, University of Helsinki and Helsinki University Hospital, Helsinki, Finland. [3] Department of Intensive Care, Austin Hospital, Melbourne, Australia. [4] Department of Intensive Care, Lapland Central Hospital, Rovaniemi, Finland.

Acknowledgements

Thank you to Sebastian Drejier for making the illustration, thank you to Jonas Björk and Anna Åkesson for guidance on statistical analyses, thank you to Niklas Nielsen for invariably sound advice and thank you to the FINNAKI Study Group: Central Finland Central Hospital: Raili Laru-Sompa, Anni Pulkkinen, Minna Saarelainen, Mikko Reilama, Sinikka Tolmunen, Ulla Rantalainen, Marja Miettinen East Savo Central Hospital: Markku Suvela, Katrine Pesola, Pekka Saastamoinen, Sirpa Kauppinen Helsinki University Hospital: Ville Pettilä, Kirsi-Maija Kaukonen, Anna-Maija Korhonen, Sara Nisula, Suvi Vaara, Raili Suojaranta-Ylinen, Leena Mildh, Mikko Haapio, Laura Nurminen, Sari Sutinen, Leena Pettilä, Helinä Laitinen, Heidi Syrjä, Kirsi Henttonen, Elina Lappi, Hillevi Boman Jorvi Central Hospital: Tero Varpula, Päivi Porkka, Mirka Sivula, Mira Rahkonen,

Anne Tsurkka, Taina Nieminen, Niina Pirttinen Kanta-Häme Central hospital: Ari Alaspää, Ville Salanto, Hanna Juntunen, Teija Sanisalo Kuopio University Hospital: Ilkka Parviainen, Ari Uusaro, Esko Ruokonen, Stepani Bendel, Niina Rissanen, Maarit Lång, Sari Rahikainen, Saija Rissanen, Merja Ahonen, Elina Halonen, Eija Vaskelainen Lapland Central Hospital: Meri Poukkanen, Esa Lintula, Sirpa Suominen Länsi-Pohja Central Hospital: Jorma Heikkinen, Timo Lavander, Kirsi Heinonen, Anne-Mari Juopperi Middle Ostrobothnia Central Hospital: Tadeusz Kaminski, Fiia Gäddnäs, Tuija Kuusela, Jane Roiko North Karelia Central Hospital: Sari Karlsson, Matti Reinikainen, Tero Surakka, Helena Jyrkönen, Tanja Eiserbeck, Jaana Kallinen Oulu University Hospital: Tero Ala-Kokko, Jouko Laurila, Sinikka Sälkiö Satakunta Hospital District: Vesa Lund, Päivi Tuominen, Pauliina Perkola, Riikka Tuominen, Marika Hietaranta, Satu Johansson South Karelia Central Hospital: Seppo Hovilehto, Anne Kirsi, Pekka Tiainen, Tuija Myllärinen, Pirjo Leino, Anne Toropainen Tampere University Hospital: Anne Kuitunen, Jyrki Tenhunen, Ilona Leppänen, Markus Levoranta, Sanna Hoppu, Jukka Sauranen, Atte Kukkurainen, Samuli Kortelainen, Simo Varila Turku University Hospital: Outi Inkinen, Niina Koivuviita, Jutta Kotamäki, Anu Laine Vaasa Central Hospital: Simo-Pekka Koivisto, Raku Hautamäki, Maria Skinnar.

Competing interests
AL is listed as an inventor on a pending patent application on the use of HBP as a diagnostic tool in sepsis. The other authors declare that they have no competing interests.

Funding
JT has received grants from the Thelma Zoégas Foundation for medical research (91282) and from the Swedish Government Research Grant (ALF). STV has received grants from the Instrumentarium Science Foundation and the Sigrid Juselius Foundation. The FINNAKI study was funded by Juselius Foundation (VP), Päivikki and Sakari Sohlberg Foundation (VP) and Helsinki University Hospital Grants (TYH 2010109/2011210, T102010070, TYH 2013343 and 2016243). AL has received grants from the Swedish Government Research Grant (ALF), Svenska Läkaresällskapet, Clas Groschinsky's foundation, Wilhelm and Martina Lundgren's foundation, Alfred Österlunds foundation and Åke Wiberg foundation. Axis-Shield Diagnostics (Dundee, UK) provided the HBP ELISA kits but where otherwise not involved in the design of the study, collection of materials, interpretation of data or writing of the manuscript.

References
1. Uchino S, Kellum JA, Bellomo R, Doig GS, Morimatsu H, Morgera S, et al. Acute renal failure in critically ill patients: a multinational, multicenter study. JAMA. 2005;294(7):813–8.
2. Group. KDIGOKAKIW. KDIGO clinical practice guideline for acute kidney injury. Kidney Int Suppl. 2012;2(Suppl.):1–138.
3. Murray PT, Mehta RL, Shaw A, Ronco C, Endre Z, Kellum JA, et al. Potential use of biomarkers in acute kidney injury: report and summary of recommendations from the 10th acute dialysis quality initiative consensus conference. Kidney Int. 2014;85(3):513–21.
4. Linder A, Christensson B, Herwald H, Bjorck L, Akesson P. Heparin-binding protein: an early marker of circulatory failure in sepsis. Clin Infect Dis. 2009;49(7):1044–50.
5. Linder A, Akesson P, Inghammar M, Treutiger CJ, Linner A, Sunden-Cullberg J. Elevated plasma levels of heparin-binding protein in intensive care unit patients with severe sepsis and septic shock. Crit Care. 2012;16(3):R90.
6. Linder A, Arnold R, Boyd JH, Zindovic M, Zindovic I, Lange A, et al. Heparin-binding protein measurement improves the prediction of severe infection with organ dysfunction in the emergency department. Crit Care Med. 2015;43(11):2378–86.
7. Fisher J, Russell JA, Bentzer P, Parsons D, Secchia S, Morgelin M, et al. Heparin-binding protein (HBP): a causative marker and potential target for heparin treatment of human sepsis-induced acute kidney injury. Shock. 2017;48(3):313–20.
8. Tyden J, Herwald H, Hultin M, Wallden J, Johansson J. Heparin-binding protein as a biomarker of acute kidney injury in critical illness. Acta Anaesthesiol Scand. 2017;61(7):797–803.
9. Nisula S, Kaukonen KM, Vaara ST, Korhonen AM, Poukkanen M, Karlsson S, et al. Incidence, risk factors and 90-day mortality of patients with acute kidney injury in Finnish intensive care units: the FINNAKI study. Intensive Care Med. 2013;39(3):420–8.
10. Levey AS, Bosch JP, Lewis JB, Greene T, Rogers N, Roth D. A more accurate method to estimate glomerular filtration rate from serum creatinine: a new prediction equation. Modification of Diet in Renal Disease Study Group. Ann Intern Med. 1999;130(6):461–70.
11. Levy MM, Fink MP, Marshall JC, Abraham E, Angus D, Cook D, et al. 2001 SCCM/ESICM/ACCP/ATS/SIS international sepsis definitions conference. Crit Care Med. 2003;31(4):1250–6.
12. DeLong ER, DeLong DM, Clarke-Pearson DL. Comparing the areas under two or more correlated receiver operating characteristic curves: a nonparametric approach. Biometrics. 1988;44(3):837–45.
13. Fisher J, Linder A. Heparin-binding protein: a key player in the pathophysiology of organ dysfunction in sepsis. J Intern Med. 2017;281(6):562–74.
14. Kolaczkowska E, Kubes P. Neutrophil recruitment and function in health and inflammation. Nat Rev Immunol. 2013;13(3):159–75.
15. Tapper H, Karlsson A, Morgelin M, Flodgaard H, Herwald H. Secretion of heparin-binding protein from human neutrophils is determined by its localization in azurophilic granules and secretory vesicles. Blood. 2002;99(5):1785–93.
16. Pereira HA, Shafer WM, Pohl J, Martin LE, Spitznagel JK. CAP37, a human neutrophil-derived chemotactic factor with monocyte specific activity. J Clin Invest. 1990;85(5):1468–76.
17. Chertov O, Ueda H, Xu LL, Tani K, Murphy WJ, Wang JM, et al. Identification of human neutrophil-derived cathepsin G and azurocidin/CAP37 as chemoattractants for mononuclear cells and neutrophils. J Exp Med. 1997;186(5):739–47.
18. Soehnlein O. Direct and alternative antimicrobial mechanisms of neutrophil-derived granule proteins. J Mol Med (Berl). 2009;87(12):1157–64.
19. Soehnlein O, Xie X, Ulbrich H, Kenne E, Rotzius P, Flodgaard H, et al. Neutrophil-derived heparin-binding protein (HBP/CAP37) deposited on endothelium enhances monocyte arrest under flow conditions. J Immunol. 2005;174(10):6399–405.
20. Chertov O, Michiel DF, Xu L, Wang JM, Tani K, Murphy WJ, et al. Identification of defensin-1, defensin-2, and CAP37/azurocidin as T-cell chemoattractant proteins released from interleukin-8-stimulated neutrophils. J Biol Chem. 1996;271(6):2935–40.
21. Gautam N, Olofsson AM, Herwald H, Iversen LF, Lundgren-Akerlund E, Hedqvist P, et al. Heparin-binding protein (HBP/CAP37): a missing link in neutrophil-evoked alteration of vascular permeability. Nat Med. 2001;7(10):1123–7.
22. Ostergaard E, Flodgaard H. A neutrophil-derived proteolytic inactive elastase homologue (hHBP) mediates reversible contraction of fibroblasts and endothelial cell monolayers and stimulates monocyte survival and thrombospondin secretion. J Leukoc Biol. 1992;51(4):316–23.
23. Bentzer P, Fisher J, Kong HJ, Morgelin M, Boyd JH, Walley KR, et al. Heparin-binding protein is important for vascular leak in sepsis. Intensive Care Med Exp. 2016;4(1):33.
24. Gomez H, Ince C, De Backer D, Pickkers P, Payen D, Hotchkiss J, et al. A unified theory of sepsis-induced acute kidney injury: inflammation, microcirculatory dysfunction, bioenergetics, and the tubular cell adaptation to injury. Shock. 2014;41(1):3–11.
25. Kashani K, Al-Khafaji A, Ardiles T, Artigas A, Bagshaw SM, Bell M, et al. Discovery and validation of cell cycle arrest biomarkers in human acute kidney injury. Crit Care. 2013;17(1):R25.
26. Honore PM, Nguyen HB, Gong M, Chawla LS, Bagshaw SM, Artigas A, et al. Urinary tissue inhibitor of metalloproteinase-2 and insulin-like growth factor-binding protein 7 for risk stratification of acute kidney injury in patients with sepsis. Crit Care Med. 2016;44(10):1851–60.
27. Russell JA, Walley KR, Singer J, Gordon AC, Hebert PC, Cooper DJ, et al. Vasopressin versus norepinephrine infusion in patients with septic shock. N Engl J Med. 2008;358(9):877–87.
28. Wang N, Jiang L, Zhu B, Wen Y, Xi XM. Beijing acute kidney injury trial W. Fluid balance and mortality in critically ill patients with acute kidney injury: a multicenter prospective epidemiological study. Crit Care. 2015;19:371.

15

The effect of multidisciplinary extracorporeal membrane oxygenation team on clinical outcomes in patients with severe acute respiratory failure

Soo Jin Na[1], Chi Ryang Chung[1], Hee Jung Choi[2], Yang Hyun Cho[3], Kiick Sung[3], Jeong Hoon Yang[1,4], Gee Young Suh[1,5] and Kyeongman Jeon[1,5]* 🄳

Abstract

Background: The Extracorporeal Life Support Organization (ELSO) has suggested that extracorporeal membrane oxygenation (ECMO) patients should be managed by a multidisciplinary team. However, there are limited data on the impact of ECMO team on the outcomes of patients with severe acute respiratory failure.

Methods: All consecutive patients with severe acute respiratory failure who underwent ECMO for respiratory support from January 2012 through December 2016 were divided into the pre-ECMO team period (before January 2014, $n = 70$) and the post-ECMO team period (after January 2014, $n = 46$). Clinical characteristics and outcomes were compared between the two groups.

Results: The mortality rates in the intensive care unit (72.9 vs. 50.0%, $P = 0.012$) and hospital (75.7 vs. 52.2%, $P = 0.009$) were significantly decreased in the post-ECMO team period compared to the pre-ECMO team period. The median duration of ECMO support was not different between the two periods. However, the proportion of patients successfully weaned off ECMO was higher in the post-ECMO team period (42.9 vs. 65.2%, $P = 0.018$). During ECMO support, the incidence of cannula problems (32.9 vs. 15.2%, $P = 0.034$) and cardiovascular events (88.6 vs. 65.2%, $P = 0.002$) was reduced after implementation of the ECMO team. The 1-year mortality was significantly different between the pre-ECMO team and post-ECMO team periods (37.8 vs. 14.3%, $P = 0.005$).

Conclusion: After implementing a multidisciplinary ECMO team, survival rate in patients treated with ECMO for severe acute respiratory failure was significantly improved.

Keywords: Extracorporeal membrane oxygenation, Patient care team, Respiratory insufficiency, Critical care outcomes, Mortality

Introduction

Recent studies showing the favorable results of extracorporeal membrane oxygenation (ECMO) have highlighted the role of ECMO in treating severe acute respiratory failure [1–4]. In addition, the number of patients receiving ECMO support in clinical practice is growing [4]. Despite the technical advances and generalization of the technique, ECMO is still a complex and costly treatment with potential adverse effects, and the clinical outcomes associated with its use are significantly different depending on the infrastructure of the providing center [5]. Therefore, the Extracorporeal Life Support Organization (ELSO) has published guidelines regarding the ideal institutional requirements for effective use of ECMO [6, 7]. In these guidelines, qualified ECMO physicians are

*Correspondence: kjeon@skku.edu
[1] Department of Critical Care Medicine, Samsung Medical Center, Sungkyunkwan University School of Medicine, 81 Irwon-ro, Gangnam-gu, Seoul 06351, Republic of Korea
Full list of author information is available at the end of the article

referred to as one of the most important components of the successful implementation of ECMO, and their various responsibilities are emphasized, from initiation of ECMO to clinical follow-up [6, 7].

Some adjunctive therapies, such as use of neuromuscular blocking agents [8] and prone positioning [9], have been shown to reduce mortality in patients with severe acute respiratory failure, and these treatments before ECMO are also associated with outcomes seen after ECMO for respiratory failure [10, 11]. Therefore, decision making about the proper indications and timing of ECMO is a challenging problem for physicians who manage patients with severe acute respiratory failure. In addition, the medical management and nursing care of patients with severe respiratory failure receiving ECMO support are complex and can be challenging; therefore, the multidisciplinary ECMO team is recommended to be incorporated into ECMO program [7].

However, there are limited data on the impact of ECMO team on the outcomes of patients with severe acute respiratory failure. The objective of this study was to investigate the association between implementation of a multidisciplinary ECMO team and clinical outcomes in adult patients with severe respiratory failure receiving ECMO support.

Methods

Study design

We conducted a retrospective cohort study between January 2012 and December 2016 at Samsung Medical Center (a 1979-bed tertiary referral hospital with tertiary-level intensive care units) in Seoul, South Korea. All patients 18 years of age or older for whom ECMO support was required for severe acute respiratory failure were enrolled in the study. A total of 136 ECMO runs in 133 patients were identified during this period. Twenty patients who were transported to our facility after initiation of ECMO in other hospitals were excluded because the decision regarding whether or not the patient was a suitable candidate for ECMO and initial management were not made by our ECMO team. The remaining 116 eligible ECMO runs were divided into the pre-ECMO team period (before January 2014, $n = 70$) and the post-ECMO team period (after January 2014, $n = 46$), according to the date of ECMO initiation (Fig. 1).

The institutional review board of the Samsung Medical Center approved this study and waived the requirement for informed consent because of the observational nature of the study. In addition, patients' information was anonymized and deidentified prior to analysis.

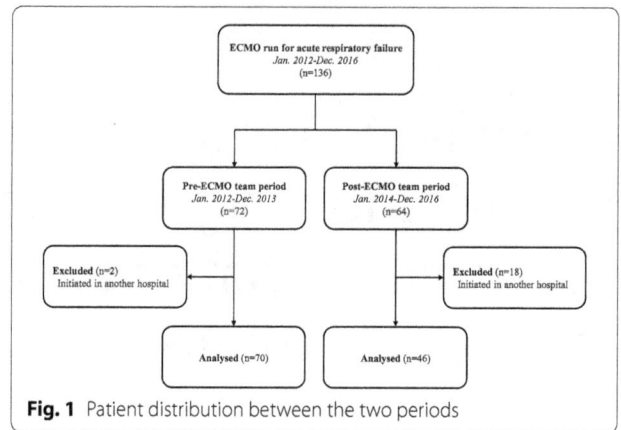

Fig. 1 Patient distribution between the two periods

ECMO team and management of ECMO

In our institution, ECMO support has been available since 2004. In the first few years, veno-arterial ECMO was primarily used in patients with cardiac failure, with veno-venous ECMO used for less than five cases per year. The incidence of ECMO runs has gradually increased, with more than 100 cases currently performed annually. The application of veno-venous ECMO for severe respiratory failure has also grown and currently represents up to 20–30% of all ECMO runs.

Before 2014, there were standard criteria for indications and contraindications of ECMO (Additional file 1), but decisions about initiation and decannulation were mostly left to the physicians that oversaw patients. Cannula- or circuit-related issues were treated through elective consultation with cardiothoracic surgeons who had experience with ECMO. In 2014, our hospital adopted a multidisciplinary ECMO team consisting of cardiovascular surgeons, cardiologists, critical care physicians, and an ECMO specialist who is a cardiovascular perfusionist trained to manage the ECMO system and clinical needs of the patients on ECMO under supervision of ECMO-trained physicians. This ECMO team was responsible for every issue related to ECMO in the hospital. Protocols for indications and contraindications, management of patients and equipment, and weaning of patients from ECMO were revised. In addition, the ECMO team was charged with educating all medical personnel including bedside nurses caring for patients on ECMO at our institution. When a patient was deemed eligible for ECMO, the final decision to initiate ECMO was made by the treating intensivist and ECMO team, consisting of two more critical care physicians who are board certified in pulmonary and critical care medicine and cardiovascular surgeon, after a comprehensive assessment based on our protocol outlining the indications and contraindications. The primary cannulation strategy for adult respiratory

ECMO was the veno-venous mode. The veno–veno-arterial mode was considered if the patient needed additional support due to hemodynamic failure. Cannulation was performed by the attending cardiothoracic surgeons using either the percutaneous method with the Seldinger technique or the surgical method at the bedside or in the operating room. Cannulation sites and cannula sizes were selected at the discretion of the cardiothoracic surgeons. Usually, a 20–28-Fr cannula was used for venous drainage via the common femoral vein, and a 14–18- or 20–24-Fr cannula was used for venous return via the internal jugular or the common femoral vein, respectively. The Prolonged Life Support System (Quadrox PLS, Maquet Inc., Rastatt, Germany) and the Capiox Emergency Bypass System (Capiox EBS; Terumo, Inc., Tokyo, Japan) were used. Pump blood flow and sweep gas flow rates were adjusted to maintain a target oxygen saturation and carbon dioxide removal rate. The mechanical ventilation (MV) strategy during ECMO was adapted from the study protocol of the CESAR trial [1], providing assisted pressure-controlled ventilation while limiting the peak inspiratory pressure to 25 cmH_2O and applying positive end-expiratory airway pressure of 10 cmH_2O, and respiratory rate of 10 breaths/min, on inspired oxygen fraction of 30%. Once the patients were stabilized and lightly sedated, spontaneous ventilation with pressure support mode was considered. In all patients, arterial catheterization was performed for continuous hemodynamic monitoring. Our ECMO team performed daily rounds and assessed the state of the ECMO circuit, development of ECMO-associated complications, and the possibility of weaning. An ECMO-trained physician provided 24-h on-call coverage, and an ECMO specialist participated in all intra-hospital transport of patients on ECMO. If a patient was considered ready to be weaned off ECMO support, decisions regarding decannulation were assessed through a protocolized weaning trial. Cannulae were removed at the bedside by cardiothoracic surgeons.

Data collection and clinical outcomes

The clinical and laboratory data from patients who were treated with ECMO have been prospectively registered in the ECMO database of our hospital since 2012. For this study, these data were supplemented with a retrospective review of all hospital medical records. Demographic data, including age, sex, comorbidity, immune state, history of cardiac arrest, diagnosis, acute physiology and chronic health evaluation (APACHE) II score, and sequential organ failure assessment (SOFA) score, were recorded at admission to the intensive care unit (ICU). Presence of an artificial airway, use of MV, ventilator setting immediately before ECMO initiation, use

of rescue and adjunctive treatment before ECMO, worst values from arterial blood gas and lactate tests within 6 h before ECMO initiation, respiratory extracorporeal membrane oxygenation survival prediction (RESP) score [11], predicting death for severe ARDS on VV-ECMO (PRESERVE) score [10], ECMO mode, and cannulation site were recorded on the first day of ECMO support.

The primary outcome in this study was in-hospital mortality. Secondary outcomes were ICU mortality, rate of weaning from ECMO, duration of ECMO support, adverse events during ECMO, rate of weaning from MV, duration of MV before weaning, ICU and hospital lengths of stay, and 1-year mortality after ECMO initiation. Adverse events during ECMO were defined as follows: cannula-related (vessel perforation with hemorrhage, arterial cannulation, malposition requiring repositioning, or accidental decannulation), other ECMO-related, hematological (gastrointestinal bleeding, cannula site bleeding, surgical site bleeding, plasma hemoglobin level > 50 mg/dL, or disseminated intravascular coagulation), neurological (brain death, seizure, cerebral infarction, or brain hemorrhage), cardiovascular (inotrope or vasopressor use, myocardial stunning, arrhythmia, cardiac tamponade, or cardiac arrest), pulmonary (pneumothorax or pulmonary hemorrhage), renal (serum creatinine level > 1.5 mg/dL or continuous renal replacement therapy), and infection (white blood cell count < 1500×10^3 cells/mm^3, culture-confirmed new infection, or ECMO-associated wound infection). Clinical outcomes were identified through medical record review. The Korean National Database, which uses citizen registration numbers, was used to obtain information about patient death at 1 year after ECMO initiation.

Statistical analysis

To compare characteristics and clinical outcomes between the two periods, we analyzed categorical variables using χ^2 tests or Fisher's exact tests, when applicable, with data presented as numbers and percentages. Continuous variables were presented as medians with interquartile ranges, and Mann–Whitney U test was used for analysis. To adjust for potential confounding factors in the association between implementation of a multidisciplinary ECMO team and in-hospital mortality, multiple logistic regression analysis was used. Data are presented as adjusted odds ratios (ORs) with 95% confidence intervals (CI). Survival curves were constructed using the Kaplan–Meier method and compared with a log-rank test. For all analyses, a two-tailed test with a P value less than 0.05 was considered statistically significant. Statistical analyses were performed using SPSS 18.0 for Windows (Chicago, IL, USA).

Results

Baseline clinical characteristics

The baseline clinical characteristics of 116 patients separated according to whether their ECMO treatment period coincided with the implementation of the specialized ECMO team are shown in Table 1. Age, sex, and comorbidities were similar between the two periods. However, patients with airway disease and malignancy were more common in the pre-ECMO team period. Bacterial pneumonia was the most common pulmonary condition causing acute respiratory failure. The proportion of patients with bacterial pneumonia was higher in the pre-ECMO team period (45.7 vs. 26.1%; $P = 0.033$), while the

proportion of patients with viral pneumonia was higher in the post-ECMO team period (2.9 vs. 17.4%, $P = 0.014$). The APACHE II (18 [15–25] vs. 25 [21–32], $P < 0.001$) and SOFA scores (6 [4–9] vs. 8 [6–14], $P = 0.003$) on the day of ICU admission were significantly higher in the post-ECMO team period compared with the pre-ECMO team period. However, the RESP and PRESERVE scores were similar between periods.

Medical management prior to ECMO

Treatment modalities for severe acute respiratory failure prior to ECMO initiation are presented in Table 2. The duration of MV prior to initiation of ECMO was similar

Table 1 Baseline patient characteristics

	Pre-ECMO team period ($n = 70$)	Post-ECMO team period ($n = 46$)	P value
Age (years)	61 (52–69)	60 (52–64)	0.672
Male	52 (74.3)	34 (73.9)	0.964
Body mass index (kg/m²)	23.1 (20.7–24.8)	23.8 (20.6–25.8)	0.163
Comorbidity			
Cardiovascular disease	7 (10.0)	5 (10.9)	>0.999
Chronic renal failure	6 (8.6)	3 (6.5)	>0.999
Asthma/COPD	12 (17.1)	2 (4.4)	0.039
Liver cirrhosis	3 (4.3)	3 (6.5)	0.680
Malignancy			0.052
Solid tumor	18 (25.7)[a]	6 (13.0)[b]	
Hematologic malignancy	11 (15.7)[c]	5 (10.9)[d]	
Immunocompromised state	23 (32.9)	17 (37.0)	0.650
Cardiac arrest before ECMO	8 (11.4)	10 (21.7)	0.134
Primary diagnosis			
Bacterial pneumonia	32 (45.7)	12 (26.1)	0.033
Viral pneumonia	2 (2.9)	8 (17.4)	0.014
Interstitial lung disease	15 (21.4)	5 (10.9)	0.141
Trauma/burn	2 (2.9)	4 (8.7)	0.212
Asphyxia	1 (1.4)	1 (2.2)	>0.999
Other[e]	18 (25.7)	16 (34.8)	0.294
Severity score on the first day in the ICU			
APACHE II	18 (15–25)	25 (21–32)	<0.001
SOFA	6 (4–9)	8 (6–14)	0.003
RESP score	1 (−1 to 2)	0 (−2 to 2)	0.171
PRESERVE score	5 (4–7)	6 (4–7)	0.664

Values are given as the median (interquartile range) or n (%)

APACHE II acute physiology and chronic health evaluation II, *COPD* chronic obstructive pulmonary disease, *ECMO* extracorporeal membrane oxygenation, *ICU* intensive care unit, *PRESERVE* predicting death for severe ARDS on VV-ECMO, *RESP* respiratory extracorporeal membrane oxygenation survival prediction, *SOFA* sequential organ failure assessment

[a] Meningioma ($n = 1$), malignant mesothelioma ($n = 1$), lung ($n = 10$), esophageal ($n = 2$), liver ($n = 2$), and colon cancer ($n = 2$)

[b] Acute myeloid leukemia ($n = 3$), acute lymphocytic leukemia ($n = 1$), chronic lymphocytic leukemia ($n = 1$), myelodysplastic syndrome ($n = 4$), and multiple myeloma ($n = 2$)

[c] Glioma ($n = 1$), lung cancer ($n = 2$), colon cancer ($n = 2$), and non-seminomatous germ cell tumor ($n = 1$)

[d] Acute myeloid leukemia ($n = 1$), multiple myeloma ($n = 1$), and lymphoma ($n = 3$)

[e] Other includes radiation therapy-induced pneumonitis, pulmonary tuberculosis, diffuse alveolar hemorrhage, pulmonary alveolar proteinosis, and airway occlusion by tumor mass or blood clot

Table 2 Medical management prior to extracorporeal membrane oxygenation

	Pre-ECMO team period ($n = 70$)	Post-ECMO team period ($n = 46$)	P value
Duration of MV before ECMO, days	2 (0–6)	2 (0–7)	0.510
Pre-ECMO ventilator settings[a]			
PaO_2/FiO_2	71.5 (56.0–96.5)	91.8 (68.3–114.3)	0.033
FiO2 (%)	100 (100–100)	100 (70–100)	0.009
PEEP (cmH_2O)	10 (5–12)	10 (5–12)	0.239
Peak inspiratory pressure (cmH_2O)	30 (24–34)	28 (23–31)	0.402
Minute volume (L)	9.1 (6.8–11.2)	9.5 (8.2–11.9)	0.420
VT/PBW (mL/kg)	6.8 (5.1–8.0)	6.8 (5.9–8.6)	0.710
Pre-ECMO treatment			
Steroid	46 (65.7)	19 (41.3)	0.010
Neuromuscular blocking agent	35 (50.0)	26 (56.5)	0.491
Inhaled nitric oxide	8 (11.4)	12 (26.1)	0.041
Prone position	4 (5.7)	10 (21.7)	0.010
Vasopressor infusion	44 (62.9)	29 (63.0)	0.984
Pre-ECMO blood gas			
pH	7.26 (7.13–7.38)	7.22 (7.09–7.35)	0.333
$PaCO_2$ (mmHg)	58.1 (45.8–73.5)	57.8 (44.7–68.5)	0.699
PaO_2 (mmHg)	61.4 (55.0–74.2)	64.2 (54.8–84.5)	0.726
HCO_3 (mmol/L)	25.8 (21.8–30.2)	23.2 (19.2–28.2)	0.063
SaO_2 (%)	89.4 (85.6–92.1)	89.4 (82.6–94.5)	0.890
Lactate before ECMO (mmol/L)	2.26 (1.53–4.80)	2.10 (1.60–5.11)	0.948

Values are given as the median (interquartile range) or n (%)

ECMO extracorporeal membrane oxygenation, *FiO₂* fraction of inspired oxygen, *MV* mechanical ventilation, *PaCO₂* partial pressure of carbon dioxide in arterial blood, *PaO₂* partial pressure of oxygen in arterial blood, *PBW* predicted body weight, *PEEP* positive end-expiratory pressure, *SaO₂* arterial oxygen saturations, *VT* tidal volume

[a] Data were available for 104 patients (66 patients in the pre-ECMO team period and 40 patients in the post-ECMO team period)

in the pre- and post-ECMO team periods. Measurements performed during MV prior to ECMO, including positive end-expiratory pressure, peak inspiratory pressure, tidal volume per predicted body weight, and the worst values of arterial blood gases, were not different between the two periods. However, the partial pressure of oxygen in the arterial blood per fraction of inspired oxygen (PaO_2/FiO_2, PF) was significantly lower in the pre-ECMO team period (71.5 [56.0–96.5]) compared to the post-ECMO team period (91.8 [68.3–114.3]) ($P = 0.033$). As an adjunctive or rescue therapy for severe respiratory failure, steroids, neuromuscular blocking agents, prone positioning, and inhaled nitric oxide were used in 56.0, 52.6, 12.1, and 17.2% of overall cases, respectively. Patients in the pre-ECMO team period were more likely to receive steroids (65.7 vs. 41.3%, $P = 0.010$) and less likely to receive inhaled nitric oxide (11.4 vs. 26.1%, $P = 0.041$) or prone positioning (5.7 vs. 21.7%, $P = 0.010$) compared to the post-ECMO team period. Neuromuscular blocking agent usage was similar between the two periods (50.0 vs. 56.5%, $P = 0.491$).

ECMO management

Details on ECMO management are summarized in Table 3. Veno-venous ECMO was planned in all patients; in one case in the pre-ECMO team period, the cannula was unintentionally inserted into the common femoral artery, and ECMO support started in the veno-arterial mode. Another veno–veno-arterial mode was used in one case for additional hemodynamic support. Femoro-jugular configuration was present in 85.7% of cases, and femoro-femoral configuration was found in 11.4% of cases in the pre-ECMO team period, but the proportion of femoro-femoral cases increased to 28.3% in the post-ECMO team period.

Compared to the pre-ECMO team period (42.9%), the proportion of cases involving successful weaning from ECMO was significantly higher in the post-ECMO team period (65.2%) ($P = 0.018$). However, the median duration of ECMO support was not different between the two periods. Cardiovascular events were the most common complication in patients treated with ECMO, followed by pulmonary, infection-related, renal, and hematological complications. However, only the incidence of cardiovascular events was significantly different between the pre-ECMO team and post-ECMO team periods (88.6 vs.

Table 3 Management of extracorporeal membrane oxygenation

	Pre-ECMO team period ($n = 70$)	Post-ECMO team period ($n = 46$)	P value
Initial ECMO configuration			0.044
Femoro-jugular veno-venous	60 (85.7)	32 (69.6)	
Femoro-femoral veno-venous	8 (11.4)	13 (28.3)	
Femoro-femoral veno-arterial	2 (2.9)	0 (0.0)	
Mixed (veno–veno-arterial)	0 (0.0)	1 (2.2)	
Successful weaning off of ECMO	30 (42.9)	30 (65.2)	0.018
Duration of ECMO support (days)	10 (7–20)	11 (4–27)	0.674
Survivors	9 (5–16)	9 (4–23)	0.755
Non-survivors	15 (8–24)	19 (3–27)	0.754
Adverse events during ECMO			
ECMO-related complications			
Cannula	23 (32.9)	7 (15.2)	0.034
Malposition requiring repositioning	21	5	
Vessel perforation	1	0	
Arterial cannulation	1	0	
Accidental decannulation	0	2	
Other	11 (15.7)	11 (23.9)	0.271
Patient complications			
Hematological	20 (28.6)	10 (21.7)	0.411
Neurological	9 (12.9)	1 (2.2)	0.086
Cardiovascular[a]	62 (88.6)	30 (65.2)	0.002
Inotrope or vasopressor use	51	30	
Myocardial stunning	3	0	
Arrhythmia	19	5	
Cardiac tamponade	1	0	
Cardiac arrest	10	1	
Pulmonary	23 (32.9)	15 (32.6)	0.978
Renal	36 (51.4)	23 (50.0)	0.880
Infection	36 (51.4)	19 (41.3)	0.285

Values are given as the median (interquartile range) or n (%)

ECMO indicates extracorporeal membrane oxygenation

[a] One or more complications may be listed

65.2%, $P = 0.002$). There were cannula-related complications in 32.9% of cases in the pre-ECMO team period and in 15.2% of cases in the post-ECMO team period ($P = 0.034$). Other technical issues were not significantly different (Additional file 2).

Clinical outcomes
Patients were followed for a median of 573 (285–1231) days or until death after ECMO initiation. Although none of patients with malignancy had limitation of care decision at the time of ECMO initiation, do-not-resuscitate order was instituted in 9 (31.0%) out of 29 patients in pre-ECMO team period and 2 (18.2%) out of 11 patients in post-ECMO team period ($P = 0.694$). Overall, out of 116 ECMO patients, 77 (66.4%) deaths occurred during

hospitalization. The ICU (72.9 vs. 50.0%, $P = 0.012$) and hospital (75.7 vs. 52.2%, $P = 0.009$) mortality rates were both significantly lower in the post-ECMO team period (Table 4). Also, the Kaplan–Meier survival curve showed a significant difference between the survival rates of the two periods during a 1-year follow-up period after ECMO initiation ($P = 0.005$) (Fig. 2). The rate of weaning from MV after ECMO was higher in the post-ECMO team period (56.5%) than in the pre-ECMO team period (30.0%) ($P = 0.004$) (Table 4). However, the median lengths of stay in the ICU and the hospital were not different between the two periods. The results of univariable and multivariable analyses with the logistic regression model are presented in Table 5. After adjusting for potential confounding factors, the post-ECMO team

Table 4 Clinical outcomes

	Pre-ECMO team period (n = 70)	Post-ECMO team period (n = 46)	P value
Mortality			
Hospital	53 (75.7)	24 (52.2)	0.009
Intensive care unit	51 (72.9)	23 (50.0)	0.012
Length of stay (days)			
Hospital	36 (19–62)	39 (31–55)	0.528
Survivors	74 (32–118)	40 (34–72)	0.394
Non-survivors	32 (17–46)	37 (24–49)	0.725
Intensive care unit	28 (14–37)	25 (7–41)	0.633
Survivors	34 (17–63)	27 (7–42)	0.395
Non-survivors	28 (14–36)	24 (11–38)	0.796
Successful weaning off of mechanical ventilation	21 (30.0)	26 (56.5)	0.004
Duration of mechanical ventilation, days	18 (9–29)	15 (4–31)	0.253
Survivors	19 (8–28)	16 (4–39)	0.439
Non-survivors	18 (10–29)	14 (5–26)	0.246

Values are given as the median (interquartile range) or n (%)

ECMO indicates extracorporeal membrane oxygenation

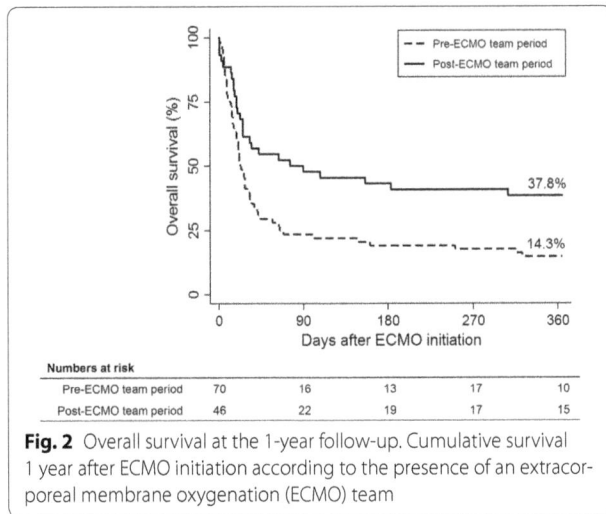

Fig. 2 Overall survival at the 1-year follow-up. Cumulative survival 1 year after ECMO initiation according to the presence of an extracorporeal membrane oxygenation (ECMO) team

period was still significantly associated with lower in-hospital mortality (adjusted OR 0.11, 95% CI 0.03–0.46, P = 0.003). Other factors independently associated with in-hospital mortality were asthma/chronic obstructive pulmonary disease, malignancy, and RESP score (Table 5).

Discussion

Our study investigated the impact of a multidisciplinary ECMO team on clinical outcomes in patients who underwent ECMO for severe acute respiratory failure and found that implementation of this ECMO team was associated with significant reductions in ICU and hospital mortalities. The improvement in survival rates was maintained at the 1-year follow-up after ECMO initiation. Furthermore, the incidence of adverse events during ECMO support was reduced, and the successful weaning from ECMO and MV significantly increased after the ECMO team was implemented.

Our findings are consistent with the results of a previous study showing the beneficial impact on mortality rates of a program dedicated to ECMO in all adult and pediatric patients undergoing veno-arterial and veno-venous ECMO [12]. Several studies have demonstrated that the survival of patients with severe acute respiratory failure was significantly improved when treated with ECMO than when treated with conventional ventilation support and suggested that such patients be referred and transferred to an ECMO center [1, 13]. Nonetheless, long-term survival in this population has been more importantly associated with pre-morbid illnesses and functional ability at hospital discharge than with acute illness factors [14, 15]. However, our study found that ECMO management by a multidisciplinary team improved long-term outcomes in patients who underwent ECMO for severe acute respiratory failure. Therefore, our findings support the establishment of ECMO referral centers that include dedicated ECMO staffing in order to enhance the effective use of ECMO to improve long-term survival as well as to overcome acute illnesses in patients with severe acute respiratory failure [6, 7].

The beneficial effects associated with a specialized ECMO team in patients receiving ECMO might be related to multiple factors. First, patient selection for ECMO can be a possible explanation for these beneficial effects. ECMO initially emerged as a salvage therapy in

Table 5 Univariable and multivariable analyses with logistic regression models for probability of in-hospital mortality

	Univariable			Multivariable		
	OR	95% CI	P value	OR	95% CI	P value
Post-ECMO team period	0.35	0.16–0.78	0.010	0.11	0.03–0.46	0.003
Asthma/COPD	7.72	0.97–61.36	0.053	10.76	1.17–99.04	0.036
Malignancy	2.76	1.12–6.78	0.027	3.97	1.21–13.01	0.023
Primary diagnosis[a]	–	–	–	–	–	–
Viral pneumonia	1.43	0.35–5.88	0.621	0.37	0.05–2.76	0.332
Others	1.30	0.33–5.12	0.706	0.76	0.12–4.97	0.773
APACHE II score	1.02	0.98–1.07	0.344	1.09	0.99–1.20	0.092
SOFA score	1.02	0.93–1.12	0.654	1.10	0.91–1.32	0.314
RESP score	0.85	0.73–0.99	0.034	0.77	0.62–0.96	0.020
PaO_2/FiO_2 prior to ECMO	1.00	0.99–1.01	0.776	1.02	1.00–1.04	0.058

APACHE II acute physiology and chronic health evaluation II, *COPD* chronic obstructive pulmonary disease, *ECMO* extracorporeal membrane oxygenation, *FiO_2* fraction of inspired oxygen, *MV* mechanical ventilation, *PaO_2* partial pressure of oxygen in arterial blood, *RESP* respiratory extracorporeal membrane oxygenation survival prediction, *SOFA* sequential organ failure assessment

[a] The reference group is bacterial pneumonia

patients with severe acute respiratory failure who cannot maintain adequate oxygenation or carbon dioxide removal despite MV; now, however, it is expanding its role beyond just being a salvage therapy, and some studies report that early initiation of ECMO is associated with lower mortality [16]. However, the disadvantages of ECMO might outweigh the advantages when implementing ECMO too early, given that complications, which can be serious and sometimes fatal, are possible throughout the entire course of ECMO support [4, 17]. Therefore, it is important to decide when and to whom we should apply ECMO for respiratory support. In this study, the proportion of patients with malignancy, which is usually considered to be a contraindication of ECMO, was higher than in previous ECMO studies. Although acute respiratory failure is one of the most common causes of ICU admission in patients with malignancies, the outcomes of ECMO in this population are disappointing [18], with only few cases reported to be successful [19, 20]. After the multidisciplinary ECMO team was implemented in our hospital, decisions about ECMO initiation were made by this ECMO team through comprehensive assessment with relevant consultants. As a result, the rate of survival to hospital discharge in patients with malignancy increased from 13.8 to 36.4% between the pre-ECMO team and post-ECMO team periods, respectively. The 1-year survival rate also increased from 3.4 to 18.2% after ECMO team implementation.

The duration and settings of MV and adjunctive therapies prior to ECMO are also known to be associated with differences in prognosis [10, 11, 21]. Although most parameters measured during ventilation were similar between the two periods in our study, the PF ratio was significantly lower in the post-ECMO team period. There was no difference in the duration of MV prior to ECMO initiation between the two periods, but it is possible that ECMO in the post-ECMO team period was started early in patients with less severe form of respiratory failure than in the pre-ECMO team period.

Next, the beneficial effects of the ECMO team can be explained by the dedication of the experienced and skilled ECMO physicians and staff members to ECMO. ELSO guidelines recommend that ECMO physicians should have sufficient experience and expertise in critical care and ECMO [6, 7]. Several previous studies revealed that a higher hospital-wide volume of ECMO cases was associated with lower mortality in patients who underwent ECMO [5, 22, 23]. Similarly, a specialized ECMO team will experience a greater volume of ECMO cases and be able to improve the skills associated with ECMO when they are responsible for ECMO throughout the entire center, rather than when managing only selected ECMO cases presented as elective consultations. The structure of an ECMO team could be similar to that of the high-intensity ICU staffing model, which is defined as mandatory intensivist consultation or the presence of a dedicated intensivist in the ICU [24]. The clinical benefit of the high-intensity staffing model over the low-intensity staffing model, which is defined as the absence of an intensivist or elective, rather than mandatory, intensivist consultation, in critically ill patients was already identified in several studies [25, 26].

Although this study provides new information on the impact of a multidisciplinary ECMO team on the clinical outcomes of adult patients with severe respiratory failure receiving ECMO support, our study has some limitations that should be considered. First, because it was conducted as a retrospective cohort study in a single center, there is a potential risk of confounding variables and selection bias. For example, the frequency of malignancy, which was considered to be a factor associated with poor outcomes, was significantly different between the two periods. Although it could also be considered as an effect of the ECMO team, however, the data regarding how many cancer patients had refused ECMO support by the team could not be extracted from the medical records during the study period. Second, the potential influence associated with the time difference between the two periods could not be excluded. Especially, growing experience with number of cases during the study period should be considered. Volume–outcome relationship in ECMO might stem from the beneficial effects of more experienced practitioners [27]. Recently, the ELSO registry has described improved outcomes in patients supported with ECMO over time, which might be attributed to the accumulation of experience [4].

In addition, the results from several studies that investigated the treatment of acute respiratory distress syndrome published during our study period might have influenced our practice, although the effects of these treatments on clinical outcomes in patients on ECMO remain unclear. Third, another research question was to identify changes in the selection of patients before and after implementation of the ECMO team. However, the data regarding how many patients with severe acute respiratory failure had been refused ECMO for respiratory support could not be extracted from the medical records during the study period before and after implementation of ECMO team. Further investigation with a larger patient population is needed to clarify the proper selection of patients for ECMO by the multidisciplinary team and the association of proper patient selection with clinical outcomes.

Conclusion

After implementing a multidisciplinary ECMO team, short- and long-term survival rates were significantly improved in patients treated with ECMO for severe acute respiratory failure. Our findings support the recommendation that ECMO centers should have a specialized organization including ECMO staff members who are well qualified and have experience in ECMO in order to maximize the beneficial effects of this treatment in patients with acute respiratory failure.

Authors' contributions
SJN collected and analyzed the data and drafted this manuscript. CRC, HJC, YHC, KS, JHY, and GYS contributed to the design of this study, analysis of the data, and writing of the manuscript. KJ conceived and designed the study, analyzed the data, and wrote the final manuscript. All authors read and approved the final manuscript.

Author details
[1] Department of Critical Care Medicine, Samsung Medical Center, Sungkyunkwan University School of Medicine, 81 Irwon-ro, Gangnam-gu, Seoul 06351, Republic of Korea. [2] Intensive Care Unit Nursing Department, Samsung Medical Center, Sungkyunkwan University School of Medicine, Seoul, Republic of Korea. [3] Department of Thoracic and Cardiovascular Surgery, Samsung Medical Center, Sungkyunkwan University School of Medicine, Seoul, Republic of Korea. [4] Division of Cardiology, Department of Medicine, Samsung Medical Center, Sungkyunkwan University School of Medicine, Seoul, Republic of Korea. [5] Division of Pulmonary and Critical Care Medicine, Department of Medicine, Samsung Medical Center, Sungkyunkwan University School of Medicine, Seoul, Republic of Korea.

Competing interests
The authors declare that they have no competing interests.

Funding
This work was supported by Samsung Medical Center grant (OTX0002901).

References
1. Peek GJ, Mugford M, Tiruvoipati R, Wilson A, Allen E, Thalanany MM, et al. Efficacy and economic assessment of conventional ventilatory support versus extracorporeal membrane oxygenation for severe adult respiratory failure (CESAR): a multicentre randomised controlled trial. Lancet. 2009;374:1351–63.
2. Patroniti N, Zangrillo A, Pappalardo F, Peris A, Cianchi G, Braschi A, et al. The Italian ECMO network experience during the 2009 influenza A(H1N1) pandemic: preparation for severe respiratory emergency outbreaks. Intensive Care Med. 2011;37:1447–57.
3. Pham T, Combes A, Roze H, Chevret S, Mercat A, Roch A, et al. Extracorporeal membrane oxygenation for pandemic influenza A(H1N1)-induced acute respiratory distress syndrome: a cohort study and propensity-matched analysis. Am J Respir Crit Care Med. 2013;187:276–85.
4. Thiagarajan RR, Barbaro RP, Rycus PT, McMullan DM, Conrad SA, Fortenberry JD, et al. Extracorporeal Life Support Organization Registry International Report 2016. ASAIO J. 2017;63:60–7.
5. Barbaro RP, Odetola FO, Kidwell KM, Paden ML, Bartlett RH, Davis MM, et al. Association of hospital-level volume of extracorporeal membrane oxygenation cases and mortality. Analysis of the extracorporeal life support organization registry. Am J Respir Crit Care Med. 2015;191:894–901.
6. ELSO Guidelines For ECMO Centers, Extracorporeal Life Support Organization. https://www.elso.org/resources/guidelines.asp. Assessed July 2017.
7. Combes A, Brodie D, Bartlett R, Brochard L, Brower R, Conrad S, et al. Position paper for the organization of extracorporeal membrane oxygenation programs for acute respiratory failure in adult patients. Am J Respir Crit Care Med. 2014;190:488–96.
8. Papazian L, Forel JM, Gacouin A, Penot-Ragon C, Perrin G, Loundou A, et al. Neuromuscular blockers in early acute respiratory distress syndrome. N Engl J Med. 2010;363:1107–16.
9. Guerin C, Reignier J, Richard JC, Beuret P, Gacouin A, Boulain T, et al. Prone positioning in severe acute respiratory distress syndrome. N Engl J Med. 2013;368:2159–68.
10. Schmidt M, Zogheib E, Roze H, Repesse X, Lebreton G, Luyt CE, et al. The PRESERVE mortality risk score and analysis of long-term outcomes after extracorporeal membrane oxygenation for severe acute respiratory distress syndrome. Intensive Care Med. 2013;39:1704–13.
11. Schmidt M, Bailey M, Sheldrake J, Hodgson C, Aubron C, Rycus PT, et al. Predicting survival after extracorporeal membrane oxygenation for severe acute respiratory failure. The Respiratory Extracorporeal Membrane Oxygenation Survival Prediction (RESP) score. Am J Respir Crit Care Med. 2014;189:1374–82.
12. Cotza M, Carboni G, Ballotta A, Kandil H, Isgro G, Carlucci C, et al. Modern ECMO: why an ECMO programme in a tertiary care hospital. Eur Heart J Suppl. 2016;18:E79–85.

13. Noah MA, Peek GJ, Finney SJ, Griffiths MJ, Harrison DA, Grieve R, et al. Referral to an extracorporeal membrane oxygenation center and mortality among patients with severe 2009 influenza A(H1N1). JAMA. 2011;306:1659–68.

14. Wang CY, Calfee CS, Paul DW, Janz DR, May AK, Zhuo H, et al. One-year mortality and predictors of death among hospital survivors of acute respiratory distress syndrome. Intensive Care Med. 2014;40:388–96.

15. Enger TB, Philipp A, Lubnow M, Fischer M, Camboni D, Lunz D, et al. Long-term survival in adult patients with severe acute lung failure receiving veno-venous extracorporeal membrane oxygenation. Crit Care Med. 2017;45:1718–25.

16. Kanji HD, McCallum J, Norena M, Wong H, Griesdale DE, Reynolds S, et al. Early veno-venous extracorporeal membrane oxygenation is associated with lower mortality in patients who have severe hypoxemic respiratory failure: a retrospective multicenter cohort study. J Crit Care. 2016;33:169–73.

17. Fan E, Gattinoni L, Combes A, Schmidt M, Peek G, Brodie D, et al. Veno-venous extracorporeal membrane oxygenation for acute respiratory failure: a clinical review from an international group of experts. Intensive Care Med. 2016;42:712–24.

18. Azoulay E, Mokart D, Pene F, Lambert J, Kouatchet A, Mayaux J, et al. Outcomes of critically ill patients with hematologic malignancies: prospective multicenter data from France and Belgium—a groupe de recherche respiratoire en reanimation onco-hematologique study. J Clin Oncol. 2013;31:2810–8.

19. Aboud A, Marx G, Sayer H, Gummert JF. Successful treatment of an aggressive non-Hodgkin's lymphoma associated with acute respiratory insufficiency using extracorporeal membrane oxygenation. Interact CardioVasc Thorac Surg. 2008;7:173–4.

20. Liao WI, Tsai SH, Chiu SK. Successful use of extracorporeal membrane oxygenation in a hematopoietic stem cell transplant patient with idiopathic pneumonia syndrome. Respir Care. 2013;58:e6–10.

21. Pranikoff T, Hirschl RB, Steimle CN, Anderson HL 3rd, Bartlett RH. Mortality is directly related to the duration of mechanical ventilation before the initiation of extracorporeal life support for severe respiratory failure. Crit Care Med. 1997;25:28–32.

22. Karamlou T, Vafaeezadeh M, Parrish AM, Cohen GA, Welke KF, Permut L, et al. Increased extracorporeal membrane oxygenation center case volume is associated with improved extracorporeal membrane oxygenation survival among pediatric patients. J Thorac Cardiovasc Surg. 2013;145:470–5.

23. Freeman CL, Bennett TD, Casper TC, Larsen GY, Hubbard A, Wilkes J, et al. Pediatric and neonatal extracorporeal membrane oxygenation: does center volume impact mortality?*. Crit Care Med. 2014;42:512–9.

24. Kim MM, Barnato AE, Angus DC, Fleisher LA, Kahn JM. The effect of multidisciplinary care teams on intensive care unit mortality. Arch Intern Med. 2010;170:369–76.

25. Pronovost PJ, Angus DC, Dorman T, Robinson KA, Dremsizov TT, Young TL. Physician staffing patterns and clinical outcomes in critically ill patients: a systematic review. JAMA. 2002;288:2151–62.

26. Wilcox ME, Chong CA, Niven DJ, Rubenfeld GD, Rowan KM, Wunsch H, et al. Do intensivist staffing patterns influence hospital mortality following ICU admission? A systematic review and meta-analyses. Crit Care Med. 2013;41:2253–74.

27. Maclaren G, Pasquali SK, Dalton HJ. Volume-outcome relationships in extracorporeal membrane oxygenation: is bigger really better?*. Crit Care Med. 2014;42:726–7.

16

Effects of combination therapy using antithrombin and thrombomodulin for sepsis-associated disseminated intravascular coagulation

Toshiaki Iba[1*], Akiyoshi Hagiwara[2], Daizoh Saitoh[3], Hideaki Anan[4], Yutaka Ueki[5], Koichi Sato[6] and Satoshi Gando[7]

Abstract

Background: No single anticoagulant has been proven effective for sepsis-associated disseminated intravascular coagulation (DIC). Thus, the concomitant use of antithrombin concentrate and recombinant thrombomodulin has been conceived. This observational study was conducted to investigate the efficacy and safety of this combination therapy.

Methods: A total of 510 septic DIC patients who received antithrombin substitution were retrospectively analyzed. Among them, 228 were treated with antithrombin and recombinant thrombomodulin (combination therapy) and the rest were treated with antithrombin alone (monotherapy). Propensity score matching created 129 matched pairs, and 28-day all-cause mortality, DIC scores, the sequential organ failure assessment (SOFA) scores, and the incidence of bleeding were compared.

Results: A log-rank test revealed a significant association between combination therapy and a lower 28-day mortality rate (hazard ratio 0.49, 95% confidence interval 0.29–0.82, $P = 0.006$) in the matched pairs. The DIC scores and the SOFA scores in the combination therapy group were significantly lower than those in the monotherapy group on Day 4 and Day 7. The incidence of bleeding did not differ between the groups (2.11 vs. 2.31%, $P = 1.000$).

Conclusions: The current study demonstrated the potential benefit of adding recombinant thrombomodulin to antithrombin. The co-administration of these two anticoagulants was associated with reduced mortality among patients with sepsis-induced DIC without increasing the risk of bleeding.

Keywords: Disseminated intravascular coagulation, Sepsis, Antithrombin, Thrombomodulin, Propensity analysis

Background

Anticoagulant therapy for sepsis-associated disseminated intravascular coagulation (DIC) is widely performed in Japan [1], and antithrombin concentrate and recombinant thrombomodulin are the two most popular agents utilized for this treatment [2]. However, not a single

anticoagulant has proven to be effective. Furthermore, neither of the above-mentioned agents has been recommended for use outside Japan [3, 4]. To examine the effects of recombinant thrombomodulin, Hayakawa et al. [5] conducted a retrospective multicenter survey examining 1784 sepsis-associated DIC cases. They created 452 propensity score-matched pairs and performed a logistic regression analysis. As a result, a significant association between recombinant thrombomodulin use and lower mortality (odds ratio [OR] 0.757; 95% confidence interval [CI] 0.574–0.999, $P = 0.049$) was recognized. The same group also performed a similar analysis on antithrombin

*Correspondence: toshiiba@cf6.so-net.ne.jp
[1] Department of Emergency and Disaster Medicine, Juntendo University Graduate School of Medicine, 2-1-1 Hongo Bunkyo-ku, Tokyo 113-8421, Japan
Full list of author information is available at the end of the article

concentrate and reported that the inverse probability of a treatment-weighted propensity score analysis indicated a statistically significant association between antithrombin supplementation and lower mortality (OR 0.748, 95% CI 0.572–0.978, $P = 0.034$). However, a propensity score-matched analysis did not show a significant association in a latter analysis [6]. In contrast to the situation in Japan, the international guidelines for sepsis do not recommend the use of antithrombin, and recombinant thrombomodulin is still not available outside Japan [7]. Despite the lack of robust evidence, the concomitant use of antithrombin and recombinant thrombomodulin has become popular in clinics, and recent post-marketing surveys have reported that combination therapy is now used in 50% of cases, at present [8]. Regarding the efficacy of combination therapy, available information remains sparse and the results are inconsistent. We formerly performed a logistic regression analysis among septic DIC patients who had undergone antithrombin supplementation and reported that the co-administration of recombinant thrombomodulin was a significant factor affecting survival [9]. Since the number of patients who received combination therapy was relatively small in that study, we repeated the survey and accumulated 159 patients in the second study [10]. This second survey demonstrated that the 28-day survival outcome in the combination therapy group was 80.5%, while it was only 63.9% in the antithrombin monotherapy group; this difference was statistically significant. Regarding the bleeding incidence, combination therapy is reportedly not associated with a risk of bleeding [10]. Since information regarding the effects and adverse effects of combination therapy is still limited [11], we planned to examine these issues in the third survey.

Methods

Patient selection

This post-marketing surveillance was performed as a multi-institutional, post-marketing survey. A total of 570 sepsis-associated DIC patients with an antithrombin activity ≦70% who were treated between June 2014 and June 2016 were registered. For the diagnosis of DIC, the Japanese Association for Acute Medicine (JAAM)-DIC criteria (Additional file 1: Supplement Table 1) [12] were utilized. Patients with a history of an allergic shock reaction to antithrombin, with major bleeding, an age of younger than 18 years old, or who were pregnant were excluded.

Ethics, consent and permissions and consent to publish

The survey was performed under the supervision of the Japanese Ministry of Health, Labour and Welfare (JMHW) and was conducted in accordance with the Declaration of Helsinki and Good Vigilance Practice and Good Post-marketing Study Practice. Since the complete anonymization of personal data was performed upon data collection, the ethical committee of Juntendo University waived the need to obtain informed consent and the patients' agreement. In the same reason, the institutional committee judged that the consent to publish was not required.

Treatment

When the patients met the JAAM-DIC criteria and had an antithrombin activity level of ≦ 70%, antithrombin concentrate (Nihon Pharmaceutical Co. Ltd, Tokyo, Japan) was administered for up to 3 consecutive days unless the patient died or treatment was stopped for any justifiable reason. The concomitant use of other anticoagulants was not prohibited, and recombinant thrombomodulin (TM-α; Asahi Kasei Parma Corporation, Tokyo, Japan) was administered intravenously according to the drug manufacturer's recommendation (0.06 mg/kg/day for 6 days by either intravenous bolus injection or intravenous infusion over 15 min via a catheter). Standard sepsis care was performed, and platelet concentrate and fresh-frozen plasma were used as substitution therapy, if necessary [13].

Data collection

The baseline data for the coagulation markers including fibrinogen/fibrin degradation products (FDP), D-dimer, prothrombin time (PT) ratio, platelet counts and antithrombin activity were measured before the treatment. Systemic inflammatory response syndrome (SIRS) score, sequential organ failure assessment (SOFA) score, and JAAM-DIC score were also calculated. Serial data for each coagulation marker, SIRS score, SOFA score and JAAM-DIC were also measured after the start of treatment (Day 2, Day 4, Day 7).

Survival was recorded until Day 28. The bleeding events were recorded throughout the observation period. Major bleeding was defined as bleeding that was either fatal, involved the failure of a critical organ, or was associated with a decrease in the hemoglobin level of 2.0 g/dL or more or required the infusion of 2 or more units of blood. The platelet count and other coagulation profiles were measured in local laboratories.

Statistical analysis

Student's t test, Mann–Whitney test, and Fisher's exact test were used to compare covariates between patients who received antithrombin alone (monotherapy group) versus antithrombin and recombinant thrombomodulin (combination therapy group). Bonferroni's correction was used to compare DIC score and SOFA score between two groups.

Cox's proportional hazards model (Cox hazard) was applied to evaluate the effectiveness of combination therapy. We selected some possible confounding covariates from the baseline characteristics and calculated a variance inflation factor (VIF). Finally, we set age, sex, baseline SOFA score, baseline DIC score, and antithrombin activity at baseline as confounding covariates. Then, a propensity score matching (PSM) was performed with these covariates.

A caliper width of s propensity score matching was set 0.06. Using this caliper width, we performed one-to-one nearest-neighbor matching without replacement between two groups.

To evaluate an effect size in the two matched groups, we calculated the standardized difference for continuous data and phi coefficient for categorical data. Log-rank test was used to compare two survival curves between monotherapy group and combination group. Data are expressed as a number (%), mean ± standard deviation (SD), or median (interquartile range), as appropriate. For all the reported results, $P < 0.05$ or $P < 0.017$ (0.05/3, Bonferroni's correction) was considered to denote statistical significance. R version 3.1.3 was used for all analysis, and SPSS 24.0 for Windows (IBM SPSS Inc., Chicago, IL) was validated for these analyses.

Results
Baseline characteristics
A total of 570 patients were registered in this survey; however, 60 cases were excluded because their treatments did not meet the study's criteria. Twenty-eight cases had an antithrombin activity > 70% when the treatment was initiated. In 16 cases, antithrombin activity was not measured. In the other 16 cases, antithrombin was not administered on the day of diagnosis. Data from 510 cases were used in the following analyses. Among them, 228 were treated with antithrombin and recombinant thrombomodulin (combination therapy group), and the remaining 282 were treated using antithrombin alone (monotherapy group). As for the infection focus, the respiratory system was the most frequent (29.6% 151/510). The baseline characteristics of the unmatched combination therapy and monotherapy groups are presented in Table 1. Propensity score matching created 129 matched pairs (Fig. 1). All the effect sizes of confounding covariates used by the propensity score were ≤ 0.1 for the matched patients, and the characteristics of the two groups were appropriately balanced (Table 2).

Effects on survival among the patients after propensity score matching
The Kaplan–Meier survival curves for the two groups are shown in Fig. 2. The hazard ratios (HRs) for 28-day mortality for combination therapy were 0.62 (95% CI 0.40–0.98, $P = 0.043$ [Cox's proportional hazards model) and 0.55 (95% CI 0.34–0.89, $P = 0.014$ [propensity score matching]), and significant associations were observed between the combination therapy and a lower 28-day mortality (Table 3).

Effects on coagulation markers, DIC score and SOFA score
The FDP level was significantly lower in the combination therapy group on Day 7 ($P = 0.002$). A significant difference in the PT ratio was observed on Day 7 between the groups ($P = 0.014$). The relative changes in JAAM-DIC score were significantly larger for the combination therapy group than for the monotherapy group on Day 4 and Day 7 ($P = 0.004$, 0.003, respectively). The relative changes in SOFA scores were significantly larger in the combination therapy group on Day 4 ($P = 0.011$) (Fig. 3).

Bleeding events
Eighty-four cases presented with bleeding at the time of the diagnosis of DIC were not included among the bleeding events. Twenty cases which have no bleeding records before or after treatment were also excluded from the analysis. Bleeding events observed after diagnosis occurred in 4 out of 190 cases (2.11% [major: 1 case, 0.53%]) in the combination therapy group and in 5 out of 216 cases (2.31% [major: 3 case, 1.39%]) in the monotherapy group. The difference in the bleeding rate was not significant between the two groups ($P = 1.000$ [major: $P = 0.626$]). The details of the bleeding events are summarized in Table 4.

Discussion
Though this study was conducted to examine the effect of combination therapy, the comparison was performed between a combination therapy group and an antithrombin monotherapy group. Hence, the effect of recombinant thrombomodulin as an addition to antithrombin treatment was examined practically. However, since previous studies have demonstrated the possible efficacy of antithrombin substitution for sepsis-associated DIC [9, 10], we think that the results of the current study support the favorable effects of combination therapy. As for the effect of antithrombin substitution, a study using real-world data from a nationwide administrative database in Japan reported a beneficial effect [14]. A total of 9075 patients with severe pneumonia-associated DIC were

Table 1 The baseline characteristics of the enrolled patients ($n = 510$)

Factors	Monotherapy group $n = 282$	Combination therapy group $n = 228$	P value	Missing value
Survival at day 28 (%)				
No	81 (28.7)	51 (22.4)	0.127	0
Yes	201 (71.3)	177 (77.6)		
Age (mean [SD])	71.7 (14.7)	72.3 (15.6)	0.663	0
Sex (%)				
Female	115 (40.8)	88 (38.6)	0.682	0
Male	167 (59.2)	140 (61.4)		
Infection focus (*n*, %)				
Respiratory system	91 (32.3)	60 (26.3)	0.172	0
Gastrointestinal system	69 (24.5)	66 (28.9)	0.268	0
Biliary system	35 (12.4)	28 (12.3)	1.000	0
Urinary system	36 (12.8)	39 (17.1)	0.208	0
Musculoskeletal	17 (6.0)	7 (3.1)	0.142	0
Skin and soft tissue	10 (3.5)	7 (3.1)	0.809	0
Central nerve system	2 (0.7)	2 (0.9)	1.000	0
Other	13 (4.6)	15 (6.6)	0.337	0
Unknown	35 (12.4)	20 (8.8)	0.199	0
Surgical intervention	23 (8.2)	34 (14.9)	0.023	0
Non-surgical drainage[#]	5 (1.8)	10 (4.4)	0.113	0
Baseline SOFA score median [25, 75%]				
Total SOFA	10.0 [7.0, 13.0]	11.0 [8.0, 13.0]	0.062	120
Coagulation	2.0 [1.0, 3.0]	2.0 [1.0, 3.0]	0.402	15
Hepatic	0.0 [0.0, 2.0]	0.0 [0.0, 1.0]	0.020	33
Cardiovascular	2.0 [0.0, 4.0]	3.0 [0.3, 4.0]	0.001	19
CNS system	2.0 [0.0, 3.0]	2.0 [1.0, 3.0]	0.312	60
Renal system	1.0 [0.0, 2.0]	1.0 [0.0, 2.0]	0.140	21
Respiratory system	2.0 [1.0, 3.0]	2.0 [1.0, 3.0]	0.038	88
Baseline DIC score median [25, 75%]				
Total DIC score	5.0 [4.0, 6.0]	5.0 [4.0, 7.0]	0.039	29
SIRS score (*n*, %)				
0 point	130 (46.4)	77 (34.4)		
1 point	150 (53.6)	147 (65.6)	0.006	6
Platelet score	3.0 [1.0, 3.0]	3.0 [1.0, 3.0]	0.182	1
FDP score	3.0 [1.0, 3.0]	3.0 [1.0, 3.0]	0.242	14
PT ratio score (*n*, %)				
0 point	53 (19.9)	33 (14.5)		
1 point	214 (80.1)	195 (85.5)	0.123	15
Baseline laboratory score median (SD)				
Platelet count ($\times 10^9$/L)	99.5 (77.6)	89.6 (68.1)	0.130	1
FDP (µg/mL)	56.6 (150.3)	48.8 (66.7)	0.526	110
D-dimer (µg/mL)	26.8 (46.7)	19.7 (29.1)	0.053	121
PT ratio	1.97 (6.08)	1.55 (0.52)	0.298	15
Antithrombin activity (%)	49.6 (13.8)	47.3 (12.7)	0.058	17

The data were shown as mean (standard deviation; SD) or median [25th percentile, 75th percentile]

As the SIRS score and the PT ratio score were composed of binary data, Fisher's exact test was performed

Non-surgical interventions are as follows: percutaneous transcatheter abscess drainage, urinary tract stenting, biliary tract stenting

n number, *SOFA* sequential organ failure assessment, *CNS* central nervous system, *DIC* disseminated intravascular coagulation, *SIRS* systemic inflammatory response syndrome, *FDP* fibrinogen/fibrin degradation products, *PT* prothrombin time

[#] For the selection of covariates, a variance inflation factor (VIF) was calculated and the covariates with VIF $\geqq$ 5 were excluded. Finally, age, sex, baseline SOFA score, baseline DIC score, and antithrombin activityused were selected.

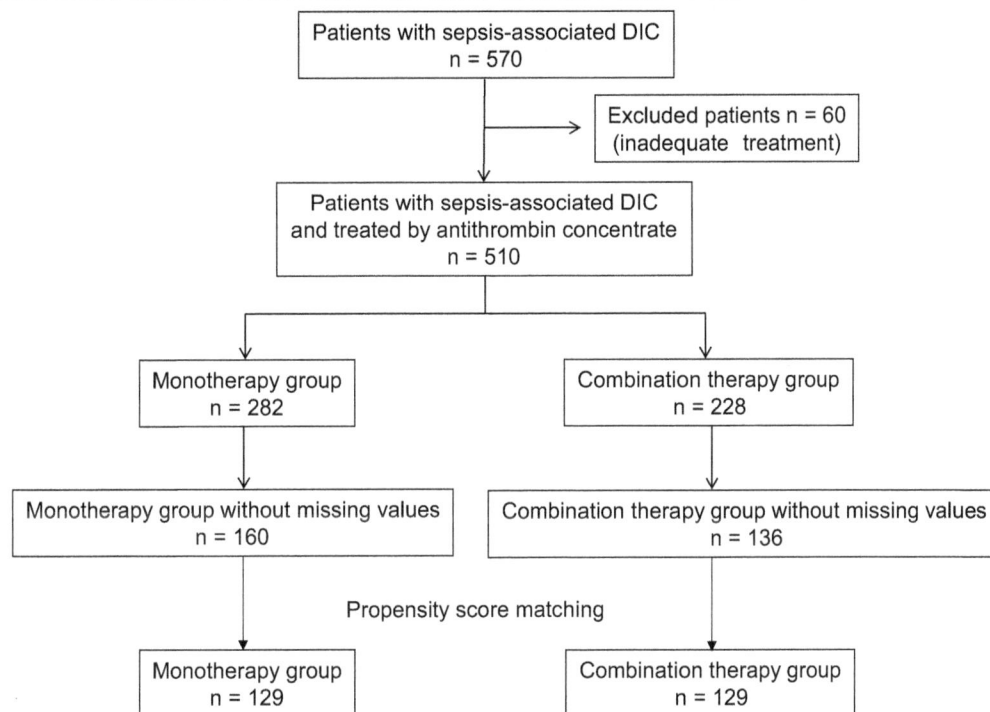

Fig. 1 Patient selection for the evaluation of antithrombin concentrate and recombinant thrombomodulin combination therapy. *DIC* disseminated intravascular coagulation

categorized into an antithrombin group (2663 cases) and a control group (6412 cases). Propensity score matching created a matched cohort of 2194 pairs of patients with and without antithrombin treatment. The results demonstrated that standard antithrombin supplementation (1500 IU/day × 3 days) was associated with a 9.9% (95% CI 3.5–16.3%) reduction in the 28-day mortality rate (with antithrombin vs. without antithrombin: 40.6 vs. 44.2%). In addition, multiple logistic regression analyses showed an association between antithrombin use and the 28-day mortality rate. Similar results in peritonitis-associated DIC patients have also been reported [15]. Based on these reports, we think that the results of the current study suggested the additive effects of recombinant thrombomodulin to antithrombin therapy in patients with sepsis-associated DIC.

With respect to the effect of recombinant thrombomodulin, a phase 3 randomized controlled trial (RCT) comparing recombinant thrombomodulin and heparin in 234 patients with DIC associated with hematologic malignancy or infection was performed in Japan [16], and a subgroup analysis for infection-based DIC revealed that although the mortality difference was 10.2% (recombinant thrombomodulin: 21.4 vs. heparin: 31.6%), the difference was not statistically significant (95% CI − 9.1 to 29.4%) [17]. Since then, the effectiveness

of this new agent has been repeatedly evaluated. For example, Yamakawa et al. [18] reported a trend toward favorable outcomes in their systematic review based on a meta-analysis. They collated data from 12 studies (838 patients from 3 RCTs and 571 patients from 9 observational studies) and reported that the relative risk of death was 0.81 (95% CI 0.62–1.06) in the RCTs and 0.59 (95% CI 0.45–0.77) in the observational studies. In contrast, Tagami et al. [19] performed propensity score and instrumental variable analyses using a Japanese nationwide administrative database (matched cohort of 1140 pairs) and reported that treatment with recombinant thrombomodulin did not reduce mortality among patients with pneumonia-associated DIC. More recently, Hagiwara et al. [20] performed an RCT at a single institute with 92 cases and reported an improved DIC resolution rate but almost identical mortality rates. The reason for these contradictory results has not yet been clarified; however, the severity of the subjects might affect the discrepancy. The beneficial effect of anticoagulants generally increases along with the severity of sepsis, and the reported effect was more evident if the study targeted severer cases [21, 22]. Yoshimura et al. [23] performed a post hoc analysis using data from a multicenter retrospective cohort study and reported that the administration of recombinant thrombomodulin was significantly

Table 2 The baseline characteristics of the patients after propensity score matching ($n = 258$)

Factors	Monotherapy group $n = 129$	Combination therapy group $n = 129$	P value	Effect size
Age, mean (SD)	73.3 (12.0)	73.8 (11.5)	0.723	0.044[a]
Sex (n, %)				
Female	54 (41.9)	52 (40.3)	0.899	0.064[a]
Male	75 (58.1)	77 (59.7)		
Infection focus (n, %)				
Respiratory system	58 (45.0)	38 (29.5)	0.014	0.160
Gastrointestinal system	22 (17.1)	34 (26.4)	0.096	0.113
Biliary system	19 (14.7)	15 (11.6)	0.581	0.046
Urinary system	12 (9.3)	23 (17.8)	0.068	0.125
Musculoskeletal	8 (6.2)	4 (3.1)	0.376	0.074
Skin and soft tissue	5 (3.9)	3 (2.3)	0.722	0.045
Central nerve system	0	1 (0.8)	1.000	0.062
Others	3 (2.3)	8 (6.2)	0.216	0.096
Unknown	14 (10.9)	12 (9.3)	0.837	0.026
Surgical intervention	8 (6.2)	19 (14.7)	0.040	0.139
Non-surgical drainage[#]	1 (0.8)	4 (3.1)	0.370	0.084
Baseline SOFA score median [25, 75%]				
Total SOFA	10.7 [2.0, 22.0]	10.8 [3.0, 19.0]	0.849[a]	0.025[a]
Hepatic	1.0 [0.0, 3.0]	0.0 [0.0, 3.0]	0.015	0.182
Cardiovascular	3.0 [0.0, 4.0]	3.0 [0.0, 4.0]	0.266	0.151
CNS system	2.0 [0.0, 4.0]	2.0 [0.0, 4.0]	0.678	0.026
Renal system	1.0 [0.0, 4.0]	1.0 [0.0, 4.0]	0.656	0.028
Respiratory system	2.0 [0.0, 4.0]	2.0 [0.0, 4.0]	0.266	0.069
Baseline DIC score Median [25, 75%]				
Total DIC score	5.7 [2.0, 8.0]	5.7 [2.0, 8.0]	0.935[a]	0.013[a]
SIRS score (n, %)				
0 point	51 (39.5)	37 (28.7)		
1 point	78 (60.5)	92 (71.3)	0.088	0.114
Platelet score	3.0 [0.0, 3.0]	3.0 [0.0, 3.0]	0.778	0.048
FDP score	3.0 [0.0, 3.0]	3.0 [0.0, 3.0]	0.829	0.105
PT ratio score (n, %)				
0 point	15 (11.6)	21 (16.3)		
1 point	114 (88.4)	108 (83.7)	0.369	0.067
Baseline laboratory score mean (SD)				
Platelet count ($\times 10^9$/L)	8.60 (6.29)	8.47 (5.04)	0.853	0.023
FDP (µg/mL)	73.9 (191.1)	51.11 (73.35)	0.206	0.158
D-dimer (µg/mL)	28.3 (48.9)	21.1 (24.3)	0.166	0.185
PT ratio	2.42 (8.68)	1.50 (0.41)	0.232	0.150
Antithrombin activity (%)	45.6 (14.1)	47.7 (11.7)	0.928	0.011[a]

[#] For the selection of covariates, a variance inflation factor (VIF) was calculated and the covariates with VIF $\geqq$ 5 were excluded. Finally, age, sex, baseline SOFA score, baseline DIC score, and antithrombin activityused were selected.

[a] Confounding covariates used by the propensity score (age, sex, baseline SOFA score, baseline DIC score, and antithrombin activity)

Non-surgical interventions are as follows: percutaneous transcatheter abscess drainage, urinary tract stenting, biliary tract stenting

When the basic assumptions of Student's t test were satisfied, data were shown mean (standard deviation) and the effect size was calculated using Cohen's d. When the basic assumptions of Student's t test were not satisfied, Mann–Whitney U test was performed and data were shown median [25 percentiles, 75 percentiles]. And the effect size was calculated using the following formula, Z-scores/a square root of sample number. For two-by-two contingency table, phi coefficient was used

n number, SD standard deviation, SOFA sequential organ failure assessment, DIC disseminated intravascular coagulation

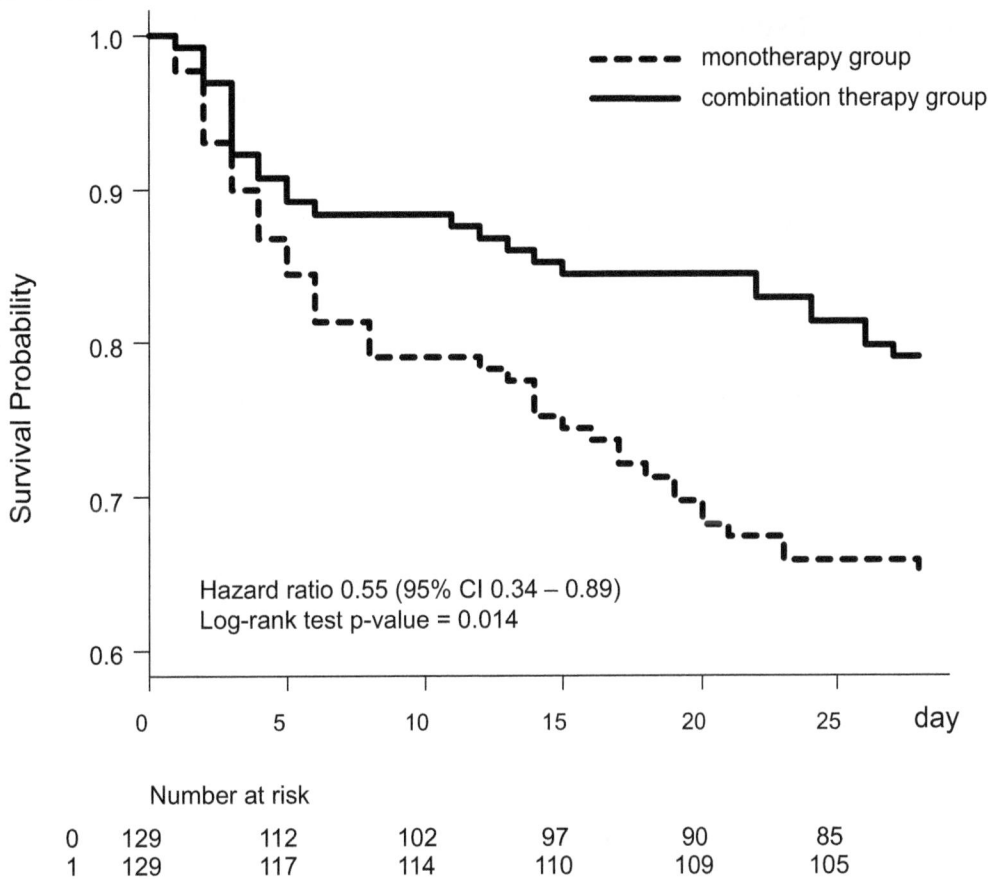

Fig. 2 Survival plots for patients in the propensity score-matched combination therapy and monotherapy groups. The 28-day survival rate was significantly higher in the combination therapy group (79.8%) than in the monotherapy group (70.0%) ($P = 0.014$, log-rank test). Hazard ratio 0.55 (0.34–0.89).

Table 3 Hazards ratio analysis in patients treated with combination therapy

Case number	Model	Hazard ratio (95% CI)	P value
510	Unadjusted	0.71 (0.45–1.11)	0.131
296[a]	Cox hazard	0.62 (0.40–0.98)	0.043
258	PS matching	0.49 (0.29–0.82)	0.006[$]

CI confidence interval, Cox hazard Cox's proportional hazards model, PS propensity score

[a] Complete case number without missing values

[$] P values were calculated using a log-rank test

associated with reduced mortality among patients with a high risk of death (APACHE II score: 24–29). Other than the above-mentioned studies, the largest RCT was conducted in 233 ICUs in 17 countries. A total of 750 patients with septic coagulopathy were randomized, and the results revealed a 3.8% reduction in the absolute risk of death (recombinant thrombomodulin group: 17.8% vs. placebo group: 21.6%, $P = 0.273$) [24]. This phase 2b study demonstrated a nonsignificant preferable effect of recombinant thrombomodulin. Regarding this study, one must keep in mind that not all patients had sepsis-associated DIC and the greatest benefit from the treatment was seen in patients with at least one organ system dysfunction and an PT international normalized ratio of greater than 1.4. In the current study, all the patients had DIC, the PT time was 1.61 ± 0.85 in the monotherapy group and 1.56 ± 0.54 in the combination therapy group, and the baseline SOFA scores were over 10 in both groups. Indeed, this was the first report to analyze matching data. As a result, a significant association between combination therapy and the 28-day mortality was recognized, and the mortality rate was significantly lower in the combination therapy group. In addition, both the JAAM-DIC score and the SOFA score were significantly lower in the combination therapy group than in the monotherapy group after the treatment (Days 4 and 7).

Regarding the safety features of recombinant thrombomodulin, a post-marketing surveillance of 2516 septic patients with DIC demonstrated that the frequency of critical bleeding was 2.6% [25], which did not differ from

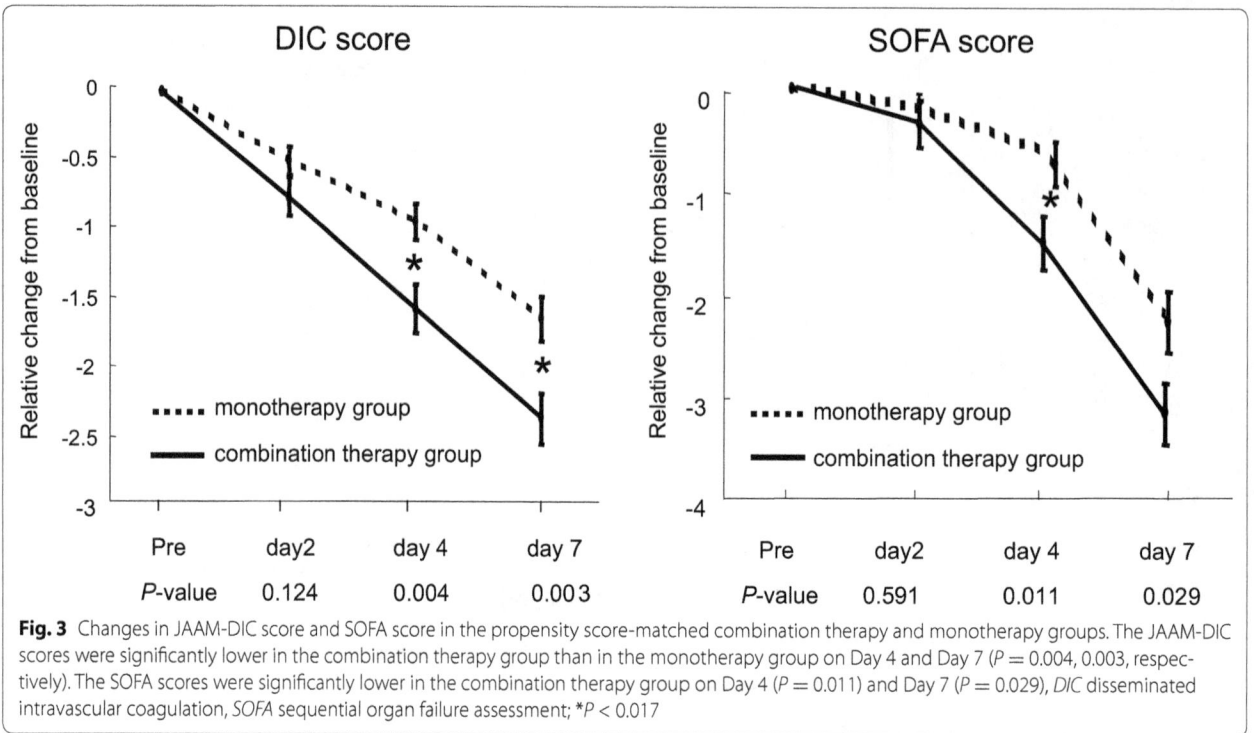

Fig. 3 Changes in JAAM-DIC score and SOFA score in the propensity score-matched combination therapy and monotherapy groups. The JAAM-DIC scores were significantly lower in the combination therapy group than in the monotherapy group on Day 4 and Day 7 ($P = 0.004$, 0.003, respectively). The SOFA scores were significantly lower in the combination therapy group on Day 4 ($P = 0.011$) and Day 7 ($P = 0.029$), *DIC* disseminated intravascular coagulation, *SOFA* sequential organ failure assessment; *$P < 0.017$

Table 4 Bleeding complications

No.	Treatment group	Bleeding site	Major/minor
Unmatched group			
1	Combination therapy	Mesenterium and intraperitoneal space	Major
2	Combination therapy	Abdominal wall, port site	Minor
3	Combination therapy	Intraperitoneal space, abdominal drain	Minor
4	Combination therapy	Urinary tract	Minor
5	Monotherapy	Intracranial space	Major
6	Monotherapy	Intraperitoneal space	Major
7	Monotherapy	Cervical spinal cord tumor	Major
8	Monotherapy	Urinary tract	Minor
9	Monotherapy	Nasal mucosa	Minor
Matched group			
5	Monotherapy	Intracranial space	Major
7	Monotherapy	Cervical spinal cord tumor	Major
9	Monotherapy	Nasal mucosa	Minor

the results of the current study, suggesting that combination therapy might not increase the incidence of bleeding. However, since a significant number of patients were excluded from this analysis, this issue should be re-examined.

The theoretical rationale for combination therapy remains to be elucidated. However, a fundamental concept is that both antithrombin and thrombomodulin activities are significantly reduced and anticoagulatory function is disrupted during sepsis. Second, antithrombin and thrombomodulin–protein C are the two major anticoagulant systems and their mechanisms of action are independent. Third, both agents are expected to have anti-inflammatory actions [26, 27]. We think that the results obtained from the current study may support the above ideas. As for preclinical studies, we have examined the additive effects of combination therapy in a lipopolysaccharide-induced rat model of septic DIC. As a result, combination therapy attenuated organ damage and histologic changes and led to an improvement in survival [28, 29]. Additional studies are required to clarify the mechanism of action.

Limitations

First, we only compared the effect between a combination therapy group and an antithrombin monotherapy group. To examine the true effect of the combination therapy, a combination therapy group, a monotherapy group, and a control group treated without anticoagulant are needed. Second, the median age of the patients was relatively higher and over 70-year-old, and thus, it might be difficult to generalize to the other countries. Finally, this was a retrospective observational study. Since the beneficial effect of combination therapy was hypothesized by the current study, a prospective randomized study is necessary as the next stage of inquiry.

Conclusion

The potential benefits of the co-administration of antithrombin and recombinant thrombomodulin were examined in a multi-institutional observation study. A propensity score-matched analysis demonstrated that the combination therapy was associated with a reduced mortality among patients with sepsis-induced DIC. Furthermore, the bleeding incidence seemed sufficiently low and the addition of recombinant thrombomodulin did not appear to increase the risk of bleeding.

Abbreviations

DIC: disseminated intravascular coagulation; OR: odds ratio; JAAM: Japanese Association for Acute Medicine; JMHW: Japanese Ministry of Health, Labour and Welfare; FDP: fibrinogen/fibrin degradation products; PT: prothrombin time; SIRS: systemic inflammatory response syndrome; SOFA: sequential organ failure assessment; VIF: variance inflation factor; IPW: inverse probability of treatment-weighted; SD: standard deviation; HR: hazard ratios; RCT: randomized controlled trial.

Authors' contributions

TI and SG conceived the study and participated in its design. TI and AH participated in the sequence alignment and drafted the manuscript. AH performed the statistical analysis. AA and KS revised the manuscript. DS and YU helped to collect and arrange the data. All authors read and approved the final manuscript.

Author details

[1] Department of Emergency and Disaster Medicine, Juntendo University Graduate School of Medicine, 2-1-1 Hongo Bunkyo-ku, Tokyo 113-8421, Japan. [2] National Center for Global Health and Medicine, Emergency Medicine and Critical Care, Tokyo, Japan. [3] Division of Traumatology, Research Institute, National Defense Medical College, Tokyo, Japan. [4] Emergency Medical Center, Fujisawa City Hospital, Fujisawa, Japan. [5] Department of Acute Critical Care and Disaster Medicine, Tokyo Medical and Dental University, Tokyo, Japan. [6] Department of Surgery, Juntendo Shizuoka Hospital, Juntendo University Graduate School of Medicine, Izunokuni-shi, Japan. [7] Division of Acute and Critical Care Medicine, Department of Anesthesiology and Critical Care Medicine, Hokkaido University Graduate School of Medicine, Sapporo, Japan.

Acknowledgements

The authors also thank all the institutes that participated in the post-marketing surveillance.

Funding

This work was supported by Ministry of Education, Culture, Sports, Science and Technology (Supported Program for the Strategic Research Foundation at Private Universities).

Competing interests

The authors declare that they have no competing interests.

References

1. Iba T, Thachil J. Present and future of anticoagulant therapy using antithrombin and thrombomodulin for sepsis-associated disseminated intravascular coagulation: a perspective from Japan. Int J Hematol. 2016;103:253–61.
2. Murata A, Okamoto K, Mayumi T, Muramatsu K, Matsuda S. Recent change in treatment of disseminated intravascular coagulation in Japan: an epidemiological study based on a National Administrative Database. Clin Appl Thromb Hemost. 2016;22:21–7.
3. Levi M, Toh CH, Thachil J, Watson HG. Guidelines for the diagnosis and management of disseminated intravascular coagulation. British Committee for Standards in Haematology. Br J Haematol. 2009;145:24–33.
4. Di Nisio M, Baudo F, Cosmi B, D'Angelo A, De Gasperi A, Malato A, et al. Diagnosis and treatment of disseminated intravascular coagulation: guidelines of the Italian Society for Haemostasis and Thrombosis (SISET). Thromb Res. 2012;129:e177–84.
5. Hayakawa M, Yamakawa K, Saito S, Uchino S, Kudo D, Iizuka Y, et al. Recombinant human soluble thrombomodulin and mortality in sepsis-induced disseminated intravascular coagulation. A multicentre retrospective study. Thromb Haemost. 2016;115:1157–66.
6. Hayakawa M, Kudo D, Saito S, Uchino S, Yamakawa K, Iizuka Y, et al. Antithrombin supplementation and mortality in sepsis-induced disseminated intravascular coagulation: a multicenter retrospective observational study. Shock. 2016;46:623–31.
7. Rhodes A, Evans LE, Alhazzani W, Levy MM, Antonelli M, Ferrer R, et al. Surviving sepsis campaign: international guidelines for management of sepsis and septic shock: 2016. Crit Care Med. 2017;45:486–552.
8. Iba T, Gando S, Saitoh D, Ikeda T, Anan H, Oda S, et al. Efficacy and bleeding risk of antithrombin supplementation in patients with septic disseminated intravascular coagulation: a third survey. Clin Appl Thromb Hemost. 2017;23:422–8.
9. Iba T, Saitoh D, Wada H, Asakura H. Efficacy and bleeding risk of antithrombin supplementation in septic disseminated intravascular coagulation: a secondary survey. Crit Care. 2014;18:497.
10. Iba T, Gando S, Saitoh D, Wada H, Di Nisio M, Thachil J. Antithrombin supplementation and risk of bleeding in patients with sepsis-associated disseminated intravascular coagulation. Thromb Res. 2016;145:46–50.
11. Yasuda N, Goto K, Ohchi Y, Abe T, Koga H, Kitano T. The efficacy and safety of antithrombin and recombinant human thrombomodulin combination therapy in patients with severe sepsis and disseminated intravascular coagulation. J Crit Care. 2016;36:29–34.
12. Gando S, Iba T, Eguchi Y, Ohtomo Y, Okamoto K, Koseki K, et al. A multicenter, prospective validation of disseminated intravascular coagulation diagnostic criteria for critically ill patients: comparing current criteria. Crit Care Med. 2006;34:625–31.
13. Wada H, Asakura H, Okamoto K, Iba T, Uchiyama T, Kawasugi K, et al. Expert consensus for the treatment of disseminated intravascular coagulation in Japan. Thromb Res. 2010;125:6–11.
14. Tagami T, Matsui H, Horiguchi H, Fushimi K, Yasunaga H. Antithrombin and mortality in severe pneumonia patients with sepsis-associated disseminated intravascular coagulation: an observational nationwide study. J Thromb Haemost. 2014;12:1470–9.
15. Tagami T, Matsui H, Fushimi K, Yasunaga H. Supplemental dose of antithrombin use in disseminated intravascular coagulation patients after abdominal sepsis. Thromb Haemost. 2015;114:537–45.
16. Saito H, Maruyama I, Shimazaki S, Yamamoto Y, Aikawa N, Ohno R, et al. Efficacy and safety of recombinant human soluble thrombomodulin (ART-123) in disseminated intravascular coagulation: results of a phase III, randomized, double-blind clinical trial. J Thromb Haemost. 2007;5:31–41.
17. Aikawa N, Shimazaki S, Yamamoto Y, Saito H, Maruyama I, Ohno R, et al. Thrombomodulin alfa in the treatment of infectious patients complicated by disseminated intravascular coagulation: subanalysis from the phase 3 trial. Shock. 2011;35:349–54.
18. Yamakawa K, Aihara M, Ogura H, Yuhara H, Hamasaki T, Shimazu T. Recombinant human soluble thrombomodulin in severe sepsis: a systematic review and meta-analysis. J Thromb Haemost. 2015;13:508–19.
19. Tagami T, Matsui H, Horiguchi H, Fushimi K, Yasunaga H. Recombinant human soluble thrombomodulin and mortality in severe pneumonia patients with sepsis-associated disseminated intravascular coagulation: an observational nationwide study. J Thromb Haemost. 2015;13:31–40.

20. Hagiwara A, Tanaka N, Uemura T, Matsuda W, Kimura A. Can recombinant human thrombomodulin increase survival among patients with severe septic-induced disseminated intravascular coagulation: a single-center, open-label, randomized controlled trial. BMJ Open. 2016;30:e012850.

21. Freeman BD, Zehnbauer BA, Buchman TG. A meta-analysis of controlled trials of anticoagulant therapies in patients with sepsis. Shock. 2003;20:5–9.

22. Dhainaut JF, Yan SB, Joyce DE, Pettilä V, Basson B, Brandt JT, et al. Treatment effects of drotrecogin alfa (activated) in patients with severe sepsis with or without overt disseminated intravascular coagulation. J Thromb Haemost. 2004;2:1924–33.

23. Yoshimura J, Yamakawa K, Ogura H, Umemura Y, Takahashi H, Morikawa M, et al. Benefit profile of recombinant human soluble thrombomodulin in sepsis-induced disseminated intravascular coagulation: a multicenter propensity score analysis. Crit Care. 2015;19:810.

24. Vincent JL, Ramesh MK, Ernest D, LaRosa SP, Pachl J, Aikawa N, et al. A randomized, double-blind, placebo-controlled, Phase 2b study to evaluate the safety and efficacy of recombinant human soluble thrombomodulin, ART-123, in patients with sepsis and suspected disseminated intravascular coagulation. Crit Care Med. 2013;41:2069–79.

25. Mimuro J, Takahashi H, Kitajima I, Tsuji H, Eguchi Y, Matsushita T, et al. Impact of recombinant soluble thrombomodulin (thrombomodulin alfa) on disseminated intravascular coagulation. Thromb Res. 2013;131:436–43.

26. Wiedermann CJ. Clinical review: molecular mechanisms underlying the role of antithrombin in sepsis. Crit Care. 2006;10:209.

27. Abeyama K, Stern DM, Ito Y, Yoshimoto Y, Tanaka M, Uchimura T, et al. The N-terminal domain of thrombomodulin sequesters high-mobility group-B1 protein, a novel antiinflammatory mechanism. J Clin Invest. 2005;15:1267–74.

28. Iba T, Nakarai E, Takayama T, Nakajima K, Sasaoka T, Ohno Y. Combination effect of antithrombin and recombinant human soluble thrombomodulin in an LPS induced rat sepsis model. Crit Care. 2009;13:R203–9.

29. Iba T, Miki T, Hashiguchi N, Yamada A, Nagaoka I. Combination of antithrombin and recombinant thrombomodulin attenuates leukocyte-endothelial interaction and suppresses the increase of intrinsic damage-associated molecular patterns in endotoxemic rats. J Surg Res. 2014;187:581–6.

17

Diaphragm function and weaning from mechanical ventilation: an ultrasound and phrenic nerve stimulation clinical study

Martin Dres[1,2]*, Ewan C. Goligher[3,4], Bruno-Pierre Dubé[1,5], Elise Morawiec[2], Laurence Dangers[1,2], Danielle Reuter[2], Julien Mayaux[2], Thomas Similowski[1,2] and Alexandre Demoule[1,2]

Abstract

Background: Diaphragm dysfunction is defined by a value of twitch tracheal pressure in response to magnetic phrenic stimulation (twitch pressure) amounting to less than 11 cmH$_2$O. This study assessed whether this threshold or a lower one would predict accurately weaning failure from mechanical ventilation. Twitch pressure was compared to ultrasound measurement of diaphragm function.

Methods: In patients undergoing a first spontaneous breathing trial, diaphragm function was evaluated by twitch pressure and by diaphragm ultrasound (thickening fraction). Receiver operating characteristics curves were computed to determine the best thresholds predicting failure of spontaneous breathing trial.

Results: Seventy-six patients were evaluated, 48 (63%) succeeded and 28 (37%) failed the spontaneous breathing trial. The optimal thresholds of twitch pressure and thickening fraction to predict failure of the spontaneous breathing trial were, respectively, 7.2 cmH$_2$O and 25.8%, respectively. The receiver operating characteristics curves were 0.80 (95% CI 0.70–0.89) for twitch pressure and 0.82 (95% CI 0.73–0.93) for thickening fraction. Both receiver operating characteristics curves were similar ($p = 0.83$). A twitch pressure value lower than 11 cmH$_2$O (the traditional cutoff for diaphragm dysfunction) predicted failure of the spontaneous breathing trial with a sensitivity of 89% (95% CI 72–98%) and a specificity of 45% (95% CI 30–60%).

Conclusions: Failure of spontaneous breathing trial can be predicted with a lower value of twitch pressure than the value defining diaphragm dysfunction. Twitch pressure and thickening fraction had similar strong performance in the prediction of failure of the spontaneous breathing trial.

Keywords: Liberation, Ventilator, Diaphragm, Weakness, Ultrasound, Extubation

Background

Diaphragm dysfunction is common in critically ill patients exposed to mechanical ventilation [1]. It can occur soon after intubation [2]. It can also occur later, where it may be a consequence of intensive care unit acquired weakness or the result of the specific time-dependent impact of mechanical ventilation on the diaphragm [3–7], a phenomenon referred to as ventilator-induced diaphragm dysfunction [8]. Diaphragm dysfunction is associated with increased mortality [2, 3, 9] and delayed liberation from mechanical ventilation [3, 4, 10, 11].

Diaphragm dysfunction manifests as a reduced capacity to generate inspiratory pressure and flow [12]. This can be assessed in term of the negative pressure swing measured at the opening of an endotracheal tube in response to bilateral phrenic nerve stimulation (Ptr,stim) [1]. Outside of the intensive care context, a Ptr,stim value amounting to less than 11 cmH$_2$O is considered indicative of diaphragm dysfunction [12–14]. In critically ill patients, this value of -11 cmH$_2$O has proven useful

*Correspondence: martin.dres@aphp.fr
[2] Service de Pneumologie et Réanimation Médicale (Département "R3S"), AP-HP, Groupe Hospitalier Pitié-Salpêtrière Charles Foix, 47-83 boulevard de l'Hôpital, 75013 Paris, France
Full list of author information is available at the end of the article

from a prognostic point of view. In a prospective study of ICU patients in whom Ptr,stim was measured at time of weaning, patients with a Ptr,stim below the 11 cmH$_2$O threshold were less likely to survive to discharge from the ICU or hospital than those with a Ptr,stim above this threshold [3]. Yet, lower Ptr,stim values are commonly encountered in ICU patients at various points of their ICU stay [2–4, 15] and two recent studies have reported successful weaning from mechanical ventilation despite lower values of Ptr,stim [3, 4]. Therefore, our hypothesis was that the Ptr,stim threshold value used to define diaphragm dysfunction (− 11 cmH$_2$O) would be not necessarily the best threshold that allows successful or failed weaning from mechanical ventilation. The present study was designed to identify the optimal Ptr,stim value to predict failure of the spontaneous breathing trial. In view of the recently reported utility of diaphragm thickening fraction (TFdi) [16] to predict failure of the spontaneous breathing trial, the predictive value of this variable was also evaluated.

Patients and methods

This study was an ancillary analysis of a study prospectively conducted over 9 months (November 1, 2014, to July 31, 2015) in a medical 10-bed ICU. Human research ethics committee approval for the study was provided by the Comité de Protection des Personnes—Ile de France 6 (ID RCB: 2014-A00715-42). Informed consent was obtained from all patients or their relatives. Data from this cohort have been previously published [3, 17].

Patients

Patients were eligible for inclusion if they had been intubated and ventilated for at least 24 h and if they met predefined readiness-to-wean criteria on daily screening [18] and were therefore ready for a first spontaneous breathing trial (Additional file 1: readiness criteria to initiate a spontaneous breathing trial). Readiness-to-wean criteria were searched for while patients were ventilated on existing mechanical ventilation setting prior to spontaneous breathing trial (SBT). Patients with clinical factors potentially interfering with phrenic nerve stimulation, who had a tracheostomy, or who were unable to follow simple orders were excluded (Additional file 1: exclusion criteria).

Measurements

All measurements were taken a few minutes before starting the SBT. Phrenic nerve stimulation was performed while patients were briefly disconnected from the ventilator (Additional file 1: description of the phrenic nerves stimulation technique), and diaphragm ultrasound (Additional file 1: description of the ultrasound

technique) was conducted while patients were mechanically ventilated under pressure support ventilation with ventilator settings decided by the attending physician. In our unit, pressure support level is set in order to provide a tidal volume of 6–8 ml/kg of ideal body weight without any sign of acute respiratory distress or discomfort. Positive end-expiratory pressure is set at 5 cmH$_2$O.

Diaphragm function was assessed in terms of changes in tracheal pressure during a magnetic stimulation (Ptr,stim), as described elsewhere [2, 4, 5, 14, 15]. Stimulations were delivered at the maximum intensity allowed by the stimulator (100%) known to result in supramaximal diaphragm contraction in most patients [2, 10, 13, 15, 19]. Diaphragm ultrasound was conducted using a 4–12-MHz linear array transducer (Sparq ultrasound system, Philips, Philips Healthcare, MA, USA). Diaphragm thickness was measured at end-expiration (Tdi,ee) and end-inspiration (Tdi,ei), and thickening fraction (TFdi) was calculated offline as (Tdi,ei–Tdi,ee)/Tdi,ee. Two observers blinded to the results of phrenic nerve stimulation performed diaphragm ultrasound. As previously reported elsewhere [3], the reproducibility of ultrasound measurements was assessed on the first 20 patients while the two observers were blinded to each other's measurements and after they performed at least 20 diaphragm ultrasounds during a 2-month training period before starting the study [3, 17]. Intra-class correlation (ICC) for Tdi,ei, Tdi,ee and TFdi were, respectively: ICC = 0.95 ($p < 0.001$), ICC = 0.96 ($p < 0.001$) and ICC = 0.87 ($p < 0.001$) [3].

Study design

After obtaining study measurements, patients underwent a SBT. During the SBT, patients were ventilated with a pressure support level 7 cmH$_2$O and 0 cmH$_2$O end-expiratory pressure for 30 min. Failure of the SBT was defined if patients developed criteria for clinical intolerance defined as follows [18]: (1) pulsed oxygen saturation < 90% with a fraction of inspired oxygen ≥ 50%, acute respiratory distress (respiratory rate ≥ 40/min with agitation or cyanosis), systolic arterial blood pressure ≥ 180 mmHg, or pH < 7.32 with an arterial carbon dioxide tension ≥ 50 mmHg. For patients with multiple failed SBT, only their first SBT was considered for the analysis.

Statistical analysis

Continuous variables are expressed as median (interquartile range), and categorical variables are expressed as absolute and relative frequency. Continuous variables were compared with Mann–Whitney U test.

The manuscript conforms to the STARD checklist for reporting of studies of diagnostic accuracy [20]. Receiver operating characteristic (ROC) curves were constructed to evaluate the performance of the two index to predict SBT failure: Ptr,stim and TFdi. Sensitivities, specificities, positive and negative predictive values, positive and negative likelihood ratios and areas under the ROC curves (AUC-ROC) were calculated. AUC-ROC were performed to identify optimal cutoff values of Ptr,stim and TFdi in predicting SBT failure, and these estimates were obtained using bootstrapping with 1000 replications. The best threshold value for each index was determined as the value associated with the best Youden index for the prediction of SBT failure. AUC-ROC were compared using the nonparametric approach of DeLong et al. [21].

Table 1 Patient's characteristics at inclusion

Characteristics	
Female, n (%)	24 (32)
Age, years	58 (48–68)
SOFA	5 (4–7)
Duration of mechanical ventilation, days	4 (2–6)
Main reason for mechanical ventilation, n (%)	
Acute respiratory failure	28 (37)
Shock	24 (32)
Coma	23 (31)
Ventilator parameters	
Pressure support level, cmH₂O	10 (8–10)
Tidal volume, ml/kg ideal body weight	7 (5–8)
PEEP, cmH₂O	5 (5–6)
Clinical parameters	
Breaths, min⁻¹	22 (20–25)
Mean arterial pressure, mmHg	80 (69–98)
Heart rate, min⁻¹	89 (78–100)
Arterial blood gases	
pH	7.44 (7.40–7.45)
PaCO₂, mmHg	38 (34–44)
PaO₂/FiO₂	279 (214–357)

Continuous variables are expressed as median (interquartile range), and categorical variables are expressed as absolute value (%)

SOFA sequential organ failure assessment, *PEEP* positive end-expiratory pressure, *PaO₂/FiO₂* ratio of arterial oxygen tension to inspired oxygen fraction

For all final comparisons, a two-tailed *p* value less than or equal to 0.05 was considered statistically significant. Statistical analyses were performed with MedCalc (MedCalc Software bvba).

Results

Between November 1, 2014, and July 31, 2015, 330 patients were admitted in our ICU. One hundred and eighty-four patients received invasive mechanical ventilation for more than 24 h leading to the enrollment of 76 consecutive patients in the study (Additional file 1: Figure E1. Flowchart of the study). The characteristics of these patients upon inclusion are given in Table 1.

Forty-eight patients (63%) passed the SBT and were subsequently extubated, while 28 patients (37%) developed criteria for SBT failure and initial ventilator settings were accordingly resumed. Of the 48 extubated patients, seven patients required resumption of ventilatory support (six were reintubated and 1 had curative noninvasive ventilation) within 48 h: five patients for respiratory distress and two patients for loss of consciousness. No stridor was reported. Prophylactic noninvasive ventilation was used in two patients.

Prediction of spontaneous breathing trial failure

Median Ptr,stim was 8.2 (5.9–12.6) cmH₂O; Ptr,stim was 10.0 (7.3–14.3) and 6.5 (3.0–8.8) cmH₂O in patients with successful and failed SBT, respectively ($p < 0.001$). The optimal threshold value of Ptr,stim to predict SBT failure was 7.2 cmH₂O (Table 2). A Ptr,stim value lower than 11 cmH₂O (the traditional cutoff for diaphragm dysfunction) predicted SBT failure with a sensitivity of 89% (95% CI 72–98%) and a specificity of 45% (95% CI 30–60%). Patients with SBT success and SBT failure according to both 7.0 and 11.0 cmH₂O thresholds of Ptr,stim are shown in Fig. 1a, b.

Median TFdi was 28% (19–35) in the whole population; TFdi was 33% (29–43) and 19% (11–25) in patients with successful SBT and SBT failure, respectively ($p < 0.001$). The optimal threshold value of TFdi to predict

Table 2 Threshold, area under the receiver operating characteristics curves (AUC-ROC), sensitivity, specificity, positive and negative likelihood ratios and positive and negative predictive values of endotracheal pressure induced by a bilateral phrenic nerve stimulation (Ptr,stim) and diaphragm thickening fraction (TFdi) to predict weaning failure from mechanical ventilation

	Threshold	AUC-ROC (95% CI)	Sensitivity (%) (95% CI)	Specificity (%) (95% CI)	Likelihood ratios (95% CI)		Predictive values (%) (95% CI)	
					Positive	Negative	Positive	Negative
Ptr,stim	7.2 cmH₂O	0.80 (0.70–0.89)	68 (47–84)	79 (64–89)	3.2 (1.7–5.8)	0.4 (0.2–0.7)	66 (51–78)	80 (70–88)
TFdi	25.8%	0.82 (0.73–0.93)	79 (59–92)	73 (58–85)	2.9 (1.8–4.8)	0.3 (0.1–0.6)	63 (51–74)	85 (74–92)

CI confidence interval

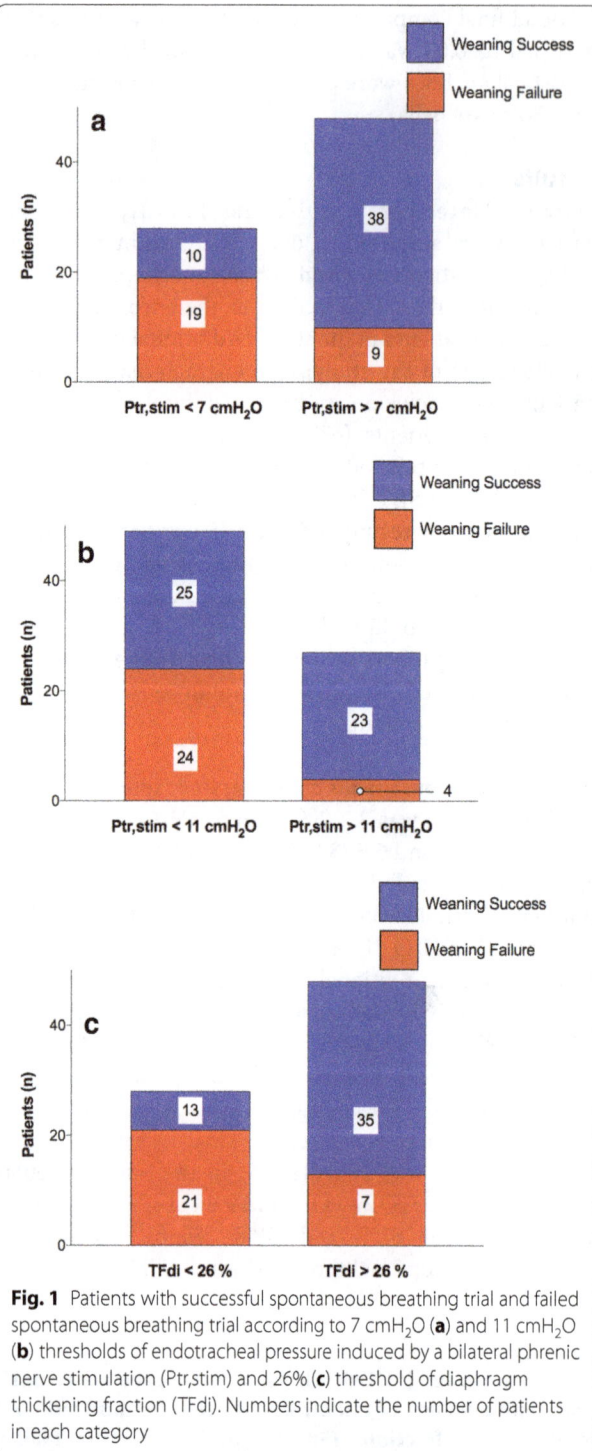

Fig. 1 Patients with successful spontaneous breathing trial and failed spontaneous breathing trial according to 7 cmH$_2$O (**a**) and 11 cmH$_2$O (**b**) thresholds of endotracheal pressure induced by a bilateral phrenic nerve stimulation (Ptr,stim) and 26% (**c**) threshold of diaphragm thickening fraction (TFdi). Numbers indicate the number of patients in each category

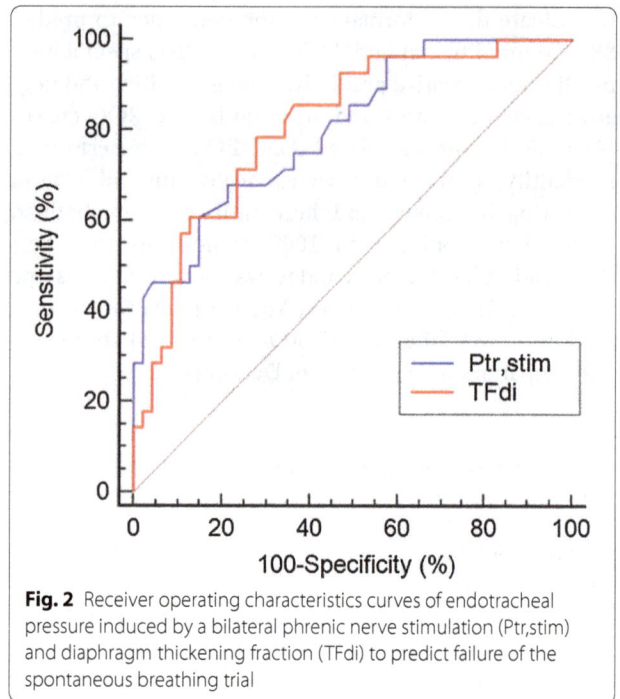

Fig. 2 Receiver operating characteristics curves of endotracheal pressure induced by a bilateral phrenic nerve stimulation (Ptr,stim) and diaphragm thickening fraction (TFdi) to predict failure of the spontaneous breathing trial

Discussion

This study reports a dual assessment of diaphragm function and its relationship with weaning outcome in mechanically ventilated medical patients undergoing a first spontaneous breathing trial. Our findings can be summarized as follows: (1) a lower value of Ptr,stim (i.e., 7.0 cmH$_2$O) than the value commonly accepted value to define diaphragm dysfunction (i.e., 11.0 cmH$_2$O) is more reliable to predict SBT failure, (2) Ptr,stim and TFdi are equivalent to predict SBT failure.

Diaphragm function and weaning from mechanical ventilation

The negative impact of diaphragm dysfunction on successful weaning from mechanical ventilation has been established by several investigations in critically ill patients [3, 4, 11, 22]. At the time of weaning, diaphragm dysfunction is highly prevalent [1] with reported rates ranging from 25–30% [11, 22] to 60–80% [3, 4]. To our knowledge, only three studies have assessed diaphragm dysfunction at the time of attempted liberation from mechanical ventilation using the gold standard technique, namely the phrenic nerves stimulation [3, 4, 23]. However, none of them provided any threshold values for Ptr,stim to predict weaning outcome. Of note, these studies including ours indicate that a substantial proportion of patients (up to 44%) can be successfully weaned from the ventilator despite having diaphragm dysfunction defined as Ptr,stim < 11 cmH$_2$O [3, 4]. Therefore,

SBT failure was 25.8%. Figure 1c shows the number of patients with SBT success and SBT failure according to 25.8%-TFdi threshold. Predictive performances of TFdi are shown in Table 2. The comparison of AUC-ROC of Ptr,stim and TFdi is displayed in Fig. 2. Ptr,stim and TFdi had similar AUC-ROC ($p = 0.83$).

normal diaphragm function according to a definition established in healthy subjects [12] is not a prerequisite for a successful SBT. This finding is not altogether surprising as many patients with chronic diaphragm dysfunction do not require mechanical ventilation [24, 25]. While diaphragm dysfunction might limit exercise capacity, the clinical consequences of diaphragm dysfunction in successfully liberated patients are uncertain. However, the impact of respiratory muscles dysfunction (not specifically the diaphragm) after critical illness may be of importance since it is associated with worse long-term outcomes [26, 27]. Overall, our findings are of importance since they highlight that presence of diaphragm dysfunction at the time of weaning should not discourage clinicians from attempting liberation from ventilation. By contrast, not all patients (23/27) with a Ptr,stim higher than 11.0 cmH$_2$O had a successfully SBT. As a matter of fact, the 11.0 cmH$_2$O threshold of Ptr,stim was associated with a lower specificity but a higher sensitivity than the 7.0 cmH$_2$O threshold in the prediction of SBT failure. The lower 7.0 cmH$_2$O Ptr,stim threshold provides the optimal combination of sensitivity and specificity in the prediction of SBT failure.

Diaphragm ultrasound in the prediction of SBT failure

The use of diaphragm ultrasound is growing in the ICU [28, 29]. It has many advantages over phrenic nerve stimulation, which requires costly equipment and extensive technical expertise. Ultrasound is a noninvasive and highly feasible bedside imaging modality, and ultrasound devices are widely available in ICUs. Several studies have proposed various ultrasound-derived markers aiming at assessing diaphragm function. Importantly, in our study, Ptr,stim and TFdi demonstrated similar performance in the prediction of weaning. Of note, the optimal TFdi cutoff (26%) identified in our study is very close to the cutoffs reported in previous investigations [16, 30, 31]. Considering ultrasound as a substitute of the phrenic nerves stimulation technique, it will make diaphragm evaluation much easier at the bedside. However, the indication of diaphragm ultrasound during the weaning process is not yet clearly defined. In addition, it is important to remind that the majority of patients are shortly and safely separated from the ventilation. As it happens, the place of diaphragm ultrasound might be viewed as a complementary investigation and not as a surrogate of clinical judgment. It may be used as a screening tool to identify patients who are at high risk of SBT failure (before conducting the SBT) or as a diagnostic method to determine the cause of SBT or extubation failure [32].

Strengths and limitations of our study

This study is the largest to report a dual approach providing comparison between the gold standard evaluation method of diaphragm function and diaphragm ultrasound during the weaning phase. However, this study has limitations. First, the generalizability of our findings may be limited by the characteristics of the patients of our cohort. Accordingly, our study might be viewed as a hypothesis generator and further trials are warranted to confirm the clinical relevance of our findings. Second, while we obtained good inter- and intra-reproducibility in the measurements of diaphragm ultrasound, centers employing the technique must also demonstrate adequate technical skill (based on reproducibility) before implementing the technique for clinical purposes. Third, we performed diaphragm ultrasound while patients were ventilated with pressure support and not during the SBT. While this approach is easier to implement (no change in ventilator setting) and less stressful for patients, it could underestimate diaphragm thickening [33]. However, the amount of pressure support was standardized in order to target a tidal volume between 6 and 8 ml/kg predicted body weight. Reassuringly, any effect of ventilatory support on TFdi is likely to introduce 'noise' in its correlation with weaning outcome and this would tend to bias the observed association toward the null. Fourth, we have assessed diaphragm function by using the changes in tracheal twitch pressure rather than the changes in transdiaphragmatic twitch pressure. This last measurement is more specific to the diaphragm function but requires the placement of two balloons, which make it more invasive. Although the two twitch pressures are not interchangeable, they are well correlated [15].

Conclusions

Diaphragm ultrasound is a reliable surrogate of the phrenic nerve stimulation method in the assessment of diaphragm function to predict weaning outcome. A multicenter investigation is now required to confirm whether the 26% value of TFdi cutoff could or could not be used widely to predict SBT outcome. Diaphragm ultrasound could be combined with cardiac echo or lung ultrasound to tailor post-extubation management according to the risk of weaning failure. Although diaphragm dysfunction did not systematically impair weaning outcome, it may behave as a marker of severity and poor prognosis. Future studies should address this hypothesis and investigate mid- and long-term consequences of diaphragm dysfunction on patient functional status and quality of life.

Abbreviations
SBT: Spontaneous breathing trial; Ptr,stim: Tracheal pressure in response to bilateral magnetic stimulation of the phrenic nerves; TFdi: Diaphragm thickening fraction; ICU: Intensive care unit; AUC-ROC: Area under the curve of receiving operating characteristics.

Authors' contributions
MD and AD designed the study. MD, AD, BPD and TS coordinated the study. MD, BPD, DR, EM, LD and JM were responsible for patient screening, enrollment, and follow-up. MD, AD, EG and TS analyzed the data. MD, AD, EG and TS wrote the manuscript. All authors had full access to all study data, contributed to drafting the manuscript or critical revision of it for important intellectual content, approved the final version of the manuscript, and took responsibility for the integrity of the data and the accuracy of the data analysis. All authors read and approved the final manuscript.

Author details
[1] UPMC Univ Paris 06, INSERM, UMRS1158, Neurophysiologie Respiratoire Expérimentale et Clinique, Sorbonne Universités, Paris, France. [2] Service de Pneumologie et Réanimation Médicale (Département "R3S"), AP-HP, Groupe Hospitalier Pitié-Salpêtrière Charles Foix, 47-83 boulevard de l'Hôpital, 75013 Paris, France. [3] Interdepartmental Division of Critical Care Medicine, University of Toronto, Toronto, Canada. [4] Division of Respirology, Department of Medicine, University Health Network and Mount Sinai Hospital, Toronto, Canada. [5] Département de Médecine, Service de Pneumologie, Hôpital Hôtel-Dieu, Centre Hospitalier de l'Université de Montréal (CHUM), Montréal, QC, Canada.

Acknowledgements
None.

Competing interests
Alexandre Demoule has signed research contracts with Medtronic, Maquet and Philips; he has also received personal fees from Medtronic, Maquet, Resmed, Fisher & Paykel and MSD. Martin Dres received personal fees from Pulsion Medical System and Lungpacer Inc. Bruno-Pierre Dubé has received honoraria from GlaxoSmithKline, Boehringer Ingelheim, Astra Zeneca and Roche. Relevant to the present study, Thomas Similowski has received personal fees from Lungpacer Inc and is a member of the board of a research association that has received, over the past 10 years, unrestricted research grants from Maquet, Hamilton, Covidien, and Philips; he is the head of a research unit (UMRS 1158) that has signed research contracts with Air Liquide Medical Systems, France; he is listed as inventor or co-inventor on several patents, granted or pending, describing a brain–ventilator interface. The other authors have no conflict of interest relevant to this study.

Funding
M.D. was supported by the French Intensive Care Society, Paris, France (bourse de mobilité 2015); The 2015 Short Term Fellowship program of the European Respiratory Society, Lausanne, Switzerland; The 2015 Bernhard Dräger Award for advanced treatment of acute respiratory failure of the European Society of Intensive Care Medicine, Brussels, Belgium; the Assistance Publique Hôpitaux de Paris, Paris, France and the Fondation pour la Recherche Médicale, Paris, France (FDM 20150734498).

References
1. Dres M, Goligher EC, Heunks LMA, Brochard LJ. Critical illness-associated diaphragm weakness. Intensive Care Med. 2017;43:1441–52.
2. Demoule A, Jung B, Prodanovic H, Molinari N, Chanques G, Coirault C, et al. Diaphragm dysfunction on admission to the intensive care unit. Prevalence, risk factors, and prognostic impact-a prospective study. Am J Respir Crit Care Med. 2013;188:213–9.
3. Dres M, Dubé B-P, Mayaux J, Delemazure J, Reuter D, Brochard L, et al. Coexistence and impact of limb muscle and diaphragm weakness at time of liberation from mechanical ventilation in medical intensive care unit patients. Am J Respir Crit Care Med. 2017;195:57–66.
4. Jung B, Moury PH, Mahul M, de Jong A, Galia F, Prades A, et al. Diaphragmatic dysfunction in patients with ICU-acquired weakness and its impact on extubation failure. Intensive Care Med. 2016;42:853–61.
5. Jaber S, Petrof BJ, Jung B, Chanques G, Berthet J-P, Rabuel C, et al. Rapidly progressive diaphragmatic weakness and injury during mechanical ventilation in humans. Am J Respir Crit Care Med. 2011;183:364–71.
6. Levine S, Nguyen T, Taylor N, Friscia ME, Budak MT, Rothenberg P, et al. Rapid disuse atrophy of diaphragm fibers in mechanically ventilated humans. N Engl J Med. 2008;358:1327–35.
7. Hermans G, Agten A, Testelmans D, Decramer M, Gayan-Ramirez G. Increased duration of mechanical ventilation is associated with decreased diaphragmatic force: a prospective observational study. Crit Care Lond Engl. 2010;14:R127.
8. Vassilakopoulos T, Petrof BJ. Ventilator-induced diaphragmatic dysfunction. Am J Respir Crit Care Med. 2004;169:336–41.
9. Heunks LMA, Doorduin J, van der Hoeven JG. Monitoring and preventing diaphragm injury. Curr Opin Crit Care. 2015;21:34–41.
10. Supinski GS, Callahan LA. Diaphragm weakness in mechanically ventilated critically ill patients. Crit Care Lond Engl. 2013;17:R120.
11. Kim WY, Suh HJ, Hong S-B, Koh Y, Lim C-M. Diaphragm dysfunction assessed by ultrasonography: influence on weaning from mechanical ventilation. Crit Care Med. 2011;39:2627–30.
12. American Thoracic Society/European Respiratory Society. ATS/ERS statement on respiratory muscle testing. Am J Respir Crit Care Med. 2002;166:518–624.
13. Mills GH, Kyroussis D, Hamnegard CH, Polkey MI, Green M, Moxham J. Bilateral magnetic stimulation of the phrenic nerves from an anterolateral approach. Am J Respir Crit Care Med. 1996;154:1099–105.
14. Mills GH, Ponte J, Hamnegard CH, Kyroussis D, Polkey MI, Moxham J, et al. Tracheal tube pressure change during magnetic stimulation of the phrenic nerves as an indicator of diaphragm strength on the intensive care unit. Br J Anaesth. 2001;87:876–84.
15. Watson AC, Hughes PD, Louise Harris M, Hart N, Ware RJ, Wendon J, et al. Measurement of twitch transdiaphragmatic, esophageal, and endotracheal tube pressure with bilateral anterolateral magnetic phrenic nerve stimulation in patients in the intensive care unit. Crit Care Med. 2001;29:1325–31.
16. DiNino E, Gartman EJ, Sethi JM, McCool FD. Diaphragm ultrasound as a predictor of successful extubation from mechanical ventilation. Thorax. 2014;69:423–7.
17. Dubé B-P, Dres M, Mayaux J, Demiri S, Similowski T, Demoule A. Ultrasound evaluation of diaphragm function in mechanically ventilated patients: comparison to phrenic stimulation and prognostic implications. Thorax. 2017;72:811–8.
18. Boles J-M, Bion J, Connors A, Herridge M, Marsh B, Melot C, et al. Weaning from mechanical ventilation. Eur Respir J Off J Eur Soc Clin Respir Physiol. 2007;29:1033–56.
19. Similowski T, Yan S, Gauthier AP, Macklem PT, Bellemare F. Contractile properties of the human diaphragm during chronic hyperinflation. N Engl J Med. 1991;325:917–23.
20. Bossuyt PM, Cohen JF, Gatsonis CA, Korevaar DA, STARD group. STARD. updated reporting guidelines for all diagnostic accuracy studies. Ann Transl Med. 2015;2016(4):85.
21. DeLong ER, DeLong DM, Clarke-Pearson DL. Comparing the areas under two or more correlated receiver operating characteristic curves: a non-parametric approach. Biometrics. 1988;44:837–45.
22. Jiang J-R, Tsai T-H, Jerng J-S, Yu C-J, Wu H-D, Yang P-C. Ultrasonographic

evaluation of liver/spleen movements and extubation outcome. Chest. 2004;126:179–85.

23. Laghi F, Cattapan SE, Jubran A, Parthasarathy S, Warshawsky P, Choi Y-SA, et al. Is weaning failure caused by low-frequency fatigue of the diaphragm? Am J Respir Crit Care Med. 2003;167:120–7.

24. Manders E, Bonta PI, Kloek JJ, Symersky P, Bogaard H-J, Hooijman PE, et al. Reduced force of diaphragm muscle fibers in patients with chronic thromboembolic pulmonary hypertension. Am J Physiol Lung Cell Mol Physiol. 2016;311:L20–8.

25. Kelley RC, Ferreira LF. Diaphragm abnormalities in heart failure and aging: mechanisms and integration of cardiovascular and respiratory pathophysiology. Heart Fail Rev. 2017;22:191–207.

26. Adler D, Dupuis-Lozeron E, Richard J-C, Janssens J-P, Brochard L. Does inspiratory muscle dysfunction predict readmission after intensive care unit discharge? Am J Respir Crit Care Med. 2014;190:347–50.

27. Medrinal C, Prieur G, Frenoy É, Robledo Quesada A, Poncet A, Bonnevie T, et al. Respiratory weakness after mechanical ventilation is associated with one-year mortality—a prospective study. Crit Care Lond Engl. 2016;20:231.

28. Zambon M, Greco M, Bocchino S, Cabrini L, Beccaria PF, Zangrillo A. Assessment of diaphragmatic dysfunction in the critically ill patient with ultrasound: a systematic review. Intensive Care Med. 2017;43:29–38.

29. Haaksma M, Tuinman PR, Heunks L. Ultrasound to assess diaphragmatic function in the critically ill-a critical perspective. Ann Transl Med. 2017;5:114.

30. Ferrari G, De Filippi G, Elia F, Panero F, Volpicelli G, Aprà F. Diaphragm ultrasound as a new index of discontinuation from mechanical ventilation. Crit Ultrasound J. 2014;6:8.

31. Dres M, Demoule A. Diaphragm dysfunction during weaning from mechanical ventilation: an underestimated phenomenon with clinical implications. Crit Care Lond Engl. 2018;22:73.

32. Mayo P, Volpicelli G, Lerolle N, Schreiber A, Doelken P, Vieillard-Baron A. Ultrasonography evaluation during the weaning process: the heart, the diaphragm, the pleura and the lung. Intensive Care Med. 2016;42:1107–17.

33. Blumhof S, Wheeler D, Thomas K, McCool FD, Mora J. Change in diaphragmatic thickness during the respiratory cycle predicts extubation success at various levels of pressure support ventilation. Lung. 2016;194:519–25.

18

Hemodynamic support in the early phase of septic shock: a review of challenges and unanswered questions

Olivier Lesur[1*], Eugénie Delile[1], Pierre Asfar[2] and Peter Radermacher[3]

Abstract

Background: Improving sepsis support is one of the three pillars of a 2017 resolution according to the World Health Organization (WHO). Septic shock is indeed a burden issue in the intensive care units. Hemodynamic stabilization is a cornerstone element in the bundle of supportive treatments recommended in the Surviving Sepsis Campaign (SSC) consecutive biannual reports.

Main body: The "Pandera's box" of septic shock hemodynamics is an eternal debate, however, with permanent contentious issues. Fluid resuscitation is a prerequisite intervention for sepsis rescue, but selection, modalities, dosage as well as duration are subject to discussion while too much fluid is associated with worsen outcome, vasopressors often need to be early introduced in addition, and catecholamines have long been recommended first in the management of septic shock. However, not all patients respond positively and controversy surrounding the efficacy-to-safety profile of catecholamines has come out. Preservation of the macrocirculation through a "best" mean arterial pressure target is the actual priority but is still contentious. Microcirculation recruitment is a novel goal to be achieved but is claiming more knowledge and monitoring standardization. Protection of the cardio-renal axis, which is prevalently injured during septic shock, is also an unavoidable objective. Several promising alternative or additive drug supporting avenues are emerging, trending toward catecholamine's sparing or even "decatecholaminization." Topics to be specifically addressed in this review are: (1) mean arterial pressure targeting, (2) fluid resuscitation, and (3) hemodynamic drug support.

Conclusion: Improving assessment and means for rescuing hemodynamics in early septic shock is still a work in progress. Indeed, the bigger the unresolved questions, the lower the quality of evidence.

Keywords: Sepsis, Septic shock, Hemodynamic support, Fluid resuscitation, Mean arterial pressure, Microcirculation, Vasopressor(s), Vasoactive drugs, Catecholamines, Decatecholaminization, Metabolic stress

Background

Sepsis is a leading cause of mortality, similar to that reported from acute myocardial infarction and lung or breast cancers in the USA [1]. This and other evidence prompted a WHO resolution in 2017 highlighting a crucial need for better recognition, assessment, and support in the near future [2]. Septic shock with multiple organ failure (i.e., the catastrophic phenotype of sepsis) represents over 50% of intensive care unit diagnostic profiles worldwide [1].

Despite advances in earlier recognition and a more effective management yielding a significant reduction in mortality rates, septic shock remains nonetheless a worrisome health care issue. The latest "Surviving Sepsis Campaign" (SSC) guidelines in 2016 were recently updated mid-2018 (supported by the SCCM and ESICM). Both 2016 and 2018 above guidelines have served as reference for the current recommendations [3, 4].

*Correspondence: Olivier.Lesur@USherbrooke.ca
[1] Division of Intensive Care Units, Department of Medicine, Faculté de Médecine et des Sciences de la Santé, Centre de Recherche du CHUS, Université de Sherbrooke, Sherbrooke, QC, Canada
Full list of author information is available at the end of the article

Hemodynamic support in the early phase of septic shock: a review of challenges...

163

This review aims to focus on the hemodynamic support in early septic shock. Three essential topics have been selected as pillar elements and are discussed: (1) targets of hemodynamic stabilization, (2) fluid resuscitation, and (3) pharmacological hemodynamic support. Recommendations, gaps and controversies, ongoing research, and unanswered questions are exposed. With specific regards to the novel 2018 SSC update and its hemodynamic bundle of recommendations, a major modification was the period of time allotted to reach the threshold of 65 mmHg of MAP and mandates to administer the first 30 mL/kg fluid resuscitation within the 1st hour of admission ("hour-1 bundle") and to introduce vasoactive agents (mainly norepinephrine—NE) sooner if this macro-circulatory goal is not achieved or not sustainably stable.

Methods

Database selection, time window, and primary search terms (MeSH) used in the present review are detailed as followed.

A search strategy on MEDLINE and PubMed was operated, looking to and prioritizing randomized clinical trials (RCTs), systematic reviews, and meta-analyses (when existing) in articles published from 2013 to mid-2018. This exhaustive review focuses on sepsis hemodynamic support, which is a wide source of debate, and was starting on the former "Surviving Sepsis Campaign (SSC) Guidelines 2016," recently updated in 2018 (supported by both SCCM and ESICM) as a central thread.

Primary search terms used (MeSH) were: sepsis, severe sepsis, septic shock, circulatory shock, distributive shock, shock, fluid resuscitation, mean arterial pressure, perfusion pressure, microcirculation, vasopressor(s), epinephrine, norepinephrine, dobutamine, decatecholaminization, beta-blocker(s), levosimendan, selepressin, arginine vasopressin, angiotensin, metabolic stress, and immunomodulation.

The highest level of evidence was used for RCTs and meta-analyses when available, using a PICO framework strategy.

Excluded were articles with data of patients under 18 years old and those relating to starch use, the latter being mostly eradicated from modern practice in this setting. The impact of the recently published Sepsis-3 definitions [5] was also not specifically explored.

Which mean arterial pressure (MAP) target to stabilize the macrocirculation?
Prognosis

Although the SSC 2016 recommends a MAP ≥ 65 mmHg during initial resuscitation (grade 1 B: strong

recommendation, moderate level of evidence) [3], there is no precise evidence-based target determined to date. These guidelines suggest that the optimal MAP should be individualized and may be higher in selected patients such as those with atherosclerosis or previous hypertension [3]. In younger patients, a lower target may be acceptable.

The time spent below different threshold values of MAP during the first days has been analyzed and correlated with survival and organ dysfunction in two similarly designed retrospective studies using MAP recordings. The best MAP threshold was 65 mmHg, and the time spent under this value was positively correlated with mortality rate [6, 7].

A large prospective observational study (FINNAKI) [8] identified 423 patients with severe sepsis and showed that those with progression of acute kidney injury (AKI) within the first 5 days of ICU admission (36.2%) had a lower time-adjusted MAP than those without progression [9]. The best time-adjusted MAP value for predicting AKI progression was 73 mmHg. However, these data were not adjusted for disease severity. A retrospective analysis of health records of 8782 septic patients in the USA found increased mortality and AKI risks with time elapsed with average MAP below 85 mmHg [10].

In daily clinical practice, the actual objectified MAP level is often higher than the recommended target. This difference is also observed in all large prospective randomized controlled trials. Indeed, MAP was measured at 80 mmHg in three recent major clinical randomized trials aiming at comparing vasoactive drugs in patients with septic shock after 24 h of treatment (CATS, VASST, SOAP) [11–13]. Another study (SEPSISPAM) suggests that a MAP target of 65 mmHg is usually sufficient in patients with septic shock. However, a higher MAP level (around 75–85 mmHg) may prevent the occurrence of AKI in patients with chronic arterial hypertension [14]. Of note, patients with a high MAP target received significantly more norepinephrine (NE) and for a longer duration, while experiencing more cardiovascular side effects, especially new more onset of atrial fibrillation.

Given the aforementioned results, the SSC 2016 and 2018 Guidelines [3, 4] as well as the ESICM recommendations suggest targeting MAP to or over 65 mmHg for the initial resuscitation and to individualize MAP according to the patient's comorbidities.

Rationale for a "best MAP," autoregulation...and microcirculation

In light of the above, MAP is commonly considered as a surrogate of global perfusion pressure, although several essential physiological particularities should be retained. Indeed, a better understanding of the autoregulatory mechanisms and microcirculatory regulation during sepsis is needed to rationally address this question. Furthermore, increasing MAP levels often (or always) imply increasing vasopressor load, raising the issue of vasopressor side effects, in addition to their action on MAP.

Autoregulation is the ability of an organ to maintain a constant blood flow entering the organ, irrespective of perfusion pressure, within a range of values called «autoregulation zone». Below this autoregulation threshold, the blood flow in the organ is directly dependent on perfusion pressure. Autoregulation is important in the brain [15], heart [16], and kidney [17], with varying autoregulation threshold values depending on the auto-regulated organ [16]. The kidney has the highest autoregulation threshold and may be considered as the first resuscitation objective, with regards to the potential impacts on the outcome [18]. Autoregulation thresholds differ with patient age and associated comorbidities (chronic hypertension). While autoregulation is a well-established key factor in acute stroke, it is still unknown whether it is maintained during sepsis and whether a traditional threshold remains unchanged [19].

Finally, perfusion pressure should not be regarded as being equivalent to MAP. Organ perfusion pressure is equal to the difference of the pressure in the artery entering the organ (usually approximated by MAP) minus the organ venous pressure. The importance of venous pressure has been shown, particularly in the kidney [20], and the relationship between a deficit of renal perfusion pressure and the risk of AKI has been reported in septic shock [21].

In addition, sepsis is associated with alterations in microcirculation characterized by increased endothelial permeability, leukocyte adhesion, and blood flow heterogeneity leading to tissue hypoxia [22, 23]. Microcirculatory blood flow may be independent from systemic hemodynamics [24]. Consequently, when systemic hemodynamic objectives (in particular MAP target) are achieved, microcirculation abnormalities may persist [23]. Hence, increasing MAP above 65 mmHg may not change microvascular perfusion. Thus, while adjusting hemodynamic objectives at the second phase of septic shock (when patients are "hemodynamically stable") is unlikely to improve installed microcirculation impairment, an early intervention with high MAP levels may prevent the onset of microcirculatory dysfunction [25–30] (Table 1). However, more knowledge and monitoring standardization are requested to secure microcirculation assessment and related support. Two trials are currently ongoing with a peripheral or targeted tissue perfusion-guided primary objective (NCT01397474, NCT02579525).

Specific effect of high vasopressor load

Increasing the MAP target to high levels often requires high vasopressor doses. Norepinephrine (NE) is the most commonly used vasopressor in septic patients. It activates both alpha- and beta-adrenergic receptors and increases systemic vascular resistance (and thus left ventricle afterload); NE usually slightly increases cardiac output due to beta-adrenergic stimulation and its effect on venous return [31]. This venous effect of NE can also impact perfusion pressure, as outlined above [20]. In addition to the consequences of excessive vasoconstriction, other effects should also be taken into account when addressing the question of optimal vasopressor load. Sympathetic overstimulation (or adrenergic stress) can be associated with numerous harmful effects such as diastolic dysfunction, tachyarrhythmia, skeletal muscle damage (e.g., apoptosis), altered coagulation or endocrinological, immunological and metabolic disturbances [32].

Fluid resuscitation: Should we do more or less, with what and when?

In the serial SSC bundles up to 2018, fluid resuscitation had been a recommended first-line cornerstone therapy to support or prevent induced cardiovascular dysfunction and for reducing in-hospital mortality in sepsis [3]. On admission obvious shortage of the effective circulatory volume in septic patients (e.g., decreased input, enhanced water loss, vascular leak or third space) is the essential premise underlying this recommendation. In this setting, fluid resuscitation must be initiated as soon as possible (ASAP) often at the emergency room, and definitely within 3–6 h, whether hypotension is obviously present or not, and to ensure optimal preload conditions for a hemodynamic homeostasis. Of note, from the original SSC 2004, derived from the protocol-based RCT (early goal-directed therapy: EGDT) which first reported an effective algorithmic approach for improving outcome in early sepsis [33], the "6 golden hours" were first abridged to "3 golden hours," the earlier always being the better form of management, as highlighted by a recent retrospective cohort study [34]. Then, the emphasis has been placed on "ASAP" fluid resuscitation support (i.e., within the 1st hour of management, 30 mL/kg!) with further dynamic assessment enabling to identify patients who require more fluids and early introduction of vasopressors to reach a MAP target in the 2018 recommendations [4].

Indeed, even with differences in timing and previous intervention(s) before randomization, three successive RCTs (ProCESS, ARISE, ProMISe) [35–37] subsequently showed no benefit in primary mortality outcomes of an EGDT-like protocol-based approach, including lack of

Table 1 Prospective studies with MAP titration and peripheral (microcirculatory) or targeted tissue/organ perfusion assessment in septic shock

Authors [ref.]	No. of patients (n)	Design of MAP titration in mmHg (time at each step, min)	Main results
Ledoux et al. [25]	10	65, 75, 85 mmHg (**105**)	CI ↑ Arterial lactates, gastric intra-mucosal-arterial P_{CO_2} difference, skin microcirculatory blood flow (skin capillary blood flow and red blood cell velocity), urine output: ns
Bourgoin et al. [26]	2 × 14	MAP 65 versus 85 mmHg (**240**) comparison of two groups	CI ↑ Arterial lactates, VO_2, and renal function: ns
Deruddre et al. [27]	11	65, 75, 85 mmHg (**120**)	65–75 mmHg: urine output ↑, RRI ↓ 75–85 mmHg: urine output, RRI: ns Creatinine clearance: ns
Jhanji et al. [28]	16	60, 70, 80, 90 mmHg (**45**)	DO_2, cutaneous PtO_2, cutaneous microvascular red blood cell flux (laser Doppler flowmetry) ↑ Sublingual capillary MFI (SDF): ns
Dubin et al. [29]	20	65, 75, 85 mmHg (**30**)	CI, systemic vascular resistance, left and right ventricular stroke work indexes ↑ Arterial lactates, DO_2, VO_2, gastric intra-mucosal-arterial P_{CO_2} difference, sublingual capillary MFI and percent of perfused capillaries (SDF imaging): ns
Thooft et al. [30]	13	65, 75, 85 mmHg (**30**)	CI, SvO_2, StO_2, sublingual perfused vessel density and MFI (SDF imaging) ↑ VO_2: ns Arterial lactates ↓

MAP mean arterial pressure, *CI* cardiac index, *VO_2* oxygen consumption, *RRI* renal resistive index, *DO_2* oxygen delivery, *MFI* microvascular flow index, *SvO_2* mixed venous oxygen saturation, *StO_2* thenar muscle oxygen saturation using near-infrared spectroscopy (NIRS), *PtO_2* tissue oxygen pressure, *SDF* side-stream dark field

ns result not significant, ↑ increase, ↓ decrease

cost-effectiveness, such that new strategies are mandatory [38].

"at least 30 mL/kg of crystalloids within the first 3 h..." (strong recommendation, low quality of evidence, SSC 2016) [3] may be within the first hour! (SSC 2018) [4].

This "fixed" minimum fluid loading is actually recommended at this step (with or without vasopressor addition) if a minimum MAP of 65 mmHg is not achieved "rapidly" (SSC 2018) [4]. The early introduction of vasopressors, which is currently observed in many studies, is not disapproved and may have outcome benefits even more [39]. Of note, about 50% of septic patients in shock are non-responsive to fluids, only half patients included in the three above cited RCTs received 30 mL/kg in this time window, and the median fluid volume infused within the first 4 h before randomization in the recent VANISH trial was below 1.7 L [35–37, 40, 41]. Of course, clinical judgment is always the rule, and the evidence of pulmonary venous congestion, for example, should waive this fluid resuscitation practice.

"..additional fluids afterward, guided by frequent reassessment of hemodynamic status..." (best practice statement 2016) [3, 4].

Because "one size does not fit all," personalized assessment is suggested after the initial fluid load, mandating identification and selection of responding patients who require more fluids.

The goals of initial resuscitation can be central venous pressure (CVP), MAP, urine output, central venous oxygen saturation ($ScvO_2$), or blood lactates, although more dynamic variables than rigid static goals are suggested and proposed (e.g., pulse pressure variation, stoke volume variation, superior vena cava collapsibility, respiratory variation of inferior vena cava, end-expiratory occlusion test, or passive leg raising test). These still need further validation because prediction of fluid responsiveness is not a current practice worldwide [42].

Indeed, too much fluid is just as detrimental as too little and *"primum non nocere."* An increased risk of death was demonstrated with > 5 L first day, as already raised in VASST, and positive fluid balance significantly associated with enhanced mortality as early as 12 h after onset of management [43, 44]. Whether this may be only a severity marker rather than a causal relationship remains to be proven, but a negative fluid balance at 72 h within a "deresuscitation" strategy is associated with lower mortality [45].

Anyway, more restrictive/conservative or "deresuscitation" fluid resuscitation strategies are currently under evaluation (ACTRN12616000006448, NCT02079402, NCT0247371).

"crystalloids are to be selected in both above steps" (strong recommendation, moderate quality of evidence) [3, 4].

The question of which crystalloid (pH balanced or not) should be preferred still remains an ongoing debate. A recent RCT, including over 15,000 patients cluster randomized in a multiple crossover trial, has challenged the use of balanced crystalloids versus normal saline (NS) in critically ill conditions [46]. Less adverse kidney events and a trend in 30-day mortality reduction were observed with balanced crystalloids, with numbers needed to treat (NNTs) of 91 and 125, respectively. However, no distinction between balanced crystalloids was mentioned and septic patients represented less than 15% of included subjects ($n = 2336$). In this latter subset, a gain in targeted outcomes in favor of balanced fluids was noted: e.g., more reductions of 30-day mortality and major renal or other events (weak recommendation, moderate quality of evidence) [46].

Several additional RCTs comparing NS versus balanced crystalloid solution are currently ongoing (NCT02875873, NCT03277677), and comparative investigations on outcomes in-between the balanced crystalloid solution portfolio (e.g., lactated Ringer vs. Plasma-Lyte A) should be mandated.

"using albumin (Alb) in addition to crystalloids when a substantial amount of fluids is needed" (weak recommendation, low quality of evidence) [3, 4].

A first subgroup analysis of septic shock patients in the SAFE study trended toward a reduction in mortality [47], while no difference in targeted mortality rates was observed in the ALBIOS as well as EARSS trials (never published!) [48, 49]. Trends toward reduced mortality in several small studies and in meta-analyses have been reported (Table 2) [50–53], although the latter suffer from differing designs, types of Alb (iso- vs. hyper-oncotic), and infusion modalities (Alb used as a resuscitation fluid vs. as a pleiotropic molecule [54]).

In addition, given the raised potential adverse impact of high chloride fluid infusion, concerns as to variable chloride contents in different commercial Alb products have recently been reported [55], and it is noteworthy in this context that in turn increasing albuminemia may decrease pH due to a higher anion gap [56].

"the frailty cardio-renal axis...."

While there is currently no strong indication as to what constitutes a "better" fluid selection in improving morbidity and mortality rates in sepsis [3], there is increasing evidence since several decades that (1) patients receiving

Table 2 Systematic reviews and meta-analyses on albumin use as a resuscitation fluid in sepsis/septic shock

Systematic reviews [ref.]	No. of patients (n)	No. of RCTs included (presented)	Intervention fluid therapy	Primary outcome	Results: albumin versus crystalloids	Comments
Bansal et al. [50]	6082	13 (6[†])	Albumin, crystalloids [HES]	Mortality	*OR 0.9 (0.8–1.01)	2 RCTs including children and 1 case mix
				RRT need	?	7 RCTs with specific comparison HES versus crystalloids
Xu et al. [51]	5838	5	Albumin, crystalloids	All-cause mortality	** OR 0.88 (0.76–1.01) $p = 0.08$ severe sepsis OR 0.81 (0.67–0.97) $p = 0.03$ Septic shock	4 of 5 RCTs not entirely dedicated to septic patients
Patel et al. [52]	4190	16[†]	Albumin, crystalloids	All-cause mortality	RR 0.93 (0.86–1.01) $p = 0.07$	~ 10 RCTs not entirely dedicated to septic patients
Rochwerg [53]	1238[††]	14 (2)	Albumin, crystalloids	All-cause mortality	NMA 0.83 (0.65–1.04) estimate	Only 2 RCTs with direct comparison and one multicentric subgroup analysis encompassing more than 98%

RCTs randomized control trials, *OR* odds ratio, *RR* relative risk, *HES* hydroxy ethyl starches, *NMA* nodal meta-analysis

*28- and 30-day mortality

**90-day mortality

[†] One EARSS from the reported conference proceedings

[††] Post hoc analyses: (1) ALBIOS trial patients ($n = 1815$) not included because Alb was not used as a resuscitation fluid; data incorporation did not affect the final results, (2) exclusion of data from the one trial encompassing less than 2% of patients did not affect the final results

the largest fluid resuscitation were those with the worse outcome [43, 44], (2) adverse events and outcomes can occur as early as 12 h after sepsis onset when fluid resuscitation is sustained [44], and (3) sepsis-associated AKI is both common and costly (e.g., renal replacement therapy—RRT). With the exception of hydroxyethyl starches (HES) (including last generation), which are associated with more frequent and severe AKI and higher RRT needs [57], protocolized resuscitation does not appear to be an influencing factor, and balanced crystalloids have either marginally or never reduced the above outcomes to date [46, 56, 58–60].

Hemodynamic drug support:... to be or not to be?

Catecholamines

According to the most recent SSC 2016–2018 Guidelines [3] *"norepinephrine (NE) is recommended as the first-choice vasopressor (strong recommendation, moderate quality of evidence)"* because of its vasopressor and positive inotropic properties as well as its effect on venous return [61]. These guidelines also *"suggest epinephrine (E) to NE with the intent of raising MAP to target (weak recommendation, low quality of evidence)."* E titrated to comparable systemic hemodynamic targets clearly results in more pronounced metabolic stress than NE [62], although to date, large RCTs have failed to show the superiority of NE alone [12] or in combination with dobutamine [11] in septic shock when compared to E. Dobutamine is frequently used as an inotropic drug, and accordingly, the SSC 2016–2018 Guidelines [3] suggest its use *"...in patients who show evidence of persistent hypoperfusion despite adequate fluid loading and the use of vasopressor agents."* However, in contrast to the use of NE this rational only represents a *"weak recommendation with low quality of evidence."* In fact, the data supporting the use of dobutamine are *"...primarily physiologic, with improved hemodynamics and some improvement in indices of perfusion...."* There are no RCT on the use of dobutamine alone, and, as mentioned above, NE in combination with dobutamine was similar to E with respect to overall outcome. Moreover, from a pharmacological point of view, the efficacy of dobutamine per se might be limited when used in combination with NE: in vitro, dobutamine is a weak β-adrenergic agonist when compared to NE [63], and a comparably lower activity of dobutamine than NE was demonstrated in healthy volunteers with respect to catecholamine-induced glucose and lactate metabolism [64]. This issue may assume particular importance in the context of the sepsis-related adrenoceptor desensitization, which is exacerbated by ongoing catecholamine treatment [65]. Furthermore, catecholamines exhibit marked immune-modulatory properties [66] and are known to profoundly affect energy, in

particular glucose metabolism [67], and inhibit gastrointestinal peristalsis (for review: see [68, 69]). In addition, *"vasopressor load"* from high-dose catecholamine infusion rates has been found to be directly related to mortality regardless of the specific MAP achieved [70] due to catecholamine-induced cardiac toxicity [71]. Therefore, the concept of *"decatecholaminization"* has been put forward in the last decade [72, 73]. Several approaches have been tested, including arginine vasopressin (AVP) or its synthetic analogs, levosimendan, angiotensin II, as well as β-blockade (Table 3). The most abundant data available is on arginine vasopressin (AVP). Albeit *"not recommended as a first line vasopressor,"* the SSC 2016–2018 Guidelines [3] in fact *"suggest adding...vasopressin (up to 0.03 U/min)...to decrease NE dosage (weak recommendation, moderate quality of evidence)."* This addition has *"catecholamine-sparing"* capacity [12] and was recently proven to lower risk of new onset atrial fibrillation in patients with distributive shock [74], which is per se a significant worsening factor of in-hospital stroke and mortality in sepsis [75]. Nevertheless, so far there has been no clear evidence from RCT that the *"decatecholaminization"* concept is really more efficient than the standard approach using NE. However, data from the VASST, ATHOS, and esmolol trials demonstrated its feasibility, safety and, moreover, suggested improved morbidity and mortality (see below).

Vasopressin (AVP) and analogs

Overall, the VASST trial more than 10 years ago did not find any outcome benefit for low-dose (0.01–0.03 U/min) AVP compared to NE [12]. However, in contrast to the underlying hypothesis that the more severe patients might benefit from this approach, the subgroup of patients with only moderate NE requirements (pre-defined as < 15 µg/min), i.e., those in whom weaning from NE was more frequent [76], presented significantly improved survival. Moreover, more patients died while still on NE in the NE group than in the AVP group. Interestingly, a post hoc analysis of the VASST database according to the Septic Shock 3.0 definition [5] showed that AVP lowered the mortality rate compared to NE in patients with lactate levels ≤ 2 mmol/L [77]. The VANISH trial, a 2×2 comparison of either AVP (up 0.06 U/min) or NE as initial vasopressor to maintain target MAP followed by hydrocortisone (HCT) or placebo, did not improve the number of kidney failure-free days, although the confidence interval did suggest a potential benefit for AVP [41]. Finally, the single-center VANCS trial showed that AVP (0.01–0.06 U/min) used as first-choice vasopressor reduced morbidity (in particular the incidence of acute renal failure and de novo atrial fibrillation) in vasoplegic patients post-cardiac surgery [78].

Table 3 Hemodynamic drug support and RCTs in septic shock

Acronym	Studied drugs	Type of study	No. of patients (n)	Primary outcome	Main results	Authors [ref.]
VASST	AVP versus NE	RCT, double blind, multi-center	778 (396 vs. 382)	Mortality at day 28	No difference; significantly lower mortality in patients with NE < 15 µg/min	Russell et al. [12]
VASST (post hoc according to sepsis 3.0)	AVP versus NE	RCT, double blind, multi-center	375 (193 vs. 182)	Mortality at day 28	Significantly lower mortality in patients with lactate ≤ 2 mmol/L	Russell et al. [77]
VANISH	AVP versus NE (subsequently HCT versus placebo)	2 × 2 RCT, double blind, multicenter	409 (104 vs. 103 vs. 101 vs. 101)	Kidney failure-free days until day 28	No difference	Gordon et al. [41]
VANC	AVP versus NE	RCT, double blind, single center	300 (149 vs. 151)	Mortality and/or severe complications	Significantly less acute renal failure and atrial fibrillation	Hajjar et al. [78]
SEPSIS-ACT	Selepressin versus NE	RCT, double blind, multi-center	53 (32 vs. 21)	MAP > 65 mmHg without NE; NE dose	Significantly lower NE load, less net fluid intake, more ventilator-free days	Russell et al. [81]
LeoPARDS	Levosimendan versus standard treatment alone	RCT, double blind, multi-center	516 (259 vs. 257)	SOFA score up to day 28	No difference; higher incidence in supraventricular tachyarrhythmia	Gordon et al. [83]
ATHOS-3	Angiotensin II versus NE	RCT, double blind, multi-center	321 (163 vs. 158)	Target MAP > 75 mmHg at 3 h	Significantly more patients with target achieved; higher reduction in SOFA score at 48 h	Khanna et al. [86]
nn	Esmolol versus conventional treatment	Open label, RCT, single center	154 (77 vs. 77)	80 < heart rate < 95 over 96 h	Significantly lower mortality at day 28	Morelli et al. [88]

RCTs randomized clinical trials, *NE* norepinephrine, *AVP* arginine vasopressin, *HCT* hydrocortisone, *nn* no name

AVP non-selectively activates all vasopressin receptor subtypes and the oxytocin receptor, thus potentially resulting in undesirable side effects (e.g., water retention, platelet aggregation) other than the hemodynamic targets [79]. Therefore, more selective V_1 agonists have been tested. While the use of terlipressin does not *"offer advantages over AVP"* [80] due to its long duration of action over several hours, the pilot SEPSIS-ACT trial of the new, short-acting selective V_{1A} receptor agonist selepressin reduced cumulative NE doses and net fluid balance, and it increased the number of ventilator-free days [81].

Levosimendan

Many patients with sepsis develop cardiac dysfunction (*"septic cardiomyopathy"* [82]), which prompted the investigation of the *"calcium sensitizer"* levosimendan. The LeoPARDS trial comparing levosimendan (0.05–0.2 µg/kg/min, depending on rate-limiting side effects) and placebo in addition to standard treatment neither reduced sepsis-induced organ failure nor affected mortality or any other secondary outcome. Levosimendan was associated, however, with a higher incidence of supraventricular tachyarrhythmia [83].

Angiotensin II

It has been known for decades that septic shock causes activation of the renin–angiotensin–aldosterone system [84], which leads to angiotensin II release [85]. The ATHOS-3 trial compared angiotensin II (1.25–40 ng/kg/min) or placebo to achieve a target MAP ≥ 75 mmHg in patients with vasodilatory shock receiving NE > 0.2 µg/kg/min [86]. This primary endpoint was reached in a significantly higher proportion of patients in the treatment versus the placebo arm (69.9 vs. 23.4%). While the number of serious adverse events and mortality at day 28 did not differ between the two groups, angiotensin II-treated patients exhibited a greater improvement in organ failure score(s) at 48 h.

β-Blockade

At first glance, β-blockade appears to be counterintuitive in patients with vasodilatory shock depending on vasopressor therapy, i.e., catecholamine treatment to achieve target MAP. However, based on the similarity in hyperadrenergic response between patients with septic shock and those with cardiac disease [87], an open-label trial in patients with septic shock requiring continuous i.v. NE and presenting with a heart rate > 95/min after 24 h of ICU care investigated the infusion of the short-acting β-blocker esmolol titrated to maintain heart rate at 80–94/min for 96 h in addition to conventional treatment

[88]. Esmolol treatment coincided with a lower area under curve for lactatemia and need of fluid resuscitation, and it was ultimately associated with a significantly lower mortality than in the conventional treatment group (49.4 vs. 80.5%).

Given the side effects of high-dose catecholamine treatment and the consequences of sympathetic overstimulation, new approaches based on the concept of *"decatecholaminization"* are being considered by the latest SSC Guidelines to treat sepsis-induced vasoplegia. On the other hand, angiotensin II and β-blockers—if used—should be handled with considerable caution and only in selected patients. New drug prospects for an optimized ventriculo-arterial coupling are currently under investigation [89].

Hydrocortisone (HCT)

Albeit HCT is not a hemodynamic drug in the sense of direct vasopressor and/or inotropic activity, since its first use in small-sized trials in the late 1990s [90, 91], the existing RCT data unanimously showed that HCT allowed accelerated resolution of shock as defined by complete weaning from vasopressor support to achieve MAP targets [92, 93]. The hastened resolution of circulatory shock was referred to attenuation of the sepsis-induced hyper-inflammatory response, inhibition of the inducible isoform of the nitric oxide (NO) synthase, thereby attenuating excess NO release, and improved adrenergic receptor responsiveness [95]. Nevertheless, since overall outcome results were equivocal, inasmuch both improved survival [94] and unchanged survival [92, 93] were reported, the use of HCT remains a matter of debate. Accordingly, the SSC 2016–2018 Guidelines [3]—which could not take into the account the more recent ADRENAL [93] and APROCCHSS [94] trials—in fact suggest *"...i.v. hydrocortisone at a dose of 200 mg per day"* only if adequate fluid resuscitation and vasopressor support do not allow restoring hemodynamic stability, however, as a weak recommendation with low quality of evidence. Clearly, HCT seems not to have any beneficial effect in the prevention of septic shock [96] and should be tapered down once resolution of shock is achieved [3]. Of note, in the context of *"decatecholaminization,"* HCT may assume particular importance: a post hoc analysis of the VASST data base demonstrated a significant interaction between AVP and HCT, inasmuch the un-protocolized use HCT was associated with attenuated mortality and morbidity in the AVP arm, whereas the opposite result was found in patients who did not receive HCT [97].

Table 4 Hemodynamics in early septic shock

Main questions	Actual recommendations*	Unanswered questions
Which MAP targets to stabilize the macrocirculation?	MAP ≥ 65 mmHg	What is the best timing for MAP intervention in sepsis? and until when? Could "permissive hypotension" be considered as in the case of trauma? for which reason(s) and target(s)?
How much fluid resuscitation and when?	From "time of presentation" or "time zero," 30 mL/kg at least within 1 h	Should we prioritize fixed minimum fluid resuscitation or dynamic personalized reassessment of circulation status?
Which fluid(s)?	Crystalloids	Beyond balanced versus unbalanced crystalloid fluid selection, should we prefer acetate- or lactate-buffered solutions?
How long?	After the initial 1-h interventions, further fluid administration needs patients' assessment for responsiveness	What "gauge for a filled tank"?
Which vasoactive (± inotropic) drug(s)?	NE is recommended as a 1st choice vasopressor. AVP or E can be added to help reaching the target (i.e., MAP) and spare NE	Within a "hour-1 bundle" strategy, should we trade-off less fluids and more vasoactive drugs to vice versa?
When?	Dobutamine only if target not reached after adequate fluid loading and use of vasoactive drugs	Are vasopressor combinations able to reach high MAP levels without detrimental cardiac side effects?
	As early as during the initial fluid resuscitation period, to achieve the target MAP ≥ 65 mmHg ASAP	With NE as the currently recommended first-line vasopressor is "decatecholaminization" feasible and safe?

MAP mean arterial pressure, NE norepinephrine, AVP arginine vasopressin, E epinephrine, ASAP as soon as possible

*According to the Surviving Sepsis Campaign 2016 and the 2018 update (Refs [3, 4])

Conclusion

Hemodynamic support in sepsis and septic shock is a perpetual work in progress.

Fluid resuscitation with crystalloids remains cornerstone of supportive therapy, *"the earlier the better,"* although *"too much is just as detrimental as too little."* Targeted goals for fluid cannot be pre-established, and dynamic monitoring and personalization are mandatory. Actual and recommended MAP target is 65 mmHg but must be adapted according to patient comorbidities (i.e., chronic hypertension) and with the understanding that convergence toward macro-to-microcirculation perfusion synchrony is difficult to reach. Vasoactive and potentially inotropic catecholamines are still (and potentially urgently) recommended for pharmacological hemodynamic support, although additional supportive molecules (e.g., vasopressin, angiotensin II) and new agents/approaches tend toward a new paradigm of "decatecholaminization."

Unanswered questions

However, while knowledge is growing and has already provided improvements toward a better assessment and monitoring of hemodynamics in patients undergoing sepsis, unresolved questions are bigger than the quality evidence, *"...a little bit does go a long way"* in this instance! Several unanswered questions with regards to the recommended SSC 2018 Guidelines are summarized in Table 4.

Abbreviations

WHO: World Health Organization; SSC: Sepsis Surviving Campaign; RCT(s): randomized clinical trial(s); PICO: patient, intervention, comparison, outcome; MAP: mean arterial pressure; AKI: acute kidney injury; ICU: intensive care unit; NE: norepinephrine; CI: cardiac index; VO$_2$: oxygen consumption; DO$_2$: oxygen delivery; MFI: microvascular flow index; SvO$_2$: mixed venous oxygen saturation; StO$_2$: tissue oxygen saturation; NIRS: near-infrared spectroscopy; Pt: tissue oxygen pressure; SDF: sidestream dark field; RRI: renal resistive index; ASAP: as soon as possible; CVP: central venous pressure; Scv: central venous oxygen saturation; NS: normal saline; NNT: number needed to treat; Alb: albumin; RTT: renal replacement therapy; HES: hydroxyethyl starches; OR: odds ratio; RR: relative risk; NMA: nodal meta-analysis; E: epinephrine; AVP: arginine vasopressin; HCT: hydrocortisone; NO: nitric oxide.

Authors' contributions

All four authors contributed to conception and design of this review, collection and interpretation of data, and writing of the manuscript. All authors read and approved the final manuscript.

Author details
[1] Division of Intensive Care Units, Department of Medicine, Faculté de Méde-cine et des Sciences de la Santé, Centre de Recherche du CHUS, Université de Sherbrooke, Sherbrooke, QC, Canada. [2] Département de Médecine Intensive-Réanimation, Centre Hospitalier Universitaire, Université d'Angers, Angers, France. [3] Institut für Anästhesiologische Pathophysiologie und Verfah-rensentwicklung, Universitätsklinikum, Ulm, Germany.

Acknowledgements
The authors thank Frederic Chagnon and Christian Audet for their help and expertise.

Competing interests
The authors declare that they have no competing interests.

Funding
CIHR (# 376770-201610PJT; 398298-201710PJT; 399567-201803PJT), Bourses du Département de Médecine FMSS-UDS (Cliniciens-Chercheurs 2018-2020: OL; Fellowship 2017-2018: ED).

References
1. Martin G, Mannino D, Eaton S, et al. The epidemiology of sepsis in the U-S from 1979 through 2000. N Engl J Med. 2003;348:1546–54.
2. Reinhart K, Daniels R, Kissoon N, et al. Recognizing sepsis as a global health priority—a WHO resolution. N Engl J Med. 2017;377:414–7.
3. Rhodes A, Evans LE, Alhazzani W, et al. Surviving Sepsis Campaign: international guidelines for management of sepsis and septic shock: 2016. Intensive Care Med. 2017;43:304–77.
4. Levy M, Evans LE, Rhodes A. The Surviving Sepsis Campaign Bundle: 2018 update. Intensive Care Med. 2018. https://doi.org/10.1007/s0013 4-018-5085-0.
5. Singer M, Deutschman CS, Seymour CW, et al. The third international consensus definitions for sepsis and septic shock (sepsis-3). JAMA. 2016;315:801–10.
6. Varpula M, Tallgren M, Saukkonen K, et al. Hemodynamic vari-ables related to outcome in septic shock. Intensive Care Med. 2005;31:1066–71.
7. Dünser MW, Takala J, Ulmer H, et al. Arterial blood pressure during early sepsis and outcome. Intensive Care Med. 2009;35:1225–33.
8. Nisula S, Kaukonen K-M, Vaara ST, The FINNAKI Study Group. Incidence, risk factors and 90-day mortality of patients with acute kidney injury in Finnish intensive care units: the FINNAKI study. Intensive Care Med. 2013;39:420–8.
9. Poukkanen M, Wilkman E, Vaara ST, The FINNAKI Study Group. Hemo-dynamic variables and progression of acute kidney injury in critically ill patients with severe sepsis: data from the prospective observational FINNAKI study. Crit Care Lond Engl. 2013;17:R295.
10. Maheshwari K, Nathanson BH, Munson SH, et al. The relationship between ICU hypotension and in-hospital mortality and morbidity in septic patients. Intensive Care Med. 2018;44:857–67.
11. Annane D, Vignon P, Renault A, The CATS Study Group. Norepinephrine plus dobutamine versus epinephrine alone for management of septic shock: a randomised trial. Lancet. 2007;370:676–84.
12. Russell JA, Walley KR, Singer J, The VASST Investigators. Vasopressin versus norepinephrine infusion in patients with septic shock. N Engl J Med. 2008;358:877–87.
13. De Backer D, Biston P, Devriendt J, The SOAP II Investigators. Comparison of dopamine and norepinephrine in the treatment of shock. N Engl J Med. 2010;362:779–89.
14. Asfar P, Meziani F, Hamel J-F, et al. High versus low blood-pressure target in patients with septic shock. N Engl J Med. 2014;370:1583–93.
15. Strandgaard S, Olesen J, Skinhoj E, et al. Autoregulation of brain circula-tion in severe arterial hypertension. Br Med J. 1973;1:507–10.
16. Berne RM. Regulation of coronary blood flow. Physiol Rev. 1964;44:1–29.
17. Cupples WA, Braam B. Assessment of renal autoregulation. Am J Physiol Renal Physiol. 2007;292:F1105–23.
18. Badin J, Boulain T, Ehrmann S, et al. Relation between mean arterial pressure and renal function in the early phase of shock: a prospective, explorative cohort study. Crit Care Lond Engl. 2011;15:R135.
19. Bellomo R, Wan L, May C. Vasoactive drugs and acute kidney injury. Crit Care Med. 2008;36(Suppl):S179–86.
20. Legrand M, Dupuis C, Simon C, et al. Association between systemic hemodynamics and septic acute kidney injury in critically ill patients: a retrospective observational study. Crit Care Lond Engl. 2013;17:R278.
21. Panwar R, Lanyon N, Davies AR, et al. Mean perfusion pressure deficit during the initial management of shock—an observational cohort study. J Crit Care. 2013;28:816–24.
22. De Backer D, Donadello K, Taccone FS, et al. Microcirculatory alterations: potential mechanisms and implications for therapy. Ann Intensive Care. 2011;1:27.
23. De Backer D, Creteur J, Preiser J-C, et al. Microvascular blood flow is altered in patients with sepsis. Am J Respir Crit Care Med. 2002;166:98–104.
24. De Backer D, Ortiz JA, Salgado D. Coupling microcirculation to systemic hemodynamics. Curr Opin Crit Care. 2010;16:250–4.
25. LeDoux D, Astiz ME, Carpati CM, et al. Effects of perfusion pressure on tissue perfusion in septic shock. Crit Care Med. 2000;28:2729–32.
26. Bourgoin A, Leone M, Delmas A, et al. Increasing mean arterial pressure in patients with septic shock: effects on oxygen variables and renal func-tion. Crit Care Med. 2005;33:780–6.
27. Deruddre S, Cheisson G, Mazoit J-X, et al. Renal arterial resistance in septic shock: effects of increasing mean arterial pressure with norepinephrine on the renal resistive index assessed with Doppler ultrasonography. Intensive Care Med. 2007;33:1557–62.
28. Jhanji S, Stirling S, Patel N, et al. The effect of increasing doses of norepi-nephrine on tissue oxygenation and microvascular flow in patients with septic shock. Crit Care Med. 2009;37:1961–6.
29. Dubin A, Pozo MO, Casabella CA, et al. Increasing arterial blood pressure with norepinephrine does not improve microcirculatory blood flow: a prospective study. Crit Care Lond Engl. 2009;13:R92.
30. Thooft A, Favory R, Salgado DR, et al. Effects of changes in arterial pressure on organ perfusion during septic shock. Crit Care Lond Engl. 2011;15:R222.
31. Hamzaoui O, Georger J-F, Monnet X, et al. Early administration of norepi-nephrine increases cardiac preload and cardiac output in septic patients with life-threatening hypotension. Crit Care Lond Engl. 2010;14:R142.
32. Dünser MW, Hasibeder WR. Sympathetic overstimulation during criti-cal illness: adverse effects of adrenergic stress. J Intensive Care Med. 2009;24:293–316.
33. Rivers E, Nguyen B, Havstad S, The Early Goal-Directed Therapy Collabora-tive Group, et al. Early goal-directed therapy in the treatment of severe sepsis and septic shock. N Engl J Med. 2001;345:1368–77.
34. Pruinelli L, Westra BL, Yadav P, et al. Delay Within the 3-hour Surviving Sepsis Campaign guideline on mortality for patients with severe sepsis and septic shock. Crit Care Med. 2018;46:500–5.
35. ProCESS Investigators, Yearly DM, Kellum JA, et al. A randomized trial of protocol-based care for early septic shock. N Engl J Med. 2014;370:1683–93.
36. ARISE Investigators, Group ACT, Peake SL, et al. Goal-directed resuscitation for patients with early septic shock. N Engl J Med. 2014;371:1496–506.
37. Mouncey PR, Osborn TM, Power GS, et al. Trial of early, goal-directed resuscitation for septic shock. N Engl J Med. 2015;372:1301–11.
38. PRISM Investigators, Rowan KM, Angus DC, et al. Early, goal-directed therapy for septic shock—a patient-level meta-analysis. N Engl J Med. 2017;376:2223–34.
39. Bai X, Yu W, Ji W, et al. Early versus delayed administration of norepineph-rine in patients with septic shock. Crit Care Lond Engl. 2014;18:532.
40. Marik PE, Cavallazzi R, Vasu T, et al. Dynamic changes in arterial waveform derived variables and fluid responsiveness in mechanically

ventilated patients: a systematic review of the literature. Crit Care Med. 2009;37:2642–7.

41. Gordon AC, Mason AJ, Thirunavukkarasu N, The VANISH Investigators. Effect of early vasopressin vs norepinephrine on kidney failure in patients with septic shock: the VANISH randomized clinical trial. JAMA. 2016;316:509–18.

42. Cecconi M, Hofer C, Teboul JL, The FENICE Investigators, ESICM Trial Group. Fluid challenges in intensive care: the FENICE study: a global inception cohort study. Intensive Care Med. 2015;41:1529–37.

43. Marik PE, Linde-Zwirble WT, Bittner EA, et al. Fluid administration in severe sepsis and septic shock, patterns and outcomes: an analysis of a large national database. Intensive Care Med. 2017;43:625–32.

44. Boyd JH, Forbes J, Nakada TA, et al. Fluid resuscitation in septic shock: a positive fluid balance and elevated central venous pressure are associated with increased mortality. Crit Care Med. 2011;39:259–65.

45. Silversides JA, Fitzgerald E, Manickavasagam US, et al. Deresuscitation of patients with iatrogenic fluid overload is associated with reduced mortality in critical illness. Crit Care Med. 2018;46:1600–7.

46. Semler MW, Self WH, Wanderer JP, et al. Balanced crystalloids versus saline in critically Ill adults. N Engl J Med. 2018;378:829–39.

47. SAFE Study Investigators, Finfer S, McEvoy S, et al. Impact of albumin compared to saline on organ function and mortality of patients with severe sepsis. Intensive Care Med. 2011;37:86–96.

48. Caironi P, Tognoni G, Masson S, The ALBIOS Study Investigators, et al. Albumin replacement in patients with severe sepsis or septic shock. N Engl J Med. 2014;370:1412–21.

49. Mira JP. Facts or myths: early albumin resuscitation during septic shock (the EARSS trial) [Internet]. Berlin [cited 2013 Jun 17]. Available from: http://www.esicm.org/flashConference/2011/Berlin/10438/swf/playe r.swf.2011.

50. Bansal M, Farrugia A, Balboni S, et al. Relative survival benefit and morbidity with fluids in severe sepsis—a network meta-analysis of alternative therapies. Curr Drug Saf. 2013;8:236–45.

51. Xu J-Y, Chen Q-H, Xie J-F, et al. Comparison of the effects of albumin and crystalloid on mortality in adult patients with severe sepsis and septic shock: a meta-analysis of randomized clinical trials. Crit Care Lond Engl. 2014;18:702.

52. Patel A, Laflan MA, Waheed U, et al. Randomised trials of human albumin for adults with sepsis: systematic review and meta-analysis with trial sequential analysis of all-cause mortality. BMJ. 2014;349:g4561.

53. Rochwerg B, Alhazzani W, Sindi A, From the Fluids in Sepsis and Septic Shock Group, et al. Fluid resuscitation in sepsis: a systematic review and network meta-analysis. Ann Intern Med. 2014;161:347–55.

54. Quinlan GJ, Martin GS, Evans TW. Albumin: biochemical properties and therapeutic potential. Hepatology. 2005;41:1211–9.

55. Lai AT, Zeller MP, Millen T, The Canadian Critical Care Trials Group, et al. Chloride and other electrolyte concentrations in commonly available 5% albumin products. Crit Care Med. 2018;46:e326–9.

56. Fencl V, Jabor A, Kazda A, et al. Diagnosis of metabolic acid-base disturbances in critically ill patients. Am J Respir Crit Care Med. 2000;162:2246–51.

57. Perner A, Haase N, Guttormsen AB, et al. Hydroxyethyl starch 130/0.42 versus Ringer's acetate in severe sepsis. N Engl J Med. 2012;367:124–34.

58. Young P, Bailey M, Beasley R, et al. Effect of a buffered crystalloid solution vs saline on acute kidney injury among patients in the intensive care unit. The SPLIT Randomized Clinical Trial. JAMA. 2015;314:1701–10.

59. Rochwerg B, Alhazzani W, Gibson A, From FISSH Group (Fluids in Sepsis and Septic Shock), et al. Fluid type and the use of renal replacement therapy in sepsis: a systematic review and network meta-analysis. Intensive Care Med. 2015;41:1561–71.

60. Kellum JA, Chawla LS, Keener C, ProCESS and ProGReSS-AKI Investigators, et al. The effects of alternative resuscitation strategies on acute kidney injury in patients with septic shock. Am J Respir Crit Care Med. 2016;193:281–7.

61. Persichini R, Silva S, Teboul JL, et al. Effects of norepinephrine on mean systemic pressure and venous return in human septic shock. Crit Care Med. 2012;40:3146–53.

62. De Backer D, Creteur J, Silva E, et al. Effects of dopamine, norepinephrine, and epinephrine on the splanchnic circulation in septic shock: which is best? Crit Care Med. 2003;31:1659–67.

63. MacGregor DA, Prielipp RC, Butterworth JF 4th, James RL, Royster RL. Relative efficacy and potency of beta-adrenoceptor agonists for generating cAMP in human lymphocytes. Chest. 1996;109(1):194–200.

64. Ensinger H, Geisser W, Brinkmann A, Wachter U, Vogt J, Radermacher P, Georgieff M, Träger K. Metabolic effects of norepinephrine and dobutamine in healthy volunteers. Shock. 2002;18(6):495–500.

65. Silverman HJ, Penaranda R, Orens JB, et al. Impaired β-adrenergic receptor stimulation of cyclic adenosine monophosphate in human septic shock: association with myocardial hyporesponsiveness to catecholamines. Crit Care Med. 1993;21:31–9.

66. Stolk RF, van der Poll T, Angus DC, et al. Potentially inadvertent immunomodulation: norepinephrine use in sepsis. Am J Respir Crit Care Med. 2016;194:550–8.

67. Barth E, Albuszies G, Baumgart K, et al. Glucose metabolism and catecholamines. Crit Care Med. 2007;35(Suppl):S508–18.

68. Andreis DT, Singer M. Catecholamines for inflammatory shock: a Jekylland-Hyde conundrum. Intensive Care Med. 2016;42:1387–97.

69. Hartmann C, Radermacher P, Wepler M, et al. Non-hemodynamic effects of catecholamines. Shock. 2017;48:390–400.

70. Dünser MW, Ruokonen E, Pettilä V, et al. Association of arterial blood pressure and vasopressor load with septic shock mortality: a post hoc analysis of a multicenter trial. Crit Care Lond Engl. 2009;13:R181.

71. Schmittinger CA, Dünser MW, Torgersen C, et al. Histologic pathologies of the myocardium in septic shock: a prospective observational study. Shock. 2013;39:329–35.

72. Singer M. Catecholamine treatment for shock–equally good or bad? Lancet. 2007;370:636–7.

73. Singer M, Matthay MA. Clinical review: thinking outside the box—an iconoclastic view of current practice. Crit Care Lond Engl. 2011;15:225.

74. McIntyre WF, Um KJ, Alhazzani W, et al. Association of vasopressin plus catecholamine vasopressors vs catecholamines alone with atrial fibrillation in patients with distributive shock. A systematic review and metanalysis. JAMA. 2018;319:1889–900.

75. Walkey AJ, Soylemez Wiener R, Ghobrial JM, et al. Incident stroke and mortality associated with new-onset atrial fibrillation in patients hospitalized with severe sepsis. JAMA. 2001;306:2248–54.

76. Bracht H, Calzia E, Georgieff M, et al. Inotropes and vasopressors: more than haemodynamics! Br J Pharmacol. 2012;165:2009–11.

77. Russell JA, Lee T, Singer J, The Vasopressin and Septic Shock Trial (VASST) Group. The septic shock 3.0 definition and trials: a Vasopressin and septic shock trial experience. Crit Care Med. 2017;45:940–8.

78. Hajjar LA, Vincent JL, Barbosa Gomes Galas FR, et al. Vasopressin versus norepinephrine in patients with vasoplegic shock after cardiac surgery: the VANCS randomized controlled trial. Anesthesiology. 2017;126:85–93.

79. Vincent JL, Su F. Physiology and pathophysiology of the vasopressinergic system. Best Pract Res Clin Anaesthesiol. 2008;22:243–52.

80. Vincent JL, De Backer D. Circulatory shock. N Engl J Med. 2013;369:1726–34.

81. Russell JA, Vincent JL, Kjølbye AL, et al. Selepressin, a novel selective vasopressin V_{1A} agonist, is an effective substitute for norepinephrine in a phase IIa randomized, placebo-controlled trial in septic shock patients. Crit Care Lond Engl. 2017;21:213.

82. Beesley SJ, Weber G, Sarge T, et al. Septic cardiomyopathy. Crit Care Med. 2018;46:625–34.

83. Gordon AC, Perkins GD, Singer M, et al. Levosimendan for the prevention of acute organ dysfunction in sepsis. N Engl J Med. 2016;375:1638–48.

84. White FN, Gold EM, Vaughn DL. Renin-aldosterone system in endotoxin shock in the dog. Am J Physiol. 1967;212:1195–8.

85. Levy B, Fritz C, Tahon E, et al. Vasoplegia treatments: the past, the present, and the future. Crit Care Lond Engl. 2018;22:52.

86. Khanna A, English SW, Wang XS, The ATHOS-3 Investigators. Angiotensin II for the Treatment of Vasodilatory Shock. N Engl J Med. 2017;377:419–30.

87. Lira A, Pinsky MR. Should β-blockers be used in septic shock? Crit Care Lond Engl. 2014;18:304.

88. Morelli A, Ertmer C, Westphal M, et al. Effect of heart rate control with esmolol on hemodynamic and clinical outcomes in patients with septic shock: a randomized clinical trial. JAMA. 2013;310:1683–91.

89. Coquerel D, Sainsily X, Dumont L, et al. The apelinergic system as an alternative to catecholamines in low-output septic shock. Crit Care Lond Engl. 2018;22:10.

90. Bollaert PE, Charpentier C, Levy B, Debouverie M, Audibert G, Larcan A. Reversal of late septic shock with supraphysiologic doses of hydrocortisone. Crit Care Med. 1998;26(4):645–50.

91. Schelling G, Stoll C, Kapfhammer HP, et al. The effect of stress doses of hydrocortisone during septic shock on posttraumatic stress disorder and health-related quality of life in survivors. Crit Care Med. 1999;27(12):2678–83.

92. Sprung CL, Annane D, Keh D, et al. Hydrocortisone therapy for patients with septic shock. N Engl J Med. 2008;358(2):111–24.

93. Venkatesh B, Finfer S, Cohen J, et al. Adjunctive glucocorticoid therapy in patients with septic shock. N Engl J Med. 2018;378(9):797–808.

94. Annane D, Renault A, Brun-Buisson C, et al. Hydrocortisone plus fludrocortisone for adults with septic shock. N Engl J Med. 2018;378(9):809–18.

95. Keh D, Boehnke T, Weber-Cartens S, et al. Immunologic and hemodynamic effects of "low-dose" hydrocortisone in septic shock: a double-blind, randomized, placebo-controlled, crossover study. Am J Respir Crit Care Med. 2003;167(4):512–20.

96. Keh D, Trips E, Marx G, et al. Effect of hydrocortisone on development of shock among patients with severe sepsis: the HYPRESS randomized clinical trial. JAMA. 2016;316(17):1775–85.

97. Russell JA, Walley KR, Gordon AC, et al. Interaction of vasopressin infusion, corticosteroid treatment, and mortality of septic shock. Crit Care Med. 2009;37(3):811–8.

19

Impact of a VAP bundle in Belgian intensive care units

Laurent Jadot[1], Luc Huyghens[2], Annick De Jaeger[3], Marc Bourgeois[4], Dominique Biarent[5], Adeline Higuet[6], Koen de Decker[7], Margot Vander Laenen[8], Baudewijn Oosterlynck[4], Patrick Ferdinande[9], Pascal Reper[10,11], Serge Brimioulle[12], Sophie Van Cromphaut[13], Stéphane Clement De Clety[14], Thierry Sottiaux[15] and Pierre Damas[1*]

Abstract

Background: In order to decrease the incidence of ventilator-associated pneumonia (VAP) in Belgium, a national campaign for implementing a VAP bundle involving assessment of sedation, cuff pressure control, oral care with chlorhexidine and semirecumbent position, was launched in 2011–2012. This report will document the impact of this campaign.

Methods: On 1 day, once a year from 2010 till 2016, except in 2012, Belgian ICUs were questioned about their ventilated patients. For each of these, data about the application of the bundle and the possible treatment for VAP were recorded.

Results: Between 36.6 and 54.8% of the 120 Belgian ICUs participated in the successive surveys. While the characteristics of ventilated patients remained similar throughout the years, the percentage of ventilated patients and especially the duration of ventilation significantly decreased before and after the national VAP bundle campaign. Ventilator care also profoundly changed: Controlling cuff pressure, head positioning above 30° were obtained in more than 90% of cases. Oral care was more frequently performed within a day, using more concentrated solutions of chlorhexidine. Subglottic suctioning also was used but in only 24.7% of the cases in the last years. Regarding the prevalence of VAP, it significantly decreased from 28% of ventilated patients in 2010 to 10.1% in 2016 ($p \leq 0.0001$).

Conclusion: Although a causal relationship cannot be inferred from these data, the successive surveys revealed a potential impact of the VAP bundle campaign on both the respiratory care of ventilated patients and the prevalence of VAP in Belgian ICUs encouraging them to follow the guidelines.

Keywords: VAP, VAP bundle, Belgian ICUs, VAP survey

Background

Ventilator-associated pneumonia (VAP) is among the most common type of intensive care unit (ICU)-acquired infection and is associated with significant morbidity and mortality [1]. In Europe, the incidence remains higher than in the USA despite the implementation of VAP bundles [2–4]. The need for the implementation of multimodal approach to decrease the incidence of VAP

has been recently reemphasized by European guidelines [5] and especially by guidelines coming from the société française d'anesthésie-réanimation and the société de réanimation de langue française [6, 7]. Besides the use of selective digestive decontamination, these guidelines support the use of 6 procedures: avoiding intubation by the use of noninvasive ventilation, avoiding nasotracheal intubation, controlling cuff pressure, reducing the level of sedation, early enteral nutrition and subglottic suctioning.

In Belgium, after having observed high rate of VAP in ICUs from previous surveys, the federal service launched a promotional campaign to implement a national VAP

*Correspondence: pdamas@chuliege.be
[1] Service de Soins Intensifs Généraux, Domaine Universitaire du Sart-Tilman, Centre Hospitalier Universitaire, 4000 Liège, Belgium
Full list of author information is available at the end of the article

bundle in 2011. This campaign involved several meetings in Brussels (attended by representatives from most Belgian ICUs) where the Belgian VAP bundle was explained and promoted. This campaign was followed by a prospective collect of all the VAP bundle data during 11 months in 2012 from voluntary participating Belgian ICUs. This collect was performed by the federal service. The national VAP bundle involved 4 items: a protocol with daily assessment of sedation, a semirecumbent position of at least 30°, the control of cuff pressure between 20 and 30 cm of H2O and the oral care with chlorhexidine. In addition, the use of subglottic suctioning was encouraged. Before and after this campaign, the college of physicians for intensive care, which also relies on the federal public service for health, food chain safety and environment, has performed surveys to evaluate the prevalence of VAP in Belgian ICUs. The present paper describes the results of the successive surveys and will examine the impact the campaign could have on the compliance of medical teams for implementing the bundle and on the prevalence of VAP. Data from the 2012 national collection study have been already published [8].

Methods

Once a year, from 2010 till 2016, except in 2012, all the 120 adult ICUs in Belgium received an invitation to participate in 1-day survey performed by the college of physicians for intensive care about ventilated patients and the occurrence of VAP. ICUs were asked about their number of beds, their occupancy, the number of ventilated patients. Ventilated patient characteristics included age, sex, primary reason for ICU admission, comorbidities, date of admission to the hospital and to the ICU, date of intubation and cause of ventilation. Regarding ventilation care, the way of intubation (nasal, oral, tracheostomy),the type of cuff (polyvinyl, polyurethane), the current cuff pressure, the type of suctioning system (opened or closed), the current head positioning, the moistening system (heat and moisture exchangers, active devices) and the use of a subglottic suctioning system were recorded for each patient. Regarding the oral care, the type of disinfection (chlorhexidine, polyvidone iodine, other), the rate of disinfection, the use of dental brushing and the type of nutrition tubing (nasogastric, orogastric, postpyloric tube, gastrostomy or jejunostomy) were also recorded for each ventilated patients. If a patient was treated for a VAP, the bacteriological results were asked for and the severity of the infection according to the grade of sepsis was recorded. No follow-up of patients was obtained.

VAP diagnosis was based on new infiltrate on chest X-ray with either fever above 38° or less than 35° or leukocytosis above 10,000 white blood cells/mm^3 and either occurrence of purulent tracheal secretions or decrease in

PaO2/FiO2. After each survey, all the ICUs, having or not participated in the survey, received a report describing the results and were encouraged to continue to implement the VAP bundle.

Statistical analysis

Quantitative data were summarized as median and interquartile (IQR) values or as mean and SD when normally distributed. Comparisons were made by the Kruskal–Wallis or Student's t test as appropriate for continuous variables and by Chi-square or Fisher's exact test for categorical variables. All tests were two-sided, and statistical significance was set at p less than 0.05.

Results

More than 60 adult ICUs participated in the surveys, except in 2016 when there were only 44. Considering that in Belgium there are 120 acute hospitals, these figures correspond to 36.6–54.8% of them. Figure 1 gives the evolution of the number of ICU beds belonging to participating ICUs, the number of patients and among them, the number of ventilated patients. As can be inferred from Fig. 1, the percentage of bed occupancy remained stable, between 75 and 80%, but the percentage of ventilated patients decreased significantly from 44.8% in 2010 to 28.7% in 2016 ($p < 0.05$). Another impressive difference between the surveys was the decrease in the duration of ventilation from the ICU admission till the day of the survey: The median was 10.5 and 13 days before the campaign, then 7, 5, 5 and 6 days after the campaign ($p < 0.001$) (Table 1).

The other characteristics of ventilated patients remained quite the same throughout the years of the surveys as shown in Table 1: age, sex, pre-ICU hospitalization stays, types of patients, underlying diseases, none of these characteristics differ between years of survey. However, regarding the causes of ventilation, the differences reached the statistical significance ($p = 0.0012$).

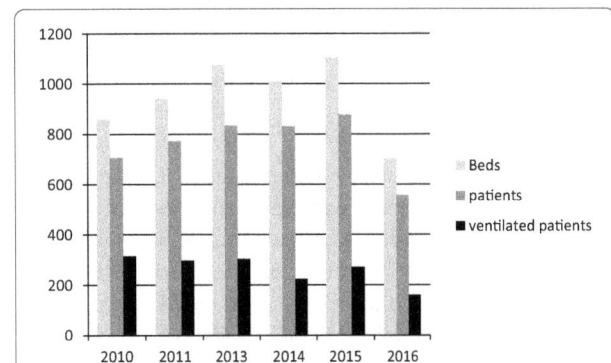

Fig. 1 Evolution of the number of ICU beds, patients and ventilated patients in participating ICUs

Table 1 Characteristics of ventilated patients

	Characteristics of patients						
	2010	2011	2013	2014	2015	2016	*p* value
Number	129	293	288	265	271	158	
Age median (IQR)	67 (54–78)	65 (54–75)	66 (54–75)	67 (57–76)	64 (54–76)	64 (50–71)	0.8412
Sex (male)	88 (68.8%)	183 (62.5%)	183 (63.5%)	162 (61.1%)	170 (62.7%)	102 (64.6%)	0.8326
Pre-ICU hosp. stay	0 (0–4)	0 (0–2)	0 (0–2)	1 (0–5)	0 (0–2)	0 (0–2)	0.3229
ICU stay median	10 (4–19)	13 (7–21)	8 (3–18)	7 (2–16)	7 (2–16)	8 (2–19)	<0.0001
Duration of ventilation median	10.5 (4–17)	13 (7–21)	7 (3–16)	5 (2–14)	5 (1–15)	6 (2–14)	<0.0001
Type of patients							0.0655
Medical	71 (55.8%)	156 (53.2%)	155 (53.2%)	138 (52.1%)	153 (56.5%)	94 (59.4%)	
Scheduled surgery	12 (9.3%)	51 (17.4%)	57 (19.8%)	52 (19.6%)	45 (16.6%)	18 (11.4%)	
Nonscheduled surgery	32 (24.8%)	51 (17.4%)	48 (16.7%)	59 (22.3%)	42 (15.5%)	30 (19%)	
Trauma	13 (10.1%)	35 (16.1%)	28 (9.7%)	16 (6%)	31 (11.4%)	16 (10.1%)	
Underlying disease							0.2724
Smoker	44 (34.1%)	102 (47%)	103 (35.7%	75 (28.3%)	81 (29.9%)	51 (32.3%)	
Asthma	7 (5.4%)	13 (4.4%)	5 (1.7%)	19 (7.2%)	9(3.3%)	5 (3.2%)	
COPD	36 (27.9%)	83 (28.3%)	89 (30.9%)	63 (23.8%)	64 (23.6%)	38 (24%)	
Solid cancer	4 (3.1%)	36 (12.3%)	28 (9.7%)	28 (10.6%)	20 (7.4%)	12 (7.6%)	
Hematological cancer	7 (5.4%)	7 (2.4%)	10 (3.5%)	4 (1.5%)	9 (3.3%)	4 (2.5%)	
Immunosuppression	12 (9.3%)	25 (8.5%)	20 (6.9%)	19 (7.2%)	16 (5.9%)	6 (3.8%)	
Corticotherapy	9 (7%)	37 (12.6%)	28 (9.7%)	39 (14.7%)	27 (10%)	15 (9.5%)	
Diabetes	13 (10.1%)	38 (13%)	42 (14.6%)	34 (12.8%)	34 (12.5%)	17 (10.8%)	
Other	NA	NA	NA	26 (9.8%)	26 (9.6%)	75 (47.4%)	
Cause of ventilation							0.0012
Hypoxia	50 (38.8%)	79 (27%)	95 (33%)	83 (31.3%)	80 (29.5%)	55 (34.8%)	
Hypercapnia	7 (5.4%)	39 (13.3%)	24 (8.3%)	19 (7.2%)	11 (4.1%)	16 (10.1%)	
Central nervous system	24 (18.6%)	47 (16%)	40 (13.9%)	32 (12.1%)	45 (16.6%)	19 (12%)	
Peripheral nervous system	0 (0%)	1 (0.3%)	2 (0.7%)	4 (1.5%)	5 (1.8%)	2 (1.3%)	
Trauma	7 (5.4%)	14 (4.8%)	12 (4.2%)	9 (3.4%)	14 (5.2%)	10 (6.3%)	
Circulatory problem	17 (13.2%)	38 (13%)	40 (17.4%)	40 (15.1%)	43 (15.9%)	17 (10.8%)	
Postoperative	17 (13.2%)	30 (10.2%)	59 (20.5%)	67 (25.2%)	63 (23.2%)	25 (15.8%)	
Other	7 (5.4%)	13 (1.1%)	16 (5.6%)	11 (4.1%)	10 (3.7%)	14 (8.9%)	

IQR Interquartile range, *ICU* intensive care unit, *COPD* chronic obstruction pulmonary disease, *NA* not available

Regarding ventilatory care, it profoundly changed before and after the national VAP bundle campaign: As shown in Table 2, the cuff pressure measurement, which was not performed in 27% of ventilated patients in 2011, was obtained in more than 90% of cases in 2015. Head positioning above 30° was seen in 2010 only in 54% of ventilated patients, and it was systematically observed in more than 90% of the patients after the campaign except in 2016, when it decreased to 88.6%. Subglottic suctioning also significantly increased, and it was however used in only 24.7% of the cases in 2016. In the same way, oral care was more frequently performed, using more concentrated solutions of chlorhexidine as shown in Table 3. Other oral disinfectants were less often used (from 15.2% in 2010 to 6.3% in 2016), polyvidone iodine

solutions remaining at a level of 34.8% in 2016. Dental brushing which was not performed in 25% of the ventilated patients in 2011 was still not done in 17.1% of the patients in 2016.

Regarding the prevalence of VAP, it significantly decreased from 28% of ventilated patients in 2010 to 10.1% in 2016 as shown in Fig. 2 ($p \leq 0.0001$). Interestingly, the associated bacteremia also decreased in absolute terms (from 7 to 2) but not relatively (from 8.9 to 12.5% of the corresponding VAP, $p = 0.9625$).

Discussion

This paper reports on the implementation of a VAP bundle in Belgium. It was indeed expected in 2012 by the federal authorities to at least halve the VAP incidence

Table 2 Ventilatory care

	2010	2011	2013	2014	2015	2016	p value
Previous NIV	25 (19.4%)	50 (17.1%)	52 (18%)	46 (17.4%)	44 (16.2%)	33 (20.9%)	0.8685
Artificial airway							0.0663
Oral intubation	95 (75.4%)	244 (83.3%)	234 (81.2%)	222 (83.8%)	226 (83.4%)	132 (83.5%)	
Nasal intubation	0	2 (0.7%)	4 (1.4%)	4 (1.6%)	6 (2.2%)	2 (1.3%)	
Tracheostomy	34 (26.4%)	47 (16%)	50 (17.4%)	39 (14.7%)	39 (14.4%)	24 (15.2%)	
Cuff							0.0318
Polyvinyl	74 (64.3%)	166 (56.6%)	170 (59%)	143 (54%)	158 (58.3%)	110 (69.6%)	
Polyurethane	41 (36.7%)	127 (43.3%)	118 (41%)	122 (46%)	113 (41.7%)	48 (30.4%)	
Cuff pressure							<0.0001
Not measured	9 (7%)	72 (24.6%)	2 (0.7%)	10 (3.8%)	4 (1.5%)	6 (3.8%)	
<20 cm H_2O	25 (19.4%)	18 (6.1%)	9 (3.1%)	9 (3.4%)	2 (0.7%)	7 (4.4%)	
20–30 cm H_2O	91 (70.5%)	196 (66.9%)	263 (91%)	228 (86%)	251 (92.6%)	137 (86.7%)	
>30 cm H_2O	4 (3.1%)	6 (2%)	10 (3.5%)	15 (5.7%)	10 (3.7%)	5 (3.2%)	
Not inflated	0	1 (0.3%)	4 (1.4%)	3 (1.1%)	(1.5%)	3 (1.9%)	
Suctioning system							<0.0001
Opened	76 (62.8%)	236 (80.5%)	204 (70.8%)	171 (64.5%)	205 (75.6%)	120 (79.7%)	
Closed	45 (37.2%)	57 (19.5%)	84 (29.2%)	94 (35.5%)	66 (24.4%)	38 (20.3%)	
Subglottic suctioning							<0.0001
Yes	7 (5.8%)	67 (22.9%)	94 (32.6%)	60 (22.6%)	70 (25.8%)	39 (24.7%)	
No	114 (94.2%)	226 (77.1%)	194 (69.2%)	205 (77.4%)	201 (74.2%)	119 (75.3%)	
Head position							<0.0001
<30°	55 (44.4%)	43 (14.7%)	21 (7.3%)	13 (4.9%)	25 (9.2%)	18 (11.4%)	
>30°	67 (54.0%)	249 (85%)	262 (91%)	249 (94%)	245 (90.4%)	140 (88.6%)	
Prone position	2 (1.6%)	1 (0.3%)	5 (1.7%)	3 (1.1%)	1 (3.7%)	0 (0%)	

NIV Noninvasive ventilation

Table 3 Oral care

Oral disinfection	2010	2011	2013	2014	2015	2016	p value
Water	1 (1%)	6 (2%)	1 (0.3%)	0 (0%)	0 (0%)	0 (0%)	
CHXD 0.2%	48 (38.4%)	126 (43%)	108 (37.5%)	132 (49.8%)	90 (33.2%)	79 (50%)	<0.0001
CHXD 0.5%	13 (10.4%)	5 (1.7%)	11 (3.8%)	7 (2.6%)	4 (1.5%)	5 (3.2%)	
CHXD 1%	0 (0%)	2 (0.7%)	26 (9%)	7 (2.6%)	16 (5.9%)	3 (1.9%)	
CHXD 2%	0 (0%)	0 (0%)	10 (3.5%)	9 (3.4%)	15 (5.5%)	7 (4.4%)	
Polyvidone iodine	44 (35.2%)	119 (40.6%)	102 (35.4%)	93 (35.1%)	124 (45.8%)	55 (34.8%)	
Other	19 (15.2%)	35 (11.9%)	30 (10.4%)	17 (6.4%)	22 (8.11%)	10 (6.3%)	
Rate of disinfection							
1/day	2 (1.6%)	31 (10.6%)	3 (1%)	9 (3.4%)	2 (0.7%)	0 (0%)	<0.0001
2/day	24 (19.2%)	41 (14%)	24 (8.3%)	27 (10.2%)	22 (8.1%)	8 (5.1%)	
3/day	36 (28.8%)	117 (39.9%)	158 (54.9%)	136 (51.3%)	116 (42.8%)	75 (47.4%)	
>3/day	63 (50.4%)	104 (35.5%)	103 (35.8%)	93 (35.1%)	131 (48.3%)	75 (47.4%)	
Dental brushing							
0/day	NK	63 (21.5%)	51 (18.7%)	32 (12.9%)	36 (13.3%)	27 (17.1%)	0.0235
1/day	NK	99 (33.8%)	103 (35.8%)	88 (33.3%)	83 (30.6%)	63 (39.9%)	
2/day	NK	70 (23.9%)	63 (21.9%)	81 (38.6%)	84 (31%)	51 (32.3%)	
2/day	NK	46 (15.7%)	47 (16.3%)	45 (17%)	53 (19.6%)	11 (7%)	
Not applicable	NK	15 (5.1%)	25 (8.7%)	19 (7.2%)	15 (5.5%)	6 (3.8%)	

CHXD Chlorhexidine, *NK*: not known

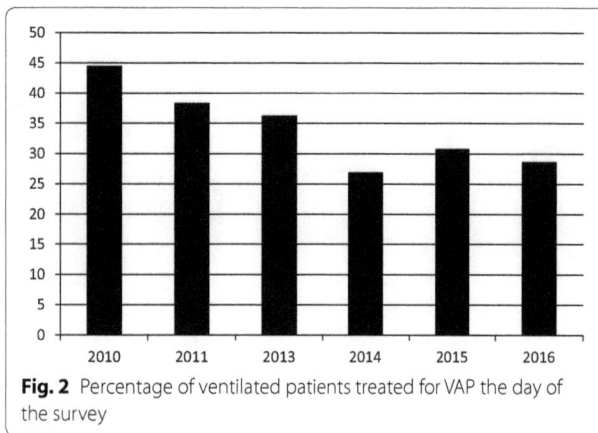

Fig. 2 Percentage of ventilated patients treated for VAP the day of the survey

encountered in Belgium. According to Fig. 2, this seems to have been reached and even exceeded, since the prevalence of VAP, as estimated by the surveys, was as high as 28% of the ventilated patients in 2010, reached 11.3% in 2014 and was maintained at this level for the next 2 years. It does not correspond to prevalence levels reported in the USA, but it corresponds to the best levels reported in European centers where VAP bundles are implemented [3, 4].

There is no clear consensus about what a VAP bundle should be [9, 10]. The first VAP bundle from the IHI includes elements which were not directly linked to the management of the airway (prevention of both thromboembolism and digestive hemorrhage) [11]. European experts proposed in 2010 only two procedures in addition to general measures such as hand hygiene, staff education and nonventilatory circuit change: control of sedation with protocol of weaning and oral care with chlorhexidine [12]. The Belgian VAP bundle [8] includes these two procedures into 4 components (sedation protocol, control of cuff pressure, oral disinfection, head of bed elevation) which were also parts of bundles recently published with reported efficacy [3, 4]. It also promotes a fifth procedure: subglottic suctioning which seems to have become the most useful procedure for the prevention of VAP [13–15].

The most striking difference between surveys appeared to be the percentage of ventilated patients and the duration of ventilation from the ICU admission till the day of the survey. Although this latter parameter was not the true duration of ventilation, it reflects a reality which means that from year to year, at one point in the year, fewer patients were ventilated and especially for less time in Belgian ICUs. Of course, this reduction of duration of ventilation reduces the risk for occurrence of VAP, estimated by these 1-day prevalence surveys. It would have been worth correlating this reduction of ventilation to

a change in sedation procedures, which, unfortunately, were not directly assessed by the surveys. It may however be inferred that the campaign had an impact because of the clear difference between the duration before and after it.

After the campaign, the compliance with head of bed elevation and control of cuff pressure increased significantly and exceeded 90%. Oral disinfection also improved. The type of antiseptic varied largely, but the rate of application increased: It was done at least 3 times a day in 79.2% in 2010 and in 94.8% in 2016 ($p < 0.0001$). Chlorhexidine concentration of 1 or 2% was more often used after the campaign, but the low concentration of 0.2% was still used in 50% in 2016. The type and the concentration of antiseptic remain a matter of debate. Chlorhexidine has been shown as effective with concentration as high as 2% in a well-conducted multicenter study in the Netherlands by Koeman in 2006 [16]. Chlorhexidine has been, however, reported to be sometimes not well tolerated by the patients [17]. More worrying is that an increase in mortality in patients receiving chlorhexidine as part of oral disinfection was recently reported by Komplas [18] although this agent is used worldwide [19]. The merit of polyvidone iodine in oral disinfection is supported by very few studies [19], although it remains used in Belgium in one-third of the patients. Regarding dental brushing, it is surprising that as many as 17.1% of patients did not benefit from this care in 2016. They were already 21.5% in 2010, though dental brushing is the only way to eliminate or reduce the dental plaque which can contain a lot of pathogenic bacteria [20]. However, even if dental brushing has been shown to reduce the rate of pneumonia in postoperative patients [21], this was curiously not yet confirmed for VAP in ventilated ICU patients [22]. Subglottic suctioning, which was promoted, remains used in Belgium in a minority of patients. This could be due to the cost of the endotracheal tube which is on average 10 times higher than conventional tubes in Belgium. However, this procedure should still be encouraged because of its efficacy reported as high as 50% reduction of VAP incidence [15].

Thus, the VAP bundle was rather correctly followed and VAP incidence decreased. Was there a clear causal relationship between these two facts? These surveys cannot ascertain that statement, but they were carried out to control the expected impact on VAP prevalence. But the question remains of the reality of this impact, especially because the effect was seen only in 2014, 2015 and 2016, while the campaign was conducted in 2012. All the improvements seen in the application of VAP bundle were, however, already obtained in 2013. Why did the reduction in VAP prevalence not occur in 2013? In fact, this question is not anecdotic, because there may have been a change in the way the VAP was diagnosed and the reduction seen in 2013 onward could be due to this change. As said by Komplas, "an apparent decrease in VAP rate could be achieved by maximally exploiting the subjectivity and inconstancies of VAP definitions" [23]. In our opinion, it was not the case, because the way of diagnosing VAP remains the same, based on radiological findings, the occurrence of fever, change in leukocytosis and bacteriological results. The surveys were answered on a voluntary basis, and there were no reasons to minimize the VAP prevalence at any time. Most medical teams were the same during the surveys. An indirect evidence of the reality in the reduction of VAP prevalence was the corresponding decrease in associated bacteremia, the rate relating to the number of VAP being stable. That means that the same type of infections was taken into account during the surveys. However, Komplas' concern regarding the data manipulation, even if unconscious, may still be real.

This report is not a true study such as the one recently published about the Spanish experience [24]. It is only a presentation of several surveys supporting the implementation of a VAP bundle in ICU ventilated patients. It gives figures from a large number of ICUs, allowing to describe the average activity of intensive care in Belgium and to encourage Belgian teams to prevent the occurrence of VAP by all valuable means. It is indeed interesting to observe the steady decline in number of ventilated patients in Belgian ICUs and duration of ventilation over time. Data quality may be, however, questioned because data could not be controlled, but remained consistent over time.

Conclusion

The occurrence of VAP was a real issue in 2010 in Belgium. The efforts made by the medical and nurses teams of the different ICUs seem to have successfully contributed to the decrease in VAP prevalence which has now reached a low plateau for several years. However, there could still be room for further improvement.

Abbreviations

VAP: ventilator-associated pneumonia; ICU: intensive care unit; IQR: interquartile range; SD: standard deviation; COPD: chronic obstruction pulmonary disease; NA: not available; NIV: noninvasive ventilation; CHXD: chlorhexidine; NK: not known.

Authors' contributions

All authors designed the study, contributed to the interpretation of the results and critically revised the manuscript. All authors made a substantial contributions to the acquisition of the data and revised the manuscript for important intellectual content. LJ and PD made a substantial contribution in writing the manuscript and interpreting the results. PD made a substantial contribution in the study design and critically revised the manuscript for important intellectual content. All authors had full access to the data, take responsibility for

the integrity of the data and the accuracy of the analysis. All authors read and approved the final manuscript.

Author details
[1] Service de Soins Intensifs Généraux, Domaine Universitaire du Sart-Tilman, Centre Hospitalier Universitaire, 4000 Liège, Belgium. [2] Dienst Intensieve Zorgen, VUB – Universitair Ziekenhuis Brussel, Campus Jette Laarbeeklaan 101, 1090 Brussels, Belgium. [3] Pediatrische Intensieve Zorgen, Universitair Ziekenhuis Gent, De Pintelaan 185, 9000 Ghent, Belgium. [4] Dienst Intensieve Zorgen, Algemeen Ziekenhuis Sint-Jan Brugge-Oostende, Ruddershove 10, 8000 Brugge, Belgium. [5] Service Soins Intensifs et Urgences, Hôpital Universitaire des Enfants Reine Fabiola, Avenue Crocq 15, 1020 Brussels, Belgium. [6] Urgentiegeneeskunde, Algemeen Ziekenhuis Sint-Maria, Ziekenhuislaan 100, 1500 Halle, Belgium. [7] Intensieve Zorgen, Universitair Ziekenhuis Onze Lieve Vrouw, Moorselbaan 164, 9300 Aalst, Belgium. [8] Anesthesiologie – Kritieke Diensten, Ziekenhuis Oost-Limburg, Campus Sint-Jan, Schiepse Bos 6, 3600 Genk, Belgium. [9] Intensieve Zorgen, Universitair Ziekenhuis Leuven, Herestraat 49, 3000 Louvain, Belgium. [10] Service de Soins Intensifs, Centre Hospitalier Universitaire Brugmann, Site Horta, Place Arthur Van Gehuchten 4, 1020 Brussels, Belgium. [11] Service de Soins Intensifs, Le Tilleriau, CHR Haute Senne, Chaussée de Braine 49, 7060 Soignies, Belgium. [12] Service de Soins Intensifs, Hôpital Erasme, Route de Lennik 808, 1070 Brussels, Belgium. [13] Intensieve Zorgen, UZA, Wilrijkstraat 10, 2650 Edegem, Belgium. [14] Service de Soins Intensifs et Urgences Pédiatriques, Cliniques Universitaires Saint-Luc, UCL, Avenue Hippocrate 10, 1200 Brussels, Belgium. [15] Soins Intensifs, Clinique Notre-Dame de Grâce, Chaussée de Nivelles, 212, 6041 Gosselies, Belgium.

Acknowledgements
None.

Competing interests
The authors declare that they have no competing interests.

References
1. Bekaert M, Timsit JF, Vansteelandt S, et al. Outcomerea Study Group. Attributable mortality of ventilator-associated pneumonia: a reappraisal using causal analysis. Am J Resp Crit Care Med. 2011;184:1133–9.
2. Hutchins K, Karras G, Erwin J, Sullivan K. Ventilator-associated pneumonia and oral care: a successful quality improvement project. Am J Infect Control. 2009;37:590–7.
3. Morris AC, Hay AW, Swann DG, et al. Reducing ventilator-associated pneumonia in intensive care: impact of implementing a care bundle. Crit Care Med. 2011;39:2218–24.
4. Bouadma L, Mourvillier B, Deiler V, et al. A multifaceted program to prevent ventilator-associated pneumonia: impact on compliance with preventive measures. Crit Care Med. 2010;38:789–96.
5. Torres A, Niederman M, Chastre J, et al. International ERS/ESICM/ESCMID/ALAT guidelines for the management of hospital-acquired pneumonia and ventilator-associated pneumonia: guidelines for the management of hospital-acquired pneumonia (HAP)/ventilator-associated pneumonia (VAP) of the European Respiratory Society (ERS), European Society of Intensive Care Medicine (ESICM), European Society of Clinical Microbiology and Infectious Diseases (ESCMID) and Asociación Latinoamericana del Tórax (ALAT). Eur Respir J. 2017;50:1700582.
6. SFAR. http://sfar.org/pneumonies-associees-aux-soins-de-reanimation/.
7. SRLF. https://www.srlf.org/wp-content/uploads/2017/09/2017_09_RFEcommune_PNEUMONIES-ASSOCIEES-AUX-SOINS-DE-REANIMATION.pdf.
8. Reper P, Dicker D, Damas P, et al. Improving the quality of the intensive care follow-up of ventilated patients during a national registration program. Public Health. 2017;148:159–66.
9. Klompas M. Ventilator-associated pneumonia: Is zero possible? Clin Inf Dis. 2010;51:1123–6.
10. O'Grady N, Murray PR, Ames N. Preventing ventilator-associated pneumonia. Does the evidence support the practice? JAMA. 2012;307:2534–9.
11. Resar R, Pronovost P, Haraden C, et al. Using a bundle approach to improve ventilator care processes and reduce ventilator-associated pneumonia. Jt Comm J Qual Patient Saf. 2005;31:243–8.

12. Rello J, Lode H, Cornaglia G, et al. The VAP care bundle contributors. A European care bundle for prevention of ventilator-associated pneumonia. Int Care Med. 2010;36:773–80.

13. Lacherade JC, De Jonghe B, Guezennec P, et al. Intermittent subglottic secretion drainage and ventilator-associated pneumonia. Am J Resp Crit Care Med. 2010;182:910–7.

14. Damas P, Frippiat F, Ancion A, et al. Prevention of ventilator-associated pneumonia and ventilator-associated conditions: a randomized controlled trial with subglottic secretion suctioning. Crit Care Med. 2015;43:22–30.

15. Caroff D, Li L, Muscedere J, Klompas M. Subglottic secretion drainage and objective outcomes: a systematic review and meta-analysis. Crit Care Med. 2016;44:830–40.

16. Koeman M, Van der Ven A, Hak E, et al. Oral decontamination with chlorhexidine reduces the incidence of ventilator-associated pneumonia. Am J Resp Crit Care Med. 2006;173:1348–55.

17. Richards D. Chlorhexidine mouthwash plaque levels and gingival health. Evid Based Dent. 2017;18:37–8.

18. Klompas M, Li L, Kleinman K, et al. Associations between ventilator bundle components and outcome JAMA. Intern Med. 2016;176:1277–83.

19. Shi Z, Xie H, Wang P, et al. Oral hygiene care for critically ill patients to prevent ventilator-associated pneumonia. Cochrane Database Syst Rev. 2013. https://doi.org/10.1002/14651858.CD00836.pub2.

20. Fourrier F, Cau-Pottier E, Boutigny H, et al. Effect of dental plaque antiseptic decontamination on bacterial colonization and nosocomial infection in critically ill patients. Int Care Med. 2000;26:1239–47.

21. Akutsu Y, Matsubara H, Shuto K, et al. Preoperative dental brushing can reduce the risk of postoperative pneumonia in esophageal cancer patients. Surgery. 2010;147:497–502.

22. Gu WJ, Gong YZ, Pan L, et al. Impact of oral care with versus without toothbrushing on the prevention of ventilator-associated pneumonia: a systematic review and meta-analysis of randomized controlled trials. Crit Care. 2012;16:R90.

23. Klompas M. What is new in the prevention of nosocomial pneumonia in the ICU? Curr Opin Crit Care. 2017;23:378–84.

24. Alvarez-Lerma F, Palomar-Martinez M, Sanchez-Garcia M, et al. Prevention of ventilator-associated pneumonia: the multimodal approach of the Spanish ICU Pneumonia Zero program. Crit Care Med. 2018;46:181–8.

20

Carotid and femoral Doppler do not allow the assessment of passive leg raising effects

Valentina Girotto[1*], Jean-Louis Teboul[1], Alexandra Beurton[1], Laura Galarza[1], Thierry Guedj[2], Christian Richard[1] and Xavier Monnet[1]

Abstract

Background: The hemodynamic effects of the passive leg raising (PLR) test must be assessed through a direct measurement of cardiac index (CI). We tested whether changes in Doppler common carotid blood flow (CBF) and common femoral artery blood flow (FBF) could detect a positive PLR test (increase in CI ≥ 10%). We also tested whether CBF and FBF changes could track simultaneous changes in CI during PLR and volume expansion. In 51 cases, we measured CI (PiCCO2), CBF and FBF before and during a PLR test (one performed for CBF and another for FBF measurements) and before and after volume expansion, which was performed if PLR was positive.

Results: Due to poor echogenicity or insufficient Doppler signal quality, CBF could be measured in 39 cases and FBF in only 14 cases. A positive PLR response could not be detected by changes in CBF, FBF, carotid nor by femoral peak systolic velocities (areas under the receiver operating characteristic curves: 0.58 ± 0.10, 0.57 ± 0.16, 0.56 ± 0.09 and 0.64 ± 10, respectively, all not different from 0.50). The correlations between simultaneous changes in CI and CBF and in CI and FBF during PLR and volume expansion were not significant ($p = 0.41$ and $p = 0.27$, respectively).

Conclusion: Doppler measurements of CBF and of FBF, as well as measurements of their peak velocities, are not reliable to assess cardiac output and its changes.

Keywords: Volume expansion, Fluid responsiveness, Hemodynamic monitoring, Cardiac output

Background

Since it has been demonstrated that fluid overload can be deleterious in patients with acute respiratory distress syndrome [1] and severe sepsis [2], it is of paramount importance to avoid excessive fluid administration in such cases. The decision to give fluids must be guided by a reliable prediction of fluid responsiveness as only 50% of patients respond to fluid administration by increasing cardiac output [3]. In order to predict the response of cardiac output to fluid infusion, the passive leg raising (PLR) test has been validated. It consists in lifting the legs passively at 45° and moving the trunk down horizontally,

starting from a semi-recumbent position. By transferring a consistent amount of venous blood from the legs and the splanchnic compartment toward the intrathoracic compartment, it increases the mean systemic pressure [4], the cardiac preload and consequently cardiac output in the case of preload responsiveness of both ventricles [5]. However, it must be coupled with a direct and real-time measurement of cardiac output, which is often invasive [6–8].

The Doppler measurement of blood flow and its velocity in the carotid as well as in the femoral arteries may be interesting for estimating the changes in cardiac output during a PLR test, since changes in arterial blood flow and in cardiac output might be proportional. Nevertheless, contradictory results have been published regarding this issue [9–14].

---

*Correspondence: girotto.valentina@gmail.com
[1] Service de Réanimation Médicale, Hôpital de Bicêtre, Hôpitaux Universitaires Paris-Sud, Insert UMR_999, Université Paris-Sud, Assistance Publique – Hôpitaux de Paris, Le Kremlin-Bicêtre, France
Full list of author information is available at the end of the article

Our study had two aims. The first was to test whether changes in carotid and femoral Doppler measurements were able to detect a positive PLR test. The second was to investigate the ability of carotid and femoral Doppler measurements to track the changes in cardiac index, during PLR and fluid administration.

Methods

Patients

Before starting the study, we obtained the agreement of our institutional review board (*Comité pour la protection des personnes Ile-de-*France VI, ref # 2016-A00959-42). All patients or their relatives accepted to participate in the study. It took place at a 25-bed medical intensive care unit of a university hospital between June and November 2016.

Patients were included in the study if they met the following criteria:

*   Age $\geq$ 18 years.
*   A PiCCO2 device (Pulsion Medical Systems, Feldkirchen, Germany) already in place for clinical purposes.
*   Decision to perform a PLR test made by the attending physicians.

Patients were excluded if the PLR maneuver was contraindicated (intracranial hypertension), if PLR was supposed to be unreliable (venous compression stocking and intraabdominal hypertension) or if it was impossible to perform vascular Doppler measurements.

Hemodynamic measurements

All patients were equipped with a jugular or subclavian venous catheter and a thermistor-tipped femoral arterial catheter (PV2024, Pulsion Medical Systems). Hemodynamic variables were recorded continuously by using a data acquisition software (HEM 4.2, Notocord, Croissy-sur-Seine, France). Cardiac Index was recorded by the PiCCO Win 4.0 software (Pulsion Medical Systems). For all thermodilution measurements, the results obtained from three consecutive saline boluses were averaged [15, 16].

Doppler measurements

One investigator (VG) performed all ultrasound measurements. Images were analyzed and measurements were performed offline by two investigators (VG and TG). Ultrasound examination was performed with a CX50 (Philips Healthcare, Eindhoven, The Netherlands) by using a 12–5 MHz flat linear probe.

At each step of the protocol, we obtained images of the common carotid artery. First, a long-axis view of the carotid artery was obtained approximately 1–2 cm before its bifurcation. We assessed pulsed wave Doppler, the sampling volume being positioned in the middle of the lumen with caliper parallel to blood flow (Fig. 1). Time average mean velocity (TAMEAN) and peak systolic velocity (PSV) were automatically estimated by the echograph software. Velocity-time integral (VTI) was measured by manually tracing the flow envelope for each image (Fig. 1). We kept an insonation angle of 60° between Doppler beam and sample. In longitudinal view, the maximal diameter was measured from intima to intima with an angle of 90° to the vessel.

To determine carotid blood flow, we used two different methods, one based on VTI (cm) and the other on TAMEAN (cm/s):

*   Carotid blood flow (mL/min) = TAMEAN × π r^2 × 60.
*   Carotid blood flow (mL/min) = VTI × π r^2 × Heart rate (beats/min).

where "*r*" (in cm) represents the radius of the vessel that was assumed to be circular.

In addition, we measured TAMEAN with both narrow and large sampling windows within the arterial lumen, in order to compare two different ways of calculating carotid blood flow.

Measurements were also performed at the level of the common femoral artery before the bifurcation into superficial femoral artery and deep femoral artery. Blood flow, peak systolic velocity and diameter were measured with the same method and formulas as described before. Nevertheless, at this level, the only method that was used to measure femoral blood flow was the one based on VTI. Indeed, the contour of the femoral velocity that was automatically traced by the device for measuring time average mean velocity included both positive and negative values of femoral velocities, eventually providing very low values of TAMEAN. We decided to trace the contour manually, including only the positive values in the measurement of VTI.

Study design

At baseline, a first set of transpulmonary thermodilution and Doppler measurements were recorded (Additional file 1: Figure S1). Two PLR tests ("PLR1" and "PLR2") were then consecutively performed because it was not feasible to simultaneously record carotid and femoral Doppler indices during the same PLR test. The PLR position was maintained until the maximal value of pulse contour analysis-derived cardiac index was reached, what always occurs within 1 min [5]. Between the two PLR tests, we waited for approximately 5 min to obtain

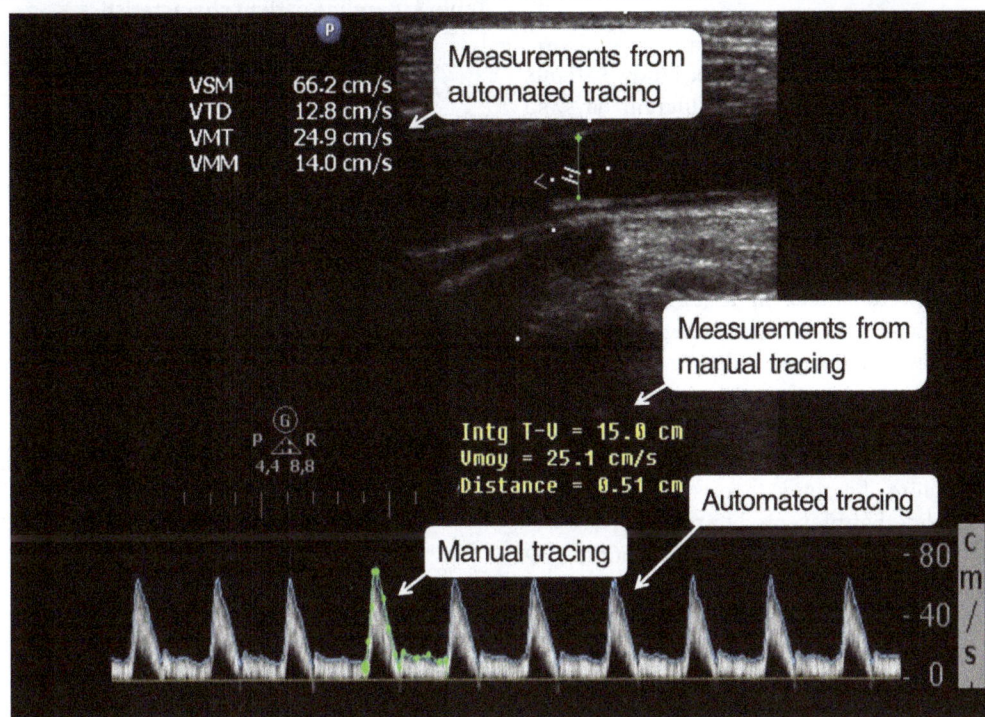

Fig. 1 Example of Doppler measurements performed in a patient

stable hemodynamic baseline values. Each PLR test was performed as previously described [6]. At its maximum effect, a second set of hemodynamic and Doppler measurements was performed (Additional file 1: Figure S1). The effects of PLR on cardiac output were measured by pulse contour analysis and not by transpulmonary thermodilution because these effects must be assessed by a real-time monitoring technique [6]. In practice, we observed the continuously changing value of pulse contour analysis-derived cardiac index while performing the Doppler measurements. As soon as the cardiac index value started to decrease, we considered that it had reached its maximum. At this precise time, we froze the image of the echograph and performed the Doppler measurements on the values displayed during the previous seconds. If pulse contour analysis-derived cardiac index increased $\geq 10\%$ during the PLR tests, compared to the baseline value, the patient was regarded as responder to the tests [8]. In total, the two PLR tests were performed within 15 min.

After the second PLR, another transpulmonary thermodilution was performed. Then, according to the decision of the clinicians in charge, only responders to the first PLR test were given 500 mL of normal saline over 10 min. All echographic and hemodynamic variables were then recorded at the end of fluid infusion, including transpulmonary thermodilution (Additional file 1: Figure

S1). Catecholamines dosages and ventilation settings were kept constant during the study period.

Data analysis

All data were normally distributed (Kolmogorov–Smirnov test for normality). Date are expressed as mean ± standard deviation (SD) or number and frequency (n, %). Comparison between time points of the study was performed using paired Student's t tests. Comparison between PLR responders and non-responders was performed using two-tailed Student's t tests. Pearson correlation coefficient was calculated to compare carotid/femoral blood flow and cardiac index as well as their relative changes following PLR and fluid infusion. A receiving operating characteristics (ROC) curve was constructed to evaluate the ability of the PLR-induced changes in carotid and femoral blood flows and velocities to detect responsiveness to PLR. The inter- and intraindividual variability of carotid Doppler measurements were also calculated. Considering a α-risk of 20% and a β-risk of 10%, to evidence an increase in 20% of carotid and femoral blood flows during PLR [9, 10], we planned to include 50 cases in the study. Statistical significance was defined by a p value < 0.05. The statistical analysis was performed using MedCalc 11.6.0 software (MedCalc, Mariakerke, Belgium).

Results

Patient characteristics

Thirty-three patients were included in the study. Patients could be included more than once at different days, so that we collected 51 cases in total, which were considered as individual cases (Fig. 2). Their characteristics are summarized in Table 1.

At the time of inclusion, in 48 (94%) cases, patients were intubated and ventilated in the volume-controlled mode. Patients received catecholamines in 46 (90%) cases (norepinephrine alone in 41 cases, dobutamine and norepinephrine in three cases, dobutamine alone in two cases).

Feasibility of carotid and femoral Doppler examination

Among all carotid Doppler measurements, two cases were excluded because of carotid stenosis and 10 because of poor image quality that prevented to reliably trace the contour of the signal (Fig. 2). Among the remaining 39 cases, in one case we could not assess carotid blood flow by TAMEAN (Fig. 2).

Among all cases, two were excluded because the femoral site was not accessible for performing Doppler measurement (obesity), 16 cases were excluded because

of a poor 2D echogenicity that prevented to precisely define the intima edge of the femoral artery and 19 cases because of poor quality of the Doppler signal (Fig. 2).

Table 1 Baseline patient characteristics

Gender (male)	22 (67%)
Age (years)	67 ± 14
Weight (kg)	68 ± 12
Height (cm)	165 ± 9
SAPS II	62 ± 19
Diagnostic	
Septic shock	16 (49%)
Cardiogenic shock	7 (21%)
ARDS	6 (18%)
Coma	2 (6%)
Pancreatitis	1 (3%)
Acute renal failure	1 (3%)
LVEF < 50%	8 (24%)

$N = 33$

Data are presented as mean ± standard deviation or number (percentage)

SAPS II simplified acute physiology score, *ARDS* acute respiratory distress syndrome, *LVEF* left ventricular ejection fraction

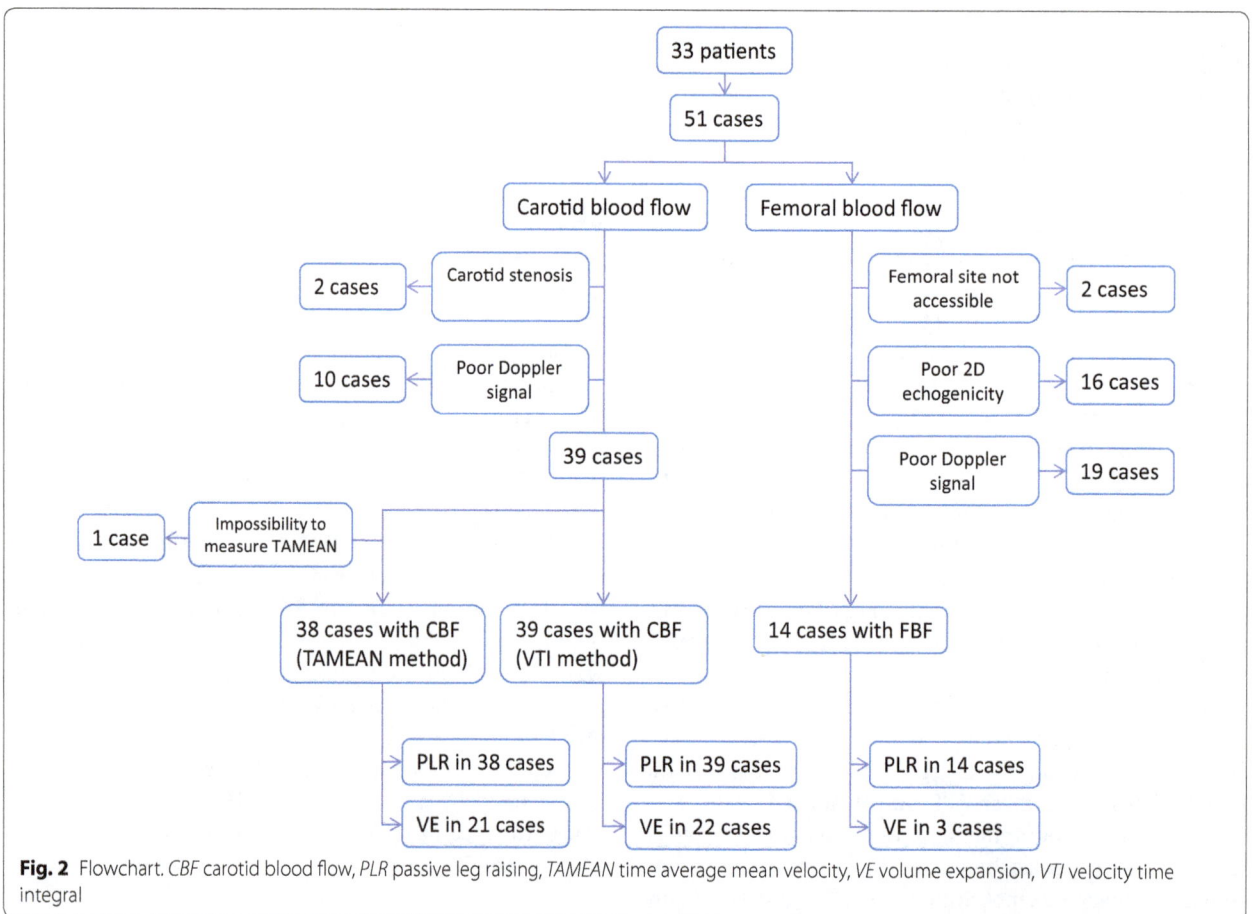

Fig. 2 Flowchart. *CBF* carotid blood flow, *PLR* passive leg raising, *TAMEAN* time average mean velocity, *VE* volume expansion, *VTI* velocity time integral

An increase in cardiac index ≥ 10% during the first PLR predicted fluid responsiveness with a positive predictive value of 93%. The specificity, sensitivity and negative predictive of PLR as a predictor of the response to fluid infusion value could not be calculated since we performed fluid infusion only in patients with a positive PLR test. An increase in cardiac index ≥ 10% during the second PLR predicted fluid responsiveness with the same positive predictive value because both PLR tests exerted similar effects on cardiac index.

The results of ROC curves analysis are presented in Additional file 1: Table S1 and Fig. 3. Neither the changes in carotid blood flow measured with the VTI method nor the carotid blood flow measured the TAMEAN method or the carotid PSV could detect a positive response to the PLR1 test. Neither the changes in femoral blood flow measured with the VTI method nor the femoral PSV could detect a positive response to the PLR2 test (Additional file 1: Table S1, Fig. 3). Results were not different when the analysis was performed with only the first case measured in each of the patients who had been included several times in the study (data not shown).

Relationship between cardiac index and carotid Doppler measurements in absolute values and relative changes

Absolute values of carotid blood flow and of PSV as well as the ratio of carotid blood flow over cardiac index during each study step are reported in Table 2.

For TAMEAN, the inter-individual variability was $8.9 \pm 8.7\%$ and the intraindividual variability was $12.7 \pm 12.2\%$. For PSV, the inter-individual variability was $5.0 \pm 4.1\%$ and the intraindividual variability was $2.2 \pm 1.7\%$. No difference was found between values of carotid blood flow calculated from TAMEAN sampled in large and narrow sampling windows ($p = 0.28$).

Considering all measurements at different study steps (Fig. 2), only weak correlations were found between absolute values of cardiac index and absolutes values of carotid blood flow calculated from TAMEAN ($n = 135$; $r = 0.54$, $p < 0.01$) (Additional file 1: Figure S2) and absolutes values of carotid PSV ($n = 139$; $r = 0.26$, $p < 0.01$). Absolute values of carotid blood flow calculated with TAMEAN were almost systematically lower than the corresponding values calculated with VTI (data not shown).

Considering all changes observed during the first PLR test ($n = 38$) and fluid infusion ($n = 21$) (Fig. 2), we found no correlation between changes in cardiac index and changes in carotid blood flow calculated from TAMEAN ($n = 59$; $r = 0.07$, $p = 0.61$) and between changes in cardiac index and changes in carotid blood flow calculated from VTI ($n = 61$; $r = 0.11$, $p = 0.41$). The ability of changes in carotid blood flow calculated from VTI and TAMEAN to detect changes in cardiac index are illustrated by 4-box tables in Additional file 1: Table S2. Results were not different when the analysis was performed with only the first case measured in each of the patients who had been included several times in the study (data not shown).

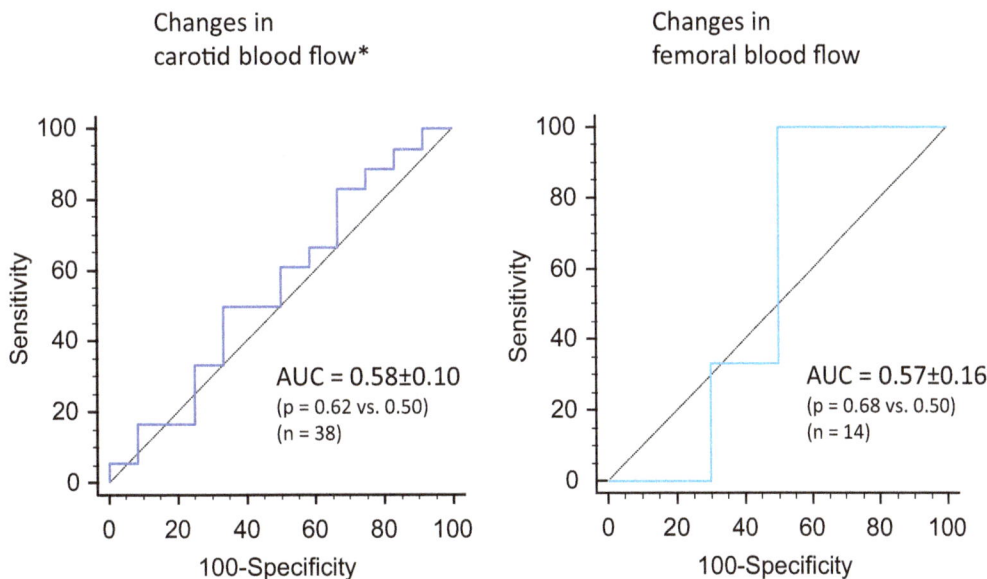

Fig. 3 Receiver operating characteristic curves describing the ability of changes in carotid femoral blood flows to detect a positive response of cardiac index to a passive leg raising test (increase ≥ 10%). *AUC* area under the curve. Asterisks results are provided for carotid blood flow measured by the velocity time integral method

Table 2 Hemodynamic and Doppler measurements

	Baseline 1	PLR1	Baseline 2	PLR2	Baseline 3	After fluid infusion
Heart rate (beats/min)						
PLR responders (n = 27)	91 ± 19	92 ± 22	89 ± 17	93 ± 17	92 ± 15	93 ± 15
PLR non-responders (n = 24)	91 ± 18	91 ± 17	87 ± 14	92 ± 14	89 ± 19	–
Systolic arterial pressure (mmHg)						
PLR responders (n = 27)	117 ± 26	129 ± 32*	115 ± 25	130 ± 34#	115 ± 32	129 ± 33$
PLR non-responders (n = 24)	125 ± 21	130 ± 24*	122 ± 18	127 ± 20#	125 ± 20	–
Diastolic arterial pressure (mmHg)						
PLR responders (n = 27)	57 ± 13	62 ± 11*	52 ± 16	62 ± 11#	57 ± 14	63 ± 18$
PLR non-responders (n = 24)	61 ± 9	64 ± 11*	60 ± 7	64 ± 9#	61 ± 10	–
Central venous pressure (mmHg)						
PLR responders (n = 27)	11 ± 4	14 ± 5*	9 ± 4	15 ± 5#	11 ± 4	12 ± 4$
PLR non-responders (n = 24)	10 ± 6	14 ± 6*	10 ± 6	13 ± 7#	10 ± 6	–
Cardiac index (L/min/m^2)						
PLR responders (n = 27)	3.11 ± 1.21	3.62 ± 1.29*	2.98 ± 1.15	3.63 ± 1.27#	2.91 ± 0.91	3.53 ± 1.16$
PLR non-responders (n = 24)	3.16 ± 1.07	3.23 ± 1.12	3.14 ± 1.10	3.23 ± 1.24#	3.17 ± 1.13	–
Carotid artery flow (TAMEAN) (mL/min)						
PLR responders (n = 21)	371 ± 138	407 ± 144	–	–	335 ± 118	390 ± 141$
PLR non-responders (n = 17)	293 ± 128	344 ± 159	–	–	321 ± 130	–
Carotid artery flow (VTI) (mL/min)						
PLR responders (n = 21)	615 ± 194	674 ± 202	–	–	601 ± 214	690 ± 221$
PLR non-responders (n = 17)	593 ± 225	617 ± 218	–	–	577 ± 227	–
Carotid PSV (cm/s)						
PLR responders (n = 22)	88 ± 23	82 ± 21	–	–	81 ± 22	88 ± 22
PLR non-responders (n = 17)	83 ± 30	77 ± 28	–	–	82 ± 23	–
Cardiac index to common carotid artery (TAMEAN) (%)						
PLR responders (n = 21)	13 ± 5	12 ± 4	–	–	12 ± 3	13 ± 5
PLR non-responders (n = 17)	9 ± 2	10 ± 3	–	–	10 ± 3	–
Femoral artery flow (VTI) (mL/min)						
PLR responders (n = 3)	–	–	408 ± 331	404 ± 319	433 ± 400	733 ± 800
PLR non-responders (n = 11)	–	–	368 ± 126	386 ± 127	382 ± 78	–
PSV femoral (cm/s)						
PLR responders (n = 17)	–	–	84 ± 28	111 ± 45#	77 ± 28	86 ± 31$
PLR non-responders (n = 18)	–	–	78 ± 17	89 ± 17	78 ± 20	–

Data are presented as mean ± standard deviation. PLR responders: cases with increase in pulse contour analysis-derived cardiac index ≥ 10% during passive leg raising, PLR non-responders: cases with increase in pulse contour analysis-derived cardiac index < 10% during passive leg raising

TAMEAN time average mean velocity, *PSV* peak systolic velocity

* $p < 0.05$ versus Baseline 1; # $p < 0.05$ versus Baseline 2; $ $p < 0.05$ versus Baseline 3

Relationship between cardiac index and femoral Doppler measurements in absolute values and relative changes

Considering all measurements at different study steps ($n = 45$, Fig. 2), a weak correlation was found between absolute values of femoral blood flow and cardiac index ($r = 0.21$, $p = 0.17$). Still considering all measurements performed at the femoral level at different study steps ($n = 118$, Fig. 2), a weak correlation was found between absolute values of PSV and cardiac index ($r = 0.32$, $p < 0.01$) (Additional file 1: Figure S3).

Considering all changes observed during the second PLR test and during fluid infusion ($n = 17$, Fig. 2), the correlation coefficient between changes in femoral blood flow and changes in cardiac index was $r = 0.28$ ($p = 0.27$). The ability of changes in carotid blood flow calculated from VTI and TAMEAN to detect changes in cardiac index are illustrated by 4-box tables in Additional file 1: Table S2. Results were not different when the analysis was performed with only the first case measured in each of the patients who had been included several times in the study (data not shown).

Discussion

The main finding of our study is that carotid and femoral blood flow and their peak velocities did not allow the detection of a positive PLR test and that their changes were not correlated with the simultaneous changes in cardiac index.

The previous results regarding the ability of Doppler measurements of peripheral arteries to estimate cardiac output and its changes are very controversial. Marik et al. [9] have demonstrated an excellent ability of changes in carotid blood flow to detect the PLR effects. Nevertheless, the authors used bioreactance as the reference for measuring cardiac output, while the accuracy of this technique has been seriously questioned [17, 18]. In a study by Préau et al. [10], the variation in femoral artery peak systolic velocity during PLR could reliably predict fluid responsiveness in critically ill patients. Nevertheless, in this study, the carotid blood flow was not investigated and, on the femoral site, only the peak systolic velocity was investigated [10]. Moreover, in this study, the diagnostic threshold that they measured for PLR-induced increases in femoral peak velocity was 8%, while the inter-observer variability of this variable was as large as $8.4 \pm 9.2\%$.

In contrast with these results, other studies in cardiac surgery patients [11, 12] and healthy volunteers [13, 14] showed that the correlation between changes in cardiac output and in common carotid blood flow either was weak or had wide limits of agreement. Our results corroborate these negative studies. Rohering et al. [12] found a strong correlation between absolute values and changes of carotid blood flow and cardiac index. However, limits of agreement in the Bland–Altman analysis ($\pm 20\%$) were so wide that they concluded that carotid Doppler should not replace direct cardiac output monitoring, especially for performing the PLR test [12]. In the study by Peatchy et al. [13], changes in carotid diameter were not measured during PLR. We measured this diameter in our study, but this did not improve the reliability of the estimation of cardiac index by carotid blood flow.

Several reasons may explain these findings. First, regarding the carotid Doppler signal, from a physiological point of view, the proportion of cardiac output that is directed toward the carotid artery may vary depending on cerebral blood flow regulation, impairing the correlation between carotid blood flow and cardiac output and controversial results have been reported regarding this point [19–24]. Second, another explanation may be the lack of reliability of the carotid and femoral Doppler measurements themselves. In the literature, we could not find a gold standard to calculate femoral and carotid blood flows. Many different methods exist [25], and they provide discordant results [26] with numerous sources of

error [27]. In our study, absolute values of carotid blood flow measured by TAMEAN were in accordance with values shown in literature [22], but they were almost systematically half of the values obtained from VTI. Even in patients that had not been excluded from the study, the echogenicity and the quality of the Doppler signal prevented to obtain precise measurements in many cases, especially at the femoral level. This likely led to errors in the measurement of the vessel diameter and hence to even larger miscalculations of blood flow values, as the squared value of arterial diameter is taken into account for measuring them. The measurement of femoral blood flow was impeded by the fact that, at this level, the anatomical landmarks tended to change with PLR. This likely explained the large intra- and inter-variability, indicating that these techniques are not suitable for the precise measurement of changes of small amplitude. Finally, access to the femoral site was difficult in obese patients, such that two of such patients were excluded. Eventually, we obtained a limited number of Doppler measurements for femoral artery. This fact may be enough to conclude that the method is not adapted to current practice in the ICU setting.

Limitations

First of all, we obtained only a limited number of measurements of Doppler variables, what has reduced the power of our analysis. Nevertheless, given the poor results we observed, it is unlikely that including more patients would have led to better results. Regarding femoral measurements, the fact that it was impossible to acquire them in a so large proportion of patients itself indicates that the technique is not appropriate. Second, some patients have been included several times in the study. Nevertheless, the analysis performed with only the first measurement performed in these patients did not show different results from the main analysis. Third, Doppler measurements were performed on one side only, while the opposite one may have provided better results. Fourth, although we took the precaution to exclude it, it is still possible that a mild degree of arterial stenosis may have influenced the relationship between cardiac output and arterial flow. Fifth, Doppler examinations were performed at the bedside in the ICU, while measurements performed in an echographic laboratory could provide more reliable measurements. Nevertheless, our methodology reflects the real-life practice. Finally, fluid infusion was not performed in non-responders, so that we could not assess the specificity and sensitivity of PLR-induced changes in arterial blood flows or velocity to assess fluid responsiveness. Nevertheless, given the poor reliability of Doppler measurements obtained in PLR responders, it is very likely that they did not perform better in PLR non-responders.

Conclusions

Carotid and femoral blood flows and peak systolic velocities were not reliable to assess the effects of a PLR test. These methods were not reliable to estimate cardiac output and its variations in intensive care patients. Many technical and physiological reasons may explain this lack of reliability.

Abbreviations
AUROC: area under the receiver operating characteristics curve; PLR: passive leg raising; PSV: peak systolic velocity; ROC: receiving operating characteristics; SD: standard deviation; TAMEAN: time average mean velocity; VTI: velocity–time integral.

Authors' contributions
VG collected the data, performed data analysis and drafted the manuscript and approved its final version. J-LT conceived the study, participated to analyzing the data and to writing the manuscript and approved its final version. LG and AB contributed to data recording and approved its final version. TG contributed to data analysis and approved its final version. CR supervised the study and approved its final version. XM conceived the study, supervised data analysis and manuscript writing and coordinated the study. All authors read and approved the final manuscript.

Author details
[1] Service de Réanimation Médicale, Hôpital de Bicêtre, Hôpitaux Universitaires Paris-Sud, Insert UMR_999, Université Paris-Sud, Assistance Publique – Hôpitaux de Paris, Le Kremlin-Bicêtre, France. [2] Service de Radiologie, Hôpital de Bicêtre, Hôpitaux Universitaires Paris-Sud, Assistance Publique – Hôpitaux de Paris, Le Kremlin-Bicêtre, France.

Acknowledgements
None.

Competing interests
Profs. Jean-Louis Teboul and Xavier Monnet are members of the Medical Advisory Board of Pulsion Medical Systems. The other authors declare that they have no competing interests.

Funding
No funding.

References
1. Wiedemann HP, Wheeler AP, Bernard GR, et al. Comparison of two fluid-management strategies in acute lung injury. N Engl J Med. 2006;354:2564–75.
2. Vincent JL, Sakr Y, Sprung CL, et al. Sepsis in European intensive care units: results of the SOAP study. Crit Care Med. 2006;34:344–53.
3. Monnet X, Marik PE, Teboul JL. Prediction of fluid responsiveness: an update. Ann Intensive Care. 2016;6:111.
4. Guérin L, Teboul JL, Persichini R, et al. Effects of passive leg raising and volume expansion on mean systemic pressure and venous return in shock in humans. Crete Care. 2015;19:411.
5. Monnet X, Rienzo M, Osman D, et al. Passive leg raising predicts fluid responsiveness in the critically ill. Crit Care Med. 2006;34:1402–7.
6. Monnet X, Teboul JL. Passive leg raising: five rules, not a drop of fluid! Crit Care. 2015;19:18.
7. Monnet X, Marik P, Teboul JL. Passive leg raising for predicting fluid responsiveness: a systematic review and meta-analysis. Intensive Care Med. 2016;42:1935–47.
8. Teboul JL, Saugel B, Cecconi M, et al. Less invasive hemodynamic monitoring in critically ill patients. Intensive Care Med. 2016;42:1350–9.
9. Marik PE, Levitov A, Young A, et al. The use of bioreactance and carotid Doppler to determine volume responsiveness and blood flow redistribution following passive leg raising in hemodynamically unstable patients. Chest. 2013;143:364–70.
10. Préau S, Saulnier F, Dewavrin F, et al. Passive leg raising is predictive of fluid responsiveness in spontaneously breathing patients with severe sepsis or acute pancreatitis. Crit Care Med. 2010;38:819–25.
11. Weber U, Glassford NJ, Eastwood GM, et al. A pilot assessment of carotid and brachial artery blood flow estimation using ultrasound Doppler in cardiac surgery patients. J Cardiothorac Vasc Anesth. 2016;30:141–8.
12. Roehrig C, Govier M, Robinson J, et al. A carotid Doppler flowmetry correlates poorly with thermodilution cardiac output following cardiac surgery. Acta Anaesthesiol Scand. 2017;61:31–8.
13. Peachey T, Tang A, Baker EC, et al. The assessment of circulating volume using inferior vena cava collapse index and carotid Doppler velocity time integral in healthy volunteers: a pilot study. Scand J Trauma Resusc Emerg Med. 2016;24:108.
14. Weber U, Glassford NJ, Eastwood GM, et al. A pilot study of the relationship between Doppler-estimated carotid and brachial artery flow and cardiac index. Anaesthesia. 2015;70:1140–7.
15. Monnet X, Teboul JL. Cardiac output monitoring: throw it out… or keep it? Crit Care. 2018;22:35.
16. Monnet X, Persichini R, Ktari M, Jozwiak M, Richard C, Teboul JL. Precision of the transpulmonary thermodilution measurements. Crit Care. 2011;27:15.
17. Kupersztych-Hagege E, Teboul JL, Artigas A, et al. Bioreactance is not reliable for estimating cardiac output and the effects of passive leg raising in critically ill patients. Br J Anaesth. 2013;111:961–6.
18. Fagnoul D, Vincent JL, De Backer D. Cardiac output measurements using the bioreactance technique in critically ill patients. Crit Care. 2012;16:460.
19. Eicke BM, von Schlichting J, Mohr-Ahaly S, et al. Lack of association between carotid artery volume blood flow and cardiac output. J Ultrasound Med. 2001;20:1293–8.
20. Gassner M, Killu K, Bauman Z, et al. Feasibility of common carotid artery point of care ultrasound in cardiac output measurements compared to invasive methods. J Ultrasound. 2014;18:127–33.
21. Tranmer BI, Keller TS, Kindt GW, et al. Loss of cerebral regulation during cardiac output variations in focal cerebral ischemia. J Neurosurg. 1992;77:253–9.
22. Yazici B, Erdoğmuş B, Tugay A. Cerebral blood flow measurements of the extracranial carotid and vertebral arteries with Doppler ultrasonography in healthy adults. Diagn Interv Radiol. 2005;11:195–8.
23. Sato K, Ogoh S, Hirasawa A, et al. The distribution of blood flow in the carotid and vertebral arteries during dynamic exercise in humans. J Physiol. 2015;589:2847–56.
24. Meng L, Hou W, Chui J, et al. Cardiac output and cerebral blood flow: the integrated regulation of brain perfusion in adult humans. Anesthesiology. 2015;123:1198–208.
25. Blanco P. Volumetric blood flow measurement using Doppler ultrasound: concerns about the technique. J Ultrasound. 2015;18:201–4.
26. Scheel P, Ruge C, Schöning M. Flow velocity and flow volume measurements in the extracranial carotid and vertebral arteries in healthy adults: reference data and the effects of age. Ultrasound Med Biol. 2000;26:1261–6.
27. Gill RW. Measurement of blood flow by ultrasound: accuracy and sources of error. Ultrasound Med Biol. 1985;11:625–41.

21

Clinical features and outcome of patients with acute respiratory failure revealing anti-synthetase or anti-MDA-5 dermato-pulmonary syndrome: a French multicenter retrospective study

Constance Vuillard[1], Marc Pineton de Chambrun[2], Nicolas de Prost[3], Claude Guérin[4,5], Matthieu Schmidt[2], Auguste Dargent[6], Jean-Pierre Quenot[6], Sébastien Préau[7], Geoffrey Ledoux[7], Mathilde Neuville[8], Guillaume Voiriot[9], Muriel Fartoukh[9], Rémi Coudroy[10], Guillaume Dumas[11], Eric Maury[11], Nicolas Terzi[12], Yacine Tandjaoui-Lambiotte[13], Francis Schneider[14], Maximilien Grall[15], Emmanuel Guérot[16], Romaric Larcher[17], Sylvie Ricome[18], Raphaël Le Mao[19], Gwenhaël Colin[20], Christophe Guitton[21], Lara Zafrani[22], Elise Morawiec[23], Marie Dubert[24], Olivier Pajot[1], Hervé Mentec[1], Gaëtan Plantefève[1] and Damien Contou[1*]

Abstract

Background: Anti-synthetase (AS) and dermato-pulmonary associated with anti-MDA-5 antibodies (aMDA-5) syndromes are near one of the other autoimmune inflammatory myopathies potentially responsible for severe acute interstitial lung disease. We undertook a 13-year retrospective multicenter study in 35 French ICUs in order to describe the clinical presentation and the outcome of patients admitted to the ICU for acute respiratory failure (ARF) revealing AS or aMDA-5 syndromes.

Results: From 2005 to 2017, 47 patients (23 males; median age 60 [1st–3rd quartiles 52–69] years, no comorbidity 85%) were admitted to the ICU for ARF revealing AS ($n = 28$, 60%) or aMDA-5 ($n = 19$, 40%) syndromes. Muscular, articular and cutaneous manifestations occurred in 11 patients (23%), 14 (30%) and 20 (43%) patients, respectively. Seventeen of them (36%) had no extra-pulmonary manifestations. C-reactive protein was increased (139 [40–208] mg/L), whereas procalcitonine was not (0.30 [0.12–0.56] ng/mL). Proportion of patients with creatine kinase $\geq 2N$ was 20% ($n = 9/47$). Forty-two patients (89%) had ARDS, which was severe in 86%, with a rate of 17% ($n = 8/47$) of extra-corporeal membrane oxygenation requirement. Proportion of patients who received corticosteroids, cyclophosphamide, rituximab, intravenous immunoglobulins and plasma exchange were 100%, 72%, 15%, 21% and 17%, respectively. ICU and hospital mortality rates were 45% ($n = 21/47$) and 51% ($n = 24/47$), respectively. Patients with aMDA-5 dermato-pulmonary syndrome had a higher hospital mortality than those with AS syndrome ($n = 16/19$, 84% vs. $n = 8/28$, 29%; $p = 0.001$).

Conclusions: Intensivists should consider inflammatory myopathies as a cause of ARF of unknown origin. Extra-pulmonary manifestations are commonly lacking. Mortality is high, especially in aMDA-5 dermato-pulmonary syndrome.

Keywords: Inflammatory myosis, Interstitial lung disease, ARDS, Acute respiratory failure, Diagnosis

*Correspondence: damien.contou@ch-argenteuil.fr
[1] Service de Réanimation Polyvalente, Centre Hospitalier Victor Dupouy, 69 rue du Lieutenant Colonel Prudhon, 95100 Argenteuil, France
Full list of author information is available at the end of the article

Background

Identifying the cause of acute respiratory distress syndrome (ARDS) is a crucial step for initiating a targeted treatment and improving prognosis [1, 2]. However, two recent studies [3, 4] showed that 8% of patients with ARDS according to the Berlin criteria [5] lacked exposure to "common" risk factors (e.g., pneumonia, acute pancreatitis, aspiration of gastric content or extra-pulmonary sepsis) with no etiology eventually retrieved in 80% of them [4]. For such atypical ARDS, a comprehensive diagnostic work-up, including specific immunologic tests, is recommended [6] so that to identify immune causes, typically amenable to specific therapeutic interventions (e.g., corticosteroids). Yet, an ancillary analysis [4] of an international, multicenter, prospective cohort study [7] reported that such immunological examinations were performed in only 5% of ARDS without common risk factors.

Anti-synthetase (AS) and anti-melanoma differentiation-associated gene 5 (aMDA-5) syndromes are near one of the other autoimmune inflammatory myopathies [8] potentially responsible for rapidly progressive interstitial lung disease leading to acute respiratory failure and ARDS [9–12]. AS and aMDA-5 dermato-pulmonary syndromes may be clinically indistinguishable one from another, with almost three-quarter of patients with aMDA-5 dermato-pulmonary syndrome exhibiting the clinical attributes of the AS syndrome [8]. When ARF is the initial presentation of AS or aMDA-5 syndromes [9–11, 13–17] or when extra-respiratory manifestations, such as muscular, cutaneous or articular signs are lacking [9, 18–22], the diagnosis is challenging, especially in the intensive care unit (ICU) setting, where many other reasons of acute respiratory failure (ARF) can be discussed. To the best of knowledge, a number of case reports of ARF revealing autoimmune inflammatory myopathies have been previously reported, but an extended case series has not been published as yet.

Therefore, we undertook this retrospective study in order to: (1) describe the clinical features and the outcome of patients admitted to the ICU for ARF revealing either an AS or an aMDA-5 dermato-pulmonary syndrome, and; (2) identify predictive factors of hospital mortality.

Patients and methods

Patients

We conducted a 13-year multicenter retrospective non-interventional study in 35 ICUs in France from January 1, 2005, to December 31, 2017. All patients older than 18 years were included if they met the following criteria:

(1) admitted to the ICU for ARF not related to cardiogenic pulmonary edema; (2) no common ARDS risk factor, among pneumonia, acute pancreatitis, aspiration of gastric content, extra-pulmonary sepsis, multiple transfusions, major trauma, pulmonary vasculitis, drowning, severe burns, identified according to the Berlin definition [5]; (3) immunologic test performed during ICU stay, which was positive for anti-synthetase (Jo-1, PL7, PL12, OJ, EJ, KS, Zo, YRS/Tyr/Ha) or anti-MDA-5 autoantibodies; and (4) no alternative diagnosis for ARF. It is worth notifying that in the present study the diagnosis of AS or aMDA-5 dermato-pulmonary syndromes had to be made during the ICU stay. Therefore, those who had a diagnosis of AS or aMDA-5 made before ICU admission were not included.

The investigator of each participating center was responsible for the identification of the patients, either from the hospital medical reports, using the function "research the files in which the key words *MDA-5* or *anti-synthetase* or *myositis* occurs" of Microsoft Windows®, or through a search using the International *Classification of Diseases* (10th Revision) following codes: M608 (autoimmune myositis), M609 (myositis), M332 (polymyositis) and M331 (dermatomyositis). The clinical charts of all identified patients were anonymized before sending to the main investigators (DC and CV). Clinical charts were reviewed in order to check the inclusion criteria.

Data collection

The following data were collected on a standardized anonymized case record form: demographic characteristics (age, gender), severity scores upon ICU admission (Sequential Organ Failure Assessment [23] and Simplified Acute Physiology Score II [24]), main comorbidities, delay between first respiratory sign and ICU admission, clinical examination (respiratory and extra-respiratory manifestations) and laboratory findings at the time of ICU admission (blood leukocytes and platelets counts, serum procalcitonin, C-reactive protein, creatine kinase and creatinine levels, PaO_2/FiO_2 with FiO_2 calculated according to the following formula [25, 26]: FiO_2 = oxygen flow in liter per minute × 0.04 + 0.21 when standard oxygen was used), radiological findings on chest X-ray and CT scan, cytological and bacteriological analyses of broncho-alveolar lavage (BAL) fluid, type of positive autoantibodies (Jo-1, PL7, PL12, OJ, EJ, KS, Zo, YRS/Tyr/Ha or aMDA-5), immunosuppressive treatments received (corticosteroids, cyclophosphamide, rituximab, basiliximab, tacrolimus, cyclosporine, methotrexate, intravenous immunoglobulins or plasma exchange), organ supports in the ICU (invasive mechanical ventilation, extra-corporeal membrane oxygenation (ECMO), renal replacement therapy, vasopressors), ICU and hospital length of stay, ICU and hospital mortality.

Written reports of chest CT scan performed at the time of ICU admission were sent to the main investigators (DC and CV) in order to individualize elementary lesions (ground-glass attenuation, alveolar consolidation, septal thickening, pleural effusion, pneumothorax, pneumomediastinum and mediastinal lymphadenopathy) and their location (lower or upper lobe predominance). Signs of lung fibrosis (honeycombing, traction bronchiectasis and reticulations) were also collected. Cytological analyses of BAL fluid collected at the time of ICU admission were reported, as well as results of open lung, skin or muscle biopsies, if performed.

Statistical analysis

Continuous variables are reported as median [1st–3rd quartiles] and compared by the Mann–Whitney U test. Categorical variables are reported as counts and percentage points in groups and compared by using the Fisher's exact test. Survival curves of patients with aMDA-5 and AS syndromes were drawn using the Kaplan–Meier method and compared using the log-rank test. All tests were two-sided, with $p < 0.05$ indicating statistical significance. The statistical analysis was performed by using the RStudio software version 0.99.441 (www.rStudio.com).

Results

Study population and clinical manifestations

From January 1, 2005, to December 31, 2017, 47 patients fulfilled the inclusion criteria, including 28 (60%) with AS syndrome (Jo-1 $n = 13/28$ (47%); PL7 $n = 9/28$ (32%); PL12 $n = 4/28$ (14%); EJ $n = 2/28$ (7%)) and 19 (40%) with aMDA-5 dermato-pulmonary syndrome. All the patients with aMDA-5 dermato-pulmonary syndrome were admitted after January 1, 2010. Demographical characteristics, main comorbidities and clinical manifestations are given in Table 1. Most of the patients had no comorbidity ($n = 40/47$, 85%). Median SAPSII and SOFA scores at the time of ICU admission were 35 [27–53] and 5 [3–8], respectively. The median delay between first respiratory sign and ICU admission was 21 [10–41] days. Most of the patients had central temperature > 38 °C ($n = 27/47$, 57%). Myalgia, arthralgia/arthritis and cutaneous manifestations occurred in 23% ($n = 11/47$), 30% ($n = 14/47$) and 43% ($n = 20/47$) of patients, respectively. About one-third of patients ($n = 17/47$, 36%) had no extra-pulmonary manifestation, in a similar proportion in aMDA-5 and AS groups.

Laboratory and radiological findings

Biological data at the time of ICU admission and radiological findings are reported in Table 2. C-reactive protein levels ($N < 5$ mg/L) were increased (139 [40–208] mg/L), while procalcitonine levels ($N < 0.5$ ng/mL) were not (0.30 [0.12–0.56] ng/mL). The rate of patients having creatine kinase plasma levels greater than 2 times the upper limit of normal laboratory range was 20% ($n = 9/47$) in the whole population, and only 31% ($n = 8/28$) in the AS group. The median PaO_2/FiO_2 ratio at ICU admission was 123 [83–147] mmHg.

Most patients ($n = 45/47$, 96%) had bilateral condensations on chest X-ray, with a predominantly lower location ($n = 46/47$, 98%) (Table 2). All patients underwent a lung CT scan, which showed ground-glass attenuation in 78% ($n = 37/47$) and alveolar condensation in 75% ($n = 35/47$). Signs of lung fibrosis were observed in 36% ($n = 17/47$), while 38% ($n = 18/47$) had mediastinal lymphadenopathies.

Broncho-alveolar fluid analysis and histological data

BAL fluid analyses were available in 89% ($n = 42/47$) of patients and are summarized in Table 2. The cell count was 250 [140–330] $\times$ 10^3/mL, and percentages of lymphocytes, neutrophils and macrophages were 11% [4–30], 38% [13–65] and 40% [20–60], respectively. BAL was performed before antibiotic therapy in only 12/42 (29%) patients and was negative for lung infection in every patient. There was no correlation between BAL findings and elementary lesions observed on chest CT scan. In particular, the proportion of patients with >40% BAL neutrophils did not differ between patients with or without elementary lesions of lung fibrosis on chest CT scan ($n = 8/19$, 42% vs. $n = 11/19$, 58%, $p = 0.72$). An open lung biopsy was performed in 4 (9%) patients and depicted findings consistent with organizing pneumonia ($n = 2$), usual interstitial pneumonitis ($n = 1$) and diffuse alveolar damage ($n = 1$) (Table 2). A total of 13 patients (28%) had a muscle ($n = 7$) or a skin ($n = 6$) biopsy performed during the ICU stay. All muscle biopsies revealed findings consistent with an inflammatory myositis, while skin biopsies were either normal ($n = 1$) or revealed findings consistent with lichenoid dermatitis ($n = 3$) or with dermatomyositis ($n = 2$) (Table 2).

ICU management and outcome

Most patients ($n = 41/47$, 89%) received an antimicrobial therapy upon ICU admission (Table 3). All patients received steroids, after a median delay of 6 [3–12] days following the ICU admission. Other immunosuppressive treatments administered are reported in Table 3.

Table 1 Demographical and clinical manifestations of patients with acute respiratory failure revealing anti-synthetase syndrome or dermato-pulmonary syndrome associated with anti-MDA-5 antibodies

	Missing data	All patients N = 47	aMDA-5 ARF N = 19	AS ARF N = 28	p
Age, years median [IQR]	0	60 [52–69]	60 [51–67]	63 [54–73]	0.51
Male, n (%)	0	23 (49)	8 (42)	15 (54)	0.64
SOFA score median [IQR]	0	5 [3–8]	4 [2–8]	5 [3–8]	0.77
SAPSII median [IQR]	0	35 [27–53]	34 [27–53]	38 [27–50]	0.94
Comorbidities, n (%)					
Chronic respiratory failure	0	1 (2)	0 (0)	1 (4)	1.00
Congestive heart failure	0	0 (0)	0 (0)	0 (0)	1.00
Cirrhosis	0	1 (2)	0 (0)	1 (4)	1.00
Chronic kidney failure	0	0 (0)	0 (0)	0 (0)	1.00
Active solid cancer or malignant hemopathy	0	0 (0)	0 (0)	0 (0)	1.00
HIV	0	0 (0)	0 (0)	0 (0)	1.00
Diabetes mellitus	0	5 (11)	1 (5)	4 (14)	0.64
Obesity (body mass index $\geq$ 30 kg/m^2)	0	1 (2)	0 (0)	1 (4)	1.00
No comorbidities	0	40 (85)	18 (95)	22 (79)	0.60
Active or former tobacco use, n (%)	0	20 (43)	7 (37)	13 (46)	0.73
Respiratory manifestations, n (%)					
Delay first respiratory sign—ICU admission, days	2	21 [10–41]	21 [11–43]	21 [10–41]	0.73
Dry cough	0	23 (49)	8 (42)	15 (54)	0.64
Chest pain	0	0 (0)	0 (0)	0 (0)	1.00
Hemoptysis	0	1 (2)	0 (0)	1 (4)	1.00
Bilateral crackles	5	34 (81)	13 (77)	21 (84)	0.69
Fever (> 38 °C)	0	27 (57)	9 (47)	18 (64)	0.40
Extra-respiratory manifestations, n (%)					
Myalgia	0	11 (23)	2 (11)	9 (32)	0.16
Muscles weakness	0	6 (13)	1 (5)	5 (18)	0.38
Arthralgia/arthritis	0	14 (30)	6 (32)	8 (29)	1.00
Cutaneous manifestations	0	20 (43)	13 (68)	7 (25)	0.008
Mechanic's hand	0	8 (17)	3 (15)	5 (19)	1.00
Raynaud's phenomenon	0	3 (6)	1 (5)	2 (7)	1.00
Facial erythema	0	12 (26)	9 (47)	3 (11)	0.007
Gottron's papules	0	5 (11)	5 (26)	0 (0)	0.008
Ulcerations	0	3 (6)	3 (16)	0 (0)	0.06
Trunk rash	0	7 (15)	5 (26)	2 (7)	0.10
No extra-respiratory manifestations	0	17 (36)	6 (31)	11 (39)	0.81

aMDA-5 anti-MDA-5 antibodies, *AS* anti-synthetase, *ARF* acute respiratory failure, *HIV* human immunodeficiency virus, *ICU* intensive care unit, *IQR* inter-quartile range, *SAPS2* simplified acute physiology score, *SOFA* sepsis-related organ failure assessment

Almost all patients ($n = 42/47$, 89%) had ARDS, categorized as severe ($PaO_2/FiO_2 \leq 100$ mmHg with PEEP ≥ 5 mmH$_2$O) in 86% ($n = 36/47$), with 17% ($n = 8/47$) of them requiring ECMO. ICU and hospital mortality rates were 45% ($n = 21/47$) and 51% ($n = 24/47$), respectively. Patients with aMDA-5 dermato-pulmonary syndrome had a higher ICU mortality than those with AS syndrome ($n = 16/19$, 84% vs. $n = 5/28$, 18%; $p < 0.001$). Among the 26 ICU survivors, 5 (19%) were diagnosed with a cancer (colorectal $n = 3$, pharyngeal $n = 1$, melanoma $n = 1$) during the 279 [158–500] days post-ICU stay follow-up.

Comparison between hospital survivors and non-survivors
Compared to patients who survived at the hospital discharge, those who died were more likely to have an aMDA-5 autoantibody ($n = 16/24$, 67% vs. $n = 3/23$, 13%; $p = 0.001$), had a higher rate of ground-glass attenuation

Table 2 Biological, radiological and cytological findings in patients with acute respiratory failure revealing anti-synthetase syndrome or dermato-pulmonary syndrome associated with anti-MDA-5 antibodies

	Missing data	All patients $N=47$	aMDA-5 ARF $N=19$	AS ARF $N=28$	p
Biological data at ICU admission, median [IQR]					
Leukocytes count (10^3/mm³)	1	11.5 [8.5–17]	8.4 [6.7–9.8]	16.0 [12.1–21.1]	< 0.001
C-reactive protein (mg/L)	9	139 [40–208]	38 [22–99]	187 [128–262]	0.30
Procalcitonine (ng/mL)	9	0.30 [0.12–0.56]	0.32 [0.11–0.48]	0.30 [0.13–1.42]	< 0.001
Creatininemia (µmol/L)	14	63 [51–78]	59 [51–73]	64 [51–80]	0.04
Creatine kinase (UI/L)	3	157 [69–256]	127 [75–186]	192 [69–932]	0.76
Creatine kinase ≥ 2N	3	9 (20)	1 (6)	8 (31)	0.02
PaCO$_2$ (mmHg)	1	34 [31–41]	34 [32–42]	33 [31–41]	0.06
PaO$_2$/FiO$_2$ (mmHg)	3	123 [83–147]	139 [91–174]	117 [78–144]	0.82
Chest X-ray, n (%)					
Bilateral opacities	0	45 (96)	19 (100)	26 (93)	0.51
Lower lobe location	0	46 (98)	19 (100)	27 (96)	1.00
Number of quadrants on chest X-ray, n					
1	0	1 (3)	0 (0)	1 (4)	0.30
2		27 (68)	10 (59)	17 (74)	
4		12 (30)	7 (41)	5 (22)	
Chest CT scan, n (%)					
Performed	0	47 (100)	19 (100)	28 (100)	1.00
Ground-glass attenuation	0	37 (78)	18 (96)	19 (68)	0.03
Alveolar consolidations	0	35 (75)	13 (68)	22 (79)	0.51
Septal thickening	0	12 (26)	8 (42)	4 (14)	0.05
Pleural effusion	0	13 (28)	3 (16)	10 (36)	0.24
Pneumothorax	0	4 (9)	3 (16)	1 (3.6)	0.29
Pneumomediastinum	0	1 (2)	1 (5)	0 (0)	0.40
Mediastinal lymphadenopathy	0	18 (38)	7 (37)	11 (39)	1.00
Signs of lung fibrosis	0	17 (36)	6 (32)	11 (39)	0.82
Traction bronchiectasis	0	17 (36)	6 (32)	11 (39)	0.82
Reticulations	0	12 (26)	4 (21)	8 (29)	0.78
Honeycombing	0	5 (10)	1 (5)	4 (14)	0.64
Broncho-alveolar lavage (BAL), n (%) or median [IQR]					
Performed	0	42 (89)	16 (84)	26 (93)	0.38
Delay ICU admission—BAL	0	1 [0–3]	0 [− 1.5–1.0]	2 [1–4]	0.08
Total cell count (10^3/mL)	8	250 [140–330]	250 [128–390]	250 [160–290]	0.42
Lymphocytes (%)	1	11 [4–30]	22 [8–34]	5 [3–17]	0.06
Neutrophils (%)	2	38 [13–65]	15 [6–36]	51 [20–80]	0.001
Macrophages (%)	2	40 [20–60]	53 [39–73]	29 [15–83]	0.009
Eosinophils (%)	6	0 [0–2]	0 [0–1]	0 [0–2]	0.154
Presence of siderophages	5	2 (4)	1 (6)	1 (4)	1.00
Lung biopsy, n (%)	0	4 (9)	1 (5)	3 (11)	–
Diffuse alveolar damage		1	0	1	
Usual interstitial pneumonitis		1	0	1	
Organizing pneumonia		2	1	1	
Skin biopsy, n (%)	0	6 (13)	5 (26)	1 (4)	–
Normal		1	0	1	
Lichenoïd dermatitis		3	3	0	
Dermatomyositis		2	2	0	
Muscle biopsy, n (%)	0	7 (15)	4 (21)	3 (11)	–
Inflammatory myositis		7	4	3	

aMDA-5 anti-MDA-5 antibodies, *AS* anti-synthetase, *ARF* acute respiratory failure, *BAL* broncho-alveolar lavage, *ICU* intensive care unit, *IQR* inter-quartile range

Table 3 ICU management and outcome of patient with acute respiratory failure revealing anti-synthetase syndrome or dermato-pulmonary syndrome associated with anti-MDA-5 antibodies

	Missing data	All patients N = 47	aMDA-5 ARF N = 19	AS ARF N = 28	p
Treatment, n (%) or median [IQR]					
Antibiotics therapy at ICU admission	0	41 (89)	15 (79)	26 (96)	0.14
Immunosuppressive treatment	0	47 (100)	19 (100)	28 (100)	1.00
Delay ICU-IS treatment (days)	0	6 [3–12]	4 [1.5–11]	6 [4–16]	0.25
Corticosteroids pulses	0	47 (100)	19 (100)	28 (100)	1.00
Cyclophosphamide	0	34 (72)	16 (84)	18 (64)	0.24
Rituximab	0	7 (15)	6 (32)	1 (4)	0.01
Cyclosporine	0	2 (4)	2 (10)	0 (0)	0.16
Tacrolimus	0	2 (4)	2 (11)	0 (0)	0.16
Basiliximab	0	2 (4)	2 (11)	0 (0)	0.16
Intravenous immunoglobulins	0	10 (21)	5 (26)	5 (18)	0.50
Plasma exchange	0	8 (17)	7 (37)	1 (4)	0.005
Number of immunosuppressive treatments	0	2 [2, 3]	3 [2–4]	2 [1, 2]	<0.001
Ventilatory support, n (%)					
Noninvasive ventilation before intubation	0	14 (30)	4 (21)	10 (36)	0.45
High-flow nasal cannula oxygen before intubation	0	21 (45)	11 (58)	10 (36)	0.23
Tracheal intubation	0	43 (92)	18 (95)	25 (89)	0.64
ARDS	0	42 (89)	18 (95)	24 (86)	0.64
Mild ($200 < PaO_2/FiO_2 \leq 300$ mmHg)	0	1 (2)	1 (6)	0 (0)	0.43
Moderate ($100 < PaO_2/FiO_2 \leq 200$ mmHg)	0	5 (12)	0 (0)	5 (21)	0.06
Severe ($PaO_2/FiO_2 \leq 100$ mmHg)	0	36 (86)	17 (94)	19 (79)	0.21
Nitric oxide inhalation	0	23 (50)	14 (74)	9 (33)	0.02
Neuromuscular blocking agents	0	36 (78)	17 (90)	19 (70)	0.16
Prone position	0	26 (57)	12 (63)	14 (52)	0.64
Veno-venous ECMO	0	8 (17)	6 (32)	2 (7)	0.05
Extra-ventilatory support, n (%)					
Renal replacement therapy	0	8 (17)	4 (21)	4 (14)	0.70
Vasopressors	0	37 (79)	17 (90)	20 (71)	0.17
Outcome, n (%) or median [IQR]					
Duration of invasive mechanical ventilation (days)	0	21 [14–35]	19 [9–26]	23 [17–37]	0.34
Length of ICU stay (days)	0	26 [19–38]	22 [17–36]	28 [21–38]	0.20
Length of hospital stay (days)	0	38 [22–67]	22 [19–44]	44 [33–70]	0.015
ICU mortality	0	21 (45)	16 (84)	5 (18)	<0.001
Hospital mortality	0	24 (51)	16 (84)	8 (29)	0.001

aMDA-5 anti-MDA-5 antibodies, *AS* anti-synthetase, *ARDS* acute respiratory distress syndrome, *ARF* acute respiratory failure, *ECMO* extra-corporal membrane oxygenation, *ICU* intensive care unit, *IQR* inter-quartile range, *IS* immunosuppressive treatment

($n = 22/24$, 92% vs. 15/23, 65%; $p = 0.04$) and a lower rate of alveolar condensation ($n = 14/24$, 58% vs. 21/23, 91%; $p = 0.02$) on chest CT scan, and were given 3 [2, 3] versus 2 [1, 2] different immunosuppressive regimens during the ICU stay ($p = 0.002$) (Table 4). After adjustment on syndrome (anti-synthetase or aMDA-5 dermato-pulmonary syndrome), the presence of ground-glass attenuations on chest CT scan was no longer associated with in-hospital mortality ($p = 0.24$). The Kaplan–Meier graph showed a lower probability of survival 90 days after ICU admission in patients with aMDA-5 antibody than in patients with AS antibody (Fig. 1; $p < 0.0001$ log-rank test).

Discussion

We are herein reporting the first large cohort of patients admitted to ICU for ARF revealing either AS or aMDA-5 dermato-pulmonary syndrome. The main findings are: (1) clinical manifestations may be nonspecific with the

Table 4 Comparison between hospital survivors and non-survivors

	Non-survivors N = 24	Survivors N = 23	p
Clinical, biological and immunological characteristics, n (%) or median [IQR]			
Age	65 [59–70]	55 [50–64]	0.062
Male	9 (38)	14 (61)	0.19
SOFA	5 [2–8]	5 [3–8]	0.73
SAPSII	32 [28–53]	41 [27–54]	0.82
Type of autoantibodies			
Anti-MDA-5	16 (67)	3 (13)	0.001
Anti-synthetase antibody	8 (33)	20 (87)	0.001
JO-1	3 (13)	10 (44)	0.04
PL7	3 (13)	6 (26)	0.28
PL12	1 (4)	3 (13)	0.35
EJ	1 (4)	1 (4)	1
Delay first respiratory sign—ICU admission, days	21 [10–43]	20 [10–39]	0.31
Creatine kinase ≥ 2N	3 (13)	6 (29)	0.27
PaO$_2$/FiO$_2$ upon ICU admission	126 [90–149]	117 [82–147]	0.65
Chest X-ray and CT scan, n (%)			
Number of quadrants on chest X-ray			
1	1 (5)	0 (0)	0.74
2	13 (62)	14 (74)	
4	7 (33)	5 (26)	
Ground-glass attenuation on chest CT scan	22 (92)	15 (65)	0.04
Alveolar consolidations on chest CT scan	14 (58)	21 (91)	0.02
Signs of lung fibrosis on chest CT scan	9 (38)	8 (35)	1.00
Broncho-alveolar lavage (BAL), n (%) or median [IQR]			
Total cell count (10^3/mL)	250 [80–370]	260 [189–293]	0.36
Lymphocytes percentage	17 [5–31]	7 [3–18]	0.33
Lymphocytes > 10%	12 (55)	9 (45)	0.76
Lymphocytes > 25%	8 (36)	4 (20)	0.41
Neutrophils percentage	20 [10–52]	49 [18–73]	0.12
Neutrophils > 40%	8 (38)	11 (55)	0.44
Neutrophils > 65%	3 (14)	7 (35)	0.16
Management in ICU, n (%) or median [IQR]			
Immunosuppressive (IS) treatment			
Delay ICU admission—IS treatment	4 [3–12]	6 [3–16]	0.63
Number of IS treatments	3 [2, 3]	2 [1, 2]	0.002
Corticosteroids	24 (100)	23 (100)	1.00
Cyclophosphamide	20 (83)	14 (61)	0.16
Rituximab	6 (25)	1 (4)	0.10
Basiliximab	2 (8)	0 (0)	0.49
Cyclosporine	1 (4)	1 (4)	1.00
Tacrolimus	2 (8)	0 (0)	0.19
Intravenous immunoglobulins	7 (29)	3 (13)	0.29
Plasma exchange	6 (25)	2 (9)	0.25
Tracheal intubation	24 (100)	19 (83)	0.05
ARDS	23 (96)	19 (83)	0.19
Severe (PaO$_2$/FiO$_2$ ≤ 100 mmHg)	22 (96)	14 (74)	0.07
Moderate (100 < PaO$_2$/FiO$_2$ ≤ 200 mmHg)	1 (4)	4 (21)	0.16
Mild (200 < PaO$_2$/FiO$_2$ ≤ 300 mmHg)	0 (0)	1 (5)	0.45
Nitric oxide inhalation	18 (78)	5 (22)	< 0.001
Veno-venous ECMO	6 (25)	2 (9)	0.25

Table 4 (continued)

	Non-survivors N = 24	Survivors N = 23	p
Vasopressors	21 (88)	16 (70)	0.17
Renal replacement therapy	5 (21)	3 (13)	0.70

ARDS acute respiratory distress syndrome, *CI* confidence interval, *ECMO* extra-corporeal membrane oxygenation, *ICU* intensive care unit, *IQR* inter-quartile range, *IS* immunosuppressive, *OR* odds ratio

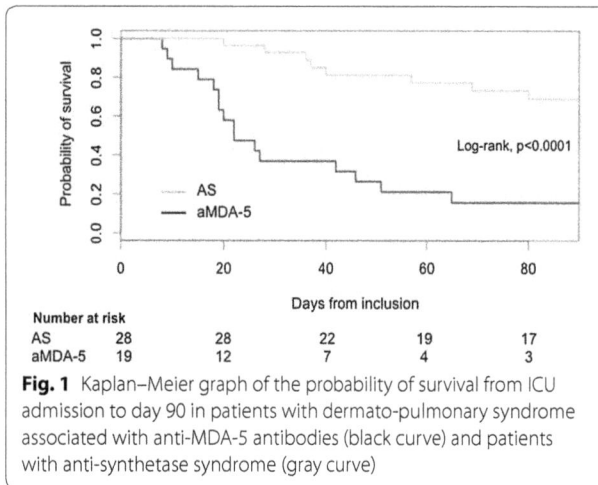

Fig. 1 Kaplan–Meier graph of the probability of survival from ICU admission to day 90 in patients with dermato-pulmonary syndrome associated with anti-MDA-5 antibodies (black curve) and patients with anti-synthetase syndrome (gray curve)

absence of extra-pulmonary manifestations of inflammatory myositis in one-third of patients; (2) hypoxemia is severe with a high rate of severe ARDS and rescue maneuvers; and (3) hospital mortality is high, especially in dermato-pulmonary syndrome associated with aMDA-5 autoantibodies.

AS and aMDA-5-associated dermato-pulmonary syndromes are two near each of the other inflammatory myopathies that may be responsible for severe acute interstitial lung diseases [9–11]. The diagnosis is easy to consider when extra-pulmonary manifestations are present. In AS syndrome, the main extra-pulmonary manifestations include myositis with elevated creatine kinase levels, non-erosive arthritis, Raynaud's phenomenon and thick cracked skin over the tips and sides of the fingers called "mechanic's hands" [27–32]. However, there is a wide heterogeneity in clinical manifestations depending on the causative AS autoantibody [33, 34]. In aMDA-5-associated dermato-pulmonary syndrome, the cutaneous manifestations (skin ulcerations or necrosis, facial erythema, mechanic's hands, periungual telangiectasia, Gottron's papules, Raynaud's phenomenon) are in the forefront [10, 11, 35] and usually contrast with the absence of clinical signs of myositis (clinically "amyopathic myositis"). Demographical and clinical findings in our patients were in line with those recently reported in

non-ICU patients with AS [22, 32, 34] or with aMDA-5 dermato-pulmonary syndromes [10].

Both in AS and aMDA-5 dermato-pulmonary syndromes, extra-pulmonary manifestations may be lacking [9, 10] rendering the diagnosis difficult to make. In our series, more than one-third of patients had no extra-pulmonary manifestations with a similar proportion in AS and aMDA-5 patients. This rate contrasts with the 10% rate recently reported [10] in patients with aMDA-5 dermato-pulmonary syndrome, reflecting the lack of training of intensivists for the clinical assessment of these patients and highlighting the need for a multidisciplinary approach. Considering the high proportion of patients lacking extra-pulmonary manifestations, the clinical presentation may mimic that of a "bilateral pneumonia without microbiological documentation." Hence, 89% of our patients received antibiotic therapy at ICU admission. The presence of an intense inflammatory syndrome with increased C-reactive protein levels contrasting with the lack of elevation of serum procalcitonin could help intensivists appreciating the probability of an infectious process, this dissociation being highly suggestive of a non-infectious inflammatory process.

In our series, BAL was performed in 89% of patients. Unlike a recent work [3] showing that a lymphocytic BAL fluid was associated with better ICU survival in ARDS patients with no common risk factor, our study failed to identify any predictive role of BAL cytology on hospital survival. BAL fluid analysis does not seem a useful diagnostic tool for AS or aMDA-5 dermato-pulmonary syndromes, but should nevertheless be performed to rule out an alternative diagnosis, such as diffuse alveolar hemorrhage or active infection.

All included patients underwent chest CT scan. Interestingly, CT chest findings predominate in the lower lobes, which is consistent with a previous report [36]. CT scan signs of lung fibrosis have been recently shown to be associated with a poor outcome in patients with ARF related to interstitial lung diseases [37]. In our study, CT scan signs of lung fibrosis were not associated with hospital mortality, probably because of a lack of adequate power. While ground-glass opacities are usually considered as potentially reversible lung lesions during idiopathic pulmonary fibrosis [38, 39], these lesions were associated with in-hospital mortality in our study, probably because they were more frequently observed during aMDA-5 dermato-pulmonary syndromes. Indeed, this association was no longer observed after adjustment on the type of positive antibody (anti-synthetase or aMDA-5).

Our series underlines the severity of AS and aMDA-5 dermato-pulmonary syndrome, since 89% of patients fulfilled the Berlin criteria for ARDS [5], categorized as severe ($PaO_2/FiO_2 \leq 100$ mmHg with PEEP ≥ 5 mmH$_2$O) in 86% of cases. Anti-MDA-5 dermato-pulmonary syndromes exhibited a significantly higher mortality than AS syndromes, with almost all these patients dying in the ICU of refractory ARDS despite a high rate of ECMO (32%). Moreover, aMDA-5 patients had a much higher mortality than those with severe ARDS included in the lung safe study [7], highlighting the irreversibility of lung lesions despite immunosuppressive treatments. These results are in line with previous series, showing that refractory ARDS is the leading cause of mortality in aMDA-5 patients [10].

Whether our patients had a true ARDS (i.e., presence of diffuse alveolar damage (DAD), the histological hallmark of ARDS) or simply fulfilled the Berlin criteria while having a non-DAD histology is unknown. In fact, the Berlin definition of ARDS is not fully reliable for diagnosing DAD, and several non-DAD histological entities (such as lung fibrosis, organizing pneumonia, diffuse alveolar hemorrhage or lung tumoral infiltration) have been reported in patients fulfilling the clinical and radiological criteria for ARDS [1, 40–42]. Regarding the onset of lung injury, the Berlin definition of ARDS stipulates that "respiratory signs should occur (or worsen) within 7 days after an exposure to a common ARDS risk factor" (e.g., pneumonia, acute pancreatitis, aspiration of gastric content or extra-pulmonary sepsis). In our patients, the absence of a common risk factor for ARDS according to the Berlin definition together with delay between first respiratory sign and ICU admission exceeding 7 days (21 days) advocate more for an ARDS mimicker rather than for a real ARDS. However, a recent histological study revealed that 50% of patients with an acute decompensation of AS syndrome due to JO-1 autoantibody exhibited histological lesions of DAD [43].

In non-ICU patients, the prognosis of inflammatory myopathies depends on the severity of lung involvement [10, 22, 32, 44]. Treatment of interstitial lung disease associated with AS and aMDA-5 dermato-pulmonary syndromes is not standardized and based on case reports. Numerous immunosuppressive therapies are available (e.g., cyclophosphamide, methotrexate, azathioprine, mycophenolate mofetil, cyclosporine, tacrolimus, rituximab, basiliximab, intravenous immunoglobulins or plasma exchange) [9, 11, 14, 21, 45, 46], but high-dose corticosteroids remain the first-line therapy. Our study underlines the wide variations in the choice of immunosuppressive treatment even if the association corticosteroids–cyclophosphamide was administered in almost 3 over 4 patients. Patients with aMDA-5 received significantly more immunosuppressive drugs highlighting a higher severity.

Of note, 19% of ICU survivors developed cancer, in line with previous series of AS patients [47].

Limitations

Our study suffers from several limitations. First, we included a limited number of patients, inherent to the rarity of the disease. However, this is the first series on ARF revealing AS or aMDA-5 syndromes in an ICU context and our findings are consistent with previous reports. This limited number of patients precluded performing multivariable analyses and thus did not allow for adjusting the observed association between some variables and mortality with potential confounders. Second, the relationship between positive AS or aMDA-5 autoantibody and ARF is not proven. We therefore cannot exclude that some patients had a fortuitously positive autoantibody and that inflammatory myopathy was not the cause of ARF. However, this hypothesis appears unlikely since an alternative diagnosis for ARF had to be excluded, and all patients were treated with immunosuppressive therapies underlining the high degree of clinician's suspicion. Third, because the patients were recruited over a 13-year period in 35 centers, ICU procedures were inevitably heterogeneous. Fourth, the prevalence of aMDA-5 dermato-pulmonary syndromes may have been underestimated during the study period since detection of aMDA-5 autoantibody was first described in 2005 [48] and was therefore routinely available only from 2010 in most of participating centers. Last, several classical predictors of mortality related to ventilation (tidal volume or driving pressure [49]) were not available as a result of a long-term retrospective design.

Clinical implications

Considering the high proportion of patients lacking extra-pulmonary manifestations and the nonspecific presentation mimicking that of a bilateral community-acquired pneumonia, we believe that ARF related to autoimmune inflammatory myopathies may be underdiagnosed. Hence, de Prost et al. recently showed that the diagnostic work-up performed in ARDS patients with no common risk factor was not comprehensive, with only 5% of patients having immunological tests [4]. The lack of screening for AS or aMDA-5 autoantibodies is probably one of the reasons why these diseases are underestimated. Therefore, when the etiology of ARF appears unclear, we recommend a more aggressive diagnostic work-up [6], including immunological tests in order to identify patients amenable to specific therapies.

A careful assessment of extra-pulmonary manifestations, such as cutaneous or articular signs, is crucial. While the presence of extra-pulmonary manifestations is highly suggestive, the 3-week delay between first respiratory signs and ICU admission, the absence of an obvious etiology for ARF, the presence of bi-basal consolidations on chest X-ray with an intense inflammatory process, contrasting with a low procalcitonin level together with the lack of microbiological documentation are the main clues to consider the diagnosis of AS or aMDA-5 syndromes in a patient without extra-pulmonary manifestation. To better assess the relevance of these signs, further prospective studies aiming at systematically screen for autoantibodies in ARDS without risk factors are needed. Once the diagnosis is made, the management is difficult and requires a multidisciplinary approach involving intensivists, pulmonologists, internists and rheumatologists in order to decide the best-individualized therapeutic strategy.

Conclusions

Intensivists should consider inflammatory myopathies, such as anti-synthetase syndrome and dermato-pulmonary syndrome associated with anti-MDA-5 antibodies, as a cause of acute respiratory failure when the etiology appears unclear. Extra-pulmonary manifestations are commonly lacking and an isolated lung involvement may reveal the disease. Hospital mortality is high, especially in aMDA-5 dermato-pulmonary syndrome.

Abbreviations
ARDS: acute respiratory distress syndrome; ARF: acute respiratory failure; AS: anti-synthetase; aMDA-5: anti-MDA-5 autoantibody; BAL: broncho-alveolar lavage; DAD: diffuse alveolar damage; ECMO: extra-corporeal membrane oxygenation; ICU: intensive care unit.

Authors' contributions
DC had full access to all the data in the study and takes responsibility for the integrity of the data and the accuracy of the data analysis. DC made substantial contribution to the study design, data collection and analysis and manuscript writing. CV contributed to data collection and interpretation, and drafting of the manuscript. MPC, NdP, AD, J-PQ, SP, GL, MN, GV, MF, RC, GD, EM, NT, YT-L, FS, MG, EG, RL, SR, RLM, GC, CG, LZ and EM contributed to patients identification in each center, data collection and manuscript writing. MD contributed to the data analysis, statistical analysis and manuscript revision. NdP, CG, OP, HM and GP contributed to the manuscript writing and revision, and provided important intellectual content. All authors read and approved the final manuscript.

Author details
[1] Service de Réanimation Polyvalente, Centre Hospitalier Victor Dupouy, 69 rue du Lieutenant Colonel Prudhon, 95100 Argenteuil, France. [2] Service de Réanimation Médicale, Centre Hospitalier Universitaire Pitié-Salpétrière – Assistance Publique Hôpitaux de Paris, 47-83 boulevard de l'Hôpital, 75013 Paris, France.

[3] Service de Réanimation Médicale, Centre Hospitalier Universitaire Henri Mondor – Assistance Publique Hôpitaux de Paris, 51 avenue du Maréchal de Lattre de Tassigny, 94010 Créteil, France. [4] Service de Réanimation Médicale, Hôpital de la Croix-Rousse, 103 Grande rue de la Croix-Rousse, 69004 Lyon, France. [5] INSERM 955, Créteil, France. [6] Service de Médecine Intensive Réanimation, Centre Hospitalier Universitaire François Mitterrand de Dijon, 14 rue Paul Gaffarel, 21000 Dijon, France. [7] Service de Réanimation, Centre Hospitalier Régional Universitaire de Lille, 2 avenue Oscar Lambret, 59000 Lille, France. [8] Service de Réanimation Médicale, Centre Hospitalier Universitaire Bichat Claude-Bernard – Assistance Publique Hôpitaux de Paris, 46 rue Henri Huchard, 75877 Paris, France. [9] Service de Réanimation médico-chirurgicale, Centre Hospitalier Universitaire Tenon – Assistance Publique Hôpitaux de Paris, 5 rue de la Chine, 75020 Paris, France. [10] Service de Réanimation médicale, Centre hospitalier universitaire de Poitiers, 2 rue de la Milétrie, 86021 Poitiers, France. [11] Service de Réanimation médicale, Centre Hospitalier Universitaire Saint-Antoine – Assistance Publique Hôpitaux de Paris, 184 rue du Faubourg Saint-Antoine, 75012 Paris, France. [12] Service de Réanimation, Centre Hospitalier Universitaire de Grenoble Alpes, avenue Maquis du Grésivaudan, 38700 La Tronche, France. [13] Service de Réanimation médico-chirurgicale, Centre Hospitalier Universitaire Avicennes – Assistance Publique Hôpitaux de Paris, 125 rue de Stalingrad, 93000 Bobigny, France. [14] Service de Réanimation, Centre Hospitalier Universitaire de Strasbourg, 1 avenue Molière, 67200 Strasbourg, France. [15] Service de Réanimation Médicale, Centre Hospitalier Universitaire de Rouen, 1 rue de Germont, 76000 Rouen, France. [16] Service de Réanimation Médicale, Centre Hospitalier Universitaire Hôpital Européen Georges-Pompidou – Assistance Publique Hôpitaux de Paris, 20 rue Leblanc, 75015 Paris, France. [17] Service de Réanimation Médicale, Centre Hospitalier Universitaire de Montpellier, 191 avenue du Doyen Gaston Giraud, 34000 Montpellier, France. [18] Service de Réanimation Polyvalente, Centre Hospitalier Robert-Ballanger, Boulevard Robert Ballanger, 93600 Aulnay-sous-Bois, France. [19] Service de Réanimation médicale, Centre Hospitalier Régional Universistaire de Brest, Site La Cavale Blanche, Boulevard Tanguy Prigent, 29200 Brest, France. [20] Service de réanimation médico-chirurgicale, Centre Hospitalier Départemental de Vendée, Les Oudairies, 85925 La Roche sur Yon Cedex 9, France. [21] Service de Réanimation médico-chirurgicale, Centre Hospitalier du Mans, 194 avenue Rubillard, 72037 Le Mans, France. [22] Service de Réanimation médicale, Hôpital Saint-Louis, Assistance Publique Hôpitaux de Paris, 1 avenue Claude Vellefaux, 75010 Paris, France. [23] Unité de Réanimation et de Surveillance continue, Service de Pneumologie et Réanimation médicale, Groupe hospitalier Pitié-Salpétrière, 47-83 bd de l'hôpital, 75651 Paris, France. [24] Service d'Immunologie Clinique, Hôpital Saint-Louis, Assistance Publique Hôpitaux de Paris, 1 avenue Claude Vellefaux, 75010 Paris, France.

Acknowledgements
We thank Jonathan Messika (Réanimation, Hôpital Louis Mourier, Colombes), Frédéric Pène (Réanimation médicale, Hôpital Cochin, Paris), Morgan Benaïs (Réanimation médico-chirurgicale, Saint Denis), Jérémy Rosman (Réanimation polyvalente, Charleville), David Schnell (Réanimation médico-chirurgicale, Angoulême), Sébastien Jochmans (Réanimation Polyvalente, Melun), Sami Hraiech and Jérémy Bourenne (Réanimations, Marseille), Guillaume Schnell (Réanimation médico-chirurgicale, Le Havre), Damien Du Cheyron (Réanimation médicale, Caen), Aude Gibelin (Réanimation médico-chirurgicale, Hôpital Tenon, Paris), Cédric Bruel (Réanimation Polyvalente, Hôpital Saint-Joseph, Paris), Kamel Toufik (Réanimation médico-chirurgicale, Orléans) and Jérémie Lemarié (Réanimation, Nancy) for having searched for eligible patients.

Competing interests
The authors declare that they have no competing interests.

Funding
This study did not receive funding from external or internal sources.

References

1. Papazian L, Doddoli C, Chetaille B, Gernez Y, Thirion X, Roch A, et al. A contributive result of open-lung biopsy improves survival in acute respiratory distress syndrome patients. Crit Care Med. 2007;35:755–62.
2. Vincent JL, Santacruz C. Do we need ARDS? Intensive Care Med. 2012;42:282–3.
3. Gibelin A, Parrot A, Maitre B, Brun-Buisson C, Mekontso Dessap A, Fartoukh M, et al. Acute respiratory distress syndrome mimickers lacking common risk factors of the Berlin definition. Intensive Care Med. 2015;42:164–72.
4. de Prost N, Pham T, Carteaux G, Mekontso Dessap A, Brun-Buisson C, Fan E, et al. Etiologies, diagnostic work-up and outcomes of acute respiratory distress syndrome with no common risk factor: a prospective multicenter study. Ann Intensive Care. 2017;7:69.
5. Ranieri VM, Rubenfeld GD, Thompson BT, Ferguson ND, Caldwell E, Fan E, et al. Acute respiratory distress syndrome: the Berlin definition. JAMA. 2012;307:2526–33.
6. Papazian L, Calfee CS, Chiumello D, Luyt CE, Meyer NJ, Sekiguchi H, et al. Diagnostic workup for ARDS patients. Intensive Care Med. 2016;42:674–85.
7. Bellani G, Laffey JG, Pham T, Fan E, Brochard L, Esteban A, et al. Epidemiology, patterns of care, and mortality for patients with acute respiratory distress syndrome in intensive care units in 50 countries. JAMA. 2016;315:788–800.
8. Hall JC, Casciola-Rosen L, Samedy LA, Werner J, Owoyemi K, Danoff SK, et al. Anti-melanoma differentiation-associated protein 5-associated dermatomyositis: expanding the clinical spectrum. Arthritis Care Res (Hoboken). 2013;65:1307–15.
9. Tillie-Leblond I, Wislez M, Valeyre D, Crestani B, Rabbat A, Israel-Biet D, et al. Interstitial lung disease and anti-Jo-1 antibodies: difference between acute and gradual onset. Thorax. 2008;63:53–9.
10. Uzunhan Y, Nunes H, Leroux G, Miyara M, Benveniste O, Allenbach Y. Dermato-pulmonary syndrome associated with MDA-5 antibodies. Eur Respir J. 2016;48(suppl 60):2138.
11. Chaisson NF, Paik J, Orbai AM, Casciola-Rosen L, Fiorentino D, Danoff S, et al. A novel dermato-pulmonary syndrome associated with MDA-5 antibodies: report of 2 cases and review of the literature. Medicine (Baltimore). 2012;91:220–8.
12. Grasselli G, Vergnano B, Pozzi MR, Sala V, D'Andrea G, Scaravilli V, et al. Interstitial pneumonia with autoimmune features: an additional risk factor for ARDS? Ann Intensive Care. 2017;7:98.
13. Bizien N, Renault A, Boles JM, Delluc A. Acute interstitial lung disease revealing antisynthetase syndrome. Rev Pneumol Clin. 2011;67:367–70.
14. Guglielmi S, Merz TM, Gugger M, Suter C, Nicod LP. Acute respiratory distress syndrome secondary to antisynthetase syndrome is reversible with tacrolimus. Eur Respir J. 2008;31:213–7.
15. Kim SH, Park IN. Acute respiratory distress syndrome as the initial clinical manifestation of an antisynthetase syndrome. Tuberc Respir Dis (Seoul). 2016;79:188–92.
16. Clawson K, Oddis CV. Adult respiratory distress syndrome in polymyositis patients with the anti-Jo-1 antibody. Arthritis Rheum. 1995;38:1519–23.
17. Piroddi IM, Ferraioli G, Barlascini C, Castagneto C, Nicolini A. Severe respiratory failure as a presenting feature of an interstitial lung disease associated with anti-synthetase syndrome (ASS). Respir Investig. 2016;54:284–8.
18. Friedman AW, Targoff IN, Arnett FC. Interstitial lung disease with autoantibodies against aminoacyl-tRNA synthetases in the absence of clinically apparent myositis. Semin Arthritis Rheum. 1996;26:459–67.
19. Shi J, Li S, Yang H, Zhang Y, Peng Q, Lu X, et al. Clinical profiles and prognosis of patients with distinct antisynthetase autoantibodies. J Rheumatol. 2017;44:1051–7.
20. Kinebuchi S, Mizuno K, Moriyama H, Ooi H, Hasegawa T, Yoshizawa H, et al. Two cases of interstitial pneumonia with anti-Jo-1 antibodies in the absence of myositis. Nihon Kokyuki Gakkai Zasshi. 2003;41:739–45.
21. Sauty A, Rochat T, Schoch OD, Hamacher J, Kurt AM, Dayer JM, et al. Pulmonary fibrosis with predominant CD8 lymphocytic alveolitis and anti-Jo-1 antibodies. Eur Respir J. 1997;10:2907–12.
22. Hervier B, Wallaert B, Hachulla E, Adoue D, Lauque D, Audrain M, et al. Clinical manifestations of anti-synthetase syndrome positive for antialanyl-tRNA synthetase (anti-PL12) antibodies: a retrospective study of 17 cases. Rheumatology (Oxford). 2010;49:972–6.
23. Vincent JL, Moreno R, Takala J, Willatts S, De Mendonca A, Bruining H, et al. The SOFA (Sepsis-related Organ Failure Assessment) score to describe organ dysfunction/failure. On behalf of the Working Group on Sepsis-Related Problems of the European Society of Intensive Care Medicine. Intensive Care Med. 1996;22:707–10.
24. Le Gall JR, Lemeshow S, Saulnier F. A new simplified acute physiology score (SAPS II) based on a European/North American multicenter study. JAMA. 1993;270:2957–63.
25. Wettstein RB, Shelledy DC, Peters JI. Delivered oxygen concentrations using low-flow and high-flow nasal cannulas. Respir Care. 2005;50:604–9.
26. Coudroy R, Frat JP, Boissier F, Contou D, Robert R, Thille AW. Early identification of acute respiratory distress disorder in the absence of positive pressure ventilation: implications for revision of the berlin criteria for acute respiratory distress syndrome. Crit Care Med. 2017;46:540–6.
27. Connors GR, Christopher-Stine L, Oddis CV, Danoff SK. Interstitial lung disease associated with the idiopathic inflammatory myopathies: what progress has been made in the past 35 years? Chest. 2010;138:1464–74.
28. Imbert-Masseau A, Hamidou M, Agard C, Grolleau JY, Cherin P. Antisynthetase syndrome. Joint Bone Spine. 2003;70:161–8.
29. Schmidt WA, Wetzel W, Friedlander R, Lange R, Sorensen HF, Lichey HJ, et al. Clinical and serological aspects of patients with anti-Jo-1 antibodies—an evolving spectrum of disease manifestations. Clin Rheumatol. 2000;19:371–7.
30. Hengstman GJ, van Engelen BG, van Venrooij WJ. Myositis specific autoantibodies: changing insights in pathophysiology and clinical associations. Curr Opin Rheumatol. 2004;16:692–9.
31. Marguerie C, Bunn CC, Beynon HL, Bernstein RM, Hughes JM, So AK, et al. Polymyositis, pulmonary fibrosis and autoantibodies to aminoacyl-tRNA synthetase enzymes. Q J Med. 1990;77:1019–38.
32. Marie I, Josse S, Decaux O, Diot E, Landron C, Roblot P, et al. Clinical manifestations and outcome of anti-PL7 positive patients with antisynthetase syndrome. Eur J Intern Med. 2013;24:474–9.
33. Vazquez-Abad D, Rothfield NF. Sensitivity and specificity of anti-Jo-1 antibodies in autoimmune diseases with myositis. Arthritis Rheum. 1996;39:292–6.
34. Marie I, Josse S, Decaux O, Dominique S, Diot E, Landron C, et al. Comparison of long-term outcome between anti-Jo1- and anti-PL7/PL12 positive patients with antisynthetase syndrome. Autoimmun Rev. 2012;11:739–45.
35. Fiorentino D, Chung L, Zwerner J, Rosen A, Casciola-Rosen L. The mucocutaneous and systemic phenotype of dermatomyositis patients with antibodies to MDA5 (CADM-140): a retrospective study. J Am Acad Dermatol. 2010;65:25–34.
36. Zamora AC, Hoskote SS, Abascal-Bolado B, White D, Cox CW, Ryu JH, et al. Clinical features and outcomes of interstitial lung disease in anti-Jo-1 positive antisynthetase syndrome. Respir Med. 2016;118:39–45.
37. Zafrani L, Lemiale V, Lapidus N, Lorillon G, Schlemmer B, Azoulay E. Acute respiratory failure in critically ill patients with interstitial lung disease. PLoS ONE. 2014;9:e104897.
38. Gay SE, Kazerooni EA, Toews GB, Lynch JP 3rd, Gross BH, Cascade PN, et al. Idiopathic pulmonary fibrosis: predicting response to therapy and survival. Am J Respir Crit Care Med. 1998;157:1063–72.
39. Wells AU, Desai SR, Rubens MB, Goh NS, Cramer D, Nicholson AG, et al. Idiopathic pulmonary fibrosis: a composite physiologic index derived from disease extent observed by computed tomography. Am J Respir Crit Care Med. 2003;167:962–9.
40. Thille AW, Esteban A, Fernandez-Segoviano P, Rodriguez JM, Aramburu JA, Penuelas O, et al. Comparison of the Berlin definition for acute respiratory distress syndrome with autopsy. Am J Respir Crit Care Med. 2013;187:761–7.
41. Patel SR, Karmpaliotis D, Ayas NT, Mark EJ, Wain J, Thompson BT, et al. The role of open-lung biopsy in ARDS. Chest. 2004;125:197–202.
42. Gerard L, Bidoul T, Castanares-Zapatero D, Wittebole X, Lacroix V, Froidure A, et al. Open lung biopsy in nonresolving acute respiratory distress syndrome commonly identifies corticosteroid-sensitive pathologies, associated with better outcome. Crit Care Med. 2018;46:907–14.

43. Yousem SA, Gibson K, Kaminski N, Oddis CV, Ascherman DP. The pulmo-
    nary histopathologic manifestations of the anti-Jo-1 tRNA synthetase
    syndrome. Mod Pathol. 2010;23:874–80.
44. Marie I, Hachulla E, Cherin P, Dominique S, Hatron PY, Hellot MF, et al.
    Interstitial lung disease in polymyositis and dermatomyositis. Arthritis
    Rheum. 2002;47:614–22.
45. Witt LJ, Curran JJ, Strek ME. The diagnosis and treatment of antisyn-
    thetase syndrome. Clin Pulm Med. 2016;23:218–26.
46. Zou J, Li T, Huang X, Chen S, Guo Q, Bao C. Basiliximab may improve the
    survival rate of rapidly progressive interstitial pneumonia in patients with
    clinically amyopathic dermatomyositis with anti-MDA5 antibody. Ann
    Rheum Dis. 2014;73:1591–3.

47. Castaneda-Pomeda M, Prieto-Gonzalez S, Grau JM. Antisynthetase syn-
    drome and malignancy: our experience. J Clin Rheumatol. 2011;17:458.
48. Sato S, Hirakata M, Kuwana M, Suwa A, Inada S, Mimori T, et al. Autoan-
    tibodies to a 140-kd polypeptide, CADM-140, in Japanese patients with
    clinically amyopathic dermatomyositis. Arthritis Rheum. 2005;52:1571–6.
49. Amato MB, Meade MO, Slutsky AS, Brochard L, Costa EL, Schoenfeld
    DA, et al. Driving pressure and survival in the acute respiratory distress
    syndrome. N Engl J Med. 2015;372:747–55.

22

Midazolam increases preload dependency during endotoxic shock in rabbits by affecting venous vascular tone

Jianxiao Chen[1], Tao Yu[1], Federico Longhini[1,2], Xiwen Zhang[1], Songqiao Liu[1], Ling Liu[1], Yi Yang[1] and Haibo Qiu[1]*

Abstract

Background: Septic patients often require sedation in intensive care unit, and midazolam is one of the most frequently used sedatives among them. But the interaction between midazolam and septic shock is not known. The aim of this study is to investigate the effects of midazolam on preload dependency in an endotoxic shock model by evaluating systemic vascular tone and cardiac function.

Methods: Eighteen rabbits were randomly divided into three groups: Control group, MID1 group and MID2 group. Rabbits underwent ketamine anaesthesia and mechanical ventilation, and haemodynamic assessments were recorded in three groups (T0). Endotoxic shock was induced by lipopolysaccharide intravenously, and fluid resuscitation and norepinephrine were administered to obtain the baseline mean arterial pressure (MAP) (T1). Rabbits received equivalent normal saline (Control) and two consecutive dosages of midazolam: $0.3 \ mg \ kg^{-1} \ h^{-1}$ (MID1) and $3 \ mg \ kg^{-1} \ h^{-1}$ (MID2) (T2). Rabbits received another round of fluid challenge and norepinephrine infusion to return the MAP to normal (T3).

Results: No significant differences in haemodynamic parameters were observed in three groups at T0, T1 or T3. Midazolam infusion significantly increased pulse pressure variation (PPV) and stroke volume variation (SVV) compared to the values in Control group, and MAP, central venous pressure (CVP), mean systemic filling pressure (Pmsf) and cardiac output (CO) decreased at T2. Same effects were observed with increasing doses of midazolam, and resistance for venous return (Rvr) decreased (MID1 vs. MID2) at T2. PPV and SVV increased significantly at T2 compared to the values at T1. MAP, CVP, Pmsf and CO decreased in MID1 and MID2 groups. Rvr also decreased in MID2 group (T2 vs. T1). Midazolam did not affect cardiac function index, systemic vascular resistance or artery resistance (T2 vs. T1).

Conclusions: Midazolam administration promoted preload dependency in septic shock models via decreased venous vascular tone without affecting cardiac function.

Keywords: Midazolam, Preload dependency, Vascular resistance, Endotoxic shock, Mean systemic filling pressure

Background

Septic shock is a deleterious systemic host response to infection characterized by hypotension that is not reversed with fluids alone. Septic shock is a common reason for admission to the intensive care unit (ICU) [1]. The response to fluid challenge is complicated by cardiovascular physiology, but it plays an important role in the resuscitation of sepsis patients [2]. However, fluid responsiveness only occurs in half of critically ill patients, including patients with sepsis [3]. Fluid resuscitation is a mainstay of early treatment, but the deleterious effects of excessive fluid administration that lead to tissue oedema are becoming clearer.

Patients with septic shock generally require mechanical ventilation, which makes the use of sedative drugs almost imperative to reduce anxiety and agitation and facilitate care. Benzodiazepines (e.g. midazolam) are commonly

*Correspondence: haiboq2000@163.com
[1] Department of Critical Care Medicine, Zhongda Hospital, School of Medicine, Southeast University, 87 Dingjiaqiao Road, Nanjing 210009, People's Republic of China
Full list of author information is available at the end of the article

used to sedate patients in the ICU, and a recent survey demonstrated that midazolam remains widely used [4]. Benzodiazepines inhibit the activity of the autonomic nervous system [5, 6]. Midazolam attenuates the release of catecholamines in vivo and induces vasoplegia, which contributes to the resulting haemodynamic changes [7, 8].

Norepinephrine, an $\alpha1$-agonist drug, is recommended as a first-line vasopressor [9]. Norepinephrine reduces the preload dependency via exertion on arterial and venous tone to increase systemic arterial resistance, primarily by recruiting blood from the large venous unstressed volume [10]. Our previous work demonstrated that propofol and dexmedetomidine increased preload dependency in an endotoxic shock model after fluid resuscitation during norepinephrine infusion, and the mechanism primarily relied on the systemic vascular system and cardiac function [11]. Few studies have reported the haemodynamic effects of midazolam infusion in endotoxic shock models during norepinephrine infusion.

In the present experimental, randomized study, we investigated the effects of midazolam on preload dependency in rabbits subjected to endotoxic shock with norepinephrine infusion by evaluating the systemic vascular system and cardiac function.

Methods

Ethics statement

New Zealand white rabbits (3.26 ± 0.14 kg body weight) were obtained from the animal centre of Southeast University and housed in a pathogen-free environment on a 12-h light/dark cycle with free food and water access for at least 5 days prior to experimentation. All animals received care according to the Helsinki convention for the use and care of animals, the "Principles of Laboratory Animal Care" formulated by the National Society for Medical Research and the "Guide for the Care and Use of Laboratory Animals" by the China National Academy of Sciences. The Academic Ethical Committee of Southeast University Medical School, Nanjing, China, approved the study protocol, which has been described previously [11].

Animal preparation

Rabbits received an intramuscular injection of ketamine (20 mg kg^{-1}) and atropine (0.15 mg kg^{-1}), which was used to reduce mucosal secretion in the airways. A marginal ear vein was cannulated to guarantee intravenous anaesthesia using ketamine (3 mg kg^{-1} h^{-1}) during the entire study protocol, as previously described [11, 12]. A tracheotomy was performed after local anaesthesia with lidocaine, and a 3.5–4-mm-inner-diameter endotracheal tube was placed. Rabbits were ventilated using a Servo-I with proper software for neonatal and paediatric

ventilation (Maquet Critical Care, Solna, Sweden). Tracheal cannulation was used to better adapt the rabbits to controlled mechanical ventilation and avoid spontaneous breathing. A continuous infusion of vecuronium (0.05 mg kg^{-1} h^{-1}) was administered for neuromuscular block, and an adjunctive bolus of 0.5–1 mg was added to optimize the animal curarization if needed.

Rabbits were ventilated via volume control ventilation with the following settings: zero end-expiratory pressure, a tidal volume equal to 8 mL kg^{-1}, an initial respiratory rate equal to 40 breath min^{-1} (modified according to the carbon dioxide partial pressure targeted to the physiological range) and an inspired fraction of oxygen of 60%. Arterial blood was sampled for gas analysis to adjust the ventilator setting in case of respiratory acidosis prior to endotoxic shock induction. The right internal jugular vein and femoral artery were surgically isolated, and a central vein catheter was placed to infuse fluids and drugs. A dedicated arterial thermodilution catheter (4 Fr, 8 cm Pulsiocath PV2014L16; Pulsion Medical Systems, Munich, Germany) was inserted to acquire the haemodynamic measurements [12]. Lactate Ringer's solution (4 mL kg^{-1} h^{-1}) was infused in the central vein catheter, and 2 mL h^{-1} of normal saline with 4 IU mL^{-1} of heparin was infused through the arterial line. Blood temperature was monitored and maintained between 38 and 39 °C via a warming lamp.

An intravenous infusion over 30 s of 0.5 mg kg^{-1} E. coli LPS (O55:B5; Sigma Chem. Co., St. Louis, MO, USA) was used to induce endotoxic shock, which was confirmed by a 25% decrease in mean arterial pressure (MAP) [13]. Fluid resuscitation (20 mL, intravenous bolus) was administered to all endotoxic rabbits, and 50 mL kg^{-1} fluid was injected for another 2 h to maintain blood pressure. Norepinephrine infusion was initiated, and the dose was titrated to maintain MAP at baseline values and remain constant throughout the entire protocol. The haemodynamic variables were allowed to stabilize, which was assessed as a variation of MAP < 10% over a 30-min period [14].

Experimental protocol

Rabbits were randomly divided into three groups ($n = 6$ in each group): Control group, MID1 group and MID2 group. Figure 1 shows the flowchart of the study protocol. Endotoxic shock was initiated after animal preparation (T0), and the following fluid resuscitation and norepinephrine infusions were administered to all three groups. Haemodynamic measurements were obtained after stabilization (T1). Rabbits received two consecutive dosages of midazolam for 30 min: 0.3 mg kg^{-1} h^{-1} (MID1 group) and 3 mg kg^{-1} h^{-1} (MID2 group). Rabbits in the Control group received equivalent doses of normal

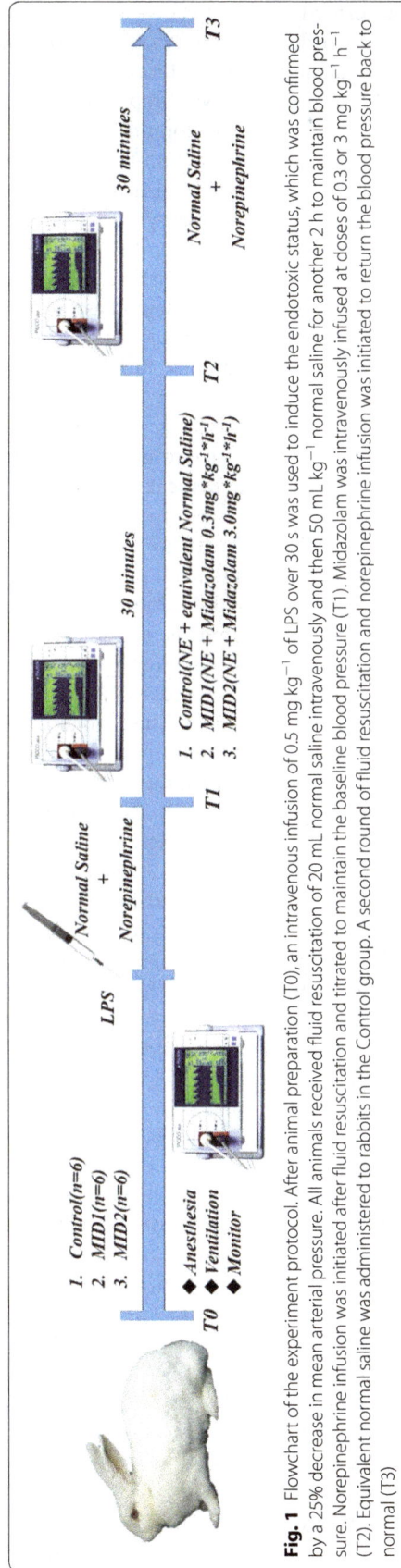

Fig. 1 Flowchart of the experiment protocol. After animal preparation (T0), an intravenous infusion of 0.5 mg kg^{-1} of LPS over 30 s was used to induce the endotoxic status, which was confirmed by a 25% decrease in mean arterial pressure. All animals received fluid resuscitation of 20 mL normal saline intravenously and then 50 mL kg^{-1} normal saline for another 2 h to maintain blood pressure. Norepinephrine infusion was initiated after fluid resuscitation and titrated to maintain the baseline blood pressure (T1). Midazolam was intravenously infused at doses of 0.3 or 3 mg kg^{-1} h^{-1} (T2). A second round of fluid resuscitation and norepinephrine infusion was initiated to return the blood pressure back to normal (T3). Equivalent normal saline was administered to rabbits in the Control group.

saline. Haemodynamic measurements were performed at the end of the 30 min trial, and the data were recorded (T2). Rabbits received another round of fluid challenge and norepinephrine infusion to return the MAP to normal (T3).

Haemodynamic measurements

Heart rate (HR), systolic blood pressure (SBP), diastolic blood pressure (DBP), MAP and central vein pressure (CVP) were continuously monitored and recorded. Haemodynamic measurements were performed using a dedicated indwelling arterial catheter for the PiCCO Plus device (Pulsion Medical Systems, Munich, Germany).

Proper calibration of the PiCCO Plus for pulse contour analysis was performed at each measurement time point using two 3-mL bolus injections of 4 °C normal saline. A third calibrating injection was performed if the first two values differed by more than 10%.

Stroke volume (SV), cardiac output (CO) and global end-diastolic volume (GEDV) were acquired via transpulmonary dilution [11, 15]. Pulse pressure variation (PPV) and stroke volume variation (SVV) were calculated for preload dependency.

Systemic vascular resistance (Rsys), mean systemic filling pressure (Pmsf), resistance to venous return (Rvr) and arterial resistance (Ra) were calculated as previously described [14, 16]. Briefly, end-inspiratory occlusions were performed at different levels of positive end-expiratory pressure (PEEP), and the extreme values of CO and CVP were recorded simultaneously. Each pair of measurements was plotted on a graph connecting CO (Y-axis) and CVP (X-axis), and the regression line was computed using the least-squares method in Microsoft Excel. Pmsf was estimated as the pressure that corresponded to the X-intercept of the regression line, and resistance to the venous return was calculated as the inverse of the slope of the line. Rsys was calculated as (MAP-CVP)/CI. Ra was estimated as (MAP-Pmsf)/CI, and Rvr was calculated as (Pmsf-CVP)/CI.

The Cardiac Function Index (CFI) was calculated as the ratio of $CO \times 1000$ to GEDV, and it was recorded as an estimate of ventricular systolic function [6, 11, 14, 17]. The ventilator settings, anaesthesia and vasoactive drugs were not modified during the study protocol.

Blood gas measurements

Blood gas measurements were obtained from the arterial and venous catheters at T0, T1, T2 and T3 to measure pH, the partial pressure of carbon dioxide (PCO_2), the ratio of alveolar oxygen partial pressure to the fraction of inspiration O_2 (P/F), lactic acid (Lac), haemoglobin (Hb), bicarbonate (HCO_3^-) and oxygen saturation of mixed venous blood (SvO_2).

Statistics

Data were analysed using SPSS 19.0 for Windows (SPSS Inc., Chicago, IL, USA) and GraphPad Prism 7 for Windows (GraphPad Prism Software Inc., La Jolla, CA, USA). We computed the descriptive statistics for all study variables. We used the Kolmogorov–Smirnov test and stratified the distribution plots to verify the distribution normality of the continuous variables. Data that were normally distributed are presented as the mean ± standard deviation (SD), and non-normally distributed data are presented as medians (interquartile, IQ). We assessed differences in the distribution normality of the continuous variables using one-way analyses of variances followed by Bonferroni corrections for multiple comparisons. We used the Mann–Whitney U test to evaluate non-normally distributed data. $p < 0.05$ was considered statistically significant for all analyses (Table 1).

Results

Eighteen rabbits were anaesthetized for the study protocol. Endotoxic shock was successfully established in all animals, as indicated by a 25% decrease in MAP. Fluid resuscitation and norepinephrine infusion (Table 2) restored MAP to the initial value prior to endotoxic shock. The rabbits received a second fluid challenge and norepinephrine infusion after midazolam infusion to return the MAP to normal. No differences were detected between the Control, MID1 and MID2 groups with respect to the time to achieve endotoxic shock (29.1 ± 6.8, 28.4 ± 7.2 and 29.0 ± 7.0 min, respectively; $p > 0.05$) or the volume of administered fluid during T0–T1 and T1–T2. The volume of administered fluid increased from T2 to T3 between the Control, MID1 and MID2 groups (29.10 ± 1.46, 45.40 ± 1.19 and 65.21 ± 1.16 mL, respectively, $p < 0.05$). No differences were detected between the Control, MID1 and MID2 groups with respect to the norepinephrine infusion rate (5.51 ± 0.23, 5.55 ± 0.21 and 5.56 ± 0.27 mcg kg^{-1} min^{-1}, respectively, $p > 0.05$). Blood gases confirmed normal baseline status, and there were no significant differences between T0, T1, T2 or T3 among all three groups (Table 3). No rabbits died.

Table 1 shows the effects of midazolam on haemodynamics. No differences between the Control, MID1 and MID2 groups were observed at T0, which demonstrates that the study population was homogeneous prior to the initiation of the sedative infusion ($p > 0.05$).

Effects of midazolam on preload dependency

Table 1 shows that no differences in PPV or SVV were observed between groups at T0. No differences in PPV or SVV were observed after modelling and resuscitation between the three groups, which demonstrates that all rabbits were without fluid responsiveness at T1.

Table 1 Haemodynamic values for each group at baseline and after fluid resuscitation and norepinephrine infusion

	T0			T1			T2			T3		
	Control	MID1	MID2	Control	MID1	MID2	Control	MID1	MID2	Control	MID1	MID2
HR (/min)	220 [213–221]	221 [219–229]	222 [219–226]	192 [190–192]△	201 [191–204]△	191 [190–194]△	188 [185–191]△	219 [215–228]*&	218 [211–224]*&	193 [191–195]△	202 [189–203]△^	192 [191–194]△^
SBP (mmHg)	131 [130–134]	130 [129–130]	130 [126–135]	142 [136–150]△	148 [141–151]△	146 [141–152]△	143 [137–150]△	129 [126–133]*&	108 [107–108]*#△&	135 [131–141]	137 [135–138]&	142 [135–147]△^
DBP (mmHg)	78 [76–80]	79 [75–80]	77 [75–80]	84 [81–85]	86 [82–88]	88 [82–89]	80 [79–84]	71 [70–77]&	57 [56–60]*#△&	79 [78–82]	80 [76–80]^	77 [76–78]&^
MAP (mmHg)	96 [92–98]	94 [93–96]	96 [92–97]	105 [98–108]△	104 [101–108]△	106 [104–110]△	103 [95–107]△	90 [87–95]*&	74 [72–76]*#△&	99 [96–103]	98 [97–99]&^	97 [96–99]&^
CVP (mmHg)	0 [0–1]	1 [0–1]	0 [0–0]	4 [3,4]△	4 [3–5]△	4 [2–4]△	4 [3–4]△	3 [3–3]△&	1 [1–2]*#△&	4 [3–4]△	5 [4–5]△^	3 [2–4]△^
CO (L/min)	0.70 [0.68–0.70]	0.71 [0.69–0.72]	0.79 [0.77–0.81]	0.97 [0.95–0.98]△	0.90 [0.89–0.96]△	0.96 [0.95–1.01]△	0.97 [0.95–1.00]△	0.83 [0.82–0.88]*△&	0.74 [0.71–0.76]*&	0.97 [0.95–0.98]△	0.90 [0.89–0.96]△^	0.96 [0.95–1.01]△^
SV (mL)	3.16 [2.97–3.42]	3.19 [3.13–3.40]	3.53 [3.46–3.64]	5.04 [4.97–5.09]△	4.77 [4.48–4.84]△	4.96 [4.82–5.28]△	5.04 [4.91–5.13]△	3.96 [3.76–4.07]*△&	3.42 [3.18–3.67]*&	4.99 [4.93–5.06]△	4.72 [4.46–4.94]△^	4.96 [4.81–5.25]△^
GEDV (mL)	51.73 [50.96,51.95]	52.61 [52.42,53.10]	52.29 [51.96,52.93]	85.10 [79.61,91.04]△	83.68 [80.95,86.80]△	84.04 [77.73,85.20]△	85.60 [79.14,90.79]△	79.88 [74.58,81.53]△	61.15 [58.22,63.21]*#△&	85.15 [79.36,90.35]△	87.28 [81.01,87.96]△^	84.84 [77.70,87.06]△^
PPV (%)	19 [17–21]	17 [16–21]	18 [17–19]	12 [9–14]△	9 [7–10]△	9 [8–10]△	12 [10–14]△	14 [12–14]△&	18 [17–20]*#&	12 [10–14]△	10 [10–11]△	11 [9–12]△^
SVV (%)	20 [18–22]	19 [17–21]	17 [16–21]	12 [11–13]△	9 [7–10]△	10 [8–10]△	11 [10–12]△	15 [14–16]*△&	19 [18–20]*#&	11 [10–12]△	10 [9–11]△^	10 [8–10]△^
Pmsf (mmHg)	11.38 [10.66–11.74]	11.25 [9.82–12.18]	10.21 [9.84–10.83]	15.10 [14.37–15.33]△	15.25 [12.80–15.90]△	13.66 [13.32–14.44]△	13.96 [12.62–15.19]△	11.99 [11.39–12.33]*&	7.47 [7.12–8.18]*#△&	15.04 [14.43–15.21]△	14.67 [13.05–16.48]△^	13.84 [11.78–14.05]△^
Rsys (mmHg min kg/L)	433.07 [407.43–467.57]	425.39 [415.13–447.27]	391.68 [385.29–396.17]	313.44 [285.22–349.96]△	344.17 [335.74–378.40]△	345.42 [329.23–359.34]△	307.07 [275.76–354.48]△	325.91 [319.91–364.31]△	321.84 [315.46–330.69]△	304.85 [277.58–330.59]△	330.35 [329.47–345.24]△	311.64 [295.34–331.80]△
Ra (mmHg min kg/L)	381.99 [359.36–415.32]	376.87 [371.82–395.45]	351.96 [348.17–354.64]	281.67 [246.52–309.64]△	309.23 [297.37–339.03]△	315.84 [291.55–322.58]△	277.14 [238.35–317.62]△	294.21 [284.26–328.25]△	295.30 [286.45–306.61]△	268.01 [240.22–293.72]△	294.57 [288.36–300.60]△	279.84 [267.47–298.88]△
Rvr (mmHg min kg/L)	50.00 [47.22–52.25]	47.09 [44.35–51.98]	42.41 [38.80–44.46]	37.02 [30.15–39.24]△	39.42 [35.58–39.94]△	37.12 [32.12–39.78]△	36.71 [26.93–37.80]△	36.04 [33.01–36.69]△	28.05 [26.93–29.48]#△&	36.80 [29.28–41.45]△	36.90 [29.71–41.42]△	32.08 [30.10–33.84]△
CFI (/min)	13.41 [13.25–13.51]	13.52 [13.22–13.55]	14.89 [14.35–15.52]	11.82 [11.33–12.46]△	10.97 [10.62–11.19]△	12.23 [11.54–12.30]△	11.86 [11.29–12.49]△	10.81 [10.25–11.29]△	12.26 [11.34–12.46]△	11.86 [11.25–12.49]△	10.81 [10.25–11.29]△	12.26 [11.34–12.46]△

The table shows the recorded haemodynamic values expressed as medians (IQR) of animal preparation at baseline (T0), after fluid resuscitation and norepinephrine infusion (T1), after midazolam infusion (T2) and after the second round of fluid resuscitation (T3) in the Control, MID1 and MID2 groups

HR heart rate, *SBP* systolic blood pressure, *DBP* diastolic blood pressure, *MAP* mean arterial pressure, *CVP* central venous pressure, *CO* cardiac output, *SV* stroke volume, *GEDV* global end-diastolic volume, *PPV* pulse pressure variation, *SVV* stroke volume variation, *Pmsf* mean systemic filling pressure, *Rsys* systemic vascular resistance, *Ra* resistance for artery, *Rvr* resistance for venous return, *CFI* Cardiac Function Index

*$p < 0.05$ versus Control, #$p < 0.05$ versus MID1, △$p < 0.05$ versus T0, &$p < 0.05$ versus T1, ^$p < 0.05$ versus T2, $n = 6$

Table 2 Fluid and norepinephrine administration during the experiment

Treatment	T0–T1			T1–T2			T2–T3		
	Control	MID1	MID2	Control	MID1	MID2	Control	MID1	MID2
Saline (mL)	343.33 ± 16.32	350.00 ± 12.64	345.00 ± 13.78	29.10 ± 1.46	29.70 ± 1.13	29.25 ± 1.24	29.10 ± 1.46	45.40 ± 1.19*	65.21 ± 1.16*#
Norepinephrine (mcg kg^{-1} min^{-1})	5.51 ± 0.23	5.55 ± 0.21	5.56 ± 0.27	5.51 ± 0.23	5.55 ± 0.21	5.56 ± 0.27	5.51 ± 0.23	5.55 ± 0.21	5.56 ± 0.27

Data are shown as the mean ± SD

T0: baseline; T1: endotoxic shock after fluid resuscitation and norepinephrine infusion; T2: after the administration of midazolam at 0.3 mg kg^{-1} h^{-1} (MID1) or 3 mg kg^{-1} h^{-1} (MID2); T3: after second round of fluid resuscitation

*$p < 0.05$ versus control, #$p < 0.05$ versus MID1

Midazolam administration significantly increased PPV in the MID2 group at T2 ($p < 0.05$), and it significantly increased SVV in the MID1 and MID2 groups ($p < 0.05$) compared to that in the Control group (Fig. 2). SVV in the MID2 group was significantly higher than that in the MID1 group at T2 ($p < 0.05$) (Fig. 1b). No differences were detected in PPV or SVV between groups at T3 ($p > 0.05$).

PPV and SVV decreased from T0 to T1 in all groups ($p < 0.05$) but increased significantly in the MID1 and MID2 groups at T2 compared to the values at T1 ($p < 0.05$). PPV and SVV decreased in the MID1 and MID2 groups from T2 to T3 ($p < 0.05$), but no differences were detected in the Control group (Table 1 and Fig. 2).

Effects of midazolam on haemodynamic parameters

As shown in Table 1, there were no significant differences in the haemodynamic parameters among the three groups at T0, T1 and T3. However, MAP and Pmsf decreased significantly in the MID1 and MID2 groups ($p < 0.05$), and CVP and CO decreased in the MID2 group compared to the values in the Control group at T2 ($p < 0.05$) (Table 1). MAP, CVP and Pmsf in the MID2 group were significantly lower than the values in the MID1 group at T2 ($p < 0.05$) (Table 1).

Midazolam dosage did not affect Rsys or Ra at T2 or T3, but Rvr deceased significantly in the MID2 group compared to that in the Control group at T2 and T3 ($p < 0.05$) (Fig. 3). There were no differences in CFI between groups at T2 or T3 ($p > 0.05$).

MAP, CVP, Pmsf, CO and SV increased from T0 to T1 and T2 to T3 in all three groups ($p < 0.05$). Rsys, Ra, Rvr, HR and CFI decreased significantly from T0 to T1 ($p < 0.05$) (Table 1). MAP, CVP, Pmsf and CO decreased in the MID1 and MID2 groups at T2 compared to the values at T1 ($p < 0.05$), and the opposite results occurred at T3 compared to the values at T2 (Table 1). Rvr only decreased in the MID2 group at T2 ($p < 0.05$). No differences were detected in Rvr from T2 to T3 (Fig. 3, $p > 0.05$).

Discussion

To our knowledge, this study is the first to investigate the effects of two midazolam doses on haemodynamics in an endotoxic shock model during norepinephrine infusion. The main results can be summarized as follows: (1) midazolam increased the preload dependency, reduced Pmsf, CVP, GEDI and Pvr and affected the SV and CO despite the increase in HR; (2) no effects on cardiac contractile function as expressed by the CFI were observed. Thus, midazolam primarily affects the heart by increasing venous capacitance.

To better elucidate the mechanism, the venous return curve of one representative rabbit was constructed from the average values obtained for right atrial pressure (a surrogate for central venous pressure) and cardiac output (Fig. 4), as previously described [18]. Three points in Fig. 4 represent the circulatory working points at T1(a), T2(c) and T3(d). The cardiac function curve did not change with increasing midazolam infusion rates (T1 and T2), but the working point left-shifted to lower values of CO and right atrial pressure. The Pmsf obtained from the venous return curve was also reduced. This Pmsf reduction may be explained by an increased vascular capacitance due to midazolam infusion, which shifted the stressed volume to the unstressed volume [19]. Vascular capacity is defined as the volume at a given pressure [19], assuming that the total intravascular volume in rabbits did not change. The recorded Pmsf reduction suggests an increase in vascular capacitance. Endotoxic rabbits with midazolam-induced haemodynamic changes were resuscitated at T3 until MAP was restored to baseline (i.e. before sedative use) to further test our hypothesis. Figure 3 shows that the C point returned to the D point, i.e. from the ascending curve to plateau status, after fluid infusion.

Augmented vascular capacitance and lower Pmsf reduced the venous return and therefore the SV and CO, despite attempts at compensation by increasing the HR. The CFI was not affected. The preload (i.e. GEDV)

Table 3 Analysis of blood gas with increasing midazolam infusion rates

	T0			T1			T2			T3		
	Control	MID1	MID2	Control	MID1	MID2	Control	MID1	MID2	Control	MID1	MID2
pHa	7.30±0.09	7.34±0.03	7.27±0.07	7.23±0.05	7.24±0.03	7.38±0.06	7.23±0.08	7.22±0.05	7.24±0.07	7.25±0.06	7.24±0.03	7.32±0.06
PCO_2 (mmHg)	33.78±9.57	33.93±5.07	33.70±6.14	35.63±7.46	33.91±4.92	34.12±5.68	33.71±6.14	34.10±5.07	36.71±6.02	33.81±5.98	33.98±5.12	35.12±5.82
P/F (mmHg)	339.65±71.59	308.55±35.01	348.02±64.01	299.75±69.52	296.15±59.58	297.68±67.35	292.51±50.51	298.30±21.10	290.51±38.62	296.62±48.91	298.50±22.30	298.36±35.72
Lac (mmol/L)	2.90±0.69	2.90±0.54	2.45±0.97	2.91±1.31	2.93±1.35	3.12±1.02	2.2±0.98	2.3±0.85	2.91±1.01	2.1±0.87	2.2±0.75	2.6±0.98
Hb (g/dL)	8.5±0.5	8.5±0.6	8.5±0.6	8.3±0.5	8.6±0.7	8.3±0.8	8.3±0.5	8.4±0.3	8.5±0.4	8.6±0.4	8.2±0.5	8.5±0.4
HCO_3^- (mmol/L)	16.2±2.4	16.1±1.6	16.7±3.3	15.79±1.9	16.25±2.3	16.35±1.8	16.68±3.42	16.31±2.31	16.31±3.06	17.08±3.06	16.52±2.11	17.31±1.98
SvO_2 (%)	88.13±2.93	88.18±2.98	85.68±4.27	85.46±3.96	85.17±3.12	86.35±3.03	85.67±4.12	85.28±3.12	85.69±3.06	86.28±4.35	86.28±4.84	85.39±2.98

Data are shown as the mean ± SD

T0: baseline; T1: endotoxic shock after the fluid resuscitation and norepinephrine infusion; T2: after the administration of midazolam at 0.3 mg kg^{-1} h^{-1} (MID1) or 3 mg kg^{-1} h^{-1} (MID2); T3: after the second round of fluid resuscitation

pHa, pH of artery; PCO_2, partial pressure of carbon dioxide; P/F, alveolar oxygen partial pressure/fraction of inspiration O_2; Lac, lactic acid; Hb, haemoglobin; HCO_3^-, bicarbonate; SvO_2, oxygen saturation of mixed venous blood; SD, standard deviation

There was no significant difference between Control, MID1 and MID2 groups at T0, T1, T2 or T3, respectively

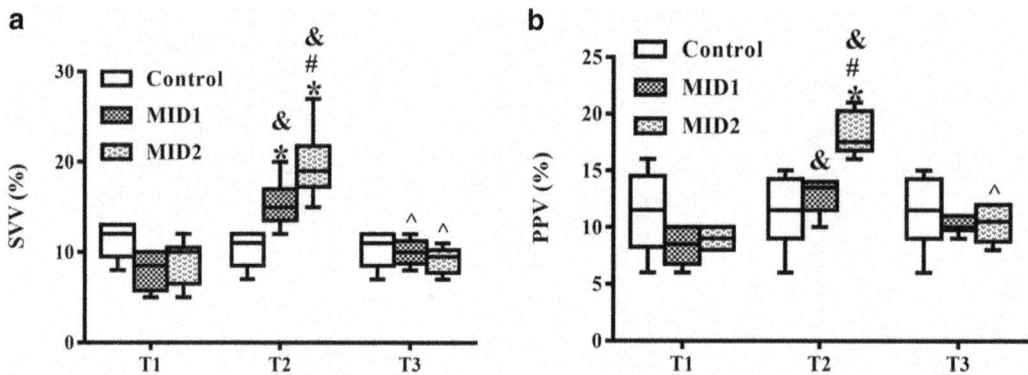

Fig. 2 Midazolam increased preload dependency of endotoxic shock rabbits. **a** The effects of midazolam on pulse pressure variation between the Control, MID1 and MID2 groups at T1, T2 and T3. **b** The effects of midazolam on stroke volume variation between the Control, MID1 and MID2 groups at T1, T2 and T3. *PPV* pulse pressure variation, *SVV* stroke volume variation; *$p < 0.05$ versus Control, #$p < 0.05$ versus MID1, &$p < 0.05$ versus T1, ^$p < 0.05$ versus T2, $n = 6$

decreased significantly because of the reduced venous return, and the preload dependency (PPV) increased significantly. The Rvr decreased significantly from T0 to T2, which confirmed midazolam-induced venous dilatation and resulted in reduced preload and increased preload dependency.

Our study demonstrates that midazolam increases preload dependency in an endotoxic shock rabbit model. This result is inconsistent with a prior clinical observational study also conducted by our work team in which midazolam use did not increase the preload dependency in septic shock patients [20]. The following reasons may explain this inconsistency. First, the midazolam dose regimen in the prior study was a bolus dose of 2.5 mg and continuous infusion of 1.5 mg h, which is equivalent to the dose in the MID1 group in our study, and the effects on vascular tone were not obvious. Second, the sedation was titrated to Ramsay 3–4 points in the prior study, and the rabbits were anaesthetized using ketamine with midazolam. These sedatives are likely not comparable.

We recorded no differences in cardiac function as expressed by the CFI, i.e. the ratio of cardiac output to global end-diastolic volume. CFI correlates with left ventricular global systolic function [21, 22], and the recorded differences in SVI and CI cannot be attributable to an effect of acidosis on contractility, or on contractility itself, but to a preload midazolam effect.

Some limitations of the present study must be mentioned. First, we used SVV and PVV to reflect volume responsiveness. Previous studies demonstrated that SVV (directly measured using different pulse contour techniques or Doppler ultrasounds) or PPV reliably predicts the response to fluids when several prerequisites are met

(e.g. absence of arrhythmias, tidal volume larger than 8 mL/kg, no respiratory movements) [23, 24]. These requirements were satisfied in the present study, and the use of SVV and PVV was likely reliable and effective.

Second, we used the end-inspiratory occlusion technique to draw the venous return curve for Pmsf computation [16]. Persichini et al. [14] recorded CO and CVP during end-inspiratory and end-expiratory ventilatory occlusions to describe a more precise curve. The description of this method was published after our study began, and our methods were chosen based on previously described literature.

In conclusion, midazolam affected the preload dependency at increasing doses in endotoxic shock rabbits undergoing norepinephrine infusion without affecting heart contractile function. These results suggest no major effects of midazolam on cardiac function in septic shock and that the haemodynamic fluctuations at large doses of midazolam were due to venous dilation. These data were derived from animal models, and further studies must be performed in humans to understand the possible interference of benzodiazepine in septic shocked patients.

Conclusions

In conclusion, a high dose of midazolam administration in a septic shock model after fluid resuscitation and norepinephrine infusion increased the preload dependency via modification of vascular resistance. No effects on cardiac function were observed. Further studies must be performed in humans to understand the possible interference of sedative drugs on haemodynamics during septic shock.

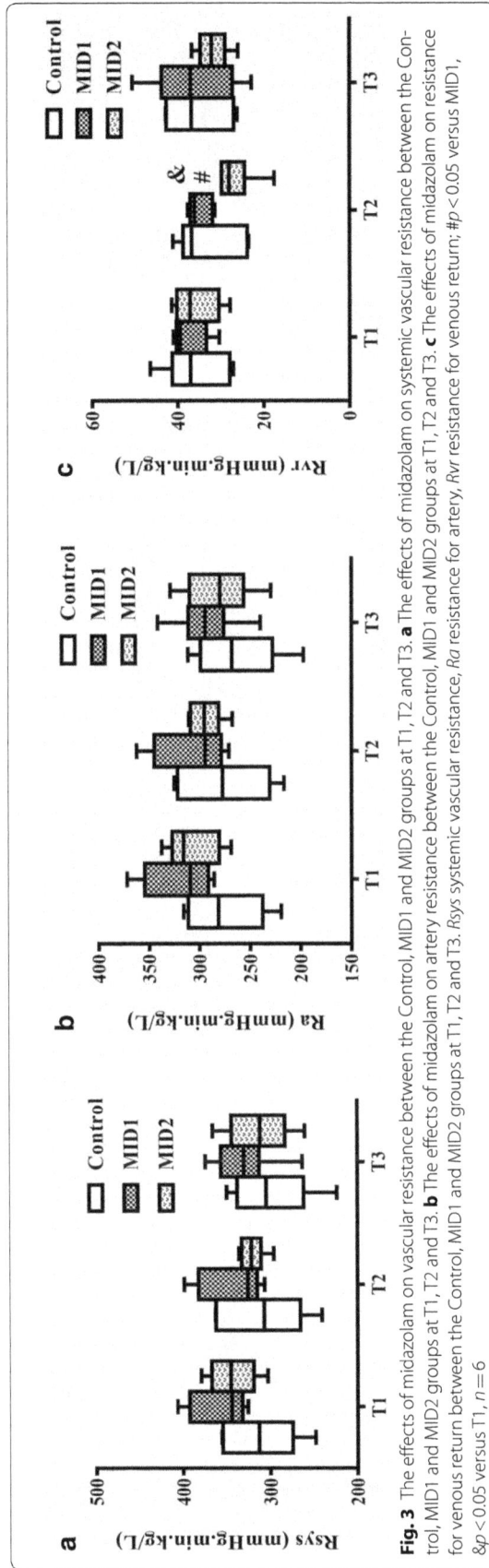

Fig. 3 The effects of midazolam on vascular resistance between the Control, MID1 and MID2 groups at T1, T2 and T3. **a** The effects of midazolam on systemic vascular resistance between the Control, MID1 and MID2 groups at T1, T2 and T3. **b** The effects of midazolam on artery resistance between the Control, MID1 and MID2 groups at T1, T2 and T3. **c** The effects of midazolam on resistance for venous return between the Control, MID1 and MID2 groups at T1, T2 and T3. *Rsys* systemic vascular resistance, *Ra* resistance for artery, *Rvr* resistance for venous return; #*p* < 0.05 versus MID1, &*p* < 0.05 versus T1, *n* = 6

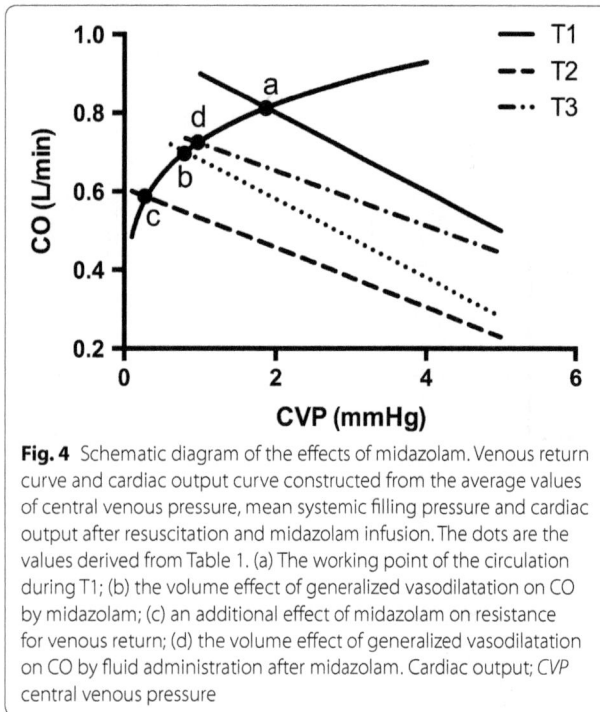

Fig. 4 Schematic diagram of the effects of midazolam. Venous return curve and cardiac output curve constructed from the average values of central venous pressure, mean systemic filling pressure and cardiac output after resuscitation and midazolam infusion. The dots are the values derived from Table 1. (a) The working point of the circulation during T1; (b) the volume effect of generalized vasodilatation on CO by midazolam; (c) an additional effect of midazolam on resistance for venous return; (d) the volume effect of generalized vasodilatation on CO by fluid administration after midazolam. Cardiac output; *CVP* central venous pressure

Authors' contributions

JX.C participated in acquisition, analysis, interpretation of data and contributed to the manuscript writing. T.Y participated in the execution of the study, data collection and analysis. F.L and XW.Z conducted the data analysis and participated in manuscript writing. SQ.L, L.L, Y.Y and HB.Q participated in the study design and reviewed the intellectual content. HB.Q participated in study design and coordination of all the study. All authors read and approved the final manuscript.

Author details
[1] Department of Critical Care Medicine, Zhongda Hospital, School of Medicine, Southeast University, 87 Dingjiaqiao Road, Nanjing 210009, People's Republic of China. [2] Anesthesia and Intensive Care, Department of Translational Medicine, Eastern Piedmont University "A. Avogadro", Novara, Italy.

Acknowledgements
Assistance with the study: there was no assistance with the study.

Competing of interests
The authors declare that they have no competing of interests.

Funding
National Natural Science Foundations of China (81501705); Projects of Jiangsu province's medical key discipline (889-KJXW11.3); Special Fund for Health-Scientific Research in the Public Interest Program (No. 201202011); Postgraduate Research and Practice Innovation Program of Jiangsu Province (KYCX17_0168).

References
1. Angus DC, van der Poll T. Severe sepsis and septic shock. N Engl J Med. 2013;369:2063.
2. Monnet X, Marik PE, Teboul JL. Prediction of fluid responsiveness: an update. Ann Intensive Care. 2016;6:111.
3. Michard F, Teboul JL. Predicting fluid responsiveness in ICU patients: a critical analysis of the evidence. Chest. 2002;121:2000–8.
4. Barr J, Fraser GL, Puntillo K, Ely EW, Gelinas C, Dasta JF, Davidson JE, Devlin JW, Kress JP, Joffe AM, Coursin DB, Herr DL, Tung A, Robinson BR, Fontaine DK, Ramsay MA, Riker RR, Sessler CN, Pun B, Skrobik Y, Jaeschke R, American College of Critical Care M. Clinical practice guidelines for the management of pain, agitation, and delirium in adult patients in the intensive care unit. Crit Care Med. 2013;41:263–306.
5. Fujiwara Y, Ito H, Asakura Y, Sato Y, Nishiwaki K, Komatsu T. Preoperative ultra short-term entropy predicts arterial blood pressure fluctuation during the induction of anesthesia. Anesth Analg. 2007;104:853–6.
6. Royse CF, Liew DF, Wright CE, Royse AG, Angus JA. Persistent depression of contractility and vasodilation with propofol but not with sevoflurane or desflurane in rabbits. Anesthesiology. 2008;108:87–93.
7. Ledowski T, Bein B, Hanss R, Paris A, Fudickar W, Scholz J, Tonner PH. Neuroendocrine stress response and heart rate variability: a comparison of total intravenous versus balanced anesthesia. Anesth Analg. 2005;101:1700–5.
8. Rutledge C, Brown B, Benner K, Prabhakaran P, Hayes L. A novel use of methylene blue in the pediatric ICU. Pediatrics. 2015;136:e1030–4.
9. Dellinger RP, Levy MM, Rhodes A, Annane D, Gerlach H, Opal SM, Sevransky JE, Sprung CL, Douglas IS, Jaeschke R, Osborn TM, Nunnally ME, Townsend SR, Reinhart K, Kleinpell RM, Angus DC, Deutschman CS, Machado FR, Rubenfeld GD, Webb SA, Beale RJ, Vincent JL, Moreno R, Surviving Sepsis Campaign Guidelines Committee including the Pediatric S. Surviving sepsis campaign: international guidelines for management of severe sepsis and septic shock: 2012. Crit Care Med. 2013;41:580–637.
10. Monnet X, Jabot J, Maizel J, Richard C, Teboul JL. Norepinephrine increases cardiac preload and reduces preload dependency assessed by passive leg raising in septic shock patients. Crit Care Med. 2011;39:689–94.
11. Yu T, Li Q, Liu L, Guo F, Longhini F, Yang Y, Qiu H. Different effects of propofol and dexmedetomidine on preload dependency in endotoxemic shock with norepinephrine infusion. J Surg Res. 2015;198:185–91.
12. Liet JM, Jacqueline C, Orsonneau JL, Gras-Leguen C, Potel G, Roze JC. The effects of milrinone on hemodynamics in an experimental septic shock model. Pediatr Crit Care Med J Soc Crit Care Med World Fed Pediatr Intensive Crit Care Soc. 2005;6:195–9.
13. Wiel E, Pu Q, Leclerc J, Corseaux D, Bordet R, Lund N, Jude B, Vallet B. Effects of the angiotensin-converting enzyme inhibitor perindopril on endothelial injury and hemostasis in rabbit endotoxic shock. Intensive Care Med. 2004;30:1652–9.
14. Persichini R, Silva S, Teboul JL, Jozwiak M, Chemla D, Richard C, Monnet X. Effects of norepinephrine on mean systemic pressure and venous return in human septic shock. Crit Care Med. 2012;40:3146–53.
15. Freitas FG, Bafi AT, Nascente AP, Assuncao M, Mazza B, Azevedo LC, Machado FR. Predictive value of pulse pressure variation for fluid responsiveness in septic patients using lung-protective ventilation strategies. Br J Anaesth. 2013;110:402–8.
16. Maas JJ, Geerts BF, van den Berg PC, Pinsky MR, Jansen JR. Assessment of venous return curve and mean systemic filling pressure in postoperative cardiac surgery patients. Crit Care Med. 2009;37:912–8.
17. Schmidt C, Roosens C, Struys M, Deryck YL, Van Nooten G, Colardyn F, Van Aken H, Poelaert JI. Contractility in humans after coronary artery surgery. Anesthesiology. 1999;91:58–70.
18. Maas JJ, Pinsky MR, de Wilde RB, de Jonge E, Jansen JR. Cardiac output response to norepinephrine in postoperative cardiac surgery patients: interpretation with venous return and cardiac function curves. Crit Care Med. 2013;41:143–50.
19. Gelman S. Venous function and central venous pressure: a physiologic story. Anesthesiology. 2008;108:735–48.
20. Yu T, Peng X, Liu L, Li Q, Huang Y, Guo F, Yang Y, Qiu H. Propofol

increases preload dependency in septic shock patients. J Surg Res. 2015;193:849–55.

21. Jabot J, Monnet X, Bouchra L, Chemla D, Richard C, Teboul JL. Cardiac function index provided by transpulmonary thermodilution behaves as an indicator of left ventricular systolic function. Crit Care Med. 2009;37:2913–8.

22. Ritter S, Rudiger A, Maggiorini M. Transpulmonary thermodilution-derived cardiac function index identifies cardiac dysfunction in acute heart failure and septic patients: an observational study. Crit Care. 2009;13:R133.

23. De Backer D, Heenen S, Piagnerelli M, Koch M, Vincent JL. Pulse pressure variations to predict fluid responsiveness: influence of tidal volume. Intensive Care Med. 2005;31:517–23.

24. De Backer D, Taccone FS, Holsten R, Ibrahimi F, Vincent JL. Influence of respiratory rate on stroke volume variation in mechanically ventilated patients. Anesthesiology. 2009;110:1092–7.

23

Artificial liver support systems: what is new over the last decade?

Juan José García Martínez[1,2]* and Karim Bendjelid[1,2,3]

Abstract

The liver is a complex organ that performs vital functions of synthesis, heat production, detoxification and regulation; its failure carries a highly critical risk. At the end of the last century, some artificial liver devices began to develop with the aim of being used as supportive therapy until liver transplantation (bridge-to-transplant) or liver regeneration (bridge-to-recovery). The well-recognized devices are the Molecular Adsorbent Recirculating System™ (MARS™), the Single-Pass Albumin Dialysis system and the Fractionated Plasma Separation and Adsorption system (Prometheus™). In the following years, experimental works and early clinical applications were reported, and to date, many thousands of patients have already been treated with these devices. The ability of artificial liver support systems to replace the liver detoxification function, at least partially, has been proven, and the correction of various biochemical parameters has been demonstrated. However, the complex tasks of regulation and synthesis must be addressed through the use of bioartificial systems, which still face several developmental problems and very high production costs. Moreover, clinical data on improved survival are conflicting. This paper reviews the progress achieved and new data published on artificial liver support systems over the past decade and the prospects for these devices.

Keywords: Acute liver failure, Acute on chronic liver failure, Artificial liver support, Albumin dialysis, MARS, Prometheus, SPAD, FPSA

Background

In 2016, liver diseases were responsible for more than one million deaths worldwide, and the trend has been clearly increasing in the last 10 years [1]. Some of these deaths occur in the context of liver failure, in the form of either acute liver failure (ALF) or acute on chronic liver failure (AoCLF). In ALF, the adult mortality is approximately 50%, despite the increase in the number of patients receiving liver transplants. Regarding AoCLF, some recent studies show that one-third of patients hospitalized for cirrhosis with an acute complication develop AoCLF, and their mortality thus increases dramatically [2]. In this context and given the shortage of organs for transplantation, efforts already have been developed to find therapeutic alternatives for patients who are waiting for a new organ (bridge-to-transplant) or who are not

candidates for transplantation but for whom recovery is considered possible (bridge-to-recovery).

From the 1990s and onwards, several systems based on the concept of albumin dialysis have been developed, the best-known being the following: the Molecular Adsorbent Recirculating System™ (MARS™), the Single-Pass Albumin Dialysis system (SPAD) and the Fractionated Plasma Separation and Adsorption system–FPSA (Prometheus™). These systems are based on the concept of albumin dialysis and therefore on the capacity to remove the albumin-bound toxins that accumulate in liver failure. These toxins are thought to be responsible for brain failure resulting from hepatic encephalopathy (HE), renal failure due to hepatorenal syndrome, cardiovascular failure and/or an immunodepression state. These devices can also remove water-soluble substances, such as ammonia, creatinine or urea and smaller proteins such as some cytokines, by standard dialysis.

Some of the substances removed by the different artificial hepatic support systems include conjugate or unconjugated bilirubin or protoporphyrin, bile acids, glycoside

*Correspondence: juanfeira@outlook.com
[1] Intensive Care Unit, Geneva University Hospitals, 4 Rue Gabrielle-Perret-Gentil, 1205 Geneva, Switzerland
Full list of author information is available at the end of the article

Artificial liver support systems: what is new over the last...

213

derivatives, phenols, short- and medium-chain fatty acids, such as octanoate, or heterocyclic organic compounds. Removal of cytokines and other recognized inducers of HE, such as ammonia or amino acids (e.g. tryptophan or glutamine), may be a valuable tool for this major complication of liver failure [3]. Some preclinical and clinical investigations also report the removal of plasmatic nitric oxide (NO) and some pro-inflammatory and anti-inflammatory cytokines, such as tumour necrosis factor alpha (TNF-α), interleukin-6 or interleukin-10 [4, 5], even though the final balance in the setting of ALF or AoCLF and its contribution to multiorgan failure are still unknown.

In the early years following the development of the different liver devices, some clinical trials demonstrated haemodynamic and neurological benefits in their use in patients with ALF and in those with AoCLF, but many of these studies were uncontrolled and included very few patients. Some randomized controlled trials showed an improvement in survival, but the small sample size, high heterogeneity of the included patients and high variability in disease severity prevented definitive conclusions from being reached [6, 7]. However, artificial liver devices have continued to be used in many hospitals, and new experimental and clinical studies on them have been published over the past decade. In the present review, the authors emphasize new data published in this field and discuss the future of these devices.

Methods and materials

We conducted research for relevant articles through Pub-Med (National Institutes of Health) and Web of Science published after 1 January 2008. The filter settings used were "English language" and "French language" and the "humans" filter. The bibliographies of the recovered articles were reviewed to identify any other relevant papers. We included randomized controlled studies preferentially, but we also discussed uncontrolled studies when the statistical comparison versus baseline was provided. We also comment on other relevant literatures.

Molecular Adsorbent Recirculating System (MARS)

The Molecular Adsorbent Recirculating System (MARS) was originally developed by Stange et al. [8]. The technique has been available for broad clinical use since 1998. The system is composed of a blood circuit, an albumin circuit and a classic "renal" circuit. Blood is dialyzed through an albumin-impregnated high-flux dialysis membrane in such a way that hydrophobic albumin-bound toxins are released through the membrane and subsequently collected by albumin in the dialyzate. The method is based on two basic thermodynamic principles: protein-binding affinity and solute movement

along a concentration gradient [9]. The elimination of toxins thus takes place through the diffusion process and depends on the free toxin concentration (which is mainly affected by the molar ratio of toxin to albumin). Toxins are cleared when passing the adsorber columns that contain activated charcoal and anion-exchange resin, and albumin is regenerated and able to accept new toxins when it passes the membrane again. Additionally, the albumin circuit itself is dialyzed in the CRRT (continuous renal replacement therapy) method, diminishing the load of water-soluble toxins.

MARS is the most widely published artificial liver support system. In the first few years following its introduction to the market, several animal and in vitro experiments and clinical studies demonstrated its capacity to remove various albumin-bound and water-soluble metabolites that accumulate in liver failure and are implicated in some of its major complications, such as HE [3, 10].

Another point of interest has been the ability of MARS to eliminate cytokines and modulate the inflammatory response involved in liver failure. Cytokines have been implicated in the development of HE, vasodilation, systemic inflammatory response syndrome (SIRS) and multiple organ failure (MOF). These proteins are believed to mediate hepatic inflammation, cholestasis and liver cell necrosis and apoptosis [11, 12]. From a theoretical standpoint, the removal of some pro-inflammatory cytokines may counteract some clinical complications of liver failure related to the inflammatory and hyperdynamic state. However, anti-inflammatory cytokines would also be removed, and the final imbalance and its contribution to multiorgan failure in the setting of ALF or AoCLF are still unknown. Old and new works show a significant elimination of some pro-inflammatory cytokines, such as TNF-α, interleukin-6 and interleukin-1 β, and anti-inflammatory cytokines, such as interleukin-10, by the MARS device [4, 5, 13]. However, other studies failed to demonstrate an effective change in the plasma cytokine concentration in patients with liver failure, perhaps due to the high rate of production in this setting [14, 15]. In 2013, Donati et al. [16] published the results of 269 MARS treatments that showed no effect on cytokine plasma levels but a significant increase in hepatic growth factor levels (a humoral hepatotrophic factor that enhances liver regeneration). Interestingly, Dominik et al. [17] demonstrated, in an in vitro study, that the removal of some cytokines could be drastically improved by using MARS with larger pore membranes, which could contribute to optimizing the cytokine plasma profile of patients. We must also consider the removal of plasmatic NO, which plays a central role in the multifactorial phenomenon of splanchnic and systemic vasodilatation and the hyperdynamic state associated with liver failure. In conclusion, the precise roles of different cytokines in the pathophysiology of liver failure and the influence of MARS on cytokine plasmatic profiles have not yet been fully elucidated over the last years. This represents undoubtedly a very interesting line of research for the future.

In recent years, some authors have been interested in other active biological substances that can also be removed by MARS. Gay et al. [18] explored the proteins dialyzed and then absorbed in the anion-exchange resin cartridge of MARS in patients with cholestasis and pruritus and found some biological relevant proteins, such as secreted Ly6/uPAR-related protein-1 (SLURP1) or defensin human neutrophil peptide–1 (HNP-1), which are involved in the inflammatory and defensive processes. In contrast, MARS does not appear to influence the plasma levels of other molecules with known immunomodulatory effects, such as neutrophil gelatinase-associated lipocalin (NGAL) or the chemokines monocyte chemoattractant protein-1 (MCP-2) and macrophage inflammatory protein-3 alpha (MIP-3α), according to some published studies [19, 20].

In vitro and in vivo studies have explored the elimination of some antibiotics by MARS, showing, for example, a significant removal of the low protein-bound antibiotics moxifloxacin and meropenem [21]. Similar results have been found with piperacillin/tazobactam. Surprisingly, one case report showed minimal removal of the highly protein-bound immunosuppressive drug tacrolimus [22]. Special attention should be paid to the dose adjustment and monitoring of some critical drugs during MARS sessions, and additional pharmacokinetic studies are required.

The optimal anticoagulation regimen during MARS has also been discussed. This is an important issue considering the difficult haemostasis balance in patients suffering from hepatic failure, who are at high risk of haemorrhagic and thrombotic phenomena. The best-known and most used method is unfractionated heparin, but there are some concerns regarding haemorrhagic risk and heparin-induced thrombocytopenia. Some studies have explored the use of continuous extracorporeal systems without anticoagulation and have found a comparable circuit lifespan [23]. In this sense, the anticoagulant-free approach may be a valid option in patients at high risk of bleeding. Local anticoagulation with citrate may also become a good option if close metabolic monitoring is exercised, and some studies have shown that it is safe and that it guarantees a longer treatment time, preventing filter loss [24, 25]. However, its widespread use cannot be recommended at this stage. In most clinical trials, unfractionated heparin was the anticoagulant of choice, but some studies have used local citrate anticoagulation,

especially trials with FPSA [26, 27], with no reported adverse effects. The use of prostacyclin can be found anecdotally in the literature.

From a technical point of view, several questions have been raised about the stability of the binding properties of albumin after passing the adsorber columns or about the influence and clinical relevance of some stabilizers (such as octanoate) used in commercial albumin preparations [28, 29]. Nevertheless, there are no definitive conclusions, and these issues should be the subject of further study in the future.

With respect to clinical outcomes, several studies were published in the first years following MARS commercial availability, mostly of a retrospective and an uncontrolled nature. Most of them demonstrated benefits in terms of encephalopathy, and some showed improvement in the haemodynamic parameters. The few randomized controlled trials (RCT) assessing survival presented conflicting results [30–32]. These trials included few patients suffering from AoCLF, which was defined in a variable way according to each study. No well-conducted RCTs were published during this period in the field of ALF.

In the last decade, new studies have been performed to help understand the potential clinical benefits of using MARS. Nevertheless, patient series remain limited, definitions and inclusion criteria are strongly variable, and randomized controlled trials are scarce. We have divided recent studies found in the literature according to whether target patients suffer exclusively from ALF or AoCLF or whether both group of patients are included together (mostly in meta-analysis studies). We also report some clinical studies that point to other medical indications for MARS (miscellaneous).

MARS for acute liver failure

Several studies on the use of MARS in the field of ALF have been published in the last decade. These studies are summarized in Table 1.

Unfortunately, only one trial, which was presented by Saliba et al. [33], was controlled and randomized. This trial included 102 patients with ALF and without an absolute contraindication for liver transplantation. Patients were recruited from 16 liver transplantation centres across France (mostly from three centres). The trial could be rated as fair, as it scored 3 on the Oxford quality scoring system [34]. We cannot consider it to be good (scores 4–5) because the trial was not blinded. Patients received conventional treatment alone or conventional treatment combined with MARS and were stratified according to whether or not the ALF was paracetamol induced. The study failed to prove a significant difference in the overall 6-month survival and in the 6-month transplant-free survival and 1-year survival. Additionally, there

Table 1 Studies with clinical endpoints for ALF using MARS

Study	Years	Design	Patients number	Outcomes	Comments	LOE
Kantola et al. [35]	2008	Controlled, non-randomized MARS + SMT vs. SMT	159	No improvement in 28-day and 6-month survivals	Trend to improved survival in unknown aetiology subgroup. Likely improvement in HE	2
Novelli et al. [45]	2008	Uncontrolled, prospective	6	Neurological and haemodynamic improvements*	Paediatric population. PELD and SOFA improvement**	3
Novelli et al. [46]	2009	Uncontrolled, retrospective	45	Number of MARS treatments associated with survival*	No improvement with MARS is a predictive factor of a fatal outcome and the need for a transplant	3
Camus et al. [47]	2009	Uncontrolled, retrospective	18	Clinical improvement. MARS therapy associated with withdrawal from the emergency transplantation list*	Clinical improvement compared to a control group obtained from a national register*	3
Saliba et al. [33]	2013	Controlled, randomized, multicentre MARS + SMT vs. SMT	102	No improvement in 6-month, 6-month transplantation-free and 1-year survivals	High transplant rate and short waiting time until transplant. Similar adverse effects	1
Lexmond et al. [36]	2015	Controlled, non-randomized MARS + SMT vs. SMT	20	No improvement in survival	Patients in MARS group were sicker. Patients in MARS group received more thrombocyte transfusion*. Paediatric population	2
Gerth et al. [37]	2017	Controlled, non-randomized MARS + SMT vs. SMT	73	No improvement in 28-day survival	Patients with graft dysfunction included. No differences in outcomes between subgroups. Biochemical improvement**	2
Hanish et al. [48]	2017	Uncontrolled, retrospective	27	Improvement in encephalopathy and in the APACHE II score**	Biochemical improvement*	3
Quintero Bernabeu et al. [49]	2018	Uncontrolled, retrospective	11	Haemodynamic improvement*	Paediatric population. No significant adverse effects	3

LOE level of evidence, determined using the strength of recommendation taxonomy (SORT) criteria [50], SMT standard medical therapy, HE hepatic encephalopathy, PELD paediatric end-stage liver disease, SOFA sequential organ failure assessment, APACHE II Acute Physiology and Chronic Health Evaluation II

*p < 0.01

**p < 0.05

was no significant improvement in encephalopathy with the MARS therapy, unlike most other published works. It is noted that the 6-month transplant-free survival was greater among the patients with paracetamol-induced ALF than that of the others (38% vs. 13%, respectively, $p < 0.01$). These disappointing results must be interpreted carefully, as the high transplantation rate and the short delay from randomization to liver transplantation in the study preclude definitive conclusions. Indeed, 14 of the 53 patients in the MARS group initially eligible for analysis were ultimately excluded because they did not receive MARS or they only received a short session of it because an organ was readily available. Sixty-six patients (64.7%) underwent transplantation, of whom 75% did so within the first 24 h following a wait-list registration. As patients with contraindication to liver transplantation were excluded from the trial, we cannot indicate whether the use of MARS might be helpful in this population and whether these patients could especially benefit from this technique (last-line treatment).

Some non-randomized controlled studies were also published, the largest being the work of Kantola et al. [35], which included 113 prospectively collected patients who received MARS and a retrospectively collected historic control group of 46 patients with whom they were compared. There was no significant difference in the 28-day and 6-month survival rates between the two groups. The native liver recovery rate of the MARS group was higher than that of the control group (49% vs. 17%, respectively, $p < 0.01$), and the transplant-free survival was also higher (66% vs. 40%, $p < 0.05$). However, the trial design and the predominantly toxic aetiology of ALF in the MARS group greatly hampered the interpretation of these results. In the most homogenous subgroup of patients with ALF of an unknown aetiology, there was a trend towards a better survival, but this was without statistical significance. The MARS patients in the other subgroups had a significantly lower model for end-stage liver disease (MELD) score compared to that of the control group, which also precludes definitive conclusions.

Two other controlled trials recently published failed to prove a survival improvement with MARS. As these are non-randomized studies, inclusion in the intervention group depended, to a large extent, on the treating physician, which is a major bias. In the work of Lexmond et al. [36], MARS treatment was reserved for the most severe patients, and these patients had a significantly higher HE grade (3.4 vs. 2, respectively, $p < 0.01$) and PELD (Paediatric End-Stage Liver Disease)/MELD score (47 vs. 38, $p < 0.05$) than those in the other group. In the study published by Gerth et al. [37], the whole cohort was composed of mildly ill patients (HE grade ≤ 1 and no vasopressor drugs). Some uncontrolled studies show

haemodynamic and neurological improvements but include few patients and are of limited quality.

MARS for acute on chronic liver failure

Trials published in the setting of AoCLF are summarized in Table 2. Only one correctly randomized controlled trial assessing survival and other clinical outcomes in this setting has been published in recent years: the RELIEF trial by Bañares et al. [38]. This relatively large multicentric trial, which scored 3 on the Oxford quality scoring system [34], failed to demonstrate a survival benefit with MARS use in both the general population included and in all of the predefined subgroups. The study showed a trend of improvement in HE in the MARS group compared to that of the control group, but this was without statistical significance. It should be pointed out that some of the exclusion criteria (platelets < 50.000/mm3, international normalized ratio > 2.3 or haemodynamic instability) could have ruled out the more severe patients. The authors also discuss the appropriateness of the schedule or dosage of the MARS sessions chosen.

In a different way, a work presented by Hessel et al. [39], which was primarily designed to explore the cost-effectiveness of MARS in patients with AoCLF, showed that the cumulative survival probability at 3 years was higher in the MARS group (logrank $p < 0.05$). However, the randomization in the study was rather unclear, and the follow-up was too long to interpret the true influence of the technique on mortality.

Recently, Gerth et al. [40] published a retrospective, controlled, non-randomized study that included 101 patients with AoCLF graded according to the new Chronic Liver Failure Consortium (CLIF-C) criteria [41]. The study showed a significant reduction in early mortality in the MARS group compared to that of the standard medical therapy (SMT) group on day 7 (0% vs. 18.5%, respectively, $p < 0.01$) and day 14 (6.4% vs. 27.8%, $p < 0.05$). This effect disappeared at day 21, which could be explained by the interruption of therapy (in the MARS group, extracorporeal therapy was performed almost daily, with a median of three sessions per patient). The 14-day mortality was especially reduced among patients with two or more organ failures (9.5% in MARS group vs. 50% in SMT group, p < 0.01). Furthermore, in Kaplan–Meier estimates of the 28-day survival rate in this subgroup of patients, MARS was associated with improvement (logrank $p < 0.05$). Similarly, the authors performed a secondary analysis of the RELIEF trial data (36) using the CLIF-C criteria and showed a benefit from MARS in regard to the 14-day mortality in the subgroup of patients with two or more organ failures, but this was without statistical significance. Despite its limitations, this study suggests the necessity for further

Table 2 Studies with clinical endpoints for AoCLF using MARS

Study	Years	Design	Patients number	Outcomes	Comments	LOE
Hessel et al. [39]	2010	Controlled, randomized MARS + SMT vs. SMT	149	3-year survival improvement*	Acceptable cost-outcome ratio (measured by cost per LYG and costs per QALY)	2
					Inadequate randomization	
Novelli et al. [51]	2010	Controlled, non-randomized MARS vs. SMT	20	MELD improvement**	Delta MELD predict survival	2
Bañares et al. [38]	2013	Controlled, randomized, multicentre MARS + SMT vs. SMT	156	No improvement in 28-day and 90-day transplant-free survivals	No differences in 28-day transplant-free survival in subgroups: MELD > 20, HRS at admission, severe HE, and progressive hyper-bilirubinemia	1
Gerth et al. [40]	2017	Controlled, non-randomized MARS + SMT vs. SMT	101	Improvement in 7-day** and 14-day*** transplant-free survivals	No differences in 21-day and 28-day transplant-free survivals	2
					Improvement in estimate 28-day transplant-free survival rate in subgroup of patients with two or more organs failure (CLIF-ACLF grade ≥ 2)*	

LOE level of evidence, determined using the strength of recommendation taxonomy (SORT) criteria [50], *SMT* standard medical therapy, *LYG* life years gained, *QALY* quality-adjusted life years, *MELD* model for end-stage liver disease, *HRS* hepatorenal syndrome, *HE* hepatic encephalopathy, *CLIF-ACLF* chronic liver failure-acute-on-chronic liver failure

*logrank $p < 0.05$

**$p < 0.01$

***$p < 0.05$

trials targeting those more severe patients suffering from AoCLF, who may especially benefit from the technique.

In addition, a meta-analysis published by Shen et al. [42] in 2016, which enrolled studies that included patients with AoCLF, showed a significative reduction in mortality with the use of artificial liver support systems. However, this meta-analysis included several non-randomized trials, and some of the studies used restrictive inclusion criteria and techniques other than MARS in the intervention group. The largest RCT used plasma exchange as liver support and included only patients with HBV-associated AoCLF [43]. These encouraging results must therefore be interpreted with caution.

Trials in the setting of AoCLF are conditioned by the absence of a worldwide recognized definition of AoCLF, which makes the selection of patients for these studies quite variable [44]. In this regard, the acceptance and use of an international definition can be a key step in optimizing future research.

MARS for acute liver failure and acute on chronic liver failure combined

The few published trials that included ALF and AoCLF patients together are uncontrolled and retrospective. Notwithstanding, several systematic reviews and meta-analyses including RCTs published over the last 20 years

have been presented recently. These studies included patients with ALF and AoCLF, and they are summarized in Table 3.

The meta-analysis published by Vaid et al. [52] in 2012 and the one published by Tsipotis et al. [53] in 2015 included quite similar trials. However, the work of Tsipotis included only RCT trials and was published 3 years later, allowing the authors to include the larger study by Saliba et al. [33] and complete data from the study by Bañares et al. [38], which had already been included in the meta-analysis by Vaid but which was reported as only a scientific abstract at the time. Both meta-analyses showed an improvement in hepatic encephalopathy with MARS (OR = 3.0, $p < 0.01$ in the Vaid study; RR = 1.5, $p < 0.01$ in the Tsipotis study). Disappointingly, neither meta-analysis showed a significant effect of MARS on mortality. Tsipotis also included some trials using Prometheus in its meta-analysis, such as the RCT published by Kribben et al. [26], which were meta-analyzed separately and combined with MARS trials with the same result.

Two systematic reviews, one published by Stutchfield et al. [54] in 2011 and the other by Guo-Lin He et al. [55] in 2015, conducted a separate meta-analysis for trials involving patients with ALF or AoCLF. In both studies, extracorporeal liver support significantly reduced

Table 3 Studies with clinical endpoints for ALF and AoCLF combined using MARS

Study	Years	Design	Patients number	Outcomes	Comments	LOE
Rusu et al. [59]	2009	Uncontrolled, retrospective	27	Improvement in HE in ALF**	Haemodynamic improvement in patients with liver failure post-transplantation**	3
				No clinical improvement in AoCLF		
Stutchfield et al. [54]	2011	Systematic review	8 RCT	ELS improved survival in ALF**	Independent meta-analysis for trials including patients with ALF or AoCLF	2
				No statistically significant reduction in mortality in AoCLF	3 trials using bioartificial devices included	
Vaid et al. [52]	2012	Meta-analysis	9 RCT 1 NRS	Improvement in HE*	No significant differences in subgroups (by age or MARS number sessions)	2
				No statistically significant reduction in overall mortality	Safety data no meta-analyzed	
Cisneros-Garza et al. [60]	2014	Uncontrolled, retrospective	70	Improvement in HE*	Patients with cholestasis disease were included. MARS associated with improved itching	3
Tsipotis et al. [53]	2015	Meta-analysis	10 RCT	Improvement in HE*	No significant differences in subgroups (by number of sessions or type of albumin dialysis technique)	2
				No statistically significant reduction in overall mortality	3 trials used Prometheus	
Guo-Lin He et al. [55]	2015	Systematic review	10 RCT	Reduction in mortality in ALF**	Independent meta-analysis for trials including patients with ALF or AoCLF	
				No statistically significant reduction in mortality in AoCLF	Very few patients with ALF included	2

LOE level of evidence, determined using the strength of recommendation taxonomy (SORT) criteria [50], *HE* hepatic encephalopathy, *RCT* randomized controlled trial, *ELS* extracorporeal liver support, *NRS* non-randomized controlled study

*$p < 0.01$

**$p < 0.05$

mortality in patients with ALF compared to SMT, and no beneficial effect on survival in AoCLF was found. However, the study of Stutchfield et al. included trials using bioartificial devices, precluding any specific conclusion for MARS.

In the systematic review by Guo-Lin He et al., only trials using MARS in the intervention group were included. In the meta-analysis of the four RCTs that involved patients with ALF, the authors compared the survival in the non-transplanted patients and found that MARS therapy significantly reduced mortality compared to SMT (RR = 0.61, $p < 0.05$). This result can be confounding because very few patients were included. Furthermore, the inclusion criteria are quite different over the studies with two trials exclusively involving patients with

liver failure secondary to cardiogenic shock. With the exception of the Saliba study [33], the other RCTs did not report on follow-up or allocation data, and scored low on the CONSORT score analysis [56]. One study did not have survival as a primary outcome. Nevertheless, the results are consistent across studies ($p = 0.52$; $I^2 = 0\%$) and suggest that MARS may be a valuable tool in the subgroup of patients with ALF who are critically ill.

Another meta-analysis published by Zheng et al. [57] in 2013 found a mortality benefit of artificial liver support systems over SMT in patients with liver failure. However, the study did not focus on albumin dialysis and included earlier studies using transfusion, haemoperfusion, haemofiltration and other outdated devices, such as the Bio-Logic-DT system.

In this regard, and in order to identify the patients who could most benefit from MARS therapy, Kantola et al. [58] analyzed 188 patients treated with MARS, most of whom suffered from ALF or AoCLF (some patients with graft failure and other liver injuries were also included). In this prospective observational study, the authors identified the aetiology of liver disease as the main factor in the survival and recovery without transplantation, with the non-transplanted patients with AoCLF having the highest mortality and probably benefitting minimally from the MARS treatment. The 1-year survival rates of all of the transplanted patients in the study were very high (91% for the ALF patients), which the authors attributed to the clinical and biochemical improvements achieved with MARS. The grade of encephalopathy prior to MARS treatment and coagulation factors levels were identified as prognostic factors in ALF.

At this time, larger RCTs with well-defined inclusion criteria are still required to confirm the benefits of MARS and to be able to widely recommend its use. In the case of ALF, which is often a life-threatening condition, the use of MARS as a bridge-to-transplant to gain time or, eventually, as a bridge-to-recovery, is warranted.

Miscellaneous

Table 4 summarizes recently published trials in which MARS was used in clinical indications other than for ALF or AoCLF. At least one ongoing RCT was identified on the US-based clinical trials registration website (Molecular Adsorbent Recirculating System (MARS®) in Hypoxic Hepatitis, clinicaltrials.gov: NCT01690845). The current status of this trial is unknown.

Single-Pass Albumin Dialysis (SPAD)

Single-Pass Albumin Dialysis was described as an alternative to more sophisticated devices, such as MARS, in the late 1990s [65]. It is the simplest artificial liver device and can be applied in any intensive care unit employing a standard CRRT. No additional adsorbent columns or circuits are required. The patient's blood is dialyzed through a high-flux hollow-fibre haemodiafilter using an albumin-containing dialyzate. After passing through the dialyzer, the dialyzate is discarded (in contrast to the MARS system, in which the albumin dialyzate is regenerated), and the toxins are thus removed from the system. High amounts of albumin are consumed with SPAD, making this treatment substantially expensive.

In 2004, Sauer et al. [66] published one of the first papers comparing the in vitro detoxification capacities of SPAD and MARS for water-soluble and protein-bound compounds (bilirubin and bile acids) and demonstrated that the performances of the two were similar and that both were superior to standard continuous venovenous haemodiafiltration (CVVHD). The authors used a 4.4% albumin dialyzate solution.

These results were partially confirmed in vivo by Kortgen et al. [67], who compared the detoxification capacity of the two techniques in patients with liver failure.

Table 4 Studies using MARS in clinical indications other than for ALF or AoCLF

Study	Years	Design	Patients number	Clinical indication	Outcomes	LOE
Wong et al. [61]	2009	Uncontrolled, prospective	6	Type 1 HRS refractory to vasoconstrictor therapy	No improvement in haemodynamics	3
					No improvement in GFR; temporary improvement of creatinine during MARS**	
					Reduction in NO levels**	
Schaefer et al. [62]	2012	Uncontrolled, retrospective	3	Severe cholestatic pruritus	Paediatric patients	3
					Significant decrease in NRS score*	
					135 MARS sessions in total, during 4, 8 and 13 months prior liver transplantation	
Lavayssière et al. [63]	2013	Uncontrolled, retrospective	32	Type 1 HRS	No improvement in renal function	3
					In patients receiving norepinephrine, significant dose reductions**	
Gilg et al. [64]	2018	Uncontrolled, prospective	10	Post-hepatectomy liver failure	No improvement in MELD	3
					No major complications reported	

LOE level of evidence, determined using the strength of recommendation taxonomy (SORT) criteria [50], *HRS* hepatorenal syndrome, *GFR* glomerular filtration rate, *NO* nitric oxide, *NRS score* numeric rating scale, NRS 0: no pruritus, NRS 10: maximal pruritus, *MELD* model for end-stage liver disease

$*p < 0.01$

$**p < 0.05$

They showed a significant decrease in the serum bilirubin level with both treatments. However, only with MARS did the creatinine and urea levels significantly decrease. There were no significant differences in the other biochemical, haemodynamic or clinical values. The study was retrospective and non-randomized, and there were far fewer patients in the SPAD arm than there were in the MARS arm. The authors performed SPAD with a 5% albumin dialyzate solution and a low dialyzate flow rate (700 mL/h), which probably influenced the results.

The determination of the optimal albumin concentration in the dialyzate solution or that of the most efficient dialyzate flow rate when carrying out SPAD was already addressed by Churchwell et al. [68] in 2009. They compared the effect of various blood flow rates, dialyzate flow rates, dialyzate albumin concentrations (0%, 2.5% and 5%) and dialyzers on the clearance of some highly protein-bound drugs (valproic acid and carbamazepine). The authors demonstrated that the highest extraction ratios were achieved using the combination of 5% albumin dialyzate and a larger polysulfone dialyzer (surface area 1.5 m^2). Two years later, Benyoub et al. [69] showed significant reductions in the bilirubin and bile acid levels in patients suffering from ALF or AoCLF from using SPAD with a 3.2% albumin dialyzate and a 1000 mL/h dialyzate flow rate. More recently, Schmuck et al. [70] found, in an in vitro model, an optimal detoxification efficiency for albumin-bound substances (bilirubin and bile acids) with a 3% albumin concentration and a dialyzate flow rate of 1000 mL/h. They used SPAD with conventional CVVHD and a high-flux polysulfone haemodiafilter.

With respect to clinical data on SPAD, only a few case reports were published in the early years, and there are currently no published studies that focus on demonstrating the clinical benefits of SPAD versus standard medical therapy (SMT) in ALF or AoCLF. Two retrospective uncontrolled studies reviewing data from patients with liver failure treated with SPAD as rescue therapy were identified. One included paediatric patients with ALF of different aetiologies [71], and the other included adults patients with severe liver dysfunction in a context of alcoholic liver disease who were treated with SPAD or Prometheus [72]. Neither of these studies allow us to draw conclusions about the clinical usefulness of SPAD, and they only show us its relative ease of use and the absence of unexpected complications from its use.

The only randomized study using SPAD was recently published by Sponholz et al. [73]. This is a randomized, controlled crossover study comparing the detoxification capacity and influence on clinical and paraclinical parameters of SPAD (4% albumin dialyzate solution; 700 mL/h dialysis flow rate) and MARS (20% albumin flow rate equal to the blood flow rate, 2000 mL/h dialysis flow rate). The authors found similar reductions in the total plasma bilirubin levels, without significant differences between the two devices. The reductions in the total bile acids and γ-glutamyl transferase levels in the SPAD arm were non-significant. The creatinine and urea levels were not significantly reduced with SPAD compared to those of MARS. In contrast to other studies, neither MARS nor SPAD induced a reduction in the systemic cytokine levels. Moreover, the patients treated with SPAD presented some metabolic derangements such as increasing lactate levels or decreasing calcium levels, which are probably explained by the preferential use of citrate anti-coagulation with a low dialysis flow rate. The effects of MARS and SPAD on the clinical parameters (HE and haemodynamic status) were small and equivalent.

Currently, SPAD may be an easy-to-use alternative to MARS, but the optimal albumin dialyzate concentration, dialyzate flow rate and treatment regimen are not yet fully established. A new randomized crossover trial comparing MARS and SPAD (with the change in the plasma levels of total bilirubin as the primary endpoint, and with tolerance, change in bile acid levels, change in conjugate bilirubin levels, pulsatility index of the middle cerebral artery and HE score as the secondary endpoints) is underway. The recruitment phase of the study has actually completed (clinicaltrials.gov: NCT02310542).

Fractionated Plasma Separation and Adsorption– FPSA (Prometheus)

The FPSA method was first described by Falkenhagen et al. [74]. While MARS uses an exogenous albumin solution, the available Prometheus machine allows for the patient's own albumin to enter the first circuit using the AlbuFlow® filter (molecular cut-off of 250 kDa). Albumin is reactivated and returned to circulation using a neutral resin adsorber (Prometh® 01) and an anion-exchange column (Prometh® 02). The blood then enters a second circuit where it is treated by conventional high-flux haemodialysis before being returned to the patient.

In the first 10 years after its appearance on the market, some studies demonstrated the in vitro and in vivo efficacy of Prometheus in clearing ammonia, bilirubin or bile acids, showing that it performs even better than MARS does [75].

These results have been confirmed in recent years. In 2009, Grodzicki el al. [76] showed significant decreases in serum ammonia, bilirubin, aspartate aminotransferase, alanine aminotransferase, urea and creatinine with the use of FPSA in patients suffering from ALF. Rifai et al. [77] demonstrated a decrease in almost all twenty-six of the amino acids measured in nine patients with liver failure (eight of them with an HE grade of 2 or more) with a single FPSA session. Some of the amino acids cleared

Artificial liver support systems: what is new over the last...

221

(such as glutamine, phenylalanine, tyrosine and tryptophan) have been directly implicated in the development of HE, suggesting that FPSA may improve this serious condition associated with liver failure. In another study involving patients with ALF monitored by cerebral microdialysis, the authors found the same trend in the removal of aromatic amino acids (especially phenylalanine) from the arterial blood after a single FPSA session, but it was surprisingly without a significant change in the concentrations measured in the microdialyzate [78]. It should be noted, in this regard, that one of the inclusion criteria was a high risk of intracranial hypertension, but the patients did not need to have clinical encephalopathy. On the same topic, we found an interesting paper published by Ryska et al. [79] that described the influence of Prometheus therapy on the evolution of intracranial pressure (ICP) in a well-conducted experimental model of ALF in pigs. The authors showed a significant reduction in the ICP in the group treated with FPSA compared to that of the control group (24 mmHg vs. 29.8 mmHg, respectively, 12 h after liver devascularization, $p < 0.05$) again indicating the probable usefulness of Prometheus in HE.

On the removal of cytokines and other molecules involved in the development and evolution of liver failure, Rocen et al. [80] measured the concentrations of cytokines, inflammatory markers (C-reactive protein and procalcitonin) and liver regeneration markers, such as hepatocyte growth factor (HGF) and α1 fetoprotein, during FPSA sessions in eleven patients with ALF of different aetiologies (nine of whom were finally transplanted). The authors showed a significant decrease in most cytokines and inflammatory marker concentrations with Prometheus, which contrasts the results of previous research [81]. Nevertheless, no clinical improvement, except for improvement of encephalopathy, was demonstrated. Surprisingly, the HGF concentration increased significantly, which could favour hepatic regeneration. As with MARS, the ability of Prometheus to influence the cytokine profile and the final clinical outcome of this action are still unclear and require further research.

Few clinical studies evaluating the survival or other clinical outcomes with Prometheus were published in the 2000s. A randomized controlled trial published during this period by Laleman et al. [81] compared SMT with MARS and Prometheus in patients presenting AoCLF, and only MARS showed benefits in some of the included haemodynamic variables, such as mean arterial pressure, stroke volume or systemic resistances. Survival was not assessed in this study. Dethloff et al. [82] showed the same tendency to improve mean arterial pressure only with MARS treatment in a randomized controlled study comparing MARS, Prometheus and conventional

haemodialysis in patients with decompensated cirrhosis. These different actions on haemodynamics of MARS and Prometheus have no obvious explanation. As described above, MARS and Prometheus may influence cytokine and inflammatory molecules concentrations, thus inducing haemodynamic changes, but the final balance for both is unknown. Several studies have demonstrated a reduction in NO levels with MARS [4, 81], which is probably removed in its main circulating complexed form, S-nitroso-serum albumin [83], but the use of Prometheus probably also influences NO levels [84]. In addition, most of the clinical trials published so far using MARS or Prometheus in AoCLF did not use haemodynamic outcomes and description of haemodynamic changes with treatment was often not included. It should also be noted that haemodynamically unstable patients were systematically excluded in these studies.

Over the last few years, only a limited number of studies have used clinical endpoints (Table 5). The most important was the HELIOS study, which was published in 2012 by Kribben et al. [26]. This is a multicentric randomized controlled trial comparing Prometheus with SMT in 145 patients with AoCLF, and the primary endpoint was the probabilities of survival at 28 days and 90 days (irrespective of liver transplantation). This RCT scored 3 on the Oxford quality scoring system. This trial failed to prove a survival benefit with Prometheus in the overall patient population, and the patient recruitment was interrupted after the interim analysis (90 patients) due to futility (204 patients were initially planned for inclusion in the study). It is important to note that in the overall population the probability of survival was slightly higher in the Prometheus group compared to the SMT group (90-day survival probability: 47% vs. 38%) but without statistical significance.

Among the predefined subgroups analyzed, the survival probability of patients with more severe liver disease (MELD > 30) treated with Prometheus was significantly higher than that of the patients treated with SMT alone (90-day survival probability: 48% vs. 9%, respectively, logrank $p < 0.05$). In the subgroups of patients with less sever disease (MELD < 20 and MELD 20–30), differences in survival are not statistically significant. This may indicate the usefulness of Prometheus when applied to more severe patients, but this conclusion is strongly limited by the small size of the subgroups.

Some other studies, although quite heterogeneous, have been published in recent years. Sentürk el al. [27] compared the biochemical and clinical parameters during FPSA in patients with ALF and AoCLF, demonstrating a significant improvement in the biochemical parameters and in HE. Survival was not assessed in this study. Komardina et al. [85] described haemodynamic

Table 5 Studies with clinical endpoints using Prometheus

Study	Years	Design	Patients number	Liver disease	Outcomes	LOE
Sentürk et al. [27]	2010	Uncontrolled, prospective	27	ALF AoCLF	Biochemical improvement Improvement in HE*	3
Kribben et al. [26]	2012	Randomized, controlled, multi-centric Prometheus + SMT vs SMT	145	AoCLF	No improvement in 28-day and 90-day survivals, except in sub-group with MELD > 30 Similar adverse effects	1
Bergis et al. [86]	2012	Controlled, non-randomized, multicentric	20	Amanitas phalloides intoxication and liver dysfunction	No statistically significance difference in survivals	2
Komardina et al. [85]	2017	Uncontrolled, prospective	39	Ischaemic ALF	Haemodynamic and biochemical improvements**	3

LOE level of evidence, determined using the strength of recommendation taxonomy (SORT) criteria [50], *HE* hepatic encephalopathy, *SMT* standard medical therapy, *MLED* model for end-stage liver disease

*$p < 0.05$

**$p < 0.01$

and biochemical improvements with Prometheus in patients with ischaemic ALF (complication after cardiac surgery), but no change in the survival was shown. Surprisingly, the overall mortality was very high in the study (only 9 of the 39 patients included were alive at day 28).

Other devices

Some new artificial devices, or modifications to currently used systems, have been developed in the past few years.

Marangoni et al. [87] presented the so-called high-efficiency MARS by inserting a double adsorption unit (double columns containing charcoal and another pair with ion-exchange resin, mounted in parallel) into the albumin circuit. The authors compared the detoxification capacity of their system with that of the "classical" MARS in four patients with liver failure and showed that the "improved" MARS was notably more effective in removing bilirubin and bile acids.

An hybrid extracorporeal protocol was presented by Akcan Arikan et al. [88], which combined high-flux CRRT for hyperammonaemia, therapeutic plasma exchange for coagulopathy and MARS for hepatic encephalopathy. They presented this protocol in a retrospective observational study that included fifteen paediatric patients with ALF or AoCLF, who were supported with this therapy and showed improvement in HE.

In 2017, one experimental study by Al-Chalabi et al. [89] using an animal model of ALF in pigs and one uncontrolled clinical trial by Huber et al. [90] including 14 patients with liver failure were published, both of which used a new device called ADVOS (ADVanced Organ Support). The laboratory prototype of ADVOS was first presented in 2013 [91] and included an extracorporeal blood circuit, a dialyzate circuit containing standard dialyzate with a 2–4% albumin concentration and a third circuit where the albumin dialyzate was divided into two parts. Before reaching the cation and anion filters, each part undergoes a change in the pH value by the addition of acid or base and is subjected to a temperature change, resulting in a release of albumin-bound toxins. The resulting dialyzates containing toxin-free albumin join with each other in order to reach the desired pH before entering the haemodialyzer again. In the animal study mentioned above, all of the animals treated by ADVOS survived (5 out of 10), whereas the pigs treated with SMT died in the 10-h observation period ($p < 0.01$). Significant haemodynamic and biochemical improvements were demonstrated with ADVOS. A significant decrease in the bilirubin level was also demonstrated in the clinical trial published by Huber et al. [90]. No further clinical studies on this promising technique have been published so far.

Some modifications of the techniques described above, such as plasma diafiltration and some protocols already used several years ago to treat liver failure, such as plasma exchange or therapeutic apheresis using a bilirubin adsorbent column, are also found anecdotally in the literature [43, 92, 93].

Conclusion

Severe liver failure is associated with high mortality, as many patients die despite undergoing optimal medical treatment. Even if liver transplantation has emerged as an essential therapy, many patients with this disease will unfortunately die while waiting for a hepatic transplant. Consequently, there is a clear need for a liver support system to provide a "bridge" to a final treatment. Over the last two decades, several artificial liver support systems with promised advances were

Artificial liver support systems: what is new over the last...

223

introduced. However, whether such improvements could be translated into survival benefit is still uncertain, given the scarcity of available results of RCTs. The present reality is probably related to several factors, including the involvement of several interconnected organs and the fact that liver failure patients constitute a heterogeneous population with severe multimorbidity [94]. Moreover, there is no precise recommendation on the effective timing of the initiation of artificial liver support systems. In this regard, the future prospects of artificial liver support systems should rely on the completion of adequately powered RCTs addressing these crucial clinical issues and endpoints. New indications for this organ support, such as post-hepatectomy liver failure, should also be explored. In the meantime, and in the absence of alternative options to support this vital organ, it is difficult to criticize the cautious use of these secured artificial liver devices as "salvage" therapy in patients suffering from ALF or severe AoCLF.

Abbreviations
MARS: Molecular Adsorbent Recirculating System; SPAD: Single-Pass Albumin Dialysis; ALF: acute liver failure; AoCLF: acute on chronic liver failure; HE: hepatic encephalopathy; NO: nitric oxide; TNF-α: tumour necrosis factor alpha; CRRT: continuous renal replacement therapy; RCT: randomized controlled trial; PELD: paediatric end-stage liver disease; MELD: model for end-stage liver disease; CLIF-C: Chronic Liver Failure Consortium; SMT: standard medical therapy; OR: odds ratio; RR: risk ratio; CVVHD: continuous venovenous haemodiafiltration; ICP: intracranial pressure; HGF: hepatocyte growth factor; ADVOS: advanced organ support.

Author details
¹ Intensive Care Unit, Geneva University Hospitals, 4 Rue Gabrielle-Perret-Gentil, 1205 Geneva, Switzerland. ² Faculty of Medicine, University of Geneva, Geneva, Switzerland. ³ Geneva Hemodynamic Research Group, Geneva, Switzerland.

Authors' contributions
JJGM drafted the majority of the manuscript. KB contributed to manuscript drafting and revised critically the manuscript. All authors read and approved the final manuscript.

Acknowledgements
Not applicable.

Competing interests
The authors declare that they have no competing interests.

Funding
No funding was obtained for the creation of this review.

References
1. Naghavi M, Abajobir AA, Abbafati C, Abbas KM, Abd-Allah F, Abera SF, et al. Global, regional, and national age-sex specific mortality for 264 causes of death, 1980–2016: a systematic analysis for the Global Burden of Disease Study 2016. Lancet. 2017;390(10100):1151–210.
2. Moreau R, Arroyo V. Acute-on-chronic liver failure: a new clinical entity. Clin Gastroenterol Hepatol. 2015;13(5):836–41.
3. Koivusalo AM, Teikari T, Hockerstedt K, Isoniemi H. Albumin dialysis has a favorable effect on amino acid profile in hepatic encephalopathy. Metab Brain Dis. 2008;23(4):387–98.
4. Guo L-MLJ-Y, Xu D-Z, Li B-S, Han H, Wang L-H, Zhang W-Y, Lu L-H, Guo X, Sun F-X, Zhang H-Y, Liu X-D, Zhang J-P, Yao Y, He Z-P, Wang M-M. Application of molecular adsorbents recirculating system to remove NO and cytokines in severe liver failure patients with multiple organ dysfunction syndrome. Liver Int. 2003;23(Suppl. 3):16–20.
5. Novelli G, Annesini MC, Morabito V, Cinti P, Pugliese F, Novelli S, et al. Cytokine level modifications: molecular adsorbent recirculating system versus standard medical therapy. Transpl Proc. 2009;41(4):1243–8.
6. Karvellas CJ, Gibney N, Kutsogiannis D, Wendon J, Bain VG. Bench-to-bedside review: current evidence for extracorporeal albumin dialysis systems in liver failure. Crit Care. 2007;11(3):215.
7. Sgroi A, Serre-Beinier V, Morel P, Buhler L. What clinical alternatives to whole liver transplantation? Current status of artificial liver devices and hepatocyte transplantation. Transplantation. 2009;87(4):457–66.
8. Stange J, Ramlow W, Mitzner S, Schmidt R, Klinkmann H. Dialysis against a recycled albumin solution enables the removal of albumin-bound toxins. Artif Organs. 1993;17(9):809–13.
9. Patzer J. Principles of bound solute dialysis. Ther Apheresis Dial. 2006;10(2):118–24.
10. Novelli G, Rossi M, Pretagostini M, Pugliese F, Ruberto F, Novelli L, et al. One hundred sixteen cases of acute liver failure treated with MARS. Transpl Proc. 2005;37(6):2557–9.
11. Liu Q. Role of cytokines in the pathophysiology of acute-on-chronic liver failure. Blood Purif. 2009;28:331–41.
12. Luo M, Guo JY, Cao WK. Inflammation: a novel target of current therapies for hepatic encephalopathy in liver cirrhosis. World J Gastroenterol. 2015;21(41):11815–24.
13. Isoniemi H, Koivusalo AM, Repo H, Ilonen I, Hockerstedt K. The effect of albumin dialysis on cytokine levels in acute liver failure and need for liver transplantation. Transpl Proc. 2005;37(2):1088–90.
14. Ilonen I, Koivusalo AM, Repo H, Hockerstedt K, Isoniemi H. Cytokine profiles in acute liver failure treated with albumin dialysis. Artif Organs. 2008;32(1):52–60.
15. Stadlbauer V, Krisper P, Aigner R, Haditsch B, Jung A, Lackner C, et al. Effect of extracorporeal liver support by MARS and Prometheus on serum cytokines in acute-on-chronic liver failure. Crit Care. 2006;10(6):R169.
16. Donati G, La Manna G, Cianciolo G, Grandinetti V, Carretta E, Cappuccilli M, et al. Extracorporeal detoxification for hepatic failure using molecular adsorbent recirculating system: depurative efficiency and clinical results in a long-term follow-up. Artif Organs. 2014;38(2):125–34.
17. Dominik A, Stange J, Pfensig C, Borufka L, Weiss-Reining H, Eggert M. Reduction of elevated cytokine levels in acute/acute-on-chronic liver failure using super-large pore albumin dialysis treatment: an in vitro study. Ther Apheresis Dial. 2014;18(4):347–52.
18. Gay M, Pares A, Carrascal M, Bosch-i-Crespo P, Gorga M, Mas A, et al. Proteomic analysis of polypeptides captured from blood during extracorporeal albumin dialysis in patients with cholestasis and resistant pruritus. PLoS ONE. 2011;6(7):e21850.
19. Roth GA, Faybik P, Hetz H, Ankersmit HJ, Hoetzenecker K, Bacher A, et al. MCP-1 and MIP3-alpha serum levels in acute liver failure and molecular adsorbent recirculating system (MARS) treatment: a pilot study. Scand J Gastroenterol. 2009;44(6):745–51.
20. Roth GA, Nickl S, Lebherz-Eichinger D, Schmidt EM, Ankersmit HJ, Faybik P, et al. Lipocalin-2 serum levels are increased in acute hepatic failure. Transpl Proc. 2013;45(1):241–4.

21. Roth GA, Sipos W, Hoferl M, Bohmdorfer M, Schmidt EM, Hetz H, et al. The effect of the molecular adsorbent recirculating system on moxifloxacin and meropenem plasma levels. Acta Anaesthesiol Scand. 2013;57(4):461–7.

22. Personett HA, Larson SL, Frazee EN, Nyberg SL, Leung N, El-Zoghby ZM. Impact of molecular adsorbent recirculating system therapy on tacrolimus elimination: a case report. Transpl Proc. 2014;46(7):2440–2.

23. Uchino S, Fealy N, Baldwin I, Morimatsu H, Bellomo R. Continuous venovenous hemofiltration without anticoagulation. ASAIO J. 2004;50(1):76–80.

24. Dyla A, Mielnicki W, Bartczak J, Zawada T, Garba P. Effectiveness and safety assessment of citrate anticoagulation during albumin dialysis in comparison to other methods of anticoagulation. Artif Organs. 2017;41(9):818–26.

25. Meijers B, Laleman W, Vermeersch P, Nevens F, Wilmer A, Evenepoel P. A prospective randomized open-label crossover trial of regional citrate anticoagulation vs. anticoagulation free liver dialysis by the Molecular Adsorbents Recirculating System. Crit Care. 2012;16(1):20.

26. Kribben A, Gerken G, Haag S, Herget-Rosenthal S, Treichel U, Betz C, et al. Effects of fractionated plasma separation and adsorption on survival in patients with acute-on-chronic liver failure. Gastroenterology. 2012;142(4):782–9.

27. Senturk E, Esen F, Ozcan PE, Rifai K, Pinarbasi B, Cakar N, et al. The treatment of acute liver failure with fractionated plasma separation and adsorption system: experience in 85 applications. J Clin Apher. 2010;25(4):195–201.

28. De Bruyn T, Meijers B, Evenepoel P, Laub R, Willems L, Augustijns P, et al. Stability of therapeutic albumin solutions used for molecular adsorbent recirculating system-based liver dialysis. Artif Organs. 2012;36(1):29–41.

29. Klammt S, Koball S, Hickstein H, Gloger M, Henschel J, Mitzner S, et al. Increase of octanoate concentrations during extracorporeal albumin dialysis treatments. Ther Apheresis Dial. 2009;13(5):437–43.

30. Heemann U, Treichel U, Loock J, Philipp T, Gerken G, Malago M, et al. Albumin dialysis in cirrhosis with superimposed acute liver injury: a prospective, controlled study. Hepatology. 2002;36(4 Pt 1):949–58.

31. Mitzner S, Stange J, Klammt S, Risler T, Erley C, Bader B, et al. Improvement of hepatorenal syndrome with extracorporeal albumin dialysis mars: results of a prospective, randomized, controlled clinical trial. Liver Transpl. 2000;6(3):277–86.

32. Sen S, Davies NA, Mookerjee RP, Cheshire LM, Hodges SJ, Williams R, et al. Pathophysiological effects of albumin dialysis in acute-on-chronic liver failure: a randomized controlled study. Liver Transpl. 2004;10(9):1109–19.

33. Saliba F, Camus C, Durand F, et al. Albumin dialysis with a noncell artificial liver support device in patients with acute liver failure: a randomized, controlled trial. Ann Intern Med. 2013;159(8):522–31.

34. Jadad ARMR, Carroll D, Jenkinson C, Reynolds DJM, Gavaghan DJ, McQuay HJ. Assessing the quality of reports of randomized clinical trials: is blinding necessary? Control Clin Trials. 1996;17(1):1–12.

35. Kantola T, Koivusalo AM, Hockerstedt K, Isoniemi H. The effect of molecular adsorbent recirculating system treatment on survival, native liver recovery, and need for liver transplantation in acute liver failure patients. Transpl Int. 2008;21(9):857–66.

36. Lexmond WS, Van Dael CM, Scheenstra R, Goorhuis JF, Sieders E, Verkade HJ, et al. Experience with molecular adsorbent recirculating system treatment in 20 children listed for high-urgency liver transplantation. Liver Transpl. 2015;21(3):369–80.

37. Gerth HU, Pohlen M, Tholking G, Pavenstadt H, Brand M, Wilms C, et al. Molecular adsorbent recirculating system (MARS) in acute liver injury and graft dysfunction: results from a case-control study. PLoS ONE. 2017;12(4):e0175529.

38. Banares R, Nevens F, Larsen FS, Jalan R, Albillos A, Dollinger M, et al. Extracorporeal albumin dialysis with the molecular adsorbent recirculating system in acute-on-chronic liver failure: the RELIEF trial. Hepatology. 2013;57(3):1153–62.

39. Hessel FP, Bramlage P, Wasem J, Mitzner SR. Cost-effectiveness of the artificial liver support system MARS in patients with acute-on-chronic liver failure. Eur J Gastroenterol Hepatol. 2010;22(2):213–20.

40. Gerth HU, Pohlen M, Tholking G, Pavenstadt H, Brand M, Husing-Kabar A, et al. Molecular adsorbent recirculating system can reduce short-term mortality among patients with acute-on-chronic liver failure-a retrospective analysis. Crit Care Med. 2017;45(10):1616–24.

41. Jalan R, Saliba F, Pavesi M, Amoros A, Moreau R, Gines P, et al. Development and validation of a prognostic score to predict mortality in patients with acute-on-chronic liver failure. J Hepatol. 2014;61(5):1038–47.

42. Shen Y, Wang XL, Wang B, Shao JG, Liu YM, Qin Y, et al. Survival benefits with artificial liver support system for acute-on-chronic liver failure: a time series-based meta-analysis. Med (Baltim). 2016;95(3):e2506.

43. Qin G, Shao JG, Wang B, Shen Y, Zheng J, Liu XJ, et al. Artificial liver support system improves short- and long-term outcomes of patients with HBV-associated acute-on-chronic liver failure: a single-center experience. Med (Baltim). 2014;93(28):e338.

44. Duseja A, Singh SP. Toward a better definition of acute-on-chronic liver failure. J Clin Exp Hepatol. 2017;7(3):262–5.

45. Novelli G, Rossi M, Morabito V, Pugliese F, Ruberto F, Perrella SM, et al. Pediatric acute liver failure with molecular adsorbent recirculating system treatment. Transpl Proc. 2008;40(6):1921–4.

46. Novelli G, Rossi M, Ferretti G, Pugliese F, Ruberto F, Lai Q, et al. Predictive criteria for the outcome of patients with acute liver failure treated with the albumin dialysis molecular adsorbent recirculating system. Ther Apheresis Dial. 2009;13(5):404–12.

47. Camus C, Lavoue S, Gacouin A, Compagnon P, Boudjema K, Jacquelinet C, et al. Liver transplantation avoided in patients with fulminant hepatic failure who received albumin dialysis with the molecular adsorbent recirculating system while on the waiting list: impact of the duration of therapy. Ther Apheresis Dial. 2009;13(6):549–55.

48. Hanish SI, Stein DM, Scalea JR, Essien EO, Thurman P, Hutson WR, et al. Molecular adsorbent recirculating system effectively replaces hepatic function in severe acute liver failure. Ann Surg. 2017;266(4):677–84.

49. Quintero Bernabeu J, Ortega Lopez J, Juamperez Goni J, Julio Tatis E, Mercadal-Hally M, Bilbao Aguirre I, et al. The role of molecular adsorbent recirculating system in pediatric acute liver failure. Liver Transpl. 2018;24(2):308–10.

50. Mark H, Ebell JS, Weiss Barry D, Woolf Steven H, Susman Jeffrey, Ewigman B, Bowman M. Strength of recommendation taxonomy (SORT): a patient-centered approach to grading evidence in the medical literature. Am Fam Physician. 2004;69:548–56.

51. Novelli G, Rossi M, Ferretti G, Pugliese F, Travaglia D, Guidi S, et al. Predictive parameters after molecular absorbent recirculating system treatment integrated with model for end stage liver disease model in patients with acute-on-chronic liver failure. Transpl Proc. 2010;42(4):1182–7.

52. Vaid A, Chweich H, Balk EM, Jaber BL. Molecular adsorbent recirculating system as artificial support therapy for liver failure: a meta-analysis. ASAIO J. 2012;58(1):51–9.

53. Tsipotis E, Shuja A, Jaber BL. Albumin dialysis for liver failure: a systematic review. Adv Chronic Kidney Dis. 2015;22(5):382–90.

54. Stutchfield BM, Simpson K, Wigmore SJ. Systematic review and meta-analysis of survival following extracorporeal liver support. Br J Surg. 2011;98(5):623–31.

55. He GL, Duan CY, Hu X, Zhou CJ, Cheng Y, Pan MX, Gao Y. Meta-analysis of survival with the molecular adsorbent recirculating system for liver failure. Int J Clin Exp Med. 2015;8(10):17046–54.

56. Moher D, Schulz KF, Altman DG. The CONSORT statement: revised recommendations for improving the quality of reports of parallel-group randomised trials. Lancet. 2001;357(9263):1191–4.

57. Zheng Z, Li X, Li Z, Ma X. Artificial and bioartificial liver support systems for acute and acute-on-chronic hepatic failure: a meta-analysis and meta-regression. Exp Ther Med. 2013;6(4):929–36.

58. Kantola T, Koivusalo A-M, Parmanen S, Höckerstedt K, Isoniemi H. Survival predictors in patients treated with a molecular adsorbent recirculating system. World J Gastroenterol. 2009;15(24):3015.

59. Rusu EE, Voiculescu M, Zilisteanu DS, Ismail G. Molecular adsorbents recirculating system in patients with severe liver failure. Experience of a single Romanian centre. J Gastrointestin Liver Dis. 2009;18(3):311–6.

60. Cisneros-Garza LE, del Rosario Muñoz-Ramírez M, Muñoz-Espinoza LE, Velasco JAVR, Moreno-Alcántar R, Marín-López E, Méndez-Sánchez N. The molecular adsorbent recirculating system as a liver support system. Summary of Mexican experience. Ann Hepatol. 2014;13(2):240–7.

61. Wong F, Raina N, Richardson R. Molecular adsorbent recirculating system is ineffective in the management of type 1 hepatorenal syndrome in patients with cirrhosis with ascites who have failed vasoconstrictor treatment. Gut. 2010;59(3):381–6.

62. Schaefer B, Schaefer F, Wittmer D, Engelmann G, Wenning D, Schmitt CP. Molecular adsorbents recirculating system dialysis in children with cholestatic pruritus. Pediatr Nephrol. 2012;27(5):829–34.

63. Lavayssiere L, Kallab S, Cardeau-Desangles I, Nogier MB, Cointault O, Barange K, et al. Impact of molecular adsorbent recirculating system on renal recovery in type-1 hepatorenal syndrome patients with chronic liver failure. J Gastroenterol Hepatol. 2013;28(6):1019–24.

64. Gilg S, Sparrelid E, Saraste L, Nowak G, Wahlin S, Stromberg C, et al. The molecular adsorbent recirculating system in posthepatectomy liver failure: results from a prospective phase I study. Hepatol Commun. 2018;2(4):445–54.

65. Seige M, Kreymann B, Jeschke B, Schweigart U, Kopp K-F, Classen M. Long term treatment of patients with acute exacerbation of chronic liver failure by albumin dialysis. Transpl Proc. 1999;31:1371–5.

66. Sauer IM, Goetz M, Steffen I, Walter G, Kehr DC, Schwartlander R, et al. In vitro comparison of the molecular adsorbent recirculation system (MARS) and single-pass albumin dialysis (SPAD). Hepatology. 2004;39(5):1408–14.

67. Kortgen A, Rauchfuss F, Gotz M, Settmacher U, Bauer M, Sponholz C. Albumin dialysis in liver failure: comparison of molecular adsorbent recirculating system and single pass albumin dialysis–a retrospective analysis. Ther Apheresis Dial. 2009;13(5):419–25.

68. Churchwell MD, Pasko DA, Smoyer WE, Mueller BA. Enhanced clearance of highly protein-bound drugs by albumin-supplemented dialysate during modeled continuous hemodialysis. Nephrol Dial Transpl. 2009;24(1):231–8.

69. Benyoub K, Muller M, Bonnet A, Simon R, Gazon M, Duperret S, Aubrun F, Viale JP. Amounts of bile acids and bilirubin removed during single-pass albumin dialysis in patients with liver failure. Ther Apheresis Dial. 2011;15(5):504–10.

70. Schmuck RB, Nawrot GH, Fikatas P, Reutzel-Selke A, Pratschke J, Sauer IM. Single pass albumin dialysis-a dose-finding study to define optimal albumin concentration and dialysate flow. Artif Organs. 2017;41(2):153–61.

71. Ringe H, Varnholt V, Zimmering M, Luck W, Gratopp A, Konig K, et al. Continuous veno-venous single-pass albumin hemodiafiltration in children with acute liver failure. Pediatr Crit Care Med. 2011;12(3):257–64.

72. Piechota M, Piechota A. An evaluation of the usefulness of extracorporeal liver support techniques in patients hospitalized in the icu for severe liver dysfunction secondary to alcoholic liver disease. Hepat Mon. 2016;16(7):e34127.

73. Sponholz C, Matthes K, Rupp D, Backaus W, Klammt S, Karailieva D, et al. Molecular adsorbent recirculating system and single-pass albumin dialysis in liver failure–a prospective, randomised crossover study. Crit Care. 2016;20:2.

74. Falkenhagen D, Strobl W, Vogt G, Schrefl A, Linsberger I, Gerner FJ, Schoenhofen M. fractionated plasma separation and adsorption system: a novel system for blood purification to remove albumin bound substances. Artif Organs. 1999;23(1):81–6.

75. Evenepoel P, Alexander W, Wilmer A, Claes K, Kuypers D, Bammens B, Nevens F, Vanrenterghem Y. Prometheus versus molecular adsorbents recirculating system: comparison of efficiency in two different liver detoxification devices. Artif Organs. 2006;30(4):276–84.

76. Grodzicki M, Kotulski M, Leonowicz D, Zieniewicz K, Krawczyk M. Results of treatment of acute liver failure patients with use of the prometheus FPSA system. Transpl Proc. 2009;41(8):3079–81.

77. Rifai K, Das A, Rosenau J, Ernst T, Kretschmer U, Haller H, et al. Changes in plasma amino acids during extracorporeal liver support by fractionated plasma separation and adsorption. Artif Organs. 2010;34(2):166–70.

78. Peter Nissen Bjerring JH, Frederiksen Hans-Jørgen, Nielsen Henning Bay, Clemmesen Jens Otto. Fin Stolze Larsen. The effect of fractionated plasma separation and adsorption on cerebral amino acid metabolism and oxidative metabolism during acute liver failure. J Hepatol. 2012;57:774–9.

79. Ryska M, Laszikova E, Pantoflicek T, Ryska O, Prazak J, Koblihova E. Fractionated plasma separation and adsorption significantly decreases intracranial pressure in acute liver failure: experimental study. Eur Surg Res. 2009;42(4):230–5.

80. Rocen M, Kieslichova E, Merta D, Uchytilova E, Pavlova Y, Cap J, et al. The effect of Prometheus device on laboratory markers of inflammation and tissue regeneration in acute liver failure management. Transpl Proc. 2010;42(9):3606–11.

81. Laleman W, Wilmer A, Evenepoel P, Elst IV, Zeegers M, Zaman Z, et al. Effect of the molecular adsorbent recirculating system and Prometheus devices on systemic haemodynamics and vasoactive agents in patients with acute-on-chronic alcoholic liver failure. Crit Care. 2006;10(4):R108.

82. Dethloff T, Tofteng F, Frederiksen H-J, Hojskov M, Hansen BA, Larsen FS. Effect of prometheus liver assist system on systemic hemodynamics in patients with cirrhosis: a randomized controlled study. World J Gastroenterol. 2008;14(13):2065.

83. Stamler JS, Jaraki O, Osborne J, Simon DI, Keaney J, Vita J, et al. Nitric oxide circulates in mammalian plasma primarily as an S-nitroso adduct of serum albumin (S-nitrosothiols/endothelium-derived relaxing factor). Proc Natl Acad Sci USA. 1992;89:7674–7.

84. Rifai K, Bode-Boeger SM, Martens-Lobenhoffer J, Ernst T, Kretschmer U, Hafer C, et al. Removal of asymmetric dimethylarginine during artificial liver support using fractionated plasma separation and adsorption. Scand J Gastroenterol. 2010;45(9):1110–5.

85. Komardina E, Yaroustovsky M, Abramyan M, Plyushch M. Prometheus therapy for the treatment of acute liver failure in patients after cardiac surgery. Kardiochir Torakochirurgia Pol. 2017;14(4):230–5.

86. Bergis D, Friedrich-Rust M, Zeuzem S, Betz C, Sarrazin C, Bojunga J. Treatment of Amanita phalloides intoxication by fractionated plasma separation and adsorption (Prometheus®). J Gastrointestin Liver Dis. 2012;21(2):171–6.

87. Marangoni R, Bellati G, Castelli A, Romagnoli E. Development of high-efficiency molecular adsorbent recirculating system: preliminary report. Artif Organs. 2014;38(10):879–83.

88. Akcan Arikan A, Srivaths P, Himes RW, Tufan Pekkucuksen N, Lam F, Nguyen T, et al. Hybrid extracorporeal therapies as a bridge to pediatric liver transplantation. Pediatr Crit Care Med. 2018;19(7):e342–9.

89. Al-Chalabi A, Matevossian E, von Thaden A, Schreiber C, Radermacher P, Huber W, et al. Evaluation of an ADVanced Organ Support (ADVOS) system in a two-hit porcine model of liver failure plus endotoxemia. Intensive Care Med Exp. 2017;5(1):31.

90. Huber W, Henschel B, Schmid R, Al-Chalabi A. First clinical experience in 14 patients treated with ADVOS: a study on feasibility, safety and efficacy of a new type of albumin dialysis. BMC Gastroenterol. 2017;17(1):32.

91. Al-Chalabi A, Matevossian E, v Thaden AK, Luppa P, Neiss A, Schuster T, et al. Evaluation of the Hepa Wash® treatment in pigs with acute liver failure. BMC Gastroenterol. 2013;13:83.

92. Viggiano D, de Pascale E, Marinelli G, Pluvio C. A comparison among three different apheretic techniques for treatment of hyperbilirubinemia. J Artif Organs. 2018;21(1):110–6.

93. Nakae H, Eguchi Y, Saotome T, Yoshioka T, Yoshimura N, Kishi Y, et al. Multicenter study of plasma diafiltration in patients with acute liver failure. Ther Apheresis Dial. 2010;14(5):444–50.

94. Bendjelid K. IABP and cardiogenic shock: a heartbreaking story. Am Heart J. 2018;199:178–80.

24

Impact of oversedation prevention in ventilated critically ill patients: a randomized trial—the AWARE study

SRLF Trial Group*

Abstract

Background: Although oversedation has been associated with increased morbidity in ventilated critically ill patients, it is unclear whether prevention of oversedation improves mortality. We aimed to assess 90-day mortality in patients receiving a bundle of interventions to prevent oversedation as compared to usual care.

Methods: In this randomized multicentre trial, all adult patients requiring mechanical ventilation for more than 48 h were included. Two groups were compared: patients managed according to usual sedation practices (control), and patients receiving sedation according to an algorithm which provided a gradual multilevel response to pain, agitation, and ventilator dyssynchrony with no specific target to alter consciousness and no use of sedation scale and promoted the use of alternatives to continuous infusion of midazolam or propofol (intervention).

Results: Inclusions were stopped before reaching the planned enrolment. Between 2012 and 2014, 584 patients were included in the intervention group and 590 in the control group. Baseline characteristics were well balanced between groups. Although the use of midazolam and propofol was significantly lower in the intervention group, 90-day mortality was not significantly lower (39.4 vs. 44.2% in the control group, $p = 0.09$). There were no significant differences in 1-year mortality between the two groups. The time to first spontaneous breathing trial and time to successful extubation were significantly shorter in the intervention group than in the control group. These last results should be interpreted with precaution regarding the several limitations of the trial including the early termination.

Conclusions: This underpowered study of severely ill patients was unable to show that a strategy to prevent oversedation could significantly reduce mortality.

Keywords: Intensive care units, Mechanical ventilation, Sedation, Mortality, Weaning

Background

Intravenous hypnotics, often combined with morphinics, are commonly used in mechanically ventilated patients in the intensive care unit (ICU) to control pain, agitation, and ensure synchrony with the ventilator [1]. However, the continuous infusion of midazolam or propofol often results in oversedation [2]. Factors involved in oversedation are multiple, including drug pharmacokinetic and pharmacodynamic properties, inadequate objectives in terms of consciousness, and lack of frequent reassessment of patient condition and hypnotic needs. Oversedation has been associated with prolonged mechanical ventilation and higher rates of nosocomial infections, ICU-acquired weakness, and delirium.

Strategies developed to avoid oversedation have been based either on (1) the use of continuous intravenous hypnotics combined with daily interruption of sedatives every 24 h [3], (2) the continuous titration of hypnotics according to predefined goals of comfort and consciousness, with frequent patient assessments and prescription changes [4–7], or (3) the first-intention use of alternatives

*Correspondence: Bdejonghe@chi-poissy-st-germain.fr
Société de Réanimation de Langue Française (SRLF), 48 Avenue Claude Vellefaux, 75010 Paris, France
Full list of author information is available at the end of the article

to continuous intravenous midazolam or propofol [8–10]. These strategies were associated with a reduction in mechanical ventilation duration. Few observational studies have assessed the impact of an oversedation prevention strategy on mortality [10–13]. In a prospective observational study, Shehabi et al. reported that patients with deep sedation (indicated by at least one measurement of Richmond Agitation Sedation Scale [RASS] −3 to −5) during the first 48 h of mechanical ventilation were more likely to die in the ICU than patients with a lighter sedation (RASS −2 to +1), independently of age, comorbidities, and severity of acute illness [11]. To the best of our knowledge, this observation has not been confirmed in a randomized trial.

The main objective of the present randomized controlled trial was to determine whether a strategy aiming to prevent oversedation could reduce 90-day mortality in critically ill patients requiring mechanical ventilation compared to usual care.

Methods

In accordance with French law, the study was approved by the institutional review board of Clermont-Ferrand, France, and by the Ethics Committee of the French Intensive Care Society (SRLF, Société de Réanimation de Langue Française). Informed consent or deferred consent was obtained from each patient or his/her legal surrogate. An independent data safety monitoring board had full access to the unblinded data.

Participants and settings

The study conducted by the SRLF Trial Group was planned as a parallel two-group individually randomized trial. Patients were eligible if they were aged 18 years or more, were receiving invasive mechanical ventilation for < 12 h, and had an expected invasive mechanical ventilation duration > 48 h after randomization. Patients admitted after cardiac arrest, those with neuromuscular disease, tracheostomy, severe intracranial hypertension, status epilepticus, decision to withdraw care, or considered moribund were not included.

Oversedation prevention (OSP)

The OSP strategy was centred on the identification of patients' level of agitation, ventilator asynchrony, and pain, on a 4-level scale, with gradual on-demand responses, frequent reassessments, and promotion of alternatives to continuous around-the-clock intravenous hypnotics infusion (Fig. 1). The alternatives to continuous infusion of midazolam or propofol in the intervention group were other benzodiazepines, antipsychotic agents, zolpidem, and hydroxyzine.

There was no aim to alter consciousness, and therefore, no sedation scale was used. However, consciousness alteration could result from treatment of existing agitation, existing ventilator dyssynchrony, or existing or anticipated pain. During two national training and education meetings, the OSP strategy was explained to investigators (usually an ICU doctor and nurse), who in turn implemented the OSP strategy in their own centre. OSP strategy posters were used at the bedside.

Usual care

Patients in the control group were treated according to the routine sedation practices used in each participating centre, reported in an pre-study survey of sedation practices in France [14]. In both intervention and control groups, the use of dexmedetomidine was not permitted. In both groups, pain was measured according to the current practice in each participating centre. Weaning was conducted according to the French ICU Society guidelines [15].

Outcomes

The primary study endpoint was 90-day mortality after randomization. Secondary endpoints were day-28, hospital and 1-year mortality, time from randomization to first spontaneous breathing trial, time to successful extubation (defined as absence of invasive mechanical ventilation for 48 consecutive hours). Other outcome criteria are reported in Additional file 1: Appendix 1.

Randomization, allocation concealment, and blinding

Using a secure, computer-generated, interactive, web-response system available at each study centre, patients were randomly assigned in a 1:1 ratio to study groups. Randomization was stratified by centre using permutation blocks of variable sizes. Sequences were generated by a biostatistician not involved in patient recruitment. Investigators had no access to the randomization list and were not aware of the size of the randomization blocks. Given the very nature of the assessed intervention, blinding of the physicians and nurses was not feasible [16–18]. However, the primary outcome (death at day 90) is an objective one, which counterbalances this lack of blinding [19].

Sample size

We assumed a mortality rate of 22% in the control group at day 90. To show a 5% absolute reduction in 90-day mortality in the OSP group, with a two-sided type I error of 5% and a power of 90%, the planned enrolment was 2720 patients.

Assessment on demand and at least every 2 to 4 hours

Clinical situation, Level 0	•No symptoms	**Therapeutic response, Level 0** **No tretament[a]**	
Clinical situation, Level 1	•Pain[b], anxiety, discomfort •Moderate agitation or ventilator dyssynchrony	**Therapeutic response, Level 1[c]** **Analgesics and/or anxiolytics (non-hypnotic) and/or neuroleptics** IV bolus (repeated as needed) or enteral route Continuous IV infusion possible only for analgesics **Level-1 symptoms not resolved**	Symptoms resolved →
Clinical situation, Level 2	•Ventilator dyssynchrony inducing or worsening a respiratory failure (desaturation, tachypnea > 40...) •Important agitation, with failed verbal reassurance	**Therapeutic response, Level 2** **Hypnotics (with or without morphinics)[d]** 1st IV bolus titration until symptoms resolved Resurgence of symptoms within the next 120 min 2nd IV bolus titration until symptoms resolved Resurgence of symptoms within the next 120 min 1st IV bolus titration followed by a continuous infusion for 6 hrs, then STOP Resurgence of symptoms within the 6 hours after STOP 2nd IV bolus titration followed by a continuous infusion for 6 hrs, then STOP **Resurgence of Level-1 or Level-2 symptoms within the 6 hours after STOP**	Resolution of symptoms for > 120 min → Resolution of symptoms for > 120 min → Resolution of symptoms for > 6 hrs after STOP → Resolution of symptoms for > 6 hrs after STOP →
Clinical situation, Level 3	•Severe ARDS (P/F < 150 & PEP ≥ 5 cm H2O)	**Therapeutic response, Level 3** **Sedation, analgesia, neuromuscular blockade** **According to the usual ICU practice in this condition;** Decrease hypnotic and morphinic dosages by 25% every 6 hours, unless otherwise specified by the attending physician or ongoing neuromuscular blokade	

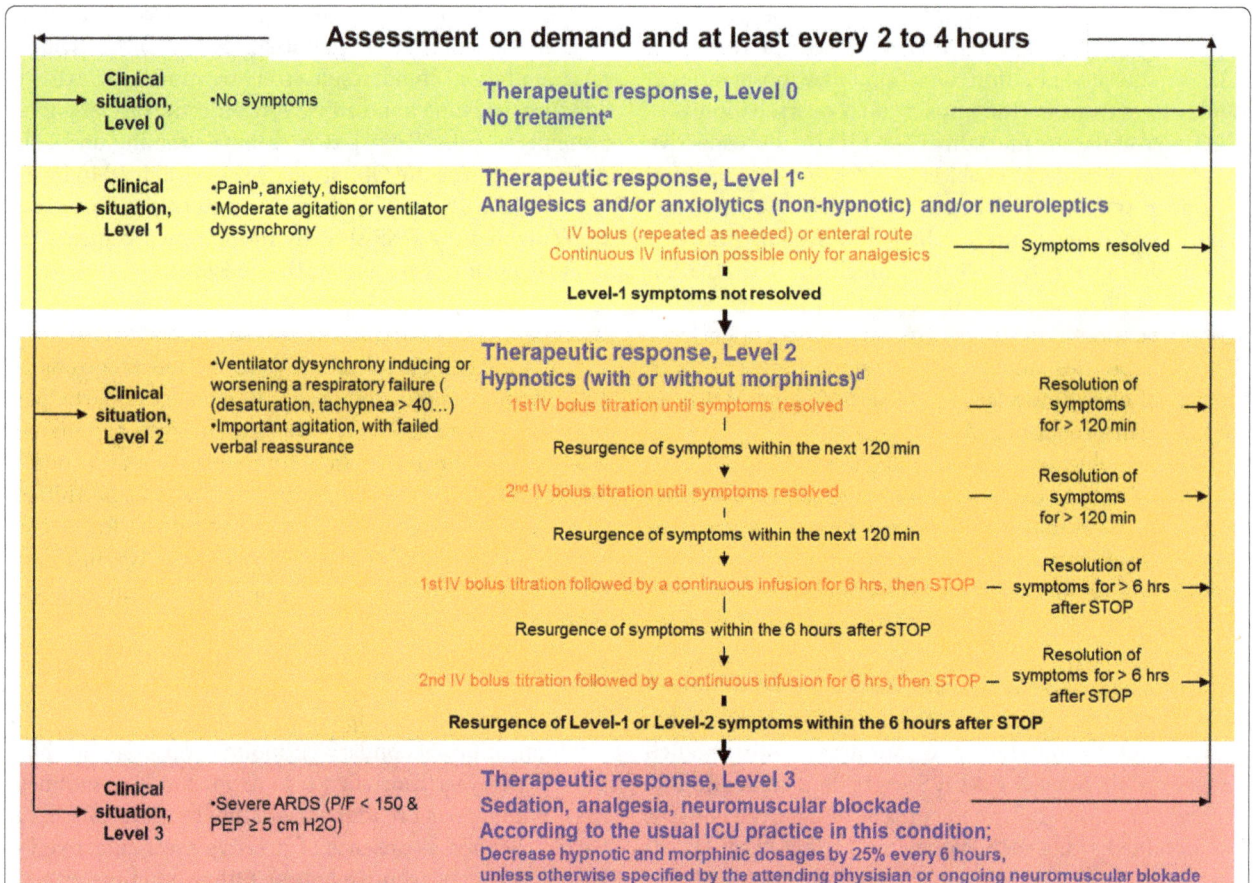

Fig. 1 Oversedation prevention (OSP) strategy was centred on patients' level of agitation, ventilator dyssynchrony, and pain, assessed on a 4-level scale, with gradual on-demand responses, frequent reassessments, and promotion of alternatives to continuous around-the-clock infusion of intravenous hypnotics. These alternatives included frequent (every 6 h) intravenous hypnotic interruptions, intravenous boluses of hypnotics without continuous intravenous infusion, and the use of non-hypnotic drugs, including neuroleptics, hydroxyzine, and anxiolytic benzodiazepines. The choice of the non-hypnotic drugs and their route of administration (intravenous boluses or nasogastric tube) were left to the preference of the attending physician. There was no restriction for the use of morphinics and non-morphinic analgesics. Patient at Level 0, who showed no discomfort, received no treatment, or continuation of a successful level-1 therapeutic response (**a**). Patient at Level 1, with only moderate discomfort, pain, or anticipated procedural pain (**b**), received any form of analgesics as deemed necessary by the attending physician and/or non-hypnotic drugs as well as verbal reassurance and, if appropriate, changing of ventilator settings (**c**). Patients at Level 2, with severe agitation or ventilator dyssynchrony first received repeated intravenous boluses of either propofol or midazolam according to physician preferences, and, if discomfort persisted, 6-h continuous intravenous infusion of midazolam or propofol. This treatment was also applied in case of Level 1 therapy failure (which was maintained or stopped according to physician preference (**d**). Patients at Level 3, with ARDS and a PaO_2/FiO_2 ratio < 150 mmHg, were treated with a continuous intravenous infusion of midazolam or propofol, with neuromuscular blocking agents administered according to physician preference. This treatment was also applied in the case of Level 2 therapy failure

Statistical analysis

Statistical analyses were conducted in the intention-to-treat population. Data were described using counts and percentages or means and standard deviations (or median and interquartile range). Death proportions were compared using the Chi-square test, and mechanical ventilation-free days were compared using the Wilcoxon test. Time-dependent events were analysed using competing risk models taking into account death and extubation. Description of the occurrence of these events was made using cumulative incidence curves. Cumulative incidence curves were compared between the two groups with the Fine and Gray test; hazard ratios (HRs) and their 95% confidence intervals (95% CIs) were estimated by the competing risk models [20]. For the two patients (one in the OSP group and one in the control group) lost to follow-up for the primary outcome (90-day mortality), imputation of missing data (alive status) was performed. A two-tailed p value < 0.05 was considered statistically significant. Statistical analyses were performed using SAS version 9.4 (SAS Institute Inc) and R version 3.2.2 [21].

Results

Baseline characteristics

Forty-six ICUs were involved in the study. Of those, 18 (39.1%) were university-affiliated, 15 (32.6%) were medical ICUs, and 31 (67.4%) medical surgical ICUs. Between July 2012 and July 2014, 1179 patients were included and randomized. The nurse/patient ratio was 2.5. The trial was stopped because of a decreasing average per centre recruitment rate, despite considerable help and encouragement. Five patients withdrew their consent and were therefore excluded from analysis, as requested by French law. Two patients (one in each group) were lost for the 90-day follow-up and were arbitrarily considered alive (Fig. 2), leaving 584 patients in the OSP group and 590 in the control group available for the main analysis.

Table 1 shows the patients' baseline characteristics, which were similar between the two groups. In the OSP and control groups, mean age (standard deviation) was 66 (13) and 67 (14), mean simplified acute physiology score II (SAPS II) was 53.6 (17.8) and 54.4 (18.6), and 54.5 and 53.0% of the patients were receiving norepinephrine at randomization, respectively. Of note, chronic psychotropic medication use did not differ between the two groups, as shown in Table 1. At randomization, more than 65% of the patients were comatose (deep sedation or unarousable), as shown in Table 1. Sedation levels at randomization are reported in Additional file 1: Appendix 2.

Outcomes

At day-90, 230 patients (39.4%) had died in the OSP group and 261 (44.2%) in the control group, $p = 0.09$. Of note those mortality rates were far higher than the initial sample size calculation of the trial. There were also no significant differences in day-28 (Table 2), in-hospital (Fig. 3), and 1-year mortality between the two groups (Table 2). Cumulative dosages of intravenous propofol and midazolam were significantly lower in the OPS group (Table 2). Cumulative dosage of intravenous sufentanil was significantly lower in the OPS group, whereas there

was no significant difference in cumulative dosages of other morphinics between the two groups (Table 2).

First spontaneous breathing trial occurred significantly earlier in the OSP group than in the control group (HR 1.18 [1.03–1.36], $p = 0.015$ (Additional file 1: Appendix 3, Figure). Similarly, successful extubation occurred significantly earlier in the OSP group than in the control group (HR 1.15 [1.02–1.31], $p = 0.03$ (Additional file 1: Appendix 3, Figure).

There was no significant difference in the other secondary outcomes, i.e. time to first sitting in a chair, time to first standing by the bed, presence of proximal muscle weakness, delirium, length of stay in the ICU (Table 2). Self-extubation was significantly more frequent in the OSP group than in the control group (70 vs. 48 events, HR 1.50 [1.04; 2.16], $p = 0.03$). Percentage of patients awake on a daily assessment between day 1 and day 7 are presented in the Additional file 1: Appendix 4.

Discussion

In this multicentre randomized study, we were unable to show that a gradual multilevel bundle strategy to prevent oversedation could significantly reduce mortality of severely ill ICU patients requiring mechanical ventilation. There were no significant differences between the two groups in in-hospital and 1-year mortality. However, oversedation prevention resulted in significantly less use of intravenous midazolam and propofol, and significantly earlier weaning initiation and extubation. Last, the numerous limitations including early termination of the trial weaken the result interpretation.

We chose an OSP strategy centred on the identification of patients' level of agitation, ventilator asynchrony, and pain, on a 4-level scale, with gradual on-demand responses, frequent reassessments, and promotion of alternatives to continuous around-the-clock intravenous hypnotics (midazolam or propofol) infusion. Interestingly, in the OSP algorithm, interventions were titrated only on patients' needs to control pain, agitation, and ventilator asynchrony (except in the level 3), with no attempt to alter consciousness, even slightly, as a specific goal. Accordingly, the OSP strategy did not include the use of any sedation scale. Cumulative dosages of propofol and midazolam were significantly lower in the OPS group. We did not use dexmedetomidine as an alternative to continuous intravenous hypnotics because at the time of study design, the very recent commercialization of dexmedetomidine in France precluded homogeneous and optimal use among the participating centres [22–25].

Our study was unable to show that the OSP strategy reduced mortality compared to standard care in critically ill patients. Furthermore, mortality was high in the study population. More than 40% of the patients had died at

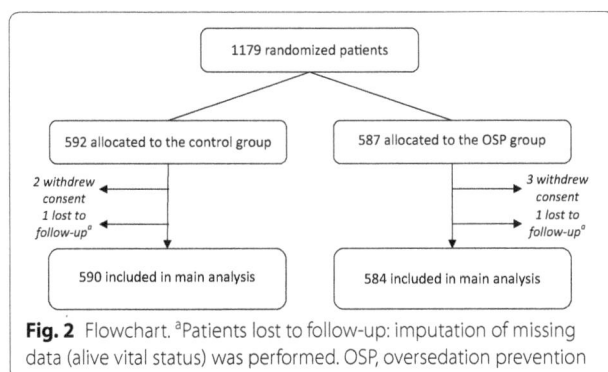

Fig. 2 Flowchart. [a]Patients lost to follow-up: imputation of missing data (alive vital status) was performed. OSP, oversedation prevention

Table 1 Demographic and baseline characteristics at randomization

	Control (n = 590)	Oversedation prevention (n = 584)
Age (years), mean (SD)	67 (14)	66 (13)
Female gender, n (%)	200 (33.9)	202 (34.6)
BMI (kilograms divided by height in metres squared), mean (SD)	26.7 (6.6)	27.4 (7.1)
Chronic alcohol use, n (%)	115 (19.5)	126 (21.6)
Chronic psychotropic medication use, n (%)	177 (30.0)	166 (28.4)
Benzodiazepine and related medications	110 (18.6)	109 (18.7)
Neuroleptics	22 (3.7)	33 (5.7)
Antidepressants	72 (12.2)	70 (12.0)
Opioid medication	42 (7.1)	35 (6.0)
Tobacco use, n (%)	156 (26.5)	169 (28.9)
Liver cirrhosis with ascites or oesophageal varices, n (%)	34 (5.8)	37 (6.3)
Chronic renal replacement therapy, n (%)	9 (1.5)	10 (1.7)
Chronic respiratory insufficiency with home oxygen therapy, n (%)	42 (7.1)	51 (8.7)
NYHA class IV chronic heart failure, n (%)	16 (2.7)	23 (3.9)
Barthel score before admission, median (Q1–Q3)	100 (100–100)	100 (95–100)
Knauss chronic health status before admission, n (%)		
Normal health status	155 (26.3)	152 (26.0)
Moderate activity limitation	285 (48.3)	267 (45.7)
Severe activity limitation due to chronic disease	139 (23.6)	157 (26.9)
Bedridden patient	11 (1.9)	8 (1.4)
MacCabe class before admission, n (%)		
No fatal disease	363 (61.5)	348 (59.6)
Ultimately fatal disease	181 (30.7)	197 (33.7)
Rapidly fatal disease	46 (7.8)	39 (6.7)
At home without assistance before current hospital admission, n (%)	373 (63.2)	367 (62.8)
ICU admission SAPS II score (first 24 h), mean (SD)	54.4 (18.6)	53.6 (17.8)
ICU admission SOFA score (first 24 h), median (Q1–Q3)	9 (7–12)	9 (7–12)
Medical admission, n (%)	520 (88.1)	530 (90.8)
Norepinephrine at randomization, n (%)	312 (53.0)	318 (54.5)
Midazolam at randomization ($n_1 = 493, n_2 = 496$), n (%)	412 (83.6)	421 (84.9)
Propofol at randomization ($n_1 = 493, n_2 = 496$), n (%)	74 (15.0)	69 (13.9)
Severe sepsis, n (%)	50 (8.5)	57 (9.8)
Septic shock, n (%)	339 (57.5)	323 (55.3)
ARDS, n (%)	186 (31.5)	187 (32.1)
ICU primary diagnosis		
Pulmonary infection, n (%)	246 (41.7)	239 (40.9)
Abdominal infection, n (%)	49 (8.3)	54 (9.3)
Other Infection, n (%)	41 (6.9)	57 (9.8)
Cardiac failure or cardiogenic pulmonary oedema, n (%)	56 (9.5)	53 (9.1)
COPD exacerbation or acute asthma, n (%)	51 (8.6)	51 (8.7)
Acute pancreatitis, n (%)	9 (1.5)	13 (2.2)
Drug intoxication, n (%)	12 (2.0)	9 (1.5)
Metabolic disorder, n (%)	18 (3.1)	7 (1.2)
Trauma, n (%)	7 (1.2)	7 (1.2)
Acute stroke, n (%)	5 (0.8)	2 (0.3)
Miscellaneous, n (%)	96 (16.3)	92 (15.8)
Sedation level on the RASS scale at randomization[a]		
Very agitated, n (%)	1 (0.4)	3 (1.1)

Impact of oversedation prevention in ventilated critically ill patients: a randomized...

231

Table 1 (continued)

	Control (n = 590)	Oversedation prevention (n = 584)
Agitated, n (%)	4 (1.5)	1 (0.4)
Restless, n (%)	3 (1.1)	5 (1.9)
Alert and calm, n (%)	12 (4.5)	12 (4.6)
Drowsy, n (%)	12 (4.5)	12 (4.6)
Light sedation, n (%)	21 (7.9)	15 (5.7)
Moderate sedation, n (%)	30 (11.3)	23 (8.8)
Deep sedation, n (%)	63 (23.8)	66 (25.2)
Unarousable, n (%)	119 (44.9)	125 (47.7)

SD, standard deviation; BMI, body mass index; NYHA, New York Heart Association; Q1–Q3, 1st and 3rd quartiles; SAPS, Simplified Acute Physiology Score, SOFA, Sequential Organ Failure Assessment; ICU, intensive care unit, COPD, chronic obstructive pulmonary disease; ARDS, acute respiratory distress syndrome

[a] Sedation was measured using the RASS scale in 268 patients in the control group and 267 patients in the oversedation prevention group. The exact level on the RASS scale was not available for 3 patients in the control group and 5 patients in the oversedation prevention group.

3 months and almost 60% at 1 year. These mortality rates were much higher than anticipated at study design and higher than those reported in previous studies on light sedation strategies [1–13]. This high mortality very likely reflects the severity of the acute conditions at ICU admission, as suggested by a SAPS II score higher than commonly reported in trials on sedation [5, 8, 10, 25, 26]. Old age and the low rate of post-operative admissions both could have contributed to the high SAPS II. Similarly, the percentage of patients on vasoactive drugs at randomization was high.

The severity of the acute conditions of our study population compared to previous studies suggests the inclusion of patients in real-life conditions. Demonstration of the positive impact of an intervention, such as a strategy to prevent oversedation, might be difficult in patients with particularly severe admission conditions and requires a larger sample of patients. In our study, less than half of the planned included patients were finally enrolled which undoubtedly makes the trial underpowered. Furthermore, the planned inclusion number was based on a mortality rate of 22% in the control group. There is such a high difference between the a priori postulated mortality rate in the control group, and the a posteriori observed one (which is much closer to 50%) that even in case we would have been able to recruit the planned 2720 patients, the real power of the trial would have been much lower than the 90% nominal power.

Despite the severity of the conditions of the study patients, and the above limitations, the OSP strategy resulted in significantly shorter mechanical ventilation duration. Similar findings have been observed in previous randomized studies on light sedation in less severely ill ICU populations. This finding is important, as physicians may be reluctant to adopt a light sedation strategy among the most severely ill patients. Indeed, as agitation and device removal may be perceived as particularly dangerous in this population, physicians may favour continuous intravenous sedation. The present trial did not show that oversedation prevention was associated with lower mortality, but it showed that it was associated with secondary benefits of faster weaning and extubation.

One explanation for shorter mechanical ventilation duration is provided in our study by a significantly shorter time to first spontaneous breathing trial. An adequate consciousness level is among the prerequisite criteria for physicians to initiate the weaning process leading to extubation, along with other criteria including absence of high-grade fever, low oxygen, positive expiratory endpressure, and vasoactive drug needs [27]. A light sedation strategy might promote preservation of consciousness or early return to consciousness when other weaning criteria are met [28].

Study limitations The numerous limitations including the early termination and associated lack of power weaken the results.

We did not design a weaning protocol in the control group; patients were treated according to usual practice in the participating ICUs. Unfortunately, we do not have any data showing that the French ICU weaning guidelines were applied similarly in both groups. Physicians in the participating study centres might have unconsciously changed their practice over the study period, with a progressive implementation of some aspects of the OSP strategy in control patients, further reducing the difference in sedation practices between the two groups. Insufficient compliance with the relatively novel multilevel gradual intervention might also have reduced the difference in sedation practices between the two groups. A cluster randomization at the ICU level would have

Table 2 Outcomes

	Control (n = 590)	Oversedation prevention (n = 584)	P value	Hazard ratio (95% confidence interval)
28-day mortality	198 (33.6)	177 (30.4)	0.24[a]	
90-day mortality	261 (44.2)	230 (39.4)	0.09[a]	
1-year mortality	296 (60.0)	267 (56.5)	0.26[a]	
Mechanical ventilation-free days at day 28 (days), median (Q1–Q3)	14 (0–24)	16 (0–24)	0.36[b]	
Ventilator-associated pneumonia, n	92	94	0.79[c]	1.04 (0.78; 1.38)
Mechanical ventilation ≥ 48 h, n (%)	425 (72.0)	418 (71.6)	0.86[a]	
Non-invasive ventilation after extubation, n (%)	152 (25.8)	177 (30.3)	0.08[a]	
Duration of non-invasive ventilation after extubation (days), median (Q1–Q3)	2 (1–4)	3 (2–4)	0.05[b]	
Tracheostomy, n	26	24	0.81[c]	0.93 (0.54; 1.62)
Delirium, n	232	230	0.99[c]	1.00 (0.84; 1.19)
Proximal weakness after awakening, n	193	208	0.26[c]	1.11 (0.92; 1.35)
Patients with intravenous midazolam, n (%)	464 (78.6)	419 (71.8)	0.01[a]	
Cumulative dosage of midazolam (mg), median (Q1–Q3)	263 (120–660)	218 (72–696)	0.03[b]	
Patients with intravenous propofol, n (%)	232 (39.3)	214 (36.6)	0.34[a]	
Cumulative dosage of propofol (mg), median (Q1–Q3)	2785 (645–7140)	1443 (120–4800)	<0.001[b]	
Patients with intravenous morphinics, n (%)	501 (84.9)	482 (82.5)	0.31[a]	
Patients with IV sufentanil, n (%)	263 (44.6)	241 (41.3)	0.28[a]	
Cumulative dosage of sufentanil (μg), median (Q1–Q3)	930 (472–2592)	870 (280-2160)	0.04[b]	
Patients with IV fentanyl, n (%)	204 (34.6)	206 (35.3)	0.8[a]	
Cumulative dosage of fentanyl (μg), median (Q1–Q3)	4985 (2400–15,445)	4656 (1340–16,200)	0.29[b]	
Patients with IV morphine, n (%)	73 (12.4)	91 (15.6)	0.1[a]	
Cumulative dosage of morphine (mg), median (Q1–Q3)	17.5 (7–55)	20 (6–43)	0.69[b]	
Patients with IV remifentanil, n (%)	49 (8.3)	45 (7.7)	0.7[a]	
Cumulative dosage of remifentanil (μg), median (Q1–Q3)	14,400 (6000–28,800)	7200 (3000-19,200)	0.05[b]	
Self-extubation, n	48	70	0.03[c]	1.50 (1.04; 2.16)
Ventricular tachycardia or fibrillation, n	18	21	0.61[c]	1.18 (0.63; 2.11)
Acute coronary syndrome or myocardial infarction, n	7	8	0.77[c]	1.16 (0.42; 3.18)
Cardiac arrest, n	20	13	0.22[c]	0.65 (0.33; 1.31)

For comparison of time dependent events analyzed using competing risks models to take into account competing risks as death or extubation (e.g. ventilator associated pneumonia), no percentages are provided

For comparison of variables in post-randomization sub-group (e.g. ICU length of stay in survivors), no P values are provided

CI, confidence interval; Q1–Q3, 1st and 3rd quartiles; MV, mechanical ventilation; VAP, ventilator-associated pneumonia; NIV, non-invasive ventilation; ICU, intensive care unit; LOS, length of stay

[a] Variables compared using the chi-square test

[b] Variables compared using the Wilcoxon test

[c] Variables analyzed using competing risks models to take into account competing risks (as death, extubation, ICU discharge, …). For each of these outcomes, Gray test P value and hazard ratio (95% confidence interval) from competing risks models were presented

limited those group contamination issues; however, the risk of a selection bias associated with such a design was deemed greater and led us to choose an individual randomization scheme [29–32]. This point remains a strong limitation to interpret the secondary endpoints in this non-blinded study.

The gap between estimated 90-day mortality used for the sample size calculation and the higher mortality rates observed also represents an important limitation study further reducing the study power.

Another limitation is that we did not use a sedation scale to measure the effect of the OSP strategy on consciousness. This option was deliberately selected to avoid that clinicians would try to titrate IV sedatives to reach the common target of slightly altered consciousness in the intervention group, in which no specific alteration of consciousness should be targeted. Unfortunately, the surrogate markers for consciousness level used in the study (amounts of sedatives used, single daily assessment

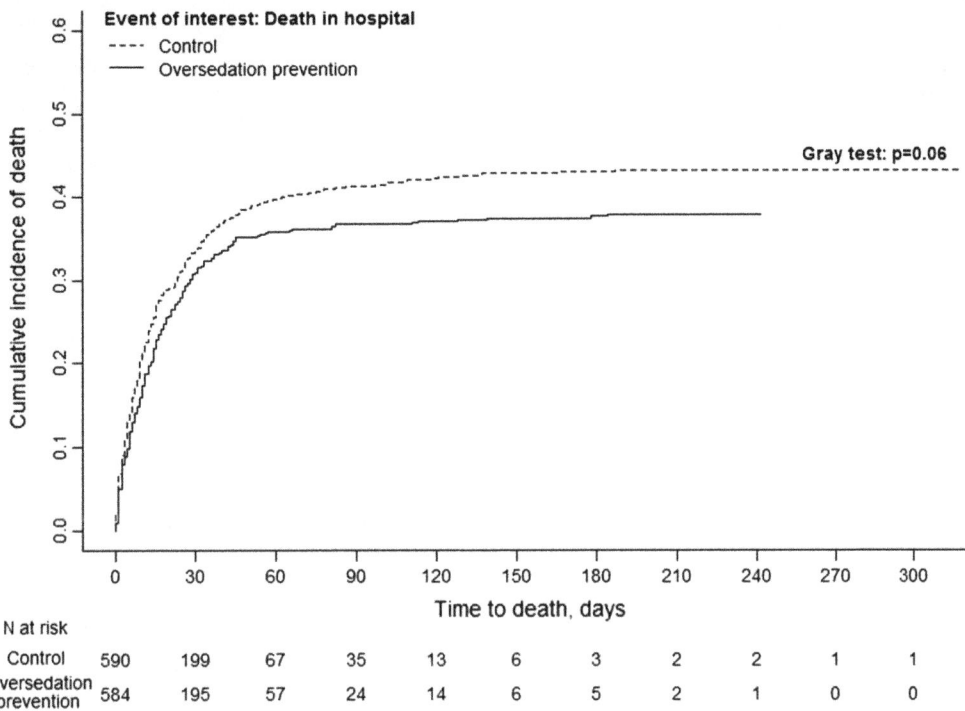

Fig. 3 Cumulative incidence of deaths in the hospital. The cumulative incidence of hospital death did not differ significantly between the two groups (220 in oversedation prevention group vs. 253 in the control group): hazard ratio for the oversedation prevention group versus the control group, 0.85; 95% confidence interval, 0.71–1.01; $p = 0.06$. For the analysis of time from randomization to death in the hospital, alive hospital discharge was handled as a competing risk

of consciousness base on a yes/no single-item scale, MV duration, etc.) all have their own limitations.

The oversedation prevention resulted in significantly less use of intravenous midazolam and propofol. Measuring doses of drug and showing a reduction in doses administered is not the same thing, but the increased rate of awake patients in the OSP group may imperfectly reflect the goal. Unfortunately, an explicit recording of implementation of multiple components of the OSP protocol could not be carried out in this large trial.

Of note, the lack of details regarding the previous alcohol consumption and the grouping within the large psychotropic category of medications with various mechanisms of action and side effects (benzodiazepines, neuroleptics, antidepressants, etc.) albeit pragmatic also represents a potential methodological limitation.

In summary, in this prospective randomized trial in severe critically ill patients requiring mechanical ventilation with early termination and under powering, we were unable to show that oversedation prevention significantly reduces mortality. However, it resulted in a significantly lower use of intravenous hypnotics, earlier time to spontaneous breathing trial, and reduced duration of mechanical ventilation. These last results should

be interpreted with precaution regarding the several limitations of the trial including the early termination.

Abbreviations
95% CI: 95% confidence interval; HR: hazard ratio; ICU: intensive care unit; OSP: oversedation prevention.

Authors' contributions
Among the writing Committee members: Bernard DE JONGHE, Julie LEGER and Bruno GIRAUDEAU wrote the manuscript. Nadia AISSAOUI and Stephan EHRMANN participated in the critical revision of the article. The writing committee members, the CERC members, the investigators, the SRLF presidents, and secretaries (Additional file 1: Appendix 3) approved the final version to be published. All authors read and approved the final manuscript.

Author details
[1] Société de Réanimation de Langue Française (SRLF), 48 Avenue Claude Vellefaux, 75010 Paris, France.

Acknowledgements
The authors are deeply indebted to the patients who agreed to participate and to all physicians who took care of them. Special thanks to all involved in the collection and analysis of the data: Louise-Marie Laisne, all CERC members, all investigators, SRLF presidents and secretaries (Additional file 1: Appendix 3).

We also thank Chantal Sevens, Florence Neels, and Mathieu Loung for their assistance.

Competing interests
The authors declare that they have no competing interests.

Funding
The study was funded by the French Intensive Care Society (Société de Réanimation de langue française: SRLF Trial Group).

References
1. Patel SB, Kress JP. Sedation and analgesia in the mechanically ventilated patient. Am J Respir Crit Care Med. 2012;185:486–97.
2. Jackson DL, Proudfoot CW, Cann KF, Walsh TS. The incidence of suboptimal sedation in the ICU: a systematic review. Crit Care. 2009;13:R204.
3. Kress J, Pohlman A, O'Connor M, Hall J. Daily interruption of sedative infusions in critically ill patients undergoing mechanical ventilation. N Engl J Med. 2000;342:1471–7.
4. Brook AD, Ahrens TS, Schaiff R, Prentice D, Sherman G, Shannon W, Kollef MH. Effect of a nursing-implemented sedation protocol on the duration of mechanical ventilation. Crit Care Med. 1999;27:2609–15.
5. De Jonghe B, Bastuji-Garin S, Fangio P, Lacherade JC, Jabot J, Appere-De-Vecchi C, Rocha N, Outin H. Sedation algorithm in critically ill patients without acute brain injury. Crit Care Med. 2005;33:120–7.
6. Quenot JP, Ladoire S, Devoucoux F, Doise JM, Cailliod R, Cunin N, Aube H, Blettery B, Charles PE. Effect of a nurse-implemented sedation protocol on the incidence of ventilator-associated pneumonia. Crit Care Med. 2007;35:2031–6.
7. Shehabi Y, Bellomo R, Reade MC, Bailey M, Bass F, Howe B, McArthur C, Murray L, Seppelt IM, Webb S, Weisbrodt L. Early goal-directed sedation versus standard sedation in mechanically ventilated critically ill patients: a pilot study*. Crit Care Med. 2013;41:1983–91.
8. Strom T, Martinussen T, Toft P. A protocol of no sedation for critically ill patients receiving mechanical ventilation: a randomised trial. Lancet. 2010;375:475–80.
9. Breen D, Karabinis A, Malbrain M, Morais R, Albrecht S, Jarnvig IL, Parkinson P, Kirkham AJ. Decreased duration of mechanical ventilation when comparing analgesia-based sedation using remifentanil with standard hypnotic-based sedation for up to 10 days in intensive care unit patients: a randomised trial. Crit Care. 2005;9:R200–10.
10. Treggiari MM, Romand JA, Yanez ND, Deem SA, Goldberg J, Hudson L, Heidegger CP, Weiss NS. Randomized trial of light versus deep sedation on mental health after critical illness. Crit Care Med. 2009;37:2527–34.
11. Shehabi Y, Bellomo R, Reade MC, Bailey M, Bass F, Howe B, McArthur CJ, Seppelt IM, Webb SA, Weisbrodt L. Early intensive care sedation predicts long-term mortality in ventilated critically ill patients. Am J Respir Crit Care Med. 2012;186:724–31.
12. Balzer F, Weiss B, Kumpf O, Treskatsch S, Spies C, Wernecke KD, Krannich A, Kastrup M. Early deep sedation is associated with decreased in-hospital and two-year follow-up survival. Crit Care. 2015;19:197.
13. Tanaka LM, Azevedo LC, Park M, Schettino G, Nassar AP, Rea-Neto A, Tannous L, de Souza-Dantas VC, Torelly A, Lisboa T, Piras C, Carvalho FB, Maia Mde O, Giannini FP, Machado FR, Dal-Pizzol F, de Carvalho AG, dos Santos RB, Tierno PF, Soares M, Salluh JI. Early sedation and clinical outcomes of mechanically ventilated patients: a prospective multicenter cohort study. Crit Care. 2014;18:R156.
14. The SRLF Trial Group. Sedation in French intensive care units: a survey of clinical practice. Ann Intensive Care. 2013;3:24.
15. Boles JM, Bion J, Connors A, et al. Weaning from mechanical ventilation. Eur Respir J. 2007;29:1933–56.
16. Eldridge S, Kerry S, Torgerson DJ. Bias in identifying and recruiting participants in cluster randomised trials: What can be done? BMJ. 2009;339:b4006.
17. Giraudeau B, Ravaud P. Preventing bias in cluster randomised trials. PLoS Med. 2009;6:e1000065.
18. Torgerson DJ. Contamination in trials: Is cluster randomisation the answer? BMJ. 2001;322:355–7.
19. Savovic J, Jones HE, Altman DG, Harris RJ, Juni P, Pildal J, Als-Nielsen B, Balk EM, Gluud C, Gluud LL, Ioannidis JP, Schulz KF, Beynon R, Welton NJ, Wood L, Moher D, Deeks JJ, Sterne JA. Influence of reported study design characteristics on intervention effect estimates from randomized, controlled trials. Ann Intern Med. 2012;157:429–38.
20. Fine JP, Gray RJ. A proportional hazards model for the subdistribution of a competing risk. J Am Stat Assoc. 1999;94:496–509.
21. R-Core-Team. R: a language and environment for statistical computing. 2015. https://www.R-project.org. Accessed 17 Sept 2018.
22. Wunsch H, Kahn JM, Kramer AA, Rubenfeld GD. Use of intravenous infusion sedation among mechanically ventilated patients in the United States. Crit Care Med. 2009;37:3031–9.
23. Pandharipande PP, Pun BT, Herr DL, Maze M, Girard TD, Miller RR, Shintani AK, Thompson JL, Jackson JC, Deppen SA, Stiles RA, Dittus RS, Bernard GR, Ely EW. Effect of sedation with dexmedetomidine vs lorazepam on acute brain dysfunction in mechanically ventilated patients: the MENDS randomized controlled trial. JAMA. 2007;298:2644–53.
24. Riker RR, Shehabi Y, Bokesch PM, Ceraso D, Wisemandle W, Koura F, Whitten P, Margolis BD, Byrne DW, Ely EW, Rocha MG. Dexmedetomidine vs midazolam for sedation of critically ill patients: a randomized trial. JAMA. 2009;301:489–99.
25. Jakob SM, Ruokonen E, Grounds RM, Sarapohja T, Garratt C, Pocock SJ, Bratty JR, Takala J. Dexmedetomidine vs. midazolam or propofol for sedation during prolonged mechanical ventilation: two randomized controlled trials. JAMA. 2012;307:1151–60.
26. Chanques G, Jaber S, Barbotte E, Violet S, Sebbane M, Perrigault PF, Mann C, Lefrant JY, Eledjam JJ. Impact of systematic evaluation of pain and agitation in an intensive care unit. Crit Care Med. 2006;34:1691–9.
27. Boles JM, Bion J, Connors A, Herridge M, Marsh B, Melot C, Pearl R, Silverman H, Stanchina M, Vieillard-Baron A, Welte T. Weaning from mechanical ventilation. Eur Respir J. 2007;29:1033–56.
28. Girard TD, Kress JP, Fuchs BD, Thomason JW, Schweickert WD, Pun BT, Taichman DB, Dunn JG, Pohlman AS, Kinniry PA, Jackson JC, Canonico AE, Light RW, Shintani AK, Thompson JL, Gordon SM, Hall JB, Dittus RS, Bernard GR, Ely EW. Efficacy and safety of a paired sedation and ventilator weaning protocol for mechanically ventilated patients in intensive care (Awakening and Breathing Controlled trial): a randomised controlled trial. Lancet. 2008;371:126–34.
29. Elliott R, McKinley S, Aitken LM, Hendrikz J. The effect of an algorithm-based sedation guideline on the duration of mechanical ventilation in an Australian intensive care unit. Intensive Care Med. 2006;32:1506–14.
30. Eldridge S, Kerry S, Torgerson DJ. Bias in identifying and recruiting participants in cluster randomised trials: What can be done? BMJ. 2009;339:b4006.
31. Giraudeau B, Ravaud P. Preventing bias in cluster randomised trials. PLoS Med. 2009;6:e1000065.
32. Torgerson DJ. Contamination in trials: Is cluster randomisation the answer? BMJ. 2001;322:355–7.

Permissions

All chapters in this book were first published in AIC, by Springer; hereby published with permission under the Creative Commons Attribution License or equivalent. Every chapter published in this book has been scrutinized by our experts. Their significance has been extensively debated. The topics covered herein carry significant findings which will fuel the growth of the discipline. They may even be implemented as practical applications or may be referred to as a beginning point for another development.

The contributors of this book come from diverse backgrounds, making this book a truly international effort. This book will bring forth new frontiers with its revolutionizing research information and detailed analysis of the nascent developments around the world.

We would like to thank all the contributing authors for lending their expertise to make the book truly unique. They have played a crucial role in the development of this book. Without their invaluable contributions this book wouldn't have been possible. They have made vital efforts to compile up to date information on the varied aspects of this subject to make this book a valuable addition to the collection of many professionals and students.

This book was conceptualized with the vision of imparting up-to-date information and advanced data in this field. To ensure the same, a matchless editorial board was set up. Every individual on the board went through rigorous rounds of assessment to prove their worth. After which they invested a large part of their time researching and compiling the most relevant data for our readers.

The editorial board has been involved in producing this book since its inception. They have spent rigorous hours researching and exploring the diverse topics which have resulted in the successful publishing of this book. They have passed on their knowledge of decades through this book. To expedite this challenging task, the publisher supported the team at every step. A small team of assistant editors was also appointed to further simplify the editing procedure and attain best results for the readers.

Apart from the editorial board, the designing team has also invested a significant amount of their time in understanding the subject and creating the most relevant covers. They scrutinized every image to scout for the most suitable representation of the subject and create an appropriate cover for the book.

The publishing team has been an ardent support to the editorial, designing and production team. Their endless efforts to recruit the best for this project, has resulted in the accomplishment of this book. They are a veteran in the field of academics and their pool of knowledge is as vast as their experience in printing. Their expertise and guidance has proved useful at every step. Their uncompromising quality standards have made this book an exceptional effort. Their encouragement from time to time has been an inspiration for everyone.

The publisher and the editorial board hope that this book will prove to be a valuable piece of knowledge for researchers, students, practitioners and scholars across the globe.

List of Contributors

Ascanio Tridente
Whiston Hospital Prescot, Merseyside and Department of Infection, Immunity and Cardiovascular Disease, The Medical School, University of Sheffield, Sheffield, UK

Julian Bion
School of Clinical and Experimental Medicine, University of Birmingham, Birmingham, UK

Gary H. Mills
University of Sheffield, Sheffield, UK

Anthony C. Gordon and Paul A. H. Holloway
Imperial College, London, UK

Geraldine. M. Clarke
The Wellcome Trust Centre for Human Genetics, University of Oxford, Oxford, UK

Andrew Walden
Intensive Care Unit, Royal Berkshire Hospital, Reading, UK

Paula Hutton and Christopher Garrard
Intensive Care Unit, John Radcliffe Hospital, Oxford, UK

Jean-Daniel Chiche
Hospital Cochin, Paris, France

Frank Stuber
Department of Anaesthesiology and Pain Medicine, Bern University Hospital and University of Bern, Bern, Switzerland

Charles Hinds
Barts and the London Queen Mary School of Medicine, London, UK

Solenn Remy, Karine Kolev-Descamps and Etienne Javouhey
Hospices Civils de Lyon, Paediatric Intensive Care Unit, Mother and Children University Hospital, 59 Boulevard Pinel, 69500 Bron, France

Morgane Gossez and Julie Demaret
Hospices Civils de Lyon, Immunology Laboratory, E. Herriot Hospital, 69003 Lyon, France

Fabienne Venet and Guillaume Monneret
Hospices Civils de Lyon, Immunology Laboratory, E. Herriot Hospital, 69003 Lyon, France.
EA 7426, Pathophysiology of Injury-Induced Immunosuppression, University Claude Bernard Lyon 1, BioMérieux Hospices Civils de Lyon, E. Herriot Hospital, 69003 Lyon, France

Alexandrine Larouche, Laurence Ducharme-Crevier, Gabrielle Constantin, Philippe Jouvet and Guillaume Emeriaud
Pediatric Intensive Care Unit, CHU Sainte-Justine, 3175 Côte Sainte-Catherine, Montreal, QC, Canada
CHU Sainte-Justine Research Center, Université de Montréal, Montreal, Canada

Guillaume Mortamet
Pediatric Intensive Care Unit, CHU Sainte-Justine, 3175 Côte Sainte-Catherine, Montreal, QC, Canada
INSERM U 955, Equipe 13, Créteil, France
CHU Sainte-Justine Research Center, Université de Montréal, Montreal, Canada

Olivier Fléchelles
Pediatric Intensive Care Unit, CHU Fort-de-France, Fort-de-France, France

Sandrine Essouri
CHU Sainte-Justine Research Center, Université de Montréal, Montreal, Canada.
Department of Pediatrics, CHU Sainte-Justine, Montreal, QC, Canada

Amélie-Ann Pellerin-Leblanc
Queen's University, Kingston, Canada

Jennifer Beck
Keenan Research Centre for Biomedical Science, Li Ka Shing Knowledge Institute, St. Michael's Hospital, Toronto, ON, Canada
Department of Pediatrics, University of Toronto, Toronto, Canada
Institute for Biomedical Engineering and Science Technology (iBEST), Ryerson University and St-Michael's Hospital, Toronto, Canada

Christer Sinderby
Keenan Research Centre for Biomedical Science, Li Ka Shing Knowledge Institute, St. Michael's Hospital, Toronto, ON, Canada
Institute for Biomedical Engineering and Science Technology (iBEST), Ryerson University and St-Michael's Hospital, Toronto, Canada
Department of Medicine, University of Toronto, Toronto, Canada

Nazzareno Fagoni and Bertilla Fiorese
Department of Anesthesia, Critical Care and Emergency, Spedali Civili University Hospital, Piazzale Ospedali Civili, 1, 23123 Brescia, Italy
Department of Molecular and Translational Medicine, University of Brescia, Brescia, Italy

Simone Piva, Elena Peli1, Fabio Turla and Elisabetta Pecci
Department of Anesthesia, Critical Care and Emergency, Spedali Civili University Hospital, Piazzale Ospedali Civili, 1, 23123 Brescia, Italy

Livio Gualdoni
School of Specialty in Anesthesia, Intensive Care and Pain Medicine, University of Brescia, Brescia, Italy

Frank Rasulo and Nicola Latronico
Department of Anesthesia, Critical Care and Emergency, Spedali Civili University Hospital, Piazzale Ospedali Civili, 1, 23123 Brescia, Italy
School of Specialty in Anesthesia, Intensive Care and Pain Medicine, University of Brescia, Brescia, Italy
Department of Medical and Surgical Specialties, Radiological Sciences and Public Health, University of Brescia, Brescia, Italy

Joo-Yeon Engelen-Lee, Matthijs C. Brouwer and Diederik van de Beek
Department of Neurology, Academic Medical Center, University of Amsterdam, Amsterdam Neuroscience, 1100 DD Amsterdam, The Netherlands

Eleonora Aronica
Department of Neuropathology, Academic Medical Center, University of Amsterdam, Amsterdam Neuroscience, Amsterdam, The Netherlands
Stichting Epilepsie Instellingen Nederland (SEIN), Cruquius, The Netherlands

Pierre Demaret
Pediatric Intensive Care Unit, Department of Pediatrics, CHC, Liège, Belgium
Université de Lille, EA 2694 - Santé Publique: épidémiologie et qualité des soins, 59000 Lille, France

Frédéric Lebrun and André Mulder
Pediatric Intensive Care Unit, Department of Pediatrics, CHC, Liège, Belgium

Oliver Karam
Pediatric Critical Care Unit, Geneva University Hospital, Geneva, Switzerland
Division of Pediatric Critical Care Medicine, Children's Hospital of Richmond at VCU, Richmond, VA, USA

Marisa Tucci and Jacques Lacroix
Division of Pediatric Critical Care Medicine, Department of Pediatrics, Sainte-Justine Hospital, Université de Montréal, Montreal, Canada

Hélène Behal and Alain Duhamel
Université de Lille, EA 2694 - Santé Publique: épidémiologie et qualité des soins, Unité de Biostatistique, 59000 Lille, France

Stéphane Leteurtre
Université de Lille, EA 2694 - Santé Publique: épidémiologie et qualité des soins, 59000 Lille, France
Pediatric Intensive Care Unit, CHU Lille, 59000 Lille, France

Marie Lecronier
Service de Pneumologie et Réanimation Médicale (Département "R3S"), Groupe Hospitalier Pitié-Salpêtrière Charles Foix, Assistance Publique-Hôpitaux de Paris, 75013 Paris, France

Sandrine Valade and Elie Azoulay
Service de Réanimation médicale, Groupe Hospitalier Saint-Louis – Lariboisière – Fernand-Widal, Assistance Publique-Hôpitaux de Paris, Paris, France

Naike Bigé and Eric Maury
Service de Réanimation médicale, Groupe Hospitalier Est Parisien, Hôpital Saint-Antoine Paris, Assistance Publique-Hôpitaux de Paris, Paris, France

Nicolas de Prost
Service de Réanimation médicale, Groupe Hospitalier Henri Mondor, Assistance Publique-Hôpitaux de Paris, Créteil, France

Damien Roux
Service de Réanimation médico-chirurgicale, Groupe Hospitalier Paris Nord, Hôpital Louis-Mourier, Assistance Publique-Hôpitaux de Paris, Colombes, France

David Lebeaux
Service de Microbiologie, Unité Mobile de Microbiologie Clinique, Hôpital Européen Georges Pompidou, Assistance Publique-Hôpitaux de Paris, Paris, France
Université Paris Descartes, Sorbonne Paris Cité, Paris, France

Alexandre Demoule and Martin Dres
Service de Pneumologie et Réanimation Médicale (Département "R3S"), Groupe Hospitalier Pitié-Salpêtrière Charles Foix, Assistance Publique-Hôpitaux de Paris, 75013 Paris, France
INSERM, UMRS1158 Neurophysiologie respiratoire expérimentale et clinique, Sorbonne Universités, UPMC Univ Paris 06, Paris, France

Clément Medrinal
Normandie Univ, UNIROUEN, EA3830 - GRHV, 76000 Rouen, France
Institute for Research and Innovation in Biomedicine (IRIB), 76000 Rouen, France
Intensive Care Unit Department, Groupe Hospitalier du Havre, Avenue Pierre Mendes France, 76290 Montivilliers, France

Aurora Robledo Quesada
Intensive Care Unit Department, Groupe Hospitalier du Havre, Avenue Pierre Mendes France, 76290 Montivilliers, France

Guillaume Prieur
Pulmonology Department, Groupe Hospitalier du Havre, Avenue Pierre Mendes France, 76290 Montivilliers, France

Yann Combret
Institut de Recherche Expérimentale et Clinique (IREC), Pôle de Pneumologie, ORL and Dermatologie, Université Catholique de Louvain, Brussels 1200, Belgium

Physiotherapy Department, Groupe Hospitalier du Havre, Avenue Pierre Mendes France, 76290 Montivilliers, France

Francis Edouard Gravier
ADIR Association, Bois Guillaume, France

Eric Frenoy
Intensive Care Unit Department, Hôpital Jacques Monod, 76290 Montivilliers, France

Olivier Contal
University of Applied Sciences and Arts Western Switzerland (HES-SO), Avenue de Beaumont, 1011 Lausanne, Switzerland

Bouchra Lamia
Normandie Univ, UNIROUEN, EA3830 - GRHV, 76000 Rouen, France
Institute for Research and Innovation in Biomedicine (IRIB), 76000 Rouen, France
Pulmonology Department, Groupe Hospitalier du Havre, Avenue Pierre Mendes France, 76290 Montivilliers, France
Intensive Care Unit, Respiratory Department, Rouen University Hospital, Rouen, France

Tristan Bonnevie
Normandie Univ, UNIROUEN, EA3830 - GRHV, 76000 Rouen, France
Institute for Research and Innovation in Biomedicine (IRIB), 76000 Rouen, France
ADIR Association, Bois Guillaume, France

Diego Orbegozo, Wasineenart Mongkolpun, Gianni Stringari, Nikolaos Markou, Jacques Creteur, Jean-Louis Vincent and Daniel De Backer
Department of Intensive Care, Erasme University Hospital, Université Libre de Bruxelles, Route de Lennik 808, 1070 Brussels, Belgium

Enrique de-Madaria and Karina Cárdenas-Jaén
Pancreatic Unit, Department of Gastroenterology, Hospital General Universitario de Alicante, Instituto de Investigación Sanitaria y Biomédica de Alicante (ISABIAL - Fundación FISABIO), Alicante, Spain

Xavier Molero and Andrea Montenegro
Exocrine Pancreatic Diseases Research Group, Hospital Universitari Vall d'Hebron, Institut de Recerca (VHIR), Universitat Autònoma de Barcelona, CIBEREHD, Barcelona, Spain

Laia Bonjoch and Daniel Closa
Department of Experimental Pathology, IIBB-CSIC, IDIBAPS, c/Rosselló 161, 7°, 08036 Barcelona, Spain

Josefina Casas
RUBAM, Department of Biomedicinal Chemistry, IQAC-CSIC, Barcelona, Spain

Giacomo Grasselli and Vittorio Scaravilli
Dipartimento di Anestesia, Rianimazione ed Emergenza-Urgenza, Fondazione IRCCS Ca' Granda, Ospedale Maggiore Policlinico, Via Francesco Sforza 35, 20122 Milan, Italy

Beatrice Vergnano and Vittoria Sala
Dipartimento di Emergenza-Urgenza, Ospedale San Gerardo, Monza, Italy

Maria Rosa Pozzi
Dipartimento di Medicina, Unità Operativa di Reumatologia, Ospedale San Gerardo, Monza, Italy

Gabriele D'Andrea
Unità Operativa di Radiodiagnostica, Ospedale San Gerardo, Monza, Italy

Marco Mantero
Dipartimento di Fisiopatologia Medico Chirurgica e dei Trapianti, Università degli Studi di Milano, Milan, Italy

Alberto Pesci
Dipartimento di Medicina e Chirurgia, Università Milano Bicocca, Monza, Italy
Clinica Pneumologica, Ospedale San Gerardo, Monza, Italy

Antonio Pesenti
Dipartimento di Anestesia, Rianimazione ed Emergenza-Urgenza, Fondazione IRCCS Ca' Granda, Ospedale Maggiore Policlinico, Via Francesco Sforza 35, 20122 Milan, Italy
Dipartimento di Fisiopatologia Medico Chirurgica e dei Trapianti, Università degli Studi di Milano, Milan, Italy

José Augusto Santos Pellegrini
Department of Critical Care Medicine, Hospital de Clínicas de Porto Alegre, Universidade Federal do Rio Grande do Sul, Porto Alegre, Brazil

Ricardo Luiz Cordioli
Department of Critical Care Medicine, Hospital Israelita Albert Einstein, São Paulo, Brazil

Department of Critical Care Medicine, Alemão Oswaldo Cruz Hospital, São Paulo, Brazil
Department of Intensive Care Unit, Hospital Israelita Albert Einstein, 627, Albert Einstein St., São Paulo 05652-900, Brazil

Ana Cristina Burigo Grumann
Department of Critical Care Medicine, Nereu Ramos Hospital, Florianópolis, Brazil

Patrícia Klarmann Ziegelmann
Statistics Department and Post-Graduation Program in Epidemiology, Universidade Federal do Rio Grande do Sul, Porto Alegre, Brazil

Leandro Utino Taniguchi
Department of Critical Care Medicine, Hospital das Clínicas de São Paulo, FMUSP, São Paulo, Brazil

Mohammed S. Alshahrani
Department of Emergency and Critical Care, King Fahad Hospital of the University-Dammam University, Al Khobar 31952, Saudi Arabia

Anees Sindi
Department of Medicine/Intensive Care, King Abdulaziz University, Jeddah, Saudi Arabia

Bayan Alahmadi and Naif Khatani
King Abdulaziz University, Jeddah, Saudi Arabia

Fahad Al-Hameed
King Abdulaziz Medical City, NGHA, Jeddah, Saudi Arabia
Intensive Care Department, King Saud bin Abdulaziz University for Health Sciences, Jeddah, Saudi Arabia

Fayez Alshamsi
Department of Internal Medicine, College of Medicine and Health Sciences, United Arab EmiratesUniversity, Al Ain, UAE

Awad Al-Omari
Medical Director of Critical Care, Dr. Suliman Al-Habib Group, AlFaisal University, Riyadh, Saudi Arabia

Mohamed El Tahan
Department of Anesthesiology, Dammam University, Dammam, Saudi Arabia

Ahmed Zein
Department of ICU, King Fahad Hospital, Jeddah, Saudi Arabia

Sultan Alamri
Department of ICU National Hospital, Internal Medicine and Critical Care, Riyadh, Saudi Arabia

Mohammed Abdelzaher
Critical Care Medicine Department, Cairo University Hospitals, Cairo, Egypt

Amenah Alghamdi and Faisal Alfousan
Department of Internal Medicine, King Abdulaziz University, Jeddah, Saudi Arabia

Adel Tash
Department of Cardiac Surgery, King Abdullah Medical City, Makkah, Saudi Arabia

Wail Tashkandi
Department of Surgery/Intensive Care, King Abdulaziz University, Jeddah, Saudi Arabia

Rajaa Alraddadi
Community Medicine Department, Ministry of Health, Jeddah, Saudi Arabia

Kim Lewis
Department of Medicine, Division of Critical Care, McMaster University, Hamilton, Canada

Mohammed Badawee
Department of Critical Care, Prince Sultan Military Medical City, Riyadh, Saudi Arabia

Yaseen M. Arabi
King Abdullah International Medical Research Center, King Saud bin Abdulaziz University for Health Sciences, Riyadh, Saudi Arabia

Eddy Fan
Interdepartmental Division of Critical Care Medicine, University of Toronto, Toronto, Canada

Waleed Alhazzani
Department of Clinical Epidemiology and Biostatistics, McMaster University, Hamilton, Canada

Jonas Tverring, Jane Fisher and Adam Linder
Division of Infection Medicine, Department of Clinical Sciences, Lund University, BMC B14, 221 84 Lund, Sweden

Ville Pettilä
Division of Intensive Care Medicine, Department of Anesthesiology, Intensive Care and Pain Medicine, University of Helsinki and Helsinki University Hospital, Helsinki, Finland

Suvi T. Vaara
Division of Intensive Care Medicine, Department of Anesthesiology, Intensive Care and Pain Medicine, University of Helsinki and Helsinki University Hospital, Helsinki, Finland
Department of Intensive Care, Austin Hospital, Melbourne, Australia

Meri Poukkanen
Department of Intensive Care, Lapland Central Hospital, Rovaniemi, Finland

Soo Jin Na and Chi Ryang Chung
Department of Critical Care Medicine, Samsung Medical Center, Sungkyunkwan University School of Medicine, 81 Irwon-ro, Gangnam-gu, Seoul 06351, Republic of Korea

Hee Jung Choi
Intensive Care Unit Nursing Department, Samsung Medical Center, Sungkyunkwan University School of Medicine, Seoul, Republic of Korea

Yang Hyun Cho and Kiick Sung
Department of Thoracic and Cardiovascular Surgery, Samsung Medical Center, Sungkyunkwan University School of Medicine, Seoul, Republic of Korea

Jeong Hoon Yang
Department of Critical Care Medicine, Samsung Medical Center, Sungkyunkwan University School of Medicine, 81 Irwon-ro, Gangnam-gu, Seoul 06351, Republic of Korea
Division of Cardiology, Department of Medicine, Samsung Medical Center, Sungkyunkwan University School of Medicine, Seoul, Republic of Korea

Gee Young Suh and Kyeongman Jeon
Department of Critical Care Medicine, Samsung Medical Center, Sungkyunkwan University School of Medicine, 81 Irwon-ro, Gangnam-gu, Seoul 06351, Republic of Korea
Division of Pulmonary and Critical Care Medicine, Department of Medicine, Samsung Medical Center, Sungkyunkwan University School of Medicine, Seoul, Republic of Korea

Toshiaki Iba
Department of Emergency and Disaster Medicine, Juntendo University Graduate School of Medicine, 2-1-1 Hongo Bunkyo-ku, Tokyo 113-8421, Japan

Akiyoshi Hagiwara
National Center for Global Health and Medicine, Emergency Medicine and Critical Care, Tokyo, Japan

Daizoh Saitoh
Division of Traumatology, Research Institute, National Defense Medical College, Tokyo, Japan

Hideaki Anan
Emergency Medical Center, Fujisawa City Hospital, Fujisawa, Japan

Yutaka Ueki
Department of Acute Critical Care and Disaster Medicine, Tokyo Medical and Dental University, Tokyo, Japan

Koichi Sato
Department of Surgery, Juntendo Shizuoka Hospital, Juntendo University Graduate School of Medicine, Izunokuni-shi, Japan

Satoshi Gando
Division of Acute and Critical Care Medicine, Department of Anesthesiology and Critical Care Medicine, Hokkaido University Graduate School of Medicine, Sapporo, Japan

Martin Dres, Laurence Dangers, Thomas Similowski and Alexandre Demoule
UPMC Univ Paris 06, INSERM, UMRS1158, Neurophysiologie Respiratoire Expérimentale et Clinique, Sorbonne Universités, Paris, France
Service de Pneumologie et Réanimation Médicale (Département "R3S"), AP-HP, Groupe
Hospitalier Pitié-Salpêtrière Charles Foix, 47-83 boulevard de l'Hôpital, 75013 Paris, France

Danielle Reuter, Julien Mayaux and Elise Morawiec
Service de Pneumologie et Réanimation Médicale (Département "R3S"), AP-HP, Groupe
Hospitalier Pitié-Salpêtrière Charles Foix, 47-83 boulevard de l'Hôpital, 75013 Paris, France

Ewan C. Goligher
Interdepartmental Division of Critical Care Medicine, University of Toronto, Toronto, Canada

Division of Respirology, Department of Medicine, University Health Network and Mount Sinai Hospital, Toronto, Canada

Bruno-Pierre Dubé
UPMC Univ Paris 06, INSERM, UMRS1158, Neurophysiologie Respiratoire Expérimentale et Clinique, Sorbonne Universités, Paris, France
Département de Médecine, Service de Pneumologie, Hôpital Hôtel-Dieu, Centre Hospitalier de l'Université de Montréal (CHUM), Montréal, QC, Canada

Olivier Lesur and Eugénie Delile
Division of Intensive Care Units, Department of Medicine, Faculté de Médecine et des Sciences de la Santé, Centre de Recherche du CHUS, Université de Sherbrooke, Sherbrooke, QC, Canada

Pierre Asfar
Département de Médecine Intensive-Reanimation, Centre Hospitalier Universitaire, Université d'Angers, Angers, France

Peter Radermacher
Institut für Anästhesiologische Pathophysiologie und Verfahrensentwicklung, Universitätsklinikum, Ulm, Germany

Laurent Jadot and Pierre Damas
Service de Soins Intensifs Généraux, Domaine Universitaire du Sart-Tilman, Centre Hospitalier Universitaire, 4000 Liège, Belgium

Luc Huyghens
Dienst Intensieve Zorgen, VUB – Universitair Ziekenhuis Brussel, Campus Jette Laarbeeklaan 101, 1090 Brussels, Belgium

Annick De Jaeger
Pediatrische Intensieve Zorgen, Universitair Ziekenhuis Gent, De Pintelaan 185, 9000 Ghent, Belgium

Marc Bourgeois and Baudewijn Oosterlynck
Dienst Intensieve Zorgen, Algemeen Ziekenhuis Sint-Jan Brugge-Oostende, Ruddershove 10, 8000 Brugge, Belgium

Dominique Biarent
Service Soins Intensifs et Urgences, Hôpital Universitaire des Enfants Reine Fabiola, Avenue Crocq 15, 1020 Brussels, Belgium

Adeline Higuet
Urgentiegeneeskunde, Algemeen Ziekenhuis Sint-Maria, Ziekenhuislaan 100, 1500 Halle, Belgium

Koen de Decker
Intensieve Zorgen, Universitair Ziekenhuis Onze Lieve Vrouw, Moorselbaan 164, 9300 Aalst, Belgium

Margot Vander Laenen
Anesthesiologie –Kritieke Diensten, Ziekenhuis Oost-Limburg, Campus Sint-Jan, Schiepse Bos 6, 3600 Genk, Belgium

Patrick Ferdinande
Intensieve Zorgen, Universitair Ziekenhuis Leuven, Herestraat 49, 3000 Louvain, Belgium

Pascal Reper
Service de Soins Intensifs, Centre Hospitalier Universitaire Brugmann, Site Horta, Place Arthur Van Gehuchten 4, 1020 Brussels, Belgium
Service de Soins Intensifs, Le Tilleriau, CHR Haute Senne, Chaussée de Braine 49, 7060 Soignies, Belgium

Serge Brimioulle
Service de Soins Intensifs, Hôpital Erasme, Route de Lennik 808, 1070 Brussels, Belgium

Sophie Van Cromphau
Intensieve Zorgen, UZA, Wilrijkstraat 10, 2650 Edegem, Belgium

Stéphane Clement De Clety
Service de Soins Intensifs et Urgences Pédiatriques, Cliniques Universitaires Saint-Luc, UCL, Avenue Hippocrate 10, 1200 Brussels, Belgium

Thierry Sottiaux
Soins Intensifs, Clinique Notre-Dame de Grâce, Chaussée de Nivelles, 212, 6041 Gosselies, Belgium

Valentina Girotto, Jean-Louis Teboul, Alexandra Beurton, Laura Galarza, Christian Richard and Xavier Monnet
Service de Réanimation Médicale, Hôpital de Bicêtre, Hôpitaux Universitaires Paris-Sud, Insert UMR_999, Université Paris-Sud, Assistance Publique – Hôpitaux de Paris, Le Kremlin-Bicêtre, France

Thierry Guedj
Service de Radiologie, Hôpital de Bicêtre, Hôpitaux Universitaires Paris-Sud, Assistance Publique – Hôpitaux de Paris, Le Kremlin-Bicêtre, France

Olivier Pajot1, Hervé Mentec, Gaëtan Plantefève, Damien Contou and Constance Vuillard
Service de Réanimation Polyvalente, Centre Hospitalier Victor Dupouy, 69 rue du Lieutenant Colonel Prudhon, 95100 Argenteuil, France

Marc Pineton de Chambrun and Matthieu Schmidt
Service de Réanimation Médicale, Centre Hospitalier Universitaire Pitié-Salpétrière – Assistance Publique Hôpitaux de Paris, 47-83 boulevard de l'Hôpital, 75013 Paris, France

Nicolas de Prost
Service de Réanimation Médicale, Centre Hospitalier Universitaire Henri Mondor – Assistance Publique Hôpitaux de Paris, 51 avenue du Maréchal de Lattre de Tassigny, 94010 Créteil, France

Claude Guérin
Service de Réanimation Médicale, Hôpital de la Croix-Rousse, 103 Grande rue de la Croix-Rousse, 69004 Lyon, France.
INSERM 955, Créteil, France

Auguste Dargent and Jean-Pierre Quenot
Service de Médecine Intensive Réanimation, Centre Hospitalier Universitaire François Mitterrand de Dijon, 14 rue Paul Gaffarel, 21000 Dijon, France

Sébastien Préau and Geoffrey Ledoux
Service de Réanimation, Centre Hospitalier Régional Universitaire de Lille, 2 avenue Oscar Lambret, 59000 Lille, France

Mathilde Neuville
Service de Réanimation Médicale, Centre Hospitalier Universitaire Bichat Claude-Bernard – Assistance Publique Hôpitaux de Paris, 46 rue Henri Huchard, 75877 Paris, France

Guillaume Voiriot and Muriel Fartoukh
Service de Réanimation médico-chirurgicale, Centre Hospitalier Universitaire Tenon – Assistance Publique Hôpitaux de Paris, 5 rue de la Chine, 75020 Paris, France

Rémi Coudroy
Service de Réanimation médicale, Centre hospitalier universitaire de Poitiers, 2 rue de la Milétrie, 86021 Poitiers, France

Guillaume Dumas and Eric Maury
11 Service de Réanimation médicale, Centre Hospitalier Universitaire Saint-Antoine – Assistance Publique Hôpitaux de Paris, 184 rue du Faubourg Saint-Antoine, 75012 Paris, France

Nicolas Terzi
Service de Réanimation, Centre Hospitalier Universitaire de Grenoble Alpes, avenue Maquis du Grésivaudan, 38700 La Tronche, France

Yacine Tandjaoui-Lambiotte
Service de Réanimation médico-chirurgicale, Centre Hospitalier Universitaire Avicennes – Assistance Publique Hôpitaux de Paris, 125 rue de Stalingrad, 93000 Bobigny, France

Francis Schneider
Service de Réanimation, Centre Hospitalier Universitaire de Strasbourg, 1 avenue Molière, 67200 Strasbourg, France

Maximilien Grall
Service de Réanimation Médicale, Centre Hospitalier Universitaire de Rouen, 1 rue de Germont, 76000 Rouen, France

Emmanuel Guérot
Service de Réanimation Médicale, Centre Hospitalier Universitaire Hôpital Européen Georges-Pompidou– Assistance Publique Hôpitaux de Paris, 20 rue Leblanc, 75015 Paris, France

Romaric Larcher
Service de Réanimation Médicale, Centre Hospitalier Universitaire de Montpellier, 191 avenue du Doyen Gaston Giraud, 34000 Montpellier, France

Sylvie Ricome
Service de Réanimation Polyvalente, Centre Hospitalier Robert-Ballanger, Boulevard Robert Ballanger, 93600 Aulnay-sous-Bois, France

Raphaël Le Mao
Service de Réanimation médicale, Centre Hospitalier Régional Universistaire de Brest, Site La Cavale Blanche, Boulevard Tanguy Prigent, 29200 Brest, France

Gwenhaël Colin
Service de réanimation médico-chirurgicale, Centre Hospitalier Départemental de Vendée, Les Oudairies, 85925 La Roche sur Yon Cedex 9, France

Christophe Guitton
Service de Réanimation médico-chirurgicale, Centre Hospitalier du Mans, 194 avenue Rubillard, 72037 Le Mans, France

Lara Zafrani
Service de Réanimation médicale, Hôpital Saint-Louis, Assistance Publique Hôpitaux de Paris, 1 avenue Claude Vellefaux, 75010 Paris, France

Elise Morawiec
Unité de Réanimation et de Surveillance continue, Service de Pneumologie et Réanimation médicale, Groupe hospitalier Pitié-Salpêtrière, 47-83 bd de l'hôpital, 75651 Paris, France

Marie Dubert
Service d'Immunologie Clinique, Hôpital Saint-Louis, Assistance Publique Hôpitaux de Paris, 1 avenue Claude Vellefaux, 75010 Paris, France

Jianxiao Chen, Tao Yu, Xiwen Zhang, Songqiao Liu, Ling Liu, Yi Yang and Haibo Qiu
Department of Critical Care Medicine, Zhongda Hospital, School of Medicine, Southeast University, 87 Dingjiaqiao Road, Nanjing 210009, People's Republic of China.

Federico Longhini
Department of Critical Care Medicine, Zhongda Hospital, School of Medicine, Southeast University, 87 Dingjiaqiao Road, Nanjing 210009, People's Republic of China
Anesthesia and Intensive Care, Department of Translational Medicine, Eastern Piedmont University "A. Avogadro", Novara, Italy

Karim Bendjelid
Intensive Care Unit, Geneva University Hospitals, 4 Rue Gabrielle-Perret-Gentil, 1205 Geneva, Switzerland
Faculty of Medicine, University of Geneva, Geneva, Switzerland
Geneva Hemodynamic Research Group, Geneva, Switzerland

Juan José García Martínez
Intensive Care Unit, Geneva University Hospitals, 4 Rue Gabrielle-Perret-Gentil, 1205 Geneva, Switzerland
Faculty of Medicine, University of Geneva, Geneva, Switzerland

Index

www.ingramcontent.com/pod-product-compliance
Lightning Source LLC
Chambersburg PA
CBHW061301190326
41458CB00011B/3738